Magnetic Resonance Imaging Handbook

Magnetic Resonance Imaging Handbook

Edited by Aaron Jackson

hayle
medical

New York

Hayle Medical,
750 Third Avenue, 9th Floor,
New York, NY 10017, USA

Visit us on the World Wide Web at:
www.haylemedical.com

ISBN: 978-1-63241-453-3

Cataloging-in-Publication Data

Magnetic resonance imaging handbook / edited by Aaron Jackson.
    p. cm.
Includes bibliographical references and index.
ISBN 978-1-63241-453-3
1. Magnetic resonance imaging. 2. Diagnostic imaging. I. Jackson, Aaron.
RC386.6.M34 M34 2017
616.075 48--dc23

Table of Contents

Preface

Magnetic resonance imaging, popularly known as MRI is an imaging technique used in radiology to image the anatomy of the body. It is widely used for medical diagnosis. The book elucidates the various sub-categories of MRI, along with its varied uses and benefits. It aims to provide a comprehensive knowledge of different types of tools and methods of magnetic resonance imaging for readers across the globe. This book is a compilation of chapters that discuss the most vital concepts and emerging trends in this field. For all those who are interested in the nuanced understanding of magnetic resonance imaging, this book can prove to be an essential guide.

The information shared in this book is based on empirical researches made by veterans in this field of study. The elaborative information provided in this book will help the readers further their scope of knowledge leading to advancements in this field.

Finally, I would like to thank my fellow researchers who gave constructive feedback and my family members who supported me at every step of my research.

Editor

Phenotype-Genotype Correlation in Wilson Disease in a Large Lebanese Family: Association of c.2299insC with Hepatic and of p. Ala1003Thr with Neurologic Phenotype

Julnar Usta[1], Antonios Wehbeh[2], Khaled Rida[1], Omar El-Rifai[1], Theresa Alicia Estiphan[2], Tamar Majarian[1], Kassem Barada[3]*

1 Department of Biochemistry and Molecular Genetics; Faculty of Medicine, American University of Beirut, Beirut, Lebanon, 2 Faculty of Medicine, American University of Beirut Medical Center, Beirut, Lebanon, 3 Division of Gastroenterology, Department of Internal Medicine, American University of Beirut Medical Center, Faculty of Medicine, Beirut, Lebanon

Abstract

Genotype phenotype correlations in Wilson disease (WD) are best established in homozygous patients or in compound heterozygous patients carrying the same set of mutations. We determined the clinical phenotype of patients with WD carrying the c.2298_2299insC in Exon 8 (c.2299insC) or the p. Ala1003Thr missense substitution in Exon 13 mutations in the homozygous or compound heterozygous state. We investigated 76 members of a single large Lebanese family. Their genotypes were determined, and clinical assessments were carried out for affected subjects. We also performed a literature search retrieving the phenotypes of patients carrying the same mutations of our patients in the homozygous or compound heterozygous state. There were 7 consanguineous marriages in this family and the prevalence of WD was 8.9% and of carriers of *ATP7B* mutation 44.7%. WD was confirmed in 9 out of 76 subjects. All 9 had the c.2299insC mutation, 5 homozygous and 4-compound heterozygous with p. Ala1003Thr. Six of our patients had hepatic, 2 had neurologic and 1 had asymptomatic phenotype. Based on our data and a literature review, clear phenotypes were reported for 38 patients worldwide carrying the c.2299insC mutation. About 53% of those have hepatic and 29% have neurologic phenotype. Furthermore, there were 10 compound heterozygous patients carrying the p. Ala1003Thr mutation. Among those, 80% having c.2299insC as the second mutation had hepatic phenotype, and all others had neurologic phenotype. We hereby report an association between the c.2299insC mutation and hepatic phenotype and between the p. Ala1003Thr mutation and neurologic phenotype.

Editor: Oleg Y. Dmitriev, University of Saskatchewan, Canada

Funding: The authors thank The Medical Practice Plan of AUB-MC and the University Research Board of the American University of Beirut for supporting the study by research grants to J. Usta. The funders had no role in study design, data collection and anlysis, decision to publish or preparation of the manuscript.

Competing Interests: The authors have declared that no competing interests exist.

* Email: kb02@aub.edu.lb

Introduction

Wilson disease (WD; MIM# 277900) is an autosomal recessive, copper transport disorder characterized by extensive phenotypic diversity [1,2]. Patients may present at any age with hepatic, neurologic, or mixed symptoms. Yet some may be asymptomatic [3]. WD is due to a defective *ATP7B* gene (OMIM*606882; Ref seq accession #: NM_000053.3); that is located on chromosome 13 (Gene map locus: 13q 14.3–921.1) that encodes a copper transporting p-type ATPase [4,5]. More than 500 mutations have been identified so far, and ongoing efforts to associate these with disease phenotypes have been inconclusive and controversial [6]. Inability to establish genotype-phenotype correlations may be attributed to the large number of mutations that occur in only few families, and to the heterogeneity of the clinical presentation of WD patients even within members of the same family. The fact that the majority of patients are compound heterozygote, having a different mutation on each allele, makes it hard to relate a

phenotype with one mutant allele. Furthermore occupational exposure to copper has been shown to cause genomic alterations and DNA damage [7]. This in combination with epigenetic modulators and environmental factors may play a role in the phenotypic heterogeneity of WD patients [8]. These difficulties may be partially overcome by studying WD in homozygous patients [9].

Specific mutations in the ATP7B gene are more frequent in populations where consanguineous marriages are prevalent. In Lebanon, consanguinity has a prevalence of 35.5%, increasing the probability of homozygozity for autosomal recessive diseases [10].

We have previously reported on multiple Lebanese families with members affected with WD. We found an association between the homozygous missense mutation p. Gly691Arg (Exon-7) with early and severe hepatic disease [11]. In addition an association between liver disease and homozygous mutations in the conserved ATP hinge region (Exon-18: p. Asn1270Ser and p. Pro1273Leu) of the *ATP7B* gene [9] was suggested. In a recent study we reported that patients with homozygous missense mutations, other than p. His1069Gln, are more likely to have a hepatic phenotype, liver failure and present at a younger age [12].

In this paper, we report on the phenotype and genotype of 9 patients with WD who belong to a single large family with extensive consanguinity. Five of our patients were homozygous for c. 2299insC (Exon-8), and four were compound heterozygous for both the c. 2299insC (Exon -8) and the missense mutation p. Ala1003Thr (Exon-13). Both mutations were previously reported as disease causing mutations [8,13,14]. A literature search retrieving reported phenotypes of all patients carrying either one or both of these two mutations was performed and compared to our own. We hereby suggest that the c. 2299insC favors a hepatic phenotype while the p. Ala1003Thr favors a neurologic phenotype.

Materials and Methods

Patients/Subjects

A total of 235 individuals distributed over 6 generations in a single extended Lebanese family, the S-family, were identified. This family came to our attention after some of its members were diagnosed with WD at the American University of Beirut Medical Center (AUBMC). Seventy six subjects (S1- S76) belonging to the S-family were enrolled in the study. Whenever an index case of WD was identified, a full clinical and genetic evaluation of that patient was conducted at AUBMC, while genotypic analysis was performed on the patient as well as all his/her family members. Out of the 76 subjects, 9 were found to have WD. Patient evaluation consisted of a full history, complete physical and neurological examination, ophthalmologic slit-lamp examination for Kayser-Fleischer (KF) rings, abdominal ultrasound, and standard biochemical tests including liver function tests, serum ceruloplasmin, serum copper and 24 hr urinary copper levels. Ceruloplasmin level was determined using immuno-nephlometric method (BN ProSpec analyzer system, from Siemen. Serum and urine copper levels were performed in a reference Laboratory (CERBA, France) as service, using Atomic absorption and ICP-MS, respectively. Five patients had brain MRI and two had EEG done as part of their evaluation.

DNA screening for exons bearing mutations or single nucleotide polymorphisms (SNPs) was performed in all recruited subjects. Cases were labeled as hepatic, neurologic, or asymptomatic following Ferenci's classification [15].

Detailed information was obtained from available family members in order to construct an accurate pedigree representing the 235 individuals of the S-family. Twelve members of the S-family died of WD according to information provided by their family members. Data pertaining to the clinical and genetic profiles of these deceased patients could not be obtained.

Ethics Statement

Written informed consent for participation in this study was obtained from all subjects or their guardians. The study protocol #: BioCh. JU.01 was approved by the International Review Board and the Research Committee at the American University of Beirut- Medical Center.

Mutation Analysis

Materials and Reagents. Various reagents used in this study were purchased from the following suppliers: IQ supermix, and Agarose from Bio-Rad; DNA purification Kit using Nucleospin Extract II columns from Machery Nagel, Germany (Cat no. 740609-50); T4 Kinase Polynucleotide from Invitrogen;

γ-^{32}P- ATP from Amersham (3000 Ci/mmol); SSDNA from Sigma Aldrich cat# D7656; Sephadex columns from GE Healthcare (Microspin G-25 column illustra 27-5325-01); and T4-Kinase from Invitrogen, Life Technology.

DNA concentration was quantified using the Gene Quant Spectrophotometer. PCR was performed using My Cycler Thermal Cycler from Bio-Rad; Membrane hybridization and crosslinking were carried out using ProBlot 12 Hybridization Oven Labnet, (31 Mayfield Avenue Edison, NJ, 08837 USA), and Spectrolinker UV Crosslinkers from Krackeler Scientific, (Inc. PO Box 1849 Albany, NY 12201-1849), respectively. Sequencing of purified DNA was carried out at the University of Saint Joseph, Department of Molecular Biology and Genetics using the Avant Genetic Analyzer (ABI 3130) machine. The sequencing reaction and subsequent purification steps were as described before [9].

Genotypic Analysis. Blood samples were collected in EDTA containing tubes, from 9 WD patients of the S-family and related members for DNA isolation. Blood samples were collected in EDTA containing tubes from 9 WD patients of the S-family and related members for DNA isolation. In brief Red Cell Lysis Buffer (RCLB composed of: 7.7 g ammonium chloride and 0.1 g potassium bicarbonate were dissolved in 1l water) was added to blood sample (2v/1v), incubated at $37°C$ for 12 min, and centrifuged (4000rpm,2 min). The resultant pellet was re-suspended in RCLB (2 ml) followed by the consecutive addition of: white cell lysis buffer (1.8 ml, WCLB composed of: 1.2 g TRIS, 1.68 g EDTA, 23.4 g sodium chloride dissolved in 1l water), SDS (24 µl of 10%) and proteinase–K (18 µl of 20 mg/ml). The suspension was incubated for 2 hrs at $55°C$ and proteins were salted out by adding 600 µl of 5 mM NaCl, followed by centrifugation at 4000 rpm for 15 min. The supernatant was transferred to a clean tube where an equal volume of ethanol (99%) was added to precipitate DNA. The flocculent DNA was transferred into 1.5 ml eppendorf tube, washed with 70% ethanol (200 µl), and centrifuged at maximum speed for 1min. The supernatant was then discarded. The pellet was allowed to air-dry and was then finally suspended in 200 µl TE buffer. DNA concentration was determined using Gene Quant Spectrophotometer at $\lambda = 260$ nm, and samples were stored at $-20°C$.

Polymerase Chain Reaction (PCR). Amplification of Exons 2–21 of WD gene were carried on all samples using My Cycler, (BIO-RAD). Primers flanking the exons' boundaries were designed (will be provided upon request) according to Petrukhin et al [16] with minor changes using primer 3 software (http://frodo.wi.mit.edu/cgibin/primer3/primer3_www.cgi). The PCR reaction mixture contained in a final volume of 50 µl: 25 µl IQ supermix (BIORAD), 22 µl H$_2$O, 1 µl of each of the primers (forward, reverse) each at a concentration of 3.4 pmoles/µl, and 1 µl DNA (250 ng). Two PCR programs were used in amplifying the exons:

Program -1 involved activation of Taq polymerase ($94°C$, 2 min), 38 cycles of denaturation ($94°C$, 30 sec), annealing ($59°C$, 30 sec), Extension ($72°C$, 40 sec) and a final extension ($72°C$, 7 min) followed by hold step. This program was used to amplify exons: 2, 4–10, 15 and 17.

Program- 2 was similar to program 1, except for the annealing temperature it was $61°C$. This program was used to amplify exons: 3, 11–14, 16, and 18–21. Amplified PCR products were then separated on 2% agarose gel, compared to DNA ladder of Molecular weight standards. DNA band corresponding to appropriate size were cut and purified using gel-extraction kits, Nucleospin Extract II columns (Machery Nagel), following Manufacturer's instructions. Sequencing of amplified exons was performed on WD patients as detailed in [9,12], compared to published normal sequences in the various databanks either Blast at National Center For Biotechnology Information (http://www.ncbi.nih.gov/Blast) or Blat at University of California Santa Cruz, Genome Bioinformatic site (http://www.genome.ucsc.edu/cgi-bin/hgBlat).

Genotypic screening of all other subjects was performed using DOT blot analysis following standard protocols [17]. Random selection of the amplified ATP7B exons: 8,10,12,13, and 16 from subjects (including WD patients) screened by Dot Blot, were sequenced to verify the Dot blot results.

Dot Blot Analysis

a. Labeling of probes. Normal and mutant probes were designed to include nucleotide base changes (mutations, SNPs) identified in patients. Probes (Table S1) were labeled using gamma ^{32}P-ATP as per instruction of the T4 kinase polynucleotide supplier. The labeled ^{32}P -probes were then denatured and centrifuged onto sephadex G-25 columns for 1min at 2400 rpm, where samples of the eluted probe were counted using liquid scintillator.

b. Membrane Preparation and Hybridization. Amplified PCR products were diluted to 0.4 ng/μl with 0.4 M NaOH − 10 mM EDTA, denatured by heating (10 min at 100°C), cooled & loaded on positively charged nitrocellulose membrane using Bio Blot machine (Bio-Rad), and washed consecutively with NaOH (100 μl, 0.4 M) followed by 2 X SSC (prepared as described in Current Protocols in Molecular Biology [17]). Briefly, the membrane was allowed to dry at room temperature and was then cross linked for 30 seconds using UV cross linker. Following pre-hybridization of membranes with aqueous prehybridization (APH) solution and denatured Salmon Sperm DNA (SSDNA) for 3hrs at 60°C, cross linked membranes were hybridized for 3–4 hours with labeled probes (10^6 cpm/300 ng) (Exons: 8,10,12,13, 16 at 45°C, 42°C, 30°C, 53°C, 43°C respectively), and were then washed at different stringencies (Table 1), dried, wrapped and exposed onto X-Ray films for 24–72 hours.

Literature Review

We conducted a comprehensive literature search of PubMed and Medline for all articles published between 1993 and 2014 using the following index terms: Wilson disease and, mutation, genotype, phenotype. We also reviewed the articles mentioned in the University of Alberta database (Wilson Disease Mutation Database: http://www.wilsondisease.med.ualberta.ca/database.asp). We included all articles that clearly stated the phenotype of patients homozygous or heterozygous for either one of these 2 mutations: c.2299 insC in Exon-8 and p. Ala1003Thr substitution in Exon-13 of the *ATP7B* gene.

Results

Clinical features

A pedigree of the S-family is presented Fig.1 showing the 235 members, and including all affected individuals and their immediate families. There were 7 consanguineous marriages in this family. Out of the 76 individuals enrolled in this study, 9 (11.8%) were diagnosed with WD (5 females & 4 males), and those are coded as: (S1, S2, S3, S4, S7, S8, S31, S41, and S59). Seven of the 9 patients belonged to 3 nuclear families, these are: (S1, S31, S59), (S7, S8) and (S3, S4). Six patients had a hepatic phenotype, two had neurologic phenotype, and one was completely asymptomatic and diagnosed by screening. Twelve out of the remaining 159 members had passed away because of WD according to their family members. Their clinical characteristics and genotype could not be determined. The prevalence of WD in the S-family, taking into account both the alive and deceased individuals, is 8.9% (21/235).

Eight patients had decreased serum ceruloplasmin level, while patient S41 had a normal level. The 24-hour urinary copper level was markedly elevated in 8 patients (average of 695.1 μg/24 hr) but was normal in one patient (S59) who was diagnosed by screening at the age of 1 year. KF rings were present in 6 affected subjects.

The clinical profiles of affected individuals are summarized in Table 2. The average age at diagnosis was **11.2** years, while the mean age of patients with hepatic and neurologic manifestation were 9.7 and 14 years, respectively.

Among the 6 patients with hepatic disease, 3 patients (S3, S4, and S7) had liver cirrhosis with portal hypertension. Patient (S3) presented with lethargy and gingival bleeding and subsequent endoscopy showed grade-3 esophageal varices. CT scan of the abdomen showed marked splenomegaly and a nodular liver consistent with cirrhosis. Patient (S4) had coarse hepatomegaly, splenomegaly, as well as a dilated portal vein by abdominal ultrasound, in addition to a prolonged INR ranging between 1.2–1.4, as well as arthropathy. Her brain MRI showed mild increase in signal intensity in the frontal lobes while her EEG was normal.

Patient (S7) presented with jaundice, increased abdominal girth, pitting edema, bleeding tendency along with generalized weakness.

Table 1. Summary of the washing stringency conditions optimized for the different normal and mutant probes.

Hybridization					
15ml APH + labeled probes for 3–4hours at specific annealing temperature					
Washings:	Volume ml/Time min/Temperature °C				
	Exon8	Exon10	Exon12	Exon13	Exon16
2XSSC-0.1%SDS	15/10/25	15/10/25	20/30/25	15/10/25	25/25/25
2XSSC-0.1%SDS	15/10/25	15/10/25	20/25/25	15/10/25	25/20/25
0.2XSSC- 0.1%SDS	15/20/25	15/15/25	20/25/34	20/20/25	20/20/25
0.2XSSC- 0.1%SDS	15/20/57	-	-	20/30/61	-
0.1XSSC-0.1%SDS	-	15/20/50	-	-	20/30/49

Radioactive ^{32}P labeled normal and mutant probes of Exons: 8, 10, 12, 13, &16 were hybridized with amplified denatured DNA loaded on positively charged membrane. Membranes were then washed under different stringency conditions with SSC- SDS. The abbreviation SSC-SDS stands for: Sodium chloride: Tri-Sodium Citrate (3 M: 0.3 M, pH 7) - Sodium Dodecyl Sulfate used at the indicated volume in ml, time in minutes and temperature °C.

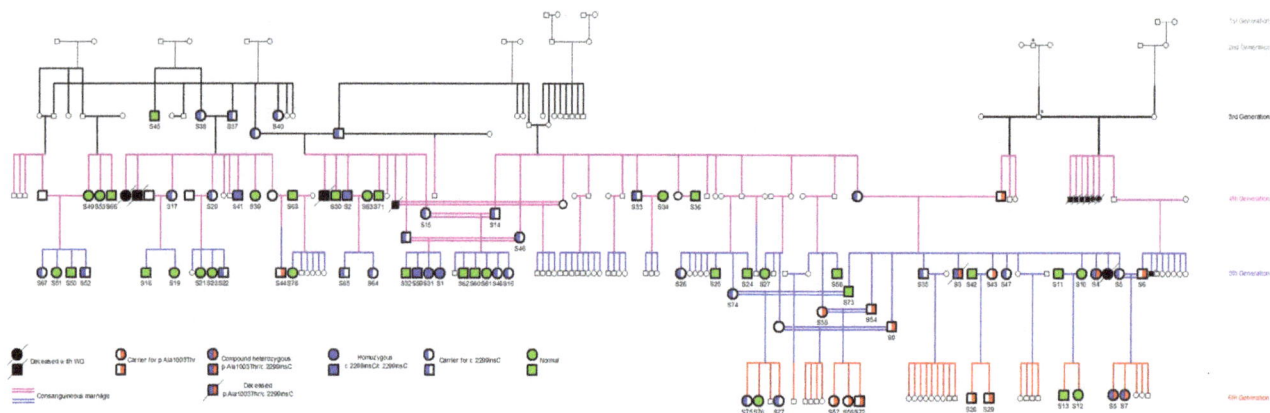

Figure 1. Pedigree of the S-family. The pedigree shows the 235 members of the S-family. The 76 members recruited in our study are highlighted. Nine members (S1, S2, S3, S4, S7, S8, S31, S41, S59) have WD. Generations were referred to by different colors: Gray for the 1st and 2nd; Black for the 3rd; Pink for the 4th; Blue for the 5th and Red for the 6th. * Refers to 2 men who were each married to 2 women.

She had no neurologic symptoms and her neurologic exam was normal. Her brain MRI showed bilateral ill-defined symmetrical areas of increased signal intensity involving Globus Pallidus and posterior limbs of internal capsule. In addition her abdominal ultrasound revealed changes of chronic liver disease as well as portal hypertension.

Patients (S1, S31) were found to have hepatomegaly by abdominal ultrasound and asymptomatic transaminitis upon diagnosis, with their alanine aminotransferase levels being elevated to 118 U/L and 105 U/L respectively. S1 had a normal Brain MRI and an EEG showing rare sharp waves in the right parietal area. Patient (S59) had hepatic involvement confirmed by ultrasonography showing fatty liver.

Two patients (S2, S41) presented with pure neurologic manifestations of WD at 12 and 16 years of age, respectively. The first presented with tremors, ataxia, slurred speech, in addition to arthropathy, while the second developed tremors, rigidity, and abnormal gait. Brain MRI of the former showed increased signal intensity in the basal ganglia and brain stem with involvement of brachium pontis bilaterally.

One patient (S8) who was asymptomatic had normal liver function tests, abdominal imaging, and brain MRI. The remaining 67 enrolled subjects were unaffected.

Mutation Analysis

The spectrum of mutations in the *ATP7B* gene of the S family was determined by sequencing exons 2–21 in WD patients (9/76) of the S family. DNA mutation numbering is based on cDNA. Genotypic findings of disease causing mutations are listed in Table 2. Five patients (S1, S2, S31, S41, and S59) were homozygous for a frame shift mutation (c. 2299insC/c. 2299insC, Exon-8/8). Four patients, (S3, S4, S7 and S8) were compound heterozygous for the frame shift in exon- 8, and missense mutation (c.3007G>A substitution) in exon-13: (c. 2299insC/p. Ala1003Thr). In addition all affected patients were simultaneously homozygous for 2 SNPs in Exon-16 (p. Val1140Ala) and Exon-12 (p. Arg 952 Lys). A SNP in Exon-10 (p. Lys832Arg) was also identified in the homozygous state in patients S1, S2, S31, S41, and S59; in the heterozygous state in S7 and S8; while it was normal in S3 and S4. Patients had normal sequences in all remaining exons: 2–7, 9, 11, 14, 15, 17, 18, 19, 20, and 21. Further screening of related family members using dot blot (Fig. 2) identified a high rate of mutant allele carriers (44.7%) distributed

as: 23/76 for the c. 2299insC (30.2%) and 11/76 for p. Ala1003Thr (14.5%). Random selection of the amplified ATP7B exons: 8, 10, 12, 13, and 16 from subjects screened by Dot Blot and including WD patients, were sequenced. Out of the 76 subjects a total of: 29 subjects for Exon-8; 19 subjects for Exon-10; 14 subjects for Exon-12; 23subjects for Exon-13, and 17 subjects for Exon-16 were sequenced confirming our Dot Blot findings.

Literature review findings

A total of 17 articles were included based on the following criteria: 1) the patient carries one of the aforementioned mutations in the homozygous or heterozygous state, or carries both of these mutations, and 2) the corresponding phenotypic presentation is stated as hepatic, neurologic, mixed or asymptomatic. Tables 3 and 4 present the number, age and nationality of patients that meet our inclusion criteria.

A total of 14 patients, including 5 of ours (this study), were homozygous for the c. 2299insC mutation (Table 3). The most common presentation was hepatic identified in 57%, while each of neurologic and asymptomatic equally presented at 21.4%. The majority of asymptomatic patients had transaminitis [18,19].

Twenty four compound heterozygous patients, carrying the c. 2299insC/allele, were identified worldwide with 12 hepatic (50%), 8 neurologic (33.3%), 3 mixed (12.5%) phenotypes and 1 asymptomatic (4%).

There were 11 patients carrying the p. Ala1003Thr mutation (c.3007G>A substitution), one of whom was homozygous and presented with hepatic phenotype at a young age (Table 4). Ten patients were compound heterozygous carrying the p. Ala1003Thr mutation on one allele. Patients with c. 2299insC on the second allele had a predominant hepatic presentation (4/5) with mean age of 13.5 yrs, whereas all patients (5/5) with non c. 2299insC on the second allele had neurologic presentation with a mean age of 22 years. One asymptomatic patient with the (c. 2299insC/p. Ala1003Thr) was diagnosed by screening at 15 years of age.

Discussion

We report in this paper the genotype-phenotype correlations in a very large single family with extensive consanguinity and a high prevalence of WD. The main finding of our study and of the literature review is an association between the c. 2299insC mutation in the homozygous and the compound heterozygous

Table 2. Clinical, biochemical and genetic profile of WD patients in the S family.

	S1	S2	S3	S4	S7	S8	S31	S41	S59
Year of birth	1993	1973	1981	1983	1993	1989	1997	1980	2007
Age (y) of symptoms onset	-	12	15	13	12	-	-	16	-
Age (y) at diagnosis	5 by screening[a]	12	16	14	12	15 by screening[a]	10 by screening[a]	16	1 by screening[a]
Clinical findings									
GI manifestations	Asymptomatic transaminitis, hepatomegaly	Absent [b]	Cirrhosis	Cirrhosis	Cirrhosis	Absent	Asymptomatic transaminitis, hepatomegaly	Absent	Asymptomatic fatty liver
Neurological	Absent	Slurred speech, ataxia, tremors	Absent	Absent	Absent	Absent	Absent	Choreo-athetosis, tremors, rigidity	Absent
Other	Absent	Arthralgia	Absent	Wilson's arthropathy	Absent	Absent	Absent	Absent	Absent
MRI of Brain	Normal	Increased signal intensity in the basal ganglia & brain stem	—	Mild increase in signal intensity in the frontal lobes	Increase in signal intensity involving globus pallidus	Normal	—	—	—
Kayser-Fleischer ring	Absent	Present	Present	Present	Present	Present	Absent	Present	Absent
Laboratory findings									
Serum ceruloplasmin g/L	<0.04	0.072	0.096	0.096	0.17	0.12	0.03	0.423[b]	<0.019
Serum Cu(µg/dL)	15	23	58	75	45	41	9	133.35	<5
24h urine Cu (µg)	99	512	775	590	645	487	152.8	230[c]	10
ALT, AST (IU/mL)	289, 167	17, 13	30, 41	30, 35	29, 45	45, 41	105, 51	3, 20	44, 37
Bilirubin T/D (mg/d)	0.3/0.1	0.4/0.2	0.5/0.2	0.4/0.1	0.7/0.3	0.7/0.2	0.2/0.1	1/0.4	0.3/0.1
Albumin (g/L)	50	43	35	43	37	40	45	45	47
INR	1	1.3	1.3	1.9	1.2	1.1	—	1	1.1
ATP7B Mutations*	2299insC/2299insC	2299insC/2299insC	2299insC/p. Ala1003Thr	2299insC/p. Ala1003Thr	2299insC/p. Ala1003Thr	2299insC/p. Ala1003Thr	2299insC/2299insC	2299insC/2299insC	2299insC/2299insC

[a]Screening refers to genetic screening of the ATP7B gene exons' by PCR followed by sequencing; [b]Few years later developed liver cirrhosis and portal hypertension;

Normal ranges of: Serum ceruloplasmin: 0.15–0.60 g/l; Serum Cu: 70–150 µg/dL; 24h urine Cu: 15–50 µg/24h; Bilirubin T/D: 0.2–1.2/0–0.5; [b]level determined after 7 years of treatment; [c]Urinary Cu level while S41was on penicillamine; * c.2298_2299insC is referred to as 2299insC. DNA Mutation numbering is based on cDNA numbering where nucleotide +1 as the A of the ATG translation initiation codon, in the reference sequence # NM_000053 with the initiation codon aa codon +1.

Exon 8 Normal N -5'-GACACGCCCCCCATGCTCTTT-3'

	1	2	3	4	5	6	7	8	9	10	11	12
A												
B		S41		S10		S23		S24		S25		
C			S26		S27		S28		S29		S33	
D		S3		S34		S35		S36		S40		
E			S42		S43		S44		S45		S49	
F		N1		S50		S51		S52		S53		
G			S54		S55		S56		S57		S58	
H												

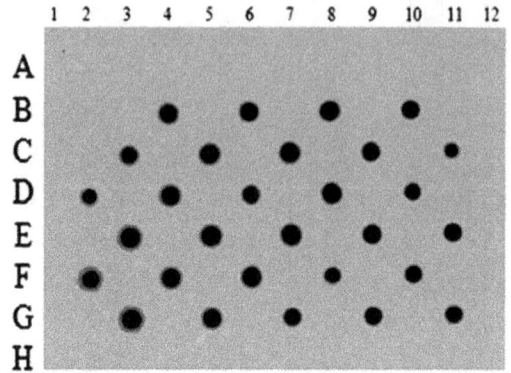

Exon 8 Mutant M-5'-GACACGCCCCCCCATGATCTTT-3'

	1	2	3	4	5	6	7	8	9	10	11	12
A												
B		S41		S10		S23		S24		S25		
C			S26		S27		S28		S29		S33	
D		S3		S34		S35		S36		S40		
E			S42		S43		S44		S45		S49	
F		N1		S50		S51		S52		S53		
G			S54		S55		S56		S57		S58	
H												

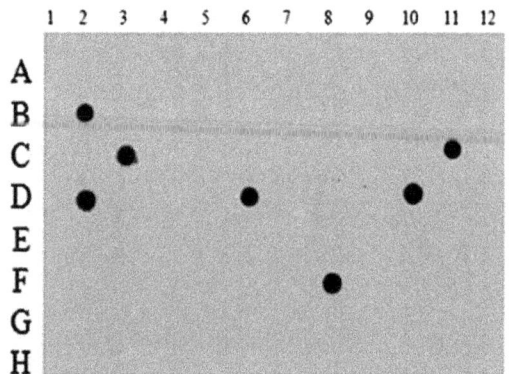

Figure 2. Dot blot image. A representative dot blot image of a membrane hybridized with normal and mutant probes of the identified exon 8 mutation. A dark spot resulting from hybridization with: Normal probe only, indicates a normal subject; Mutant probe only, indicates a homozygous subject; both normal and mutant probes indicate a carrier or heterozygous subject.

state and hepatic phenotype. On the other hand, there is an association with the mutation p. Ala1003Thr in the compound heterozygous state with a neurologic phenotype. Based on the most recent EASL practice guidelines, all patients in our study have definite Wilson disease [20].

More than 500 mutations have been described in WD, and missense ones are the most common. The majority of those mutations are rare and most patients are compound heterozygote. Hence, establishment of convincing genotype correlations has been difficult and results inconclusive [8,21–25]. In addition, other epigenetic and environmental factors play a role in disease presentation. Thus, conducting large consanguineous family studies in homogenous populations would facilitate establishment of genotype phenotype correlations as members of those families are more likely to share the same genetic and environmental factors and to be homozygous [9,26]. Finally, high concordance of the clinical and biochemical manifestations of WD among siblings suggests that members of the same family may have similar phenotypes [6], and that the influence of other genetic, epigenetic, and environmental factors may be similar in those members. As shown in the pedigree, 7 of our patients belonged to 3 nuclear sub-families reflecting the extensive consanguinity.

This is the largest single family ever reported with such a high prevalence of WD and of carriers of *ATP7B* mutations. All members of the family belong to the same village and ethnic group, with many members sharing a common household. Hence they had common environmental and dietary habits. Furthermore,

consanguineous marriage is the norm in this family as can be seen in the pedigree (Fig. 1). In addition, the 9 patients with WD are being taken care of in single tertiary care center, and thus all diagnostic procedures are uniformly standardized.

Six of our patients had liver disease, and three of those had full blown cirrhosis and portal hypertension. No liver biopsy was performed, but the diagnosis of liver cirrhosis was firmly established based on clinical, laboratory and imaging grounds as suggested elsewhere [27,28]. All six patients had the c. 2299insC mutation in the homozygous or compound heterozygous state, and 3 of them were females. However, two male patients that were homozygous for the c. 2299insC mutation had neurologic manifestations of Wilson disease, and one of them developed cirrhosis and portal hypertension years later. No liver biopsy was done on either.

As seen in table 3, there were 38 patients carrying the c. 2299insC mutation in the homozygous or compound heterozygous state worldwide. The frequencies of the hepatic, neurologic, mixed and asymptomatic phenotype was 53%, 29%, 11% and 8%, respectively. Four of the patients who had neurologic phenotype were compound heterozygous for p. His1069Gln which is known to be associated with neurologic phenotype [29]. Conversely, there were 10 compound heterozygous patients carrying the p. Ala1003Thr mutation (Table 4). For those carrying the c. 2299insC as the second mutation, hepatic phenotype was predominant, while for all others (5 out of 5), neurologic phenotype was predominant. Thus, an important question arises

Table 3. Phenotypes of patients homozygous and/or heterozygous for the c. 2299insC reported in the literature.

Genotype	Exons	No. of patients (age years)	Phenotype	Nationality	References
c.2299insC/c.2299insC[a]	8/8	1 (7)	Hepatic	Greek	Panagiotakaki et al. [34]
		2 (NA)	Hepatic	Egyptian	Abdelghaffar et al. [35]
		1 (8)	Hepatic	Cypriot	Butler et al. [36]
		1 (6)	Hepatic	Iranian	Dastsooz et al. [37]
		1 (10)	Neurologic	Chinese	Gu et al. [38]
		2 (1.3)	Asymptomatic[b]	Italian	Nicastro et al. [18]
		1 (NA)	Asymptomatic[b]	Egyptian	Abdel Ghaffar et al. [19]
		2 (7.5)	Hepatic[c]	Lebanese	Our study
		1 (1)	Hepatic[d]	Lebanese	Our study
		2 (14)	Neurologic	Lebanese	Our study
p.Arg616Gln/c.2299insC	5/8	1 (34)	Hepatic	Yugoslavian	Loudianos et al. [39]
		1 (22)	Neurologic	Bulgarian	Mihaylova et al. [40]
		1 (21)	Mixed	Bulgarian	Mihaylova et al. [40]
p.Met645Arg/c.2299insC	6/8	1 (10)	Hepatic	Spanish	Margarit et al. [23]
c.2299insC/p.Arg816Ser	8/9	1 (26)	Neurologic	Austrian	Hofer et al. [41]
c.2299insC/p.Val949Gly	8/12	1 (26)	Neurologic	Brazilian	Deguti et al. [42]
c.2299insC/p.Ala1003Thr	8/13	1 (15)	Hepatic	Yugoslavian	Loudianos et al. [39]
		3(14)	Hepatic	Lebanese	Our study
		1 (15)	Asymptomatic	Lebanese	Our study
c.2299insC/p.His1069Gln	8/14	4 (23.75)	Neurologic	Yugoslavian	Loudianos et al. [39]
		1 (10)	Hepatic	Turkish	Simsek Papur et al. [43]
c.2299insC/3402delC	8/15	1 (33)	Neurologic	Yugoslavian	Loudianos et al. [39]
		1 (9)	Hepatic	Brazilian	Deguti et al. [42]
c.2299insC/p.Leu1255Ile	8/18	1 (10)	Hepatic	Korean	Yoo [2]
c.2299insC/NA[e]	8/NA	2 (21)	Mixed	Thai	Keandaungjuntr et al. [44]
		1 (NA)	Hepatic	Egyptian	Abdelghaffar et al. [35]
		1 (19)	Hepatic	Yugoslavian	Loudianos et al. [39]
		1 (10)	Hepatic	Brazilian	Deguti et al. [42]

a. The identified c.2298–2299insC is referred to as c.2299insC.
b. The majority of asymptomatic patients in this study had transaminitis or hepatomegaly.
c. Asymptomatic transaminitis.
d. Asymptomatic fatty liver.
e. Unidentified or not reported.

Table 4. Phenotypes of patients homozygous and/or heterozygous for the p. Ala1003Thr missense mutation reported in the literature.

Genotype	Exons	No. of patients (age years)	Phenotype	Nationality	References
p.Ala1003Thr/p.Ala1003Thr	13/13	1 (<8)	Hepatic	Indian	Kumar et al. [13]
c.2299insC/p. Ala1003Thr	8/13	1 (15)	Hepatic	Yugoslavian	Loudianos et al. [39]
		3 (14)	Hepatic	Lebanese	Our study
		1 (15)	Asymptomatic	Lebanese	Our study
p.Ala1003Thr/p.His1069Gln	13/14	1 (23)	Neurologic	Yugoslavian	Loudianos et al. [39]
		1 (26)	Neurologic	Danish	Moller et al. [30]
p.Ala1003Thr/p.Val1036Ile	13/14	1 (25)	Neurologic	Turkish	Simsek Papur et al. [43]
p.Ala1003Thr/NA[a]	13/NA	1 (16)	Neurologic	Yugoslavian	Loudianos et al. [39]
		1 (20)	Neurologic	Greek	Butler et al. [36]

in compound heterozygous patients: which mutation dictates the phenotype of the patient? In view of the small number of patients and large number of mutations, this question may be difficult to answer. A suggestion by MØller LB et al [30] was made that the milder mutation dictates the age of onset and possibly the phenotype. She considered both c. 2299insC and p. His1069Gln to be severe mutations based on earlier onset of symptoms. In our study, the mean age of patients carrying the c. 2299insC mutation is 14.4 years and of those carrying the p. Ala1003Thr mutation is 17 years. Based on that, both mutations would be considered "severe". However, extensive heterogeneity exists in age of onset as shown in Tables 3 and 4.

In an ongoing study on genotype-phenotype correlations in Caucasian patients, preliminary results suggest that hepatic phenotype is present in 69% of patients who are compound heterozygous c.2299 insC/p. His1069Gln [8]. This is consistent with our suggestion that c. 2299insC is associated with hepatic phenotype, even when it is combined with another mutation that is associated with neurologic phenotype.

What then could explain the severe hepatic phenotype of a patient who is homozygous for p. Ala1003Thr as reported by Kumar et al [13]? We had reported before a strong association between hepatic phenotype, hepatic failure and homozygosity for missense mutations other than p. His1069Gln [12]. Thus, it looks like there are multiple genetic determinants of phenotype in WD, including homozygosity, the type of mutation and its severity, the weight of individual mutations in those who are compound heterozygote, as well as other known and unknown genetic and epigenetic factors.

Establishing genotype–phenotype correlations is clearly important for appropriate patient management, for initiation of early therapy in asymptomatic patients to prevent certain complications, and for monitoring the efficacy of treatment. Furthermore, it enhances understanding of the molecular pathogenesis of the disease. However, it is still fraught with extensive difficulties. In addition to the complex genetic factors, the extensive phenotypic heterogeneity of WD, and the small number of patients, other factors seem to be important in determining phenotype in WD. These include sex, ethnicity, environmental and dietary factors as well as percentage residual activity of the translated protein. Furthermore, younger age of onset of symptoms may contribute to the phenotype as well.

In the absence of a purified protein, our current understanding of how mutations and SNPs affect protein function, and therefore phenotype, remains speculative. It is plausible to assume that derangement in protein function varies with nature and position of mutation. Discordance in monozygotic twins suggests that environmental, dietary, and epigenetic factors including copper chaperones may contribute to the phenotype [31]. In addition, the expression of the *ATP7B* gene product and/or its isoforms is another factor [32]. Alternative splicing of the ATP7B gene is tissue specific. Whereas all exons are expressed in the translated liver protein, several alternatively spliced isoforms are expressed in the brain; resulting from skipping certain exons [33]. Thus translation of the *ATP7B* gene, carrying a mutation in an alternatively spliced exon, may have no phenotypic effect or manifest clinical dysfunction of that organ. Though difficult to perform *in vivo*, variation in the expression level of the different *ATP7B* isoforms in liver and brain might help in explaining the phenotypic diversity in subjects with identical genotype.

Our study has several strengths. The family we evaluated is very large and has extensive consanguinity. Its members belong to the same ethnic group and they have the same environmental exposure and similar dietary habits. Thus, potentially compounding factors on the effect of genotype on phenotype are eliminated or reduced. There are also limitations to our study. Twelve members of this family died apparently of WD. We have no way of ascertaining their phenotype. In addition, individuals belonging to such a poor family may not seek medical attention if they develop mild symptoms, due to financial limitations. Furthermore manifestations of mild phenotypes may not be easily recognized. Finally, we depended in our literature review on cases where the phenotypes are clearly indicated.

In conclusion, phenotype-genotype correlations in WD patients remain a challenge as long as diagnosis at the asymptomatic stage is not possible and functional assay of purified normal and mutant protein is still unavailable.

Acknowledgments

The authors are thankful to all patients who accepted to participate in this study.

Author Contributions

Contributed reagents/materials/analysis tools: O ER: pedigree and consent forms, figures. Conceived and designed the experiments: JU KB. Performed the experiments: KR OER. Analyzed the data: JU KB TM TAE. Wrote the paper: JU KB TM TAE.

References

1. Sternlieb I (1993) The outlook for the diagnosis of Wilson's disease. J Hepatol 17: 263–264.
2. Yoo HW (2002) Identification of novel mutations and the three most common mutations in the human ATP7B gene of Korean patients with Wilson disease. Genet Med 4: 43S–48S.
3. Bruha R, Marecek Z, Pospisilova L, Nevsimalova S, Vitek L, et al. (2011) Long-term follow-up of Wilson disease: natural history, treatment, mutations analysis and phenotypic correlation. Liver Int 31: 83–91.
4. Harada M (2002) Wilson disease. Med Electron Microsc 35: 61–66.
5. Gow PJ, Smallwood RA, Angus PW, Smith AL, Wall AJ, et al. (2000) Diagnosis of Wilson's disease: an experience over three decades. Gut 46: 415–419.
6. Chabik G, Litwin T, Czlonkowska A (2014) Concordance rates of Wilson's disease phenotype among siblings. J Inherit Metab Dis 37: 131–135.
7. Cheng TF, Choudhuri S, Muldoon-Jacobs K (2012) Epigenetic targets of some toxicologically relevant metals: a review of the literature. J Appl Toxicol 32: 643–653.
8. Ferenci P (2014) Phenotype-genotype correlations in patients with Wilson's disease. Ann N Y Acad Sci. 1315: 1–5.
9. Barada K, El-Atrache M, El H II, Rida K, El-Hajjar J, et al. (2010) Homozygous mutations in the conserved ATP hinge region of the Wilson disease gene: association with liver disease. J Clin Gastroenterol 44: 432–439.
10. Barbour B, Salameh P (2009) Consanguinity in Lebanon: prevalence, distribution and determinants. J Biosoc Sci 41: 505–517.
11. Barada K, Nemer G, ElHajj, II, Touma J, Cortas N, et al. (2007) Early and severe liver disease associated with homozygosity for an exon 7 mutation, G691R, in Wilson's disease. Clin Genet 72: 264–267.
12. Usta J, Abu Daya H, Halawi H, Al-Shareef I, El-Rifai O, et al. (2012) Homozygosity for Non-H1069Q Missense Mutations in ATP7B Gene and Early Severe Liver Disease: Report of Two Families and a Meta-analysis. JIMD Rep 4: 129–137.
13. Kumar S, Thapa BR, Kaur G, Prasad R (2006) Familial gene analysis for Wilson disease from north-west Indian patients. Ann Hum Biol 33: 177–186.
14. Gupta A, Aikath D, Neogi R, Datta S, Basu K, et al. (2005) Molecular pathogenesis of Wilson disease: haplotype analysis, detection of prevalent mutations and genotype-phenotype correlation in Indian patients. Hum Genet 118: 49–57.

15. Ferenci P, Caca K, Loudianos G, Mieli-Vergani G, Tanner S, et al. (2003) Diagnosis and phenotypic classification of Wilson disease. Liver Int 23: 139–142.

16. Petrukhin K, Lutsenko S, Chernov I, Ross BM, Kaplan JH, et al. (1994) Characterization of the Wilson disease gene encoding a P-type copper transporting ATPase: genomic organization, alternative splicing, and structure/function predictions. Hum Mol Genet 3: 1647–1656.

17. Ausubel FM (1988) Current protocols in molecular biology. New York: Published by Greene Pub.Associates and Wiley-Interscience: J. Wiley.

18. Nicastro E, Loudianos G, Zancan L, D'Antiga L, Maggiore G, et al. (2009) Genotype-phenotype correlation in Italian children with Wilson's disease. J Hepatol 50: 555–561.

19. Abdel Ghaffar TY, Elsayed SM, Elnaghy S, Shadeed A, Elsobky ES, et al. (2011) Phenotypic and genetic characterization of a cohort of pediatric Wilson disease patients. BMC Pediatr 11: 56.

20. Ferenci P, Czlonkowska A, Stremmel W, Houwen R, Rosenberg W, et al. (2012) EASL Clinical Practice Guidelines: Wilson's disease. J Hepatol 56: 671–685.

21. Curtis D, Durkie M, Balac P, Sheard D, Goodeve A, et al. (1999) A study of Wilson disease mutations in Britain. Hum Mutat 14: 304–311.

22. Kalinsky H, Funes A, Zeldin A, Pel-Or Y, Korostishevsky M, et al. (1998) Novel ATP7B mutations causing Wilson disease in several Israeli ethnic groups. Hum Mutat 11: 145–151.

23. Margarit E, Bach V, Gomez D, Bruguera M, Jara P, et al. (2005) Mutation analysis of Wilson disease in the Spanish population — identification of a prevalent substitution and eight novel mutations in the ATP7B gene. Clin Genet 68: 61–68.

24. Shah AB, Chernov I, Zhang HT, Ross BM, Das K, et al. (1997) Identification and analysis of mutations in the Wilson disease gene (ATP7B): population frequencies, genotype-phenotype correlation, and functional analyses. Am J Hum Genet 61: 317–328.

25. Kegley KM, Sellers MA, Ferber MJ, Johnson MW, Joelson DW, et al. (2010) Fulminant Wilson's disease requiring liver transplantation in one monozygotic twin despite identical genetic mutation. Am J Transplant 10: 1325–1329.

26. Thomas GR, Forbes JR, Roberts EA, Walshe JM, Cox DW (1995) The Wilson disease gene: spectrum of mutations and their consequences. Nat Genet 9: 210–217.

27. Obrador BD, Prades MG, Gomez MV, Domingo JP, Cueto RB, et al. (2006) A predictive index for the diagnosis of cirrhosis in hepatitis C based on clinical, laboratory, and ultrasound findings. Eur J Gastroenterol Hepatol 18: 57–62.

28. Pinzani M, Rombouts K, Colagrande S (2005) Fibrosis in chronic liver diseases: diagnosis and management. J Hepatol 42 Suppl: S22–36.

29. Stapelbroek JM, Bollen CW, van Amstel JK, van Erpecum KJ, van Hattum J, et al. (2004) The H1069Q mutation in ATP7B is associated with late and neurologic presentation in Wilson disease: results of a meta-analysis. J Hepatol 41: 758–763.

30. Moller LB, Horn N, Jeppesen TD, Vissing J, Wibrand F, et al. (2011) Clinical presentation and mutations in Danish patients with Wilson disease. Eur J Hum Genet 19: 935–941.

31. Huffman DL, O'Halloran TV (2001) Function, structure, and mechanism of intracellular copper trafficking proteins. Annu Rev Biochem 70: 677–701.

32. Wilson AM, Schlade-Bartusiak K, Tison JL, Macintyre G, Cox DW (2009) A minigene approach for analysis of ATP7B splice variants in patients with Wilson disease. Biochimie 91: 1342–1345.

33. Wan L, Tsai CH, Hsu CM, Huang CC, Yang CC, et al. (2010) Mutation analysis and characterization of alternative splice variants of the Wilson disease gene ATP7B. Hepatology 52: 1662–1670.

34. Panagiotakaki E, Tzetis M, Manolaki N, Loudianos G, Papatheodorou A, et al. (2004) Genotype-phenotype correlations for a wide spectrum of mutations in the Wilson disease gene (ATP7B). Am J Med Genet A 131: 168–173.

35. Abdelghaffar TY, Elsayed SM, Elsobky E, Bochow B, Buttner J, et al. (2008) Mutational analysis of ATP7B gene in Egyptian children with Wilson disease: 12 novel mutations. J Hum Genet 53: 681–687.

36. Butler P, McIntyre N, Mistry PK (2001) Molecular diagnosis of Wilson disease. Mol Genet Metab 72: 223–230.

37. Dastsooz H, Dehghani SM, Imanieh MH, Haghighat M, Moini M, et al. (2013) A new ATP7B gene mutation with severe condition in two unrelated Iranian families with Wilson disease. Gene 514: 48–53.

38. Gu YH, Kodama H, Du SL, Gu QJ, Sun HJ, et al. (2003) Mutation spectrum and polymorphisms in ATP7B identified on direct sequencing of all exons in Chinese Han and Hui ethnic patients with Wilson's disease. Clin Genet 64: 479–484.

39. Loudianos G, Kostic V, Solinas P, Lovicu M, Dessi V, et al. (2003) Characterization of the molecular defect in the ATP7B gene in Wilson disease patients from Yugoslavia. Genet Test 7: 107–112.

40. Mihaylova V, Todorov T, Jelev H, Kotsev I, Angelova L, et al. (2012) Neurological symptoms, genotype-phenotype correlations and ethnic-specific differences in Bulgarian patients with Wilson disease. Neurologist 18: 184–189.

41. Hofer H, Willheim-Polli C, Knoflach P, Gabriel C, Vogel W, et al. (2012) Identification of a novel Wilson disease gene mutation frequent in Upper Austria: a genetic and clinical study. J Hum Genet 57: 564–567.

42. Deguti MM, Genschel J, Cancado EL, Barbosa ER, Bochow B, et al. (2004) Wilson disease: novel mutations in the ATP7B gene and clinical correlation in Brazilian patients. Hum Mutat 23: 398.

43. Simsek Papur O, Akman SA, Cakmur R, Terzioglu O (2013) Mutation analysis of ATP7B gene in Turkish Wilson disease patients: identification of five novel mutations. Eur J Med Genet 56: 175–179.

44. Keandaungjuntr J, Busabaratana M, Kositchaiwat C, Sura T, Pulkes T (2011) Analysis of exon 8 of ATP7B gene in Thai patients with Wilson disease. J Med Assoc Thai 94: 1184–1188.

2

Evaluation of the Diagnostic Performance of Magnetic Resonance Spectroscopy in Brain Tumors

Wenzhi Wang, Yumin Hu, Peiou Lu, Yingci Li, Yunfu Chen, Mohan Tian*, Lijuan Yu*

Center of PET/CT-MRI, Cancer Hospital of Harbin Medical University, Harbin, 150081, China

Abstract

Object: The aim of this study was to determine the suitability of magnetic resonance spectroscopy (MRS) for screening brain tumors, based on a systematic review and meta-analysis of published data on the diagnostic performance of MRS.

Methods: The PubMed and PHMC databases were systematically searched for relevant studies up to December 2013. The sensitivities and specificities of MRS in individual studies were calculated and the pooled diagnostic accuracies, with 95% confidence intervals (CI), were assessed under a fixed-effects model.

Results: Twenty-four studies were included, comprising a total of 1013 participants. Overall, no heterogeneity of diagnostic effects was observed between studies. The pooled sensitivity and specificity of MRS were 80.05% (95% CI = 75.97%–83.59%) and 78.46% (95% CI: 73.40%–82.78%), respectively. The area under the summary receiver operating characteristic curve was 0.78. Stratified meta analysis showed higher sensitivity and specificity in child than adult. CSI had higher sensitivity and SV had higher specificity. Higher sensitivity and specificity were obtained in short TE value.

Conclusion: Although the qualities of the studies included in the meta-analysis were moderate, current evidence suggests that MRS may be a valuable adjunct to magnetic resonance imaging for diagnosing brain tumors, but requires selection of suitable technique and TE value.

Editor: Daniel Monleon, Instituto de Investigación Sanitaria INCLIVA, Spain

Funding: The authors received no specific funding for this work.

Competing Interests: The authors have declared that no competing interests exist.

* Email: tianmohan2000@126.com (MT); yulijuan2003@126.com (LY)

Introduction

The early detection of brain tumors is associated with significant clinical benefits, but presents a diagnostic challenge. A total of 57,100 new cases of brain tumors were diagnosed in Europe in 2012, and 45,000 deaths were attributed to brain tumors, half of which were glioblastomas [1]. Information on histological grade and tissue diagnosis are important for the clinical management of brain cancers, and are closely related to survival probability. However, there are two major limitations to the histopathological grading of brain tumors, especially gliomas. Firstly, although stereotactic biopsy can adequately represent pathological grading of the whole tumor, potential sampling error of biopsy was inherent. Secondly, it is very difficult to accurate assess residual tumor tissue after cytoreductive surgery [2]. Contrast-enhanced magnetic resonance imaging (MRI) is the current gold standard for guiding neurosurgeons when obtaining biopsy tissue for the diagnosis of brain tumors. However, the results of this technique can sometimes be ambiguous, and differentiating progressive or recurrent brain tumors from radiation-induced injury is difficult using MRI [3]. Proton magnetic resonance spectroscopy (MRS) provides important metabolic information of tumours, such as N-acetyl-aspartate (NAA), choline (Cho), creatine (Cr) at different MRS echo times (TEs), and showed a major advantage without electromagnetic radiation exposure as an imaging technique for guiding brain tumor biopsy procedures [4].

Several recent studies have reported the utility of MRS for brain tumor assessment, with the ability to differentiate between high-grade and low-grade gliomas [5], and between neoplastic and non-neoplastic brain lesions [6]. However, it is difficult to draw conclusions based on individual studies because variations in study qualities, and different inpatient populations and study designs may cause heterogeneity among study results. To overcome the shortcomings of individual studies, we performed a systematic review and meta-analysis of published data on the diagnostic performance of MRS for detecting, differentiating, and grading brain tumors, especially gliomas, to determine the diagnostic value of MRS.

Identification

Articles identified through key words : magnetic resonance spectroscopy, brain tumor or gliomas, sensitivity and specificty.
PubMed, N=291; PHMC, N=774

Articles identified through key words : magnetic resonance spectroscopy, brain tumor or gliomas, multi-centre study.
PubMed, N=4

868search results retrieved after 197duplicates removed

Screening

Article exclusion by title and abstract(n=814)
PubMed (n=123); PHMC (n=691)

Title and abstract screened, N=54

Eligibility

Full-text articles were accessed for eligibility, N=48

Article exclusion with reason:(n=24)
-review (n=2)
-not relevant outcome (5)
-not magnetic resonance spectroscopy diagnosis(17)

Included

n=24 articles were included in qualitative synthesis
605cases and 408 controls

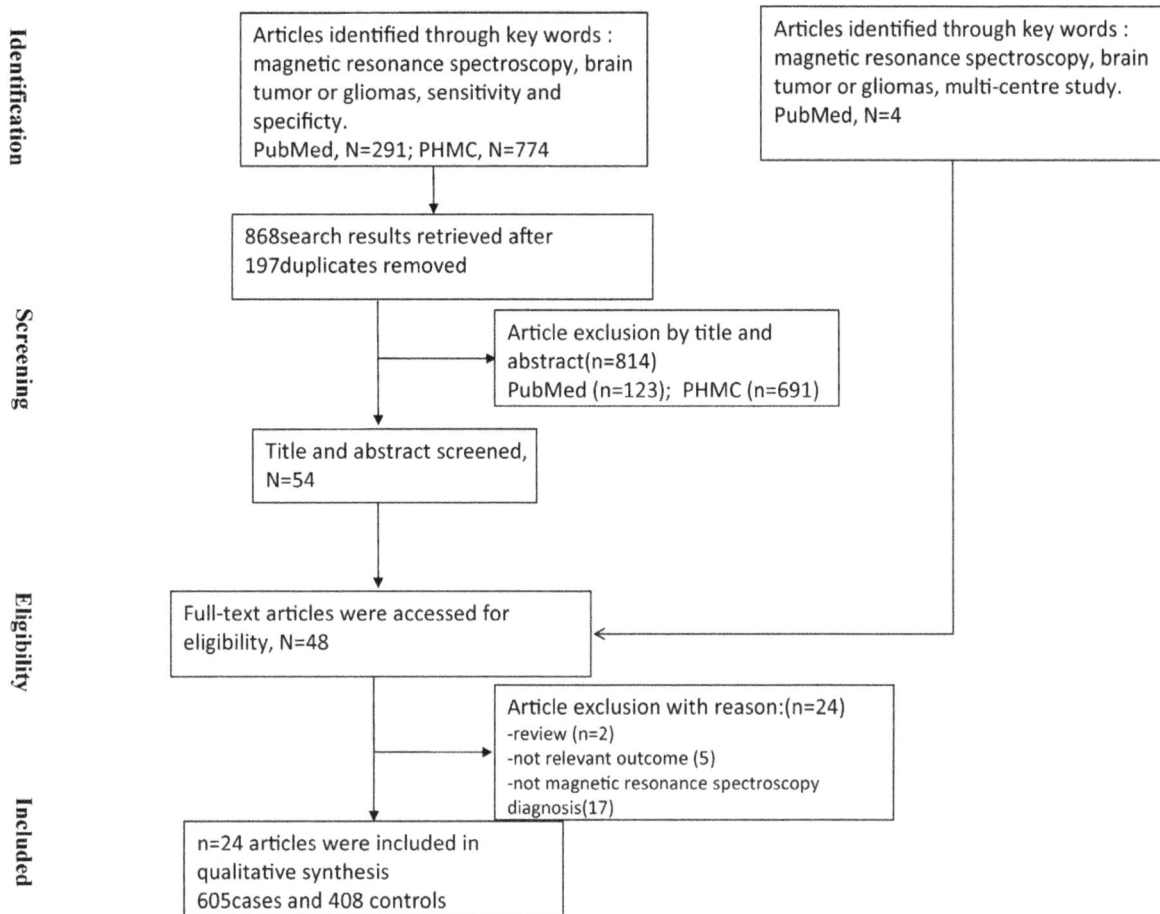

Figure 1. Flow chart showing the process of studies retrieved.

Materials and Methods

Data sources and search strategy

Electronic searches of the Medline (using PubMed as the search engine) and ProQuest Health & Medical Complete databases were conducted using the terms 'magnetic resonance spectroscopy', 'brain tumor or gliomas' and 'sensitivity and specificity' to identify appropriate studies published in English prior to December 30, 2013. Included studies must have used MRS to detect the occurrence, grade, recurrence, or transformation of brain tumors.

Study selection

Two authors independently screened the search results by title and abstract. They obtained the full text of each manuscript and excluded studies with overlapping data and studies that did not provide both sensitivity and specificity information for MRS evaluation of brain tumors. Author names, institutions, publication dates, tumor and assessment types were collected for all studies. All the studies were evaluated independently and discussed by the authors until a consensus was reached.

Data extraction and quality assessment

Two authors independently extracted the data from each study, including information on the first author, year of publication, country, sample size, tumor and assessment type, and sensitivity and specificity of MRS for brain tumors, as well as the risk of bias according to pre-specified criteria from the Cochrane Collabora-

tion's tool for assessing risk of bias [7]. The following risk-of-bias items were evaluated independently by two authors using standardized methods: sequencing generation, allocation concealment, blinding of patients and study personnel, blinding of outcome assessment, incomplete outcome data, selective reporting, and other biases.

Data synthesis and statistical analysis

In order to evaluate the diagnostic accuracy of MRS for brain tumors, we calculated the sensitivity, specificity, positive likelihood ratio (PLR), negative likelihood ratio (NLR), diagnostic odds ratio (DOR) and 95% confidence intervals (CI). The result of pathologic tissue diagnosis was the reference standard in all cases. Due to the different diagnostic purpose in multiple studies, different positive sets were defined. For tumor recurrence studies, recurrence was considered as positive and postoperative necrosis was negative. For tumor grading studies, high-grade gliomas (III–IV grade) were positive and low-grade gliomas (I–II) were negative. Statistical heterogeneities in summary effects of PLR, NLR, and DOR were tested in all data using Cochran's Q test, which approximately follows a χ^2 distribution with $k-1$ degrees of freedom (where k is the number of studies included) [8]. The statistic $I^2 = ((Q-(k-1))/Q) \times 100\%$ was also assessed. I^2 ranged from 0–100%, with 0–25%, 25–50%, 50–75%, and 75–100% indicating low, moderate, high, and very high degrees of heterogeneity, respectively [9]. We considered a p value <0.05 to indicate significant heterogeneity. Values of diagnostic effects were evaluated usinga fixed-effects or

Table 1. Characteristics of all included studies.

Study	Center	Period	Cancer	Type	TP	FP	FN	TN	Technique	Method(ms)	Cutoff
Reddy et al (2013)	Single	Adult	Gliomas	Recurrent	2	1	2	7	-	-	-
Pamir et al (2013)	Single	Adult	Gliomas	Residual	12	0	2	6	SV	LTE=135	Cho/Cr ↑ 20%
Sahin et al (2013)	Single	Adult	Gliomas	Grade	6	4	0	10	CSI	STE=30	Cho/Cr=1.3
Seeger et al (2013)	Single	Adult	Gliomas	Recurrent	16	4	7	13	CSI	LTE=135	Cho/Cr=2.33
Amin et al (2012)	Single	Adult	Gliomas	Recurrent	11	0	7	6	SV	STE=30	Cho/Cr=1.5
Crisi et al (2013)	Single	Adult	Gliomas	Detection	18	3	5	15	SV	STE=35	-
Liu et al (2012)	Single	Adult	Gliomas	Grade	19	1	3	9	SV	LTE=144	Cho/Cr=2.01
Liu et al (2012)	Single	Adult	Gliomas	Grade	16	1	6	9	SV	LTE=144	Cho/NAA=2.49
Liu et al (2012)	Single	Adult	Gliomas	Grade	17	3	5	7	SV	LTE=144	NAA/Cr=0.97
Peng et al (2012)	Single	Adult	Gliomas	Detection	19	6	3	13	CSI	LTE=144	Cho/Cr=3.16
Peng et al (2012)	Single	Adult	Gliomas	Detection	18	2	4	17	CSI	LTE=144	Cho/NAA=2.13
Peng et al (2012)	Single	Adult	Gliomas	Detection	14	2	8	17	CSI	LTE=144	Cho/Cho-n=1.28
Guillevin et al (2011)	Single	Adult	Gliomas	Recurrent	5	0	3	13	SV	TE=35/144	(Cho/NAA-Cho/Cr)/(Cho/NAA)=0.046
Zou et al (2011)	Single	Adult	Gliomas	Grade	15	0	3	12	CSI	LTE=135	NAA/Cho=0.265, ADC=1118.1×10^{-6} mm^2/s
Server et al (2011)	Single	Adult	Gliomas	Grade	54	0	5	15	CSI	LTE=135	Cho/NAA=1.78
Prat et al (2010)	Single	Adult	Gliomas	Recurrent	11	1	0	12	-	-	-
Zeng et al (2011)	Single	Adult	Gliomas	Grade	21	2	4	10	CSI	LTE=144	Cho/Cr=2.04
Zeng et al (2011)	Single	Adult	Gliomas	Grade	22	4	3	8	CSI	LTE=144	Cho/NAA=2.20
Zeng et al (2011)	Single	Adult	Gliomas	Grade	19	4	6	8	CSI	LTE=144	NAA/Cr=0.72
Senft et al (2009)	Single	Adult	Gliomas	Grade	28	17	8	10	CSI	LTE=144	Cho$_{mean}$=1.51
Senft et al (2009)	Single	Adult	Gliomas	Grade	31	6	5	21	CSI	LTE=144	Cho$_{max}$=2.02
Senft et al (2009)	Single	Adult	Gliomas	Grade	26	14	10	13	CSI	LTE=144	CE
Senft et al (2009)	Single	Adult	Gliomas	Grade	28	9	8	18	CSI	LTE=144	Cho/Cr=0.58
Hlaihel et al (2009)	Single	Adult	Gliomas	Metastases	4	1	1	15	SV/CSI	LTE/STE=32/136	Cho/Cr=2.4
Hlaihel et al (2009)	Single	Adult	Gliomas	Metastases	5	8	0	8	SV/CSI	LTE/STE=32/136	Cho/Cr=1.7
Hlaihel et al (2009)	Single	Adult	Gliomas	Metastases	2	5	3	11	SV/CSI	LTE/STE=32/136	rCBV=2
Hlaihel et al (2009)	Single	Adult	Gliomas	Metastases	2	7	3	9	SV/CSI	LTE/STE=32/136	rCBV=1.75
Hlaihel et al (2009)	Single	Adult	Gliomas	Metastases	4	7	1	9	SV/CSI	LTE/STE=32/136	rCBV=1.5
Zeng et al (2007)	Single	Adult	Gliomas	Recurrent	18	0	1	9	CSI	LTE=144	Cho/Cr=1.71
Palumbo et al (2006)	Single	Adult	Gliomas	Recurrent	17	1	2	10	SV	LTE=144	Cho/Cr=2.0
Fayed et al (2006)	Single	Adult	Gliomas	Grade	17	2	1	10	SV	STE=30	Cho/Cr=1.56
Floeth et al (2005)	Single	Adult	Gliomas	Detection	34	3	0	13	SV	LTE=135	-
Law et al (2003)	Single	Adult/Child	Gliomas	Grade	117	6	3	44	CSI	STE=6	Cho/Cr=1.08
Wang et al (1995)	Single	Child	Astrocytoma	Detection	10	1	1	14	SV	LTE=135/270	-

Table 1. Cont.

Study	Center	Period	Cancer	Type	TP	FP	FN	TN	Technique	Method(ms)	Cutoff
Wang et al (1995)	Single	Child	Ependymoma	Detection	3	2	1	20	SV	LTE = 135/270	–
Wang et al (1995)	Single	Child	Neuroectodermal tumor	Detection	9	1	2	14	SV	LTE = 135/270	–
Vellido et al (2012)	Multiple	Adult	Gliomas	Metastases	7	3	3	27	SV	STE/LTE = 20/135	–
Vellido et al (2012)	Multiple	Adult	Gliomas	Metastases	9	5	1	25	SV	STE/LTE = 20/135	–
Vellido et al (2012)	Multiple	Adult	Gliomas	Metastases	6	2	4	28	SV	STE/LTE = 20/135	–
Vellido et al (2012)	Multiple	Adult	Gliomas	Metastases	9	5	1	25	SV	STE/LTE = 20/135	–
Tate et al (2006)	Multiple	Adult	Gliomas	Grade	44	2	5	12	SV	STE = 20	–
Davies et al (2008)	Single	Child	Astrocytoma	Detection	16	0	0	18	SV	STE = 30	–

random-effects model, depending on the p value of the heterogeneity test. A summary receiver operating characteristic (SROC) curve was generated based on the sensitivity and specificity of each study for assessing the diagnostic accuracy. Linear regression of the logits of the sensitivity (Se) and specificity (Sp) was used to fit the SROC curve, through the equation $D = a+b \times S$, where $D = logit(Se) - logit(1-Sp) = log(OR)$ and $S = logit(Se) + logit(1 - Sp)$, a is the intercept and b is the regression coefficient estimated in the regression equation. D represents the diagnostic log-odds ratio that relates to the test's diagnostic accuracy for discriminating between disease-positivity and negativity, depending on the threshold used. S represents the threshold for classifying a test as positive. The closer b is to 0, the more evidence exists for a lack of significant heterogeneity with respect to OR. If b differs from 0, the OR is dependent on the threshold used. The SROC curve can be fit weighted by the inverse of the variance of the logarithm of OR from the individual studies corresponding to the area under the SROC curve (AUC). Based on the SROC, when Se equals Sp, where $Se = exp(a/2)/[1+exp(a/2)]$ and $1-Sp = 1/[1+exp(a/2)]$, $Q* = Se = 1-Sp$ was estimated to represent the diagnostic threshold at which the probability of a correct diagnosis was constant for all subjects. Funnel plot analyses and Egg's test were used to evaluate publication bias. All statistical tests were performed using mada package in R [10].

Results

Study characteristics

A total of 54 studies were identified after filtering titles and abstracts, and four multi-centre studies including pattern recognition studies was retrieved from PubMed. Finally, full texts of 48 studies were obtained. 24 studies were excluded based on the inclusion criteria, including two studies that were reviews, five studies that did not report the sensitivity and specificity of MRS for brain tumor diagnosis, and seventeen studies that did not use MRS to assess the tumor. The systematic literature search yielded 24 studies including 1013 participants (605 cases and 408 controls, Figure 1). The studies originated from 10 countries or regions (including the USA, Turkey, China, Japan, Norway, Spain, France, Germany, Italy and Egypt) and were published between 1995 and 2013. The sample sizes of the included studies ranged from 12–160 (mean 40).

All the included studies evaluated the diagnostic accuracy of MRS for the detection or grading of brain tumors. Twenty-two studies assessed gliomas [2,11,12,13,14,15,16,17,18,19,20,21,22, 23,24,25,26,27,28,29,30,31], two study assessed ependymomas and primitive neuroectodermal tumors [32,33]. Seven studies evaluated the diagnostic power of recurrence [11,14,15,19,22, 26,27], nine studies evaluated the grade [2,13,17,20,21,23,24, 28,31], five studies evaluated the detection [16,18,29,32,33], one evaluated residual tumor [12], and two evaluated tumor metastases [25,30]. The detailed diagnostic power are shown in Table 1.

Exploration of heterogeneity and sensitivity analysis

We assessed the risk of bias for each study, and the detailed standard and results for each item of bias are shown in Table S1 and Figure S1. The risk of bias is summarized in Figure 2A. In general, the risk of bias was low or unclear in most studies for many assessed items. Six studies stated that the sequences of participants were generated randomly and were therefore defined as low risk. The sponsors of 30%–67% of studies had authorship and were not involved in data collection, assessment of tumors, or interpretation of the outcomes. The sensitivities and specificities of all the different diagnostic methods were reported in 50% of

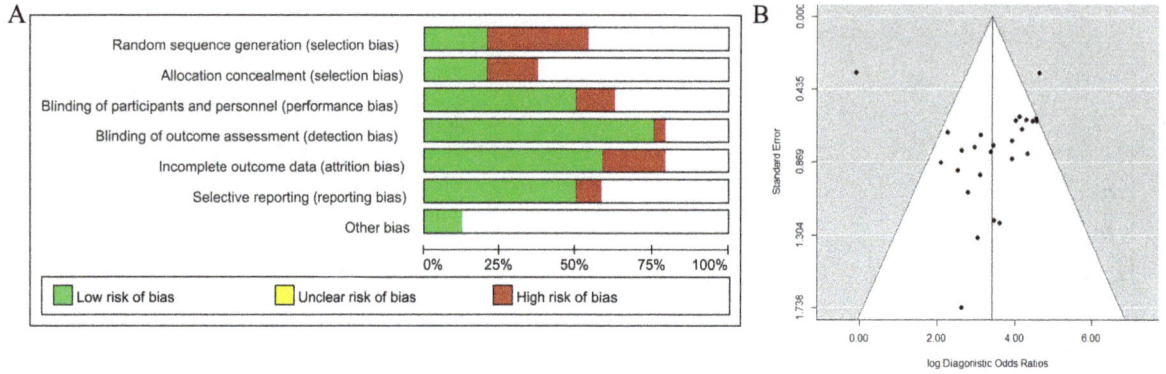

Figure 2. Methodological quality and publish bias assessment. (A) Risk of bias graph. The items of bias were independently evaluated by two authors. If the study reported all of the sensitivities and specificities of genes which were measured DNA methylation status, selective reporting was defined as low risk. (B) Funnel plot to assess bias in estimates of diagnostic odds ratio caused by small-study effects.

studies, indicating no selective reporting. Three studies were reported to be free of other sources of bias.

In order to evaluate the heterogeneity of the diagnostic effects of MRS, we performed heterogeneity tests for PLR, NLR, and DOR (Table 2). No significant heterogeneity of diagnostic effects was observed ($p>0.05$, $I^2 = 0\%$), as described in Table 2. We therefore adopted a fixed-effects model for all measures in the meta-analysis.

Funnel plots were used to demonstrate the effects of small study size for each diagnostic imaging modality, to assess publication bias by examining the relationship between the effect measure (log DOR) and its standard error. As shown in Figure 2B, relatively symmetrical funnel plots suggested potential publication bias in five of the 24 studies, which fell outside the funnel. Publication bias was evaluated using Egg's test, which found no significant differences ($p = 0.40$). This suggests that there was no trend towards higher levels of test accuracy among studies with smaller sample sizes.

Meta-regression analysis was used to assess factors affecting the diagnostic accuracy of MRS. We suspected that different tumor types, diagnostic purposes, patient period, technique of MRS and TE could affect the sensitivity and false positive rate of tumor diagnosis. We therefore used true and false positive rates as responses and studied whether the above five factors can affect the diagnostic accuracy through meta-regression analyses, respectively. As shown in Table 3, the p values for the tumor type, diagnostic purpose, MRS technique and TE in the fixed-effects model were not significant for true positive rate or false positive rate. However, periods of patient had significant effects on sensitivity and false positive rate of MRS (p value<0.001 respectively). In addition, differential of tumor grad had significant correlation with false positive rate of MRS (p value = 0.01). We

therefore concluded that the diagnostic accuracy of MRS was robust for different types, MRS technique and TE in brain tumors.

Meta-analysis and diagnostic accuracy

Meta-analysis revealed that the overall sensitivity and specificity of MRS were 80.05% (95% CI: 75.97–83.59%) and 78.46% (95% CI: 73.40%–82.78%, Figure 3A), respectively. The overall PLR after logarithmic transformation was 1.28 (95% CI: 1.05–1.52) corresponding to 3.53 (95% CI: 2.71–4.60, Table 2 and Figure 3B). The NLR after logarithmic transformation was −1.31 (95% CI: −1.53 to −1.09) corresponding to 0.29 (95% CI: 0.24–0.36, Table 2 and Figure 3B). The DOR after logarithmic transformation was 2.86 (95% CI: 2.42–3.30) corresponding to 14.66 (95% CI: 9.81–21.92, Table 2 and Figure 3B). In general, MRS thus demonstrated high diagnostic accuracy.

We generated an SROC curve based on the sensitivity and specificity of each study. The regression coefficient b was 0.002 (95% CI: −0.37–0.37), where b was close to 0 indicating a lack of heterogeneity, which was consistent with the results of heterogeneity analysis of diagnostic effects. The AUC showed relatively high diagnostic accuracy (Figure 3C, AUC = 0.78). Based on the SROC curve, the Q* metric was calculated as 84.22% (95% CI: 80.69%–87.21%), when the sensitivity equaled the specificity. These results suggest that MRS can be used for screening brain tumors with good diagnostic accuracy.

Stratified meta analysis

In order to further detailed analyze the diagnostic power of MRS, we performed Stratified meat analysis based on the period of patients, MRS technique and TE value. Diagnostic power of MRS between adult and child showed that child had more high

Table 2. The heterogeneity analysis of diagnostic effects.

	Estimate [95% CI]	Log(Estimate) [95% CI]	df	Q	P-value	I^2
PLR	3.53 [2.71–4.60]	1.28 [1.05–1.52]	41	29.77	0.90	0%
NLR	0.29 [0.24–0.36]	−1.31 [−1.53–1.09]	41	41.03	0.47	0.062%
DOR	14.66 [9.81–21.92]	2.86 [2.42–3.30]	41	41.22	0.46	0.54%

PLR: positive likelihood ratio. NLR: negative likelihood ratio. DOR: diagonistics odd ratio. Estimate [95% CI]: the pooled effect measure with the corresponding 95% confidence interval. Log(Estimate) [95% CI]: logarithmic transformation of the pooled effect measure with the corresponding 95% confidence interval. df: degrees of freedom. Q and P-value were the Q value and p value of Cochran's Q test.

Table 3. Meta-regression of potential risk of bias of methodological characteristics affecting the diagnostic sensitivity of MRS.

Factor	Label	Sensitivity		False positive rate	
		Coefficient	P value	Coefficient	P value
Cancer	Gliomas	−1.04	0.22	1.57	0.11
	Ependymoma	−1.54	0.26	0.59	0.68
	Neuroectodermal tumor	−1.06	0.38	0.43	0.78
Diagnose	Grade	0.22	0.49	1.05	0.01
	Metastases	−0.58	0.16	0.62	0.17
	Recurrent	−0.38	0.35	−0.17	0.77
	Residual	0.22	0.80	−0.80	0.63
Period	Adult	2.23	<0.001	3.04	<0.001
	Child	0.34	0.48	−1.20	0.03
Technique	SV	0.43	0.62	0.03	0.97
	CSI	0.56	0.51	1.22	0.12
TE	STE	1.19	0.20	0.26	0.81
	LTE	0.73	0.38	0.14	0.87

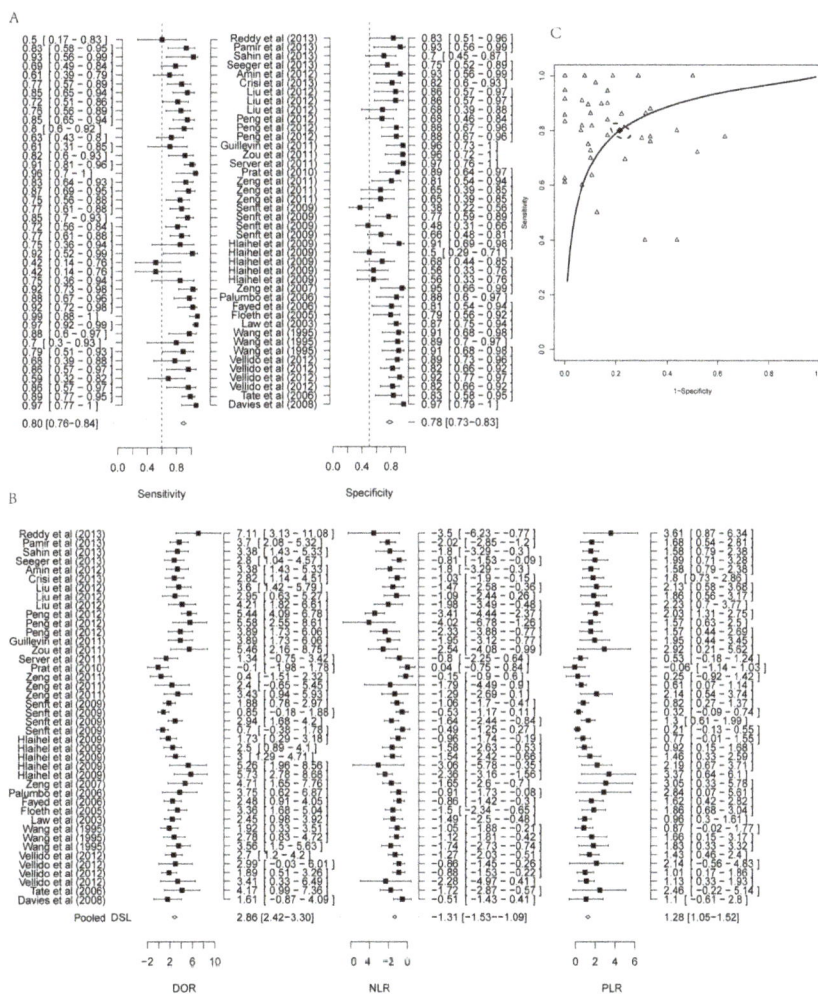

Figure 3. Forest plot of estimate of diagnostic accuracy of MRS. (A) Forest plot of estimate of sensitivity and specificity of MRS. (B) Forest plot estimate of PLR, NLR and DOR of MRS. (C) SROC curve of diagnostic performance of MRS from all studies. Solid line represents the ROC curve, and dotted line represented 95% confidence ellipse. Hollow triangle represented observed data from each study and solid rhombus represented the summary estimate.

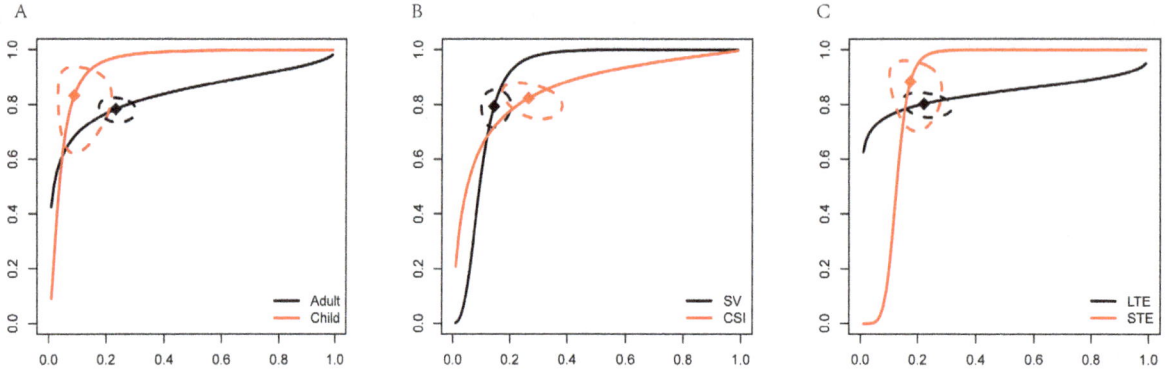

Figure 4. SROC curve of diagnostic performance of stratified meta-analysis. (A) Adult and child. (B) SV and CSI. (C) LTE and STE.

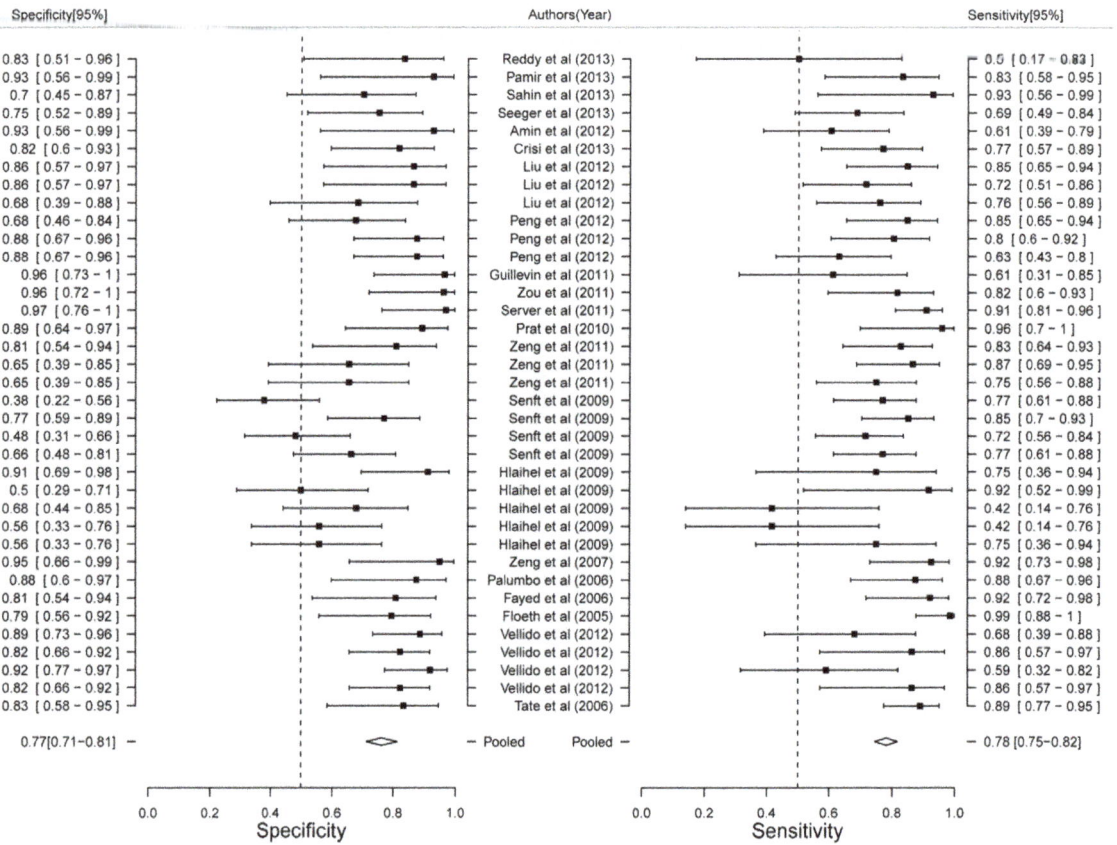

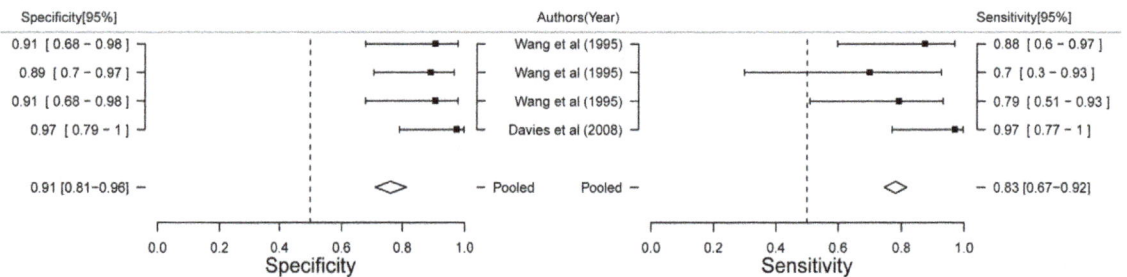

Figure 5. Forest plot of estimate of diagnostic accuracy of adult and child stratified meta-analysis.

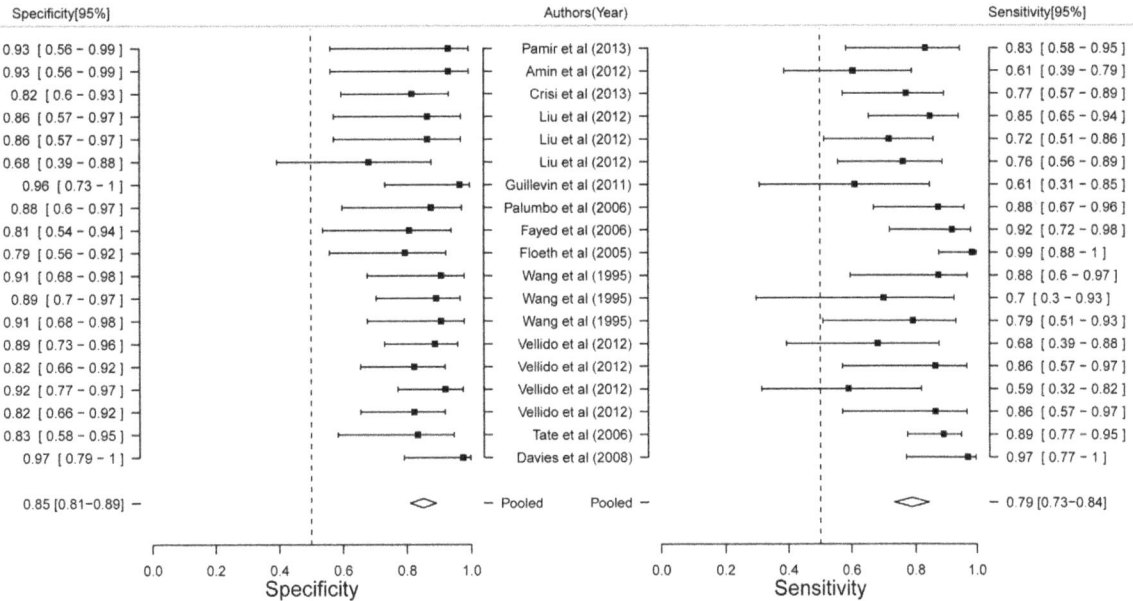

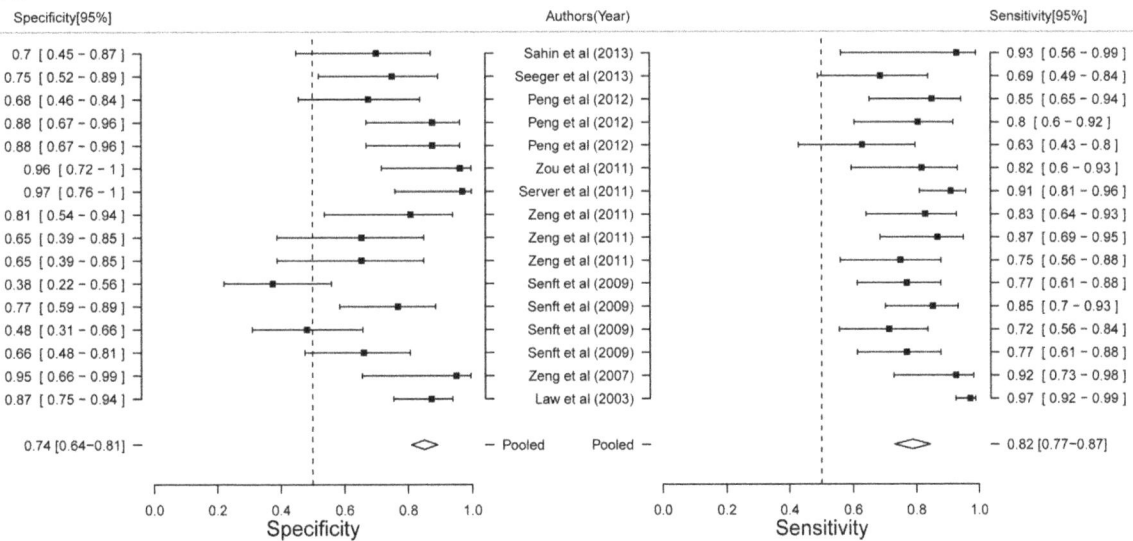

Figure 6. Forest plot of estimate of diagnostic accuracy of SV and CSI stratified meta-analysis.

accuracy than adult (AUC 0.89 VS. 0.77, Figure 4A). Diagnostic performance of MRS showed both higher sensitivity (83.37% VS. 78.38%) and specificity (91.06% VS. 76.60%) in child (Figure 5). Our results limited the very few studies on child, that will be more accurate with the increase of the number of studies. Although AUC value of SV was higher than CSI (0.89 VS. 0.79, Figure 4B), CSI had higher sensitivity (82.39% VS. 79.35%) and SV had higher specificity (85.49% VS. 73.52%, Figure 6). Two techniques of MRS has its own advantage. Finally, we analyzed the diagnostic power of LTE and STE. STE showed slightly higher AUC (0.79 VS. 0.73, Figure 4C), and had higher sensitivity (88.40% VS. 80.23%) and specificity (77.86% VS. 73.52%, Figure 7). Although some studies adopted double standard including both LTE and STE, diagnostic power has not been improved (sensitivity = 80.05% [95% CI: 75.97%–83.59%] and specificity 78.46% [95% CI: 73.40%–82.78%], respectively).

Discussion

Contrast-enhanced structural MRI is the method of choice for diagnosing brain tumors, especially follow-up of brain metastasis. However, the differentiation of locally-recurrent brain metastasis in many patients is difficult using contrast-enhanced structural MRI [34]. Various imaging techniques such as positron-emission-tomography (PET), single-photon emission computed tomography (SPECT), MRS and perfusion-weighted MRI (PWI) have been used to differentiate tumors. PET has been used to diagnose brain metastases [35], but it limits to small lesion size [36], long time interval between PET scans [37] and requiring of ionising radiation source [4]. Although SPECT provided higher sensitivity (90%) and specificity (92%) than PET, the major disadvantage of SPECT over PET was lower spatial resolution [38]. PWI and MRS as advanced MRI techniques can be successfully used to

LTE

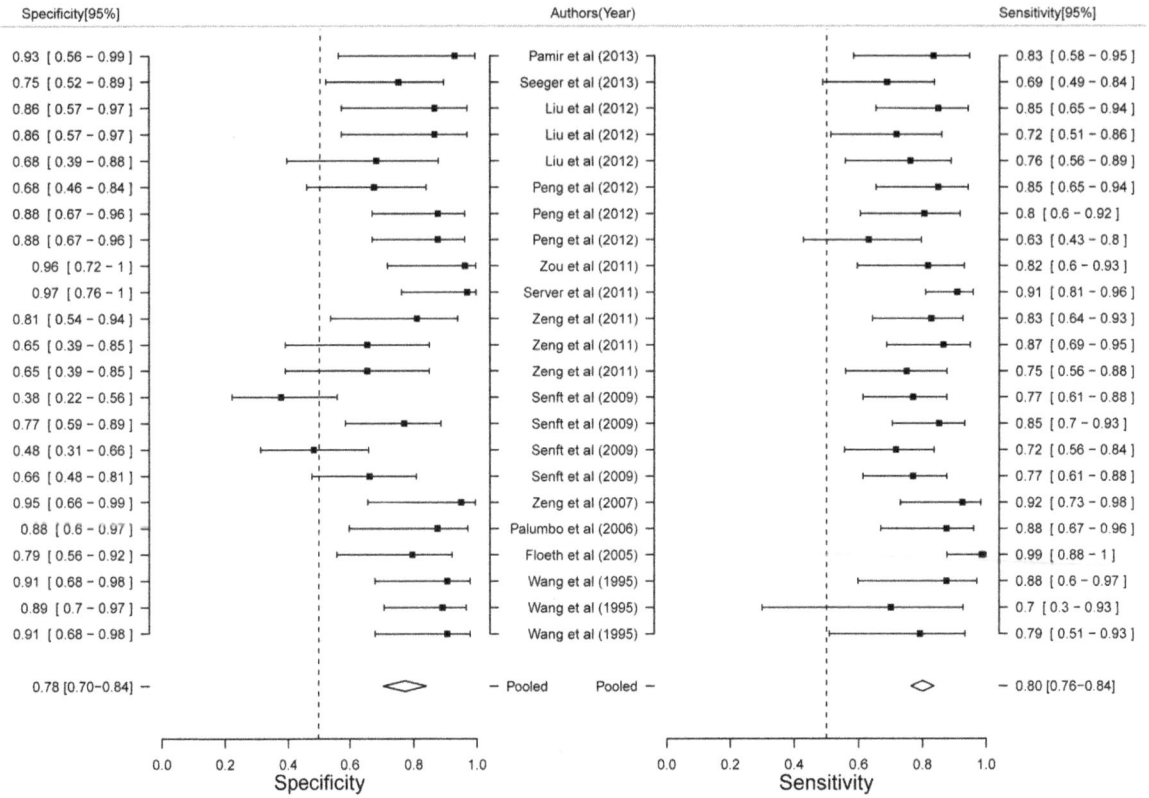

STE

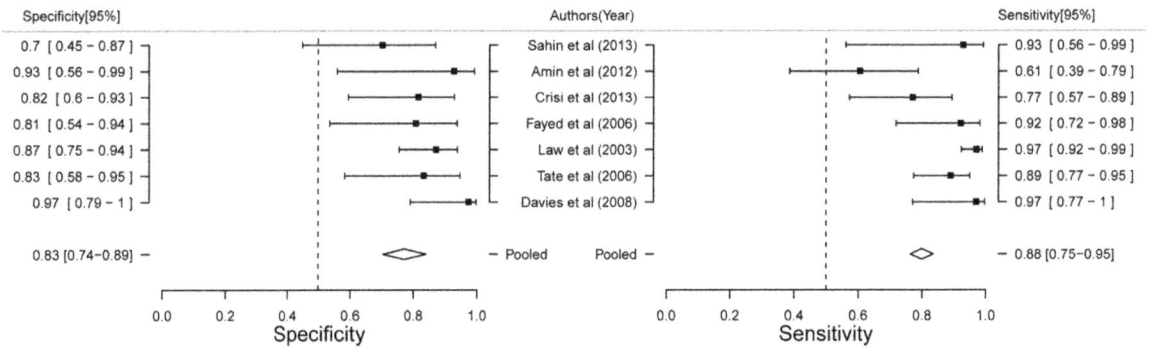

Figure 7. Forest plot of estimate of diagnostic accuracy of LTE and STE stratified meta-analysis.

differentiate brain tumors. PWI provided high sensitivity (70%–100%) and specificity (95%–100%) [37]. MRS even reached sensitivity and specificity of 100% [39]. However, these studies investigating advanced MRI techniques have mostly been based on limited numbers of patients. In addition, small size of the lesion, or susceptibility artifacts near to the lesion may negatively affect the analysis and interpretation of MRS data [40,41], thus limiting its diagnostic accuracy. It is difficult to draw conclusions about the diagnostic accuracy of MRS for brain tumors based on individual studies, and pooled studies thus represent a useful approach for assessing its diagnostic performance.

The present systematic review and meta-analysis included 24 studies, comprising a total of 1013 participants, with 605 cases and 408 controls. Overall, the methodological quality of the included studies was moderate, with no heterogeneity or publication bias, despite the fact that the different studies used different criteria for

positivity. Meta-analytically, MRS demonstrated slightly high sensitivity and specificity for discriminating brain tumors (pooled estimates of 80.58% and 78.46%, respectively), suggesting that it is a suitable and accurate diagnostic technique for brain tumors. Based on stratified meta analysis, MRS showed higher sensitivity and specificity in STE than LTE. CSI had higher sensitivity and SV had higher specificity. Diagnostic accuracy of MRS between adult and child need to increase the number of studies on child.

The present meta-analysis had several limitations. First, no large-scale prospective validation studies have been carried out by stereotactic biopsy. Second, the included studies did not provide sufficient information to assess the diagnostic values of other imaging techniques for comparison with multimodal imaging studies. Third, the included studies used a combination of different controls (normal, necrosis, and low-grade, respectively) as reference standards for determining diagnostic accuracy. Fourth, although we evaluated the diagnostic accuracy of MRS for brain tumors, more gliomas were included.

In conclusion, despite the limitations of this systematic review and meta-analysis, current evidence suggests that MRS may be an appropriate, non-invasive method for diagnosing brain tumors.

Acknowledgments

We thank Li Bai for her assistance with the statistical analysis.

Author Contributions

Conceived and designed the experiments: MT LY. Performed the experiments: YH PL. Analyzed the data: WW. Contributed reagents/materials/analysis tools: YH PL. Contributed to the writing of the manuscript: WW MT LY. Checked the literature: YC. Examined the evaluation of risk of bias: YL.

References

1. Ferlay J, Steliarova-Foucher E, Lortet-Tieulent J, Rosso S, Coebergh JW, et al. (2013) Cancer incidence and mortality patterns in Europe: estimates for 40 countries in 2012. Eur J Cancer 49: 1374–1403.

2. Law M, Yang S, Wang H, Babb JS, Johnson G, et al. (2003) Glioma grading: sensitivity, specificity, and predictive values of perfusion MR imaging and proton MR spectroscopic imaging compared with conventional MR imaging. AJNR Am J Neuroradiol 24: 1989–1998.

3. Schlemmer HP, Bachert P, Henze M, Buslei R, Herfarth KK, et al. (2002) Differentiation of radiation necrosis from tumor progression using proton magnetic resonance spectroscopy. Neuroradiology 44: 216–222.

4. Kwock L, Smith JK, Castillo M, Ewend MG, Collichio F, et al. (2006) Clinical role of proton magnetic resonance spectroscopy in oncology: brain, breast, and prostate cancer. Lancet Oncol 7: 859–868.

5. Moller-Hartmann W, Herminghaus S, Krings T, Marquardt G, Lanfermann H, et al. (2002) Clinical application of proton magnetic resonance spectroscopy in the diagnosis of intracranial mass lesions. Neuroradiology 44: 371–381.

6. Martin AJ, Liu H, Hall WA, Truwit CL (2001) Preliminary assessment of turbo spectroscopic imaging for targeting in brain biopsy. AJNR Am J Neuroradiol 22: 959–968.

7. Higgins JPT Green S (2011) Cochrane Handbook for Systematic Reviews of Interventions Version 5.1.0 [updated March 2011]. The Cochrane Collaboration. Available: www.cochrane-handbook.org. Accessed 2014 October 27.

8. Jiang Y, Zhang R, Zheng J, Liu P, Tang G, et al. (2012) Meta-analysis of 125 rheumatoid arthritis-related single nucleotide polymorphisms studied in the past two decades. PLoS One 7: e51571.

9. Walter SD (2002) Properties of the summary receiver operating characteristic (SROC) curve for diagnostic test data. Stat Med 21: 1237–1256.

10. Thorlund K, Imberger G, Johnston BC, Walsh M, Awad T, et al. (2012) Evolution of heterogeneity (I2) estimates and their 95% confidence intervals in large meta-analyses. PLoS One 7: e39471.

11. Reddy K, Westerly D, Chen C (2013) MRI patterns of T1 enhancing radiation necrosis versus tumour recurrence in high-grade gliomas. J Med Imaging Radiat Oncol 57: 349–355.

12. Pamir MN, Ozduman K, Yildiz E, Sav A, Dincer A (2013) Intraoperative magnetic resonance spectroscopy for identification of residual tumor during low-grade glioma surgery: clinical article. J Neurosurg 118: 1191–1198.

13. Sahin N, Melhem ER, Wang S, Krejza J, Poptani H, et al. (2013) Advanced MR imaging techniques in the evaluation of nonenhancing gliomas: perfusion-weighted imaging compared with proton MR spectroscopy and tumor grade. Neuroradiol J 26: 531–541.

14. Seeger A, Braun C, Skardelly M, Paulsen F, Schittenhelm J, et al. (2013) Comparison of three different MR perfusion techniques and MR spectroscopy for multiparametric assessment in distinguishing recurrent high-grade gliomas from stable disease. Acad Radiol 20: 1557–1565.

15. Amin A, Moustafa H, Ahmed E, El-Toukhy M (2012) Glioma residual or recurrence versus radiation necrosis: accuracy of pentavalent technetium-99m-dimercaptosuccinic acid [Tc-99m (V) DMSA] brain SPECT compared to proton magnetic resonance spectroscopy (1H-MRS): initial results. J Neurooncol 106: 579–587.

16. Crisi G, Orsingher L, Filice S (2013) Lipid and macromolecules quantitation in differentiating glioblastoma from solitary metastasis: a short-echo time single-voxel magnetic resonance spectroscopy study at 3 T. J Comput Assist Tomogr 37: 265–271.

17. Liu ZL, Zhou Q, Zeng QS, Li CF, Zhang K (2012) Noninvasive evaluation of cerebral glioma grade by using diffusion-weighted imaging-guided single-voxel proton magnetic resonance spectroscopy. J Int Med Res 40: 76–84.

18. Peng J, Ouyang Y, Fang WD, Luo TY, Li YM, et al. (2012) Differentiation of intracranial tuberculomas and high grade gliomas using proton MR spectroscopy and diffusion MR imaging. Eur J Radiol 81: 4057–4063.

19. Guillevin R, Menuel C, Taillibert S, Capelle L, Costalat R, et al. (2011) Predicting the outcome of grade II glioma treated with temozolomide using proton magnetic resonance spectroscopy. Br J Cancer 104: 1854–1861.

20. Zou QG, Xu HB, Liu F, Guo W, Kong XC, et al. (2011) In the assessment of supratentorial glioma grade: the combined role of multivoxel proton MR spectroscopy and diffusion tensor imaging. Clin Radiol 66: 953–960.

21. Server A, Kulle B, Gadmar OB, Josefsen R, Kumar T, et al. (2011) Measurements of diagnostic examination performance using quantitative apparent diffusion coefficient and proton MR spectroscopic imaging in the preoperative evaluation of tumor grade in cerebral gliomas. Eur J Radiol 80: 462–470.

22. Prat R, Galeano I, Lucas A, Martinez JC, Martin M, et al. (2010) Relative value of magnetic resonance spectroscopy, magnetic resonance perfusion, and 2-(18F)fluoro-2-deoxy-D-glucose positron emission tomography for detection of recurrence or grade increase in gliomas. J Clin Neurosci 17: 50–53.

23. Zeng Q, Liu H, Zhang K, Li C, Zhou G (2011) Noninvasive evaluation of cerebral glioma grade by using multivoxel 3D proton MR spectroscopy. Magn Reson Imaging 29: 25–31.

24. Senft C, Hattingen E, Pilatus U, Franz K, Schanzer A, et al. (2009) Diagnostic value of proton magnetic resonance spectroscopy in the noninvasive grading of solid gliomas: comparison of maximum and mean choline values. Neurosurgery 65: 908–913; discussion 913.

25. Hlaihel C, Guilloton L, Guyotat J, Streichenberger N, Honnorat J, et al. (2010) Predictive value of multimodality MRI using conventional, perfusion, and spectroscopy MR in anaplastic transformation of low-grade oligodendrogliomas. J Neurooncol 97: 73–80.

26. Zeng QS, Li CF, Zhang K, Liu H, Kang XS, et al. (2007) Multivoxel 3D proton MR spectroscopy in the distinction of recurrent glioma from radiation injury. J Neurooncol 84: 63–69.

27. Palumbo B, Lupattelli M, Pelliccioli GP, Chiarini P, Moschini TO, et al. (2006) Association of 99mTc-MIBI brain SPECT and proton magnetic resonance spectroscopy (1H-MRS) to assess glioma recurrence after radiotherapy. Q J Nucl Med Mol Imaging 50: 88–93.

28. Fayed N, Morales H, Modrego PJ, Pina MA (2006) Contrast/Noise ratio on conventional MRI and choline/creatine ratio on proton MRI spectroscopy accurately discriminate low-grade from high-grade cerebral gliomas. Acad Radiol 13: 728–737.

29. Floeth FW, Pauleit D, Wittsack HJ, Langen KJ, Reifenberger G, et al. (2005) Multimodal metabolic imaging of cerebral gliomas: positron emission tomography with [18F]fluoroethyl-L-tyrosine and magnetic resonance spectroscopy. J Neurosurg 102: 318–327.

30. Vellido A, Romero E, Julia-Sape M, Majos C, Moreno-Torres A, et al. (2012) Robust discrimination of glioblastomas from metastatic brain tumors on the basis of single-voxel (1)H MRS. NMR Biomed 25: 819–828.

31. Tate AR, Underwood J, Acosta DM, Julia-Sape M, Majos C, et al. (2006) Development of a decision support system for diagnosis and grading of brain tumours using in vivo magnetic resonance single voxel spectra. NMR Biomed 19: 411–434.

32. Wang Z, Sutton LN, Cnaan A, Haselgrove JC, Rorke LB, et al. (1995) Proton MR spectroscopy of pediatric cerebellar tumors. AJNR Am J Neuroradiol 16: 1821–1833.

33. Davies NP, Wilson M, Harris LM, Natarajan K, Lateef S, et al. (2008) Identification and characterisation of childhood cerebellar tumours by in vivo proton MRS. NMR Biomed 21: 908–918.

34. Dooms GC, Hecht S, Brant-Zawadzki M, Berthiaume Y, Norman D, et al. (1986) Brain radiation lesions: MR imaging. Radiology 158: 149–155.

35. Di Chiro G, DeLaPaz RL, Brooks RA, Sokoloff L, Kornblith PL, et al. (1982) Glucose utilization of cerebral gliomas measured by [18F] fluorodeoxyglucose and positron emission tomography. Neurology 32: 1323–1329.

36. Thompson TP, Lunsford LD, Kondziolka D (1999) Distinguishing recurrent tumor and radiation necrosis with positron emission tomography versus stereotactic biopsy. Stereotact Funct Neurosurg 73: 9–14.

37. Kickingereder P, Dorn F, Blau T, Schmidt M, Kocher M, et al. (2013) Differentiation of local tumor recurrence from radiation-induced changes after stereotactic radiosurgery for treatment of brain metastasis: case report and review of the literature. Radiat Oncol 8: 52.

38. Serizawa T, Saeki N, Higuchi Y, Ono J, Matsuda S, et al. (2005) Diagnostic value of thallium-201 chloride single-photon emission computerized tomography in differentiating tumor recurrence from radiation injury after gamma knife surgery for metastatic brain tumors. J Neurosurg 102 Suppl: 266–271.

39. Chernov M, Hayashi M, Izawa M, Ochiai T, Usukura M, et al. (2005) Differentiation of the radiation-induced necrosis and tumor recurrence after gamma knife radiosurgery for brain metastases: importance of multi-voxel proton MRS. Minim Invasive Neurosurg 48: 228–234.

40. Truong MT, St Clair EG, Donahue BR, Rush SC, Miller DC, et al. (2006) Results of surgical resection for progression of brain metastases previously treated by gamma knife radiosurgery. Neurosurgery 59: 86–97; discussion 86–97.

41. Haroon HA, Patankar TF, Zhu XP, Li KL, Thacker NA, et al. (2007) Comparison of cerebral blood volume maps generated from T2* and T1 weighted MRI data in intra-axial cerebral tumours. Br J Radiol 80: 161–168.

3

MR-Based Morphometry of the Posterior Fossa in Fetuses with Neural Tube Defects of the Spine

Ramona Woitek[1]*, Anton Dvorak[2], Michael Weber[1], Rainer Seidl[3], Dieter Bettelheim[4], Veronika Schöpf[1], Gabriele Amann[5], Peter C. Brugger[6], Julia Furtner[1], Ulrika Asenbaum[1], Daniela Prayer[1], Gregor Kasprian[1]

1 Department of Biomedical Imaging and Image-guided Therapy, Medical University of Vienna, Vienna, Austria, 2 Public Hospital Wiener Neustadt, Wiener Neustadt, Austria, 3 Department of Paediatrics and Adolescent Medicine, Medical University of Vienna, Vienna, Austria, 4 Department of Obstetrics and Gynecology, Medical University of Vienna, Vienna, Austria, 5 Department of Clinical Pathology, Medical University of Vienna, Vienna, Austria, 6 Center for Anatomy and Cell Biology, Medical University of Vienna, Vienna, Austria

Abstract

Objectives: In cases of "spina bifida," a detailed prenatal imaging assessment of the exact morphology of neural tube defects (NTD) is often limited. Due to the diverse clinical prognosis and prenatal treatment options, imaging parameters that support the prenatal differentiation between open and closed neural tube defects (ONTDs and CNTDs) are required. This fetal MR study aims to evaluate the clivus-supraocciput angle (CSA) and the maximum transverse diameter of the posterior fossa (TDPF) as morphometric parameters to aid in the reliable diagnosis of either ONTDs or CNTDs.

Methods: The TDPF and the CSA of 238 fetuses (20–37 GW, mean: 28.36 GW) with a normal central nervous system, 44 with ONTDS, and 13 with CNTDs (18–37 GW, mean: 24.3 GW) were retrospectively measured using T2-weighted 1.5 Tesla MR - sequences.

Results: Normal fetuses showed a significant increase in the TDPF (r=.956; p<.001) and CSA (r=.714; p<.001) with gestational age. In ONTDs the CSA was significantly smaller (p<.001) than in normal controls and CNTDs, whereas in CNTDs the CSA was not significantly smaller than in controls (p=.160). In both ONTDs and in CNTDs the TDPF was significantly different from controls (p<.001).

Conclusions: The skull base morphology in fetuses with ONTDs differs significantly from cases with CNTDs and normal controls. This is the first study to show that the CSA changes during gestation and that it is a reliable imaging biomarker to distinguish between ONTDs and CNTDs, independent of the morphology of the spinal defect.

Editor: Amanda Bruce, The University of Kansas Medical Center, United States of America

Funding: Funding was supported by the Austrian National Bank (OeNB 14812, "Quantitative Morphometrie der fetalen Gehirnentwicklung für Pathologiemodellierung und Diagnose"). The funders had no role in study design, data collection and analysis, decision to publish, or preparation of the manuscript.

* Email: ramona.woitek@meduniwien.ac.at

Introduction

The prenatal differentiation between open (ONTDs) and closed neural tube defects (CNTDs) of the spine is crucial because postnatal prognoses differ considerably. The differentiation based on MRI findings of the neural tube defect (NTD) can be impeded by limited depiction and distinction of the anatomical structures at the site of the NTD, especially in early second-trimester fetuses due to limited spatial resolution. As a generally accepted rule, ONTDs are almost always associated with Chiari II malformations, except for very few cases where CNTDs have been reported in association with Chiari II malformations [1–3]. In a fetus with Chiari II malformation the posterior fossa is small due to hypoplasia of the supraoccipital, exoccipital and basioccipital parts of the occipital bone resulting in caudal displacement of the

vermis cerebelli and the brainstem. Associated supratentorial abnormalities are dysgenesis of the corpus callosum, enlarged massa intermedia, hydrocephalic lateral ventricles, polymicrogyria, tectal beaking, hemispheric interdigitations and cortical heterotopias, and the so-called Luckenschaedel or lacunar skull [4–6]. Currently, various imaging signs of a morphologically abnormal posterior fossa have been described by ultrasound. These non-quantitative criteria comprise the banana sign [7–9], an effaced cisterna magna [10], bilateral downward-triangle shape (triangle sign), quadrilateral angular shape (square sign) of the lateral ventricles, [11] and absence of the translucency of the fourth ventricle [12].

Only few studies exist that report quantifiable criteria on prenatal ultrasound or MRI in large numbers of fetuses: the clivus-supraocciput angle (CSA) (evaluated on ultrasound in normally

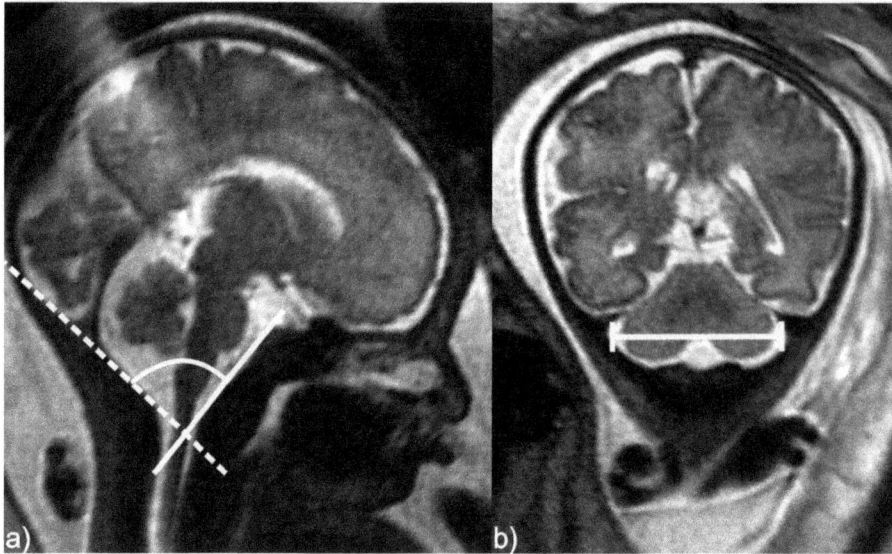

Figure 1. Schematic drawings of the CSA and the TDPF a) Measurement of the CSA. Midsagittal T2-weighted SSFSE MR image of a fetus at 33 GW. Continuous line along the postero-superior surface of the clivus connecting the most cranial part of the clivus with the anterior border of the foramen magnum (basion). Dashed line along the antero-superior surface of the supraocciput cutting the posterior border of the foramen magnum (opisthon). The angle between these two lines is the CSA. b) Measurement of the TDPF. Coronal T2-weighted MR image of a fetus at 33 GW. The distance between the medial surfaces of the lateral bony margins of the posterior fossa at the level of the lateral insertions of the tentorium cerebelli was measured.

developing fetuses and in fetuses with Chiari II malformations) [10,13], calculation of the posterior fossa volume (MRI-based, investigated in normally developing fetuses only) [14], the sagittal diameter of the brainstem, the brainstem to occipital bone diameter, and the ratio of the first to the latter (examined in normally developing fetuses and in fetuses with Chiari II malformations on ultrasound) [15].

This fetal MR study aims to evaluate the formerly described CSA [10,13] and the maximum transverse diameter of the posterior fossa (TDPF) as morphometric parameters to aid in the reliable diagnosis of either ONTDs or CNTDs. The two parameters CSA and TDPF were chosen as they can both be easily measured by prenatal ultrasound or MRI.

Methods

The Ethics Committee of the Medical University of Vienna approved the protocol for this study and we conducted the study according to the Declaration of Helsinki. Written informed consent was waived by the ethics committee due to the retrospective study design.

Patients

All 289 patients were referred to our department for fetal MRI between 2006 and 2014 to rule out or to confirm suspicious findings on fetal ultrasound. The established gestational age was based on ultrasound examinations during the first trimester. MRI revealed no pathology or isolated congenital pathologies that did not affect the CNS (n = 238). The most common pathologies were congenital diaphragmatic hernia, gastroschisis, cleft lip and palate, esophageal atresia, and cystic adenomatous malformation of the lung. Patient data were anonymized and de-identified prior to analysis.

MRI

MRI examinations were performed on a 1.5 Tesla system (Philips Medical Systems, Best, The Netherlands) with a five-element, phased-array cardiac coil. No contrast agents or sedation were used.

The MRI protocol included axial, and coronal T2-weighted single-shot fast spin-echo (SSFSE) sequences, and/or steady-state free precession (SSFP) sequences. All sequences were acquired as previously proposed [16] and adjusted according to the changing structural composition of the fetal brain during gestation.

Image Evaluation

Image evaluation was performed separately for each fetus by one reader, in fetuses with NTDs (resident with experience in fetal MRI and in neuroimaging) and in the cohort of 238 fetuses with a normal CNS (medical student extensively trained by a professor of radiology with the subspecialties of neuroradiology and fetal MRI). A sample of 75 fetuses with normal CNS was evaluated by both readers blinded for results not obtained by themselves. On midsagittal slices of T2-weighted SSFSE or SSFP MR sequences, the CSA was measured using two lines: The first line was placed along the postero-superior surface of the clivus, connecting the most cranial part of the clivus and the anterior border of the foramen magnum (basion) (continuous line in Figure 1a). The second line was placed along the superior surface of the supraocciput, cutting the posterior border of the foramen magnum (opisthon) (dashed line in Figure 1a). These anatomical structures could be easily identified, as there is high contrast between the hypointense bony clivus and supraocciput and the adjacent hyperintense cerebrospinal fluid (CSF) on these sequences. The angle at which the continuous and the dashed lines intersected was measured as the CSA. The angle was measured on up to three midsagittal images, each from a different MR sequence, depending on the number of acquired sagittal T2-weighted SSFSE or

SSFP sequences. Consequently, the mean value of all measurements was used for statistical evaluations.

To measure the distance between the medial surfaces of the lateral bony margins of the posterior fossa at the level of the lateral insertions of the tentorium cerebelli (Figure 1b), the largest distance between the lateral borders of the posterior cranial fossa at the level of the insertion of the tentorium cerebelli was depicted (TDPF) on coronal T2-weighted SSFSE or SSFP sequences. In each fetus, the distance was measured on up to three images, each from a different MR sequence, depending on the number of acquired MR sequences. The mean value of all measurements in one fetus was then used for statistical evaluations.

Three fetuses at similar gestational ages are shown in Figure 2 in order to illustrate the way the measurements of the CSA and TDPF were performed in fetuses with normal CNS development, with an ONTD or CNTD.

Inclusion criteria

Only fetuses with unequivocal imaging results with regard to the presence of either an ONTD or CNTD were included in our study.

Exclusion criteria

MR sequences with severe fetal head movement were excluded. If the CSA or the TDPF could not be measured on midsagittal or coronal images, respectively, the entire sequence was excluded from analysis. Fetuses of multiple pregnancies, with intrauterine growth restriction, or with neural pathologies other than those related to neural tube defects of the spine, were excluded.

Statistical Evaluation

Statistical planning and analysis were performed by a statistician (M.W.) using the SPSS 17.0 software package for Microsoft Windows, SPSS, Chicago, Ill). The study cohort was divided into three groups: fetuses with ONTDs of the spine; fetuses with CNTDs of the spine; and fetuses with normal CNS development. For each of those fetuses with NTDs of the spine, an age-matched control fetus was selected from the group of fetuses with normal neural development, with a maximum difference of +/−3 days of gestation. This age-based matching was performed because both the CSA and the TDPF increased with gestational age. To estimate interrater reliability the differences between the measurements performed by the two readers in a sample of 75 fetuses with normal CNS were calculated for the CSA and DTPF. Pearson correlation coefficients were computed to estimate consistency between the two readers.

The minimum and maximum values for the clivus-supraocciput angle and the TDPF were assessed, and mean values were calculated, as well as standard deviations and the 10th and 90th percentiles for both measurements. Pearson correlation was used to calculate correlations of gestational age with the CSA or TDPF in fetuses with normal CNS development and in fetuses with NTDs. A mixed model analysis of variance and student's t-tests for dependent samples were used to calculate differences between fetuses with normal CNS development and fetuses with ONTDs or CNTDs, respectively. Student's t-tests for independent samples were used to calculate differences between fetuses with ONTDs and with CNTDs. A p-value equal to or below 0.05 was considered statistically significant.

Results

Between 2006 and 2014 a NTD has been diagnosed in 65 fetuses based on MRI at our institution. The diagnoses could be confirmed in 44 cases of ONTDs and in 13 cases of CNTDs by postnatal surgery or postmortem examination. In 6 fetuses no follow up information was available, therefore they were excluded from our study.

Terminations of pregnancy were performed in 24 fetuses with ONTDs between 18 and 35 GW based on the diagnoses established using fetal ultrasound and MRI and on maternal α-fetoprotein levels. Due to the retrospective study design no measurements comparable to our MR-based morphometry were

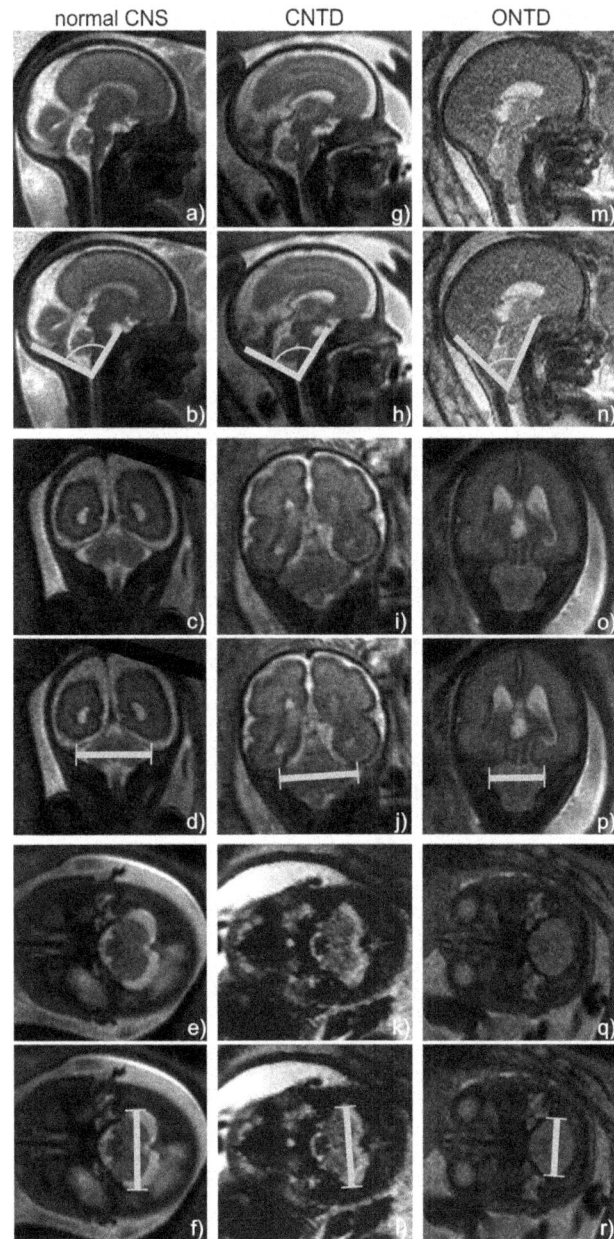

Figure 2. Line drawings show measurements of the CSA and TDPF performed on MR images of three exemplar fetuses: one fetus with normal CNS development at 27 GW (a–f), one fetus with a CNTD at 28GW (g–l) and one fetus with an ONTD at 27 GW (m–r). The CSA was measured on midsagittal T2-weighted SSFSE MR images (a+b, g+h, m+n). The TDPF was measured on coronal T2-weighted MR images (c+d, i+j, o+p) or on axial T2-weighted MR images (e+f, k+l, q+r).

Table 1. Descriptive statistics of groups of fetuses with ONTDs and CNTDs and their respective control fetuses with normal CNS development.

| | n | gestational age [weeks] | | clivus-supraocciput angle [°] | max. DM of the posterior fossa [mm] |
		mean ± std dev	min–max		
ONTDs	44	24.7±5.1	17–37	53.4±10.4	22.4±5.8
controls	44	24.7±5.2	17–37	78.0±8.5	32.3±9.0
CNTDs	13	26.2±2	19–33	75.0±11.1	25.1±6.5
controls	13	26.3±5.3	19–33	80.0±8.8	37.2±8.7

n = number of fetuses, std dev = standard deviation, min = minimum, max = maximum, DM = diameter.

performed during postmortem examination. 33 fetuses with NTDs were born alive after cesarian section.

Two fetuses with ONTDs had to be entirely excluded due to severe head motion and insufficient overall image quality in one case, and due to twin pregnancy in another case. In one ONTD the CSA was not reliably measurable retrospectively and in three ONTDs the DMPF was not reliably measurable retrospectively, all due to motion artifacts on those sequences necessary to perform measurement. Descriptive statistics for the subgroups of included fetuses with ONTDs (n = 44), CNTDs (n = 13), and normal CNS development (n = 238) are shown in Table 1.

In an exemplar subgroup of 75 fetuses with normal CNS TDPF and CSA were measured by two readers (R.W., A.D.) and assessed for interrater reliability (Figure 3; Table 2). Correlations between the two readers with regards to the CSA and the TDPF were high (r = .95; p<.001).

When we began evaluating fetuses with NTDs (17–37 GW, mean: 24.3 GW), we observed a significant correlation between gestational age and the TDPF (r = .943, p<.000) (Figure 4a), and a lower and insignificant correlation between the CSA and gestational age (r = .103, p = .452) (Figure 4b). As the finding concerning the CSA was in contrast to previously published results [10], we subsequently evaluated 238 fetuses with normal CNS development to obtain their CSA and TDPF (20–37 GW, mean:

28.36 GW) to confirm whether there was an increase in the CSA during gestation. These 238 fetuses were homogeneously distributed with regard to their gestational age, with 13–15 fetuses in each gestational week except for the 21st and 37th gestational weeks, in which there were only 10 and nine fetuses, respectively. Mean values, standard deviations, 10th and 90th percentiles for each gestational week between the 21st and 37th gestational week, and mean and standard deviations for all fetuses with a normal CNS development are shown in Table 3. In this cohort of fetuses, we found a significant and very high correlation between gestational age and the TDPF (r = .956; p<.001) (Figure 5a), and a significant correlation between gestational age and the CSA (r = .714; p<.001) (Figure 5b).

In both groups of fetuses with ONTDs and CNTDs, the TDPF was significantly different from their age-matched control fetuses (p<.001 for both groups) (Figure 6). The TDPF was not significantly different when directly comparing fetuses with ONTDs to fetuses with CNTDs of the spine (p = .677) (Figure 7).

Only in fetuses with ONTDs was the CSA significantly different from their age-matched control fetuses (p<.001), whereas, in CNTDs, it was not (p = .163). The CSA was also significantly different when comparing fetuses with ONTDs to those with CNTDs of the spine (p<.001) (Figure 7). Gestational age did not significantly differ in groups of ONTDs and CNTDs (p = .623).

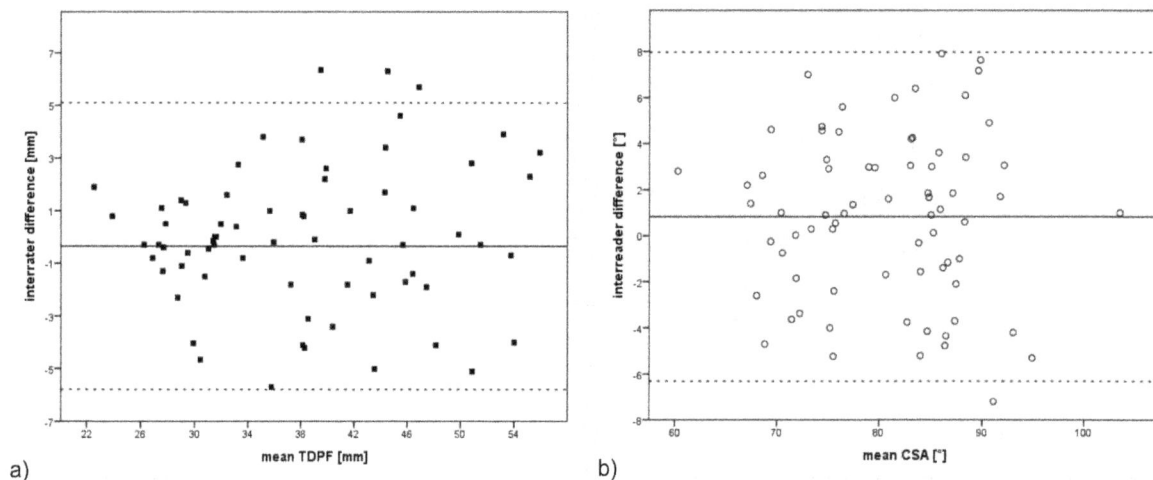

a)   b)

Figure 3. Measurements of the TDPF and CSA by two readers. a) Mean TDPF measured by the two readers plotted against the interrater difference. Continuous line represents overall mean difference (0.4 mm). Dashed lines represent 95% confidence intervals. b) Mean CSA measured by the two readers plotted against the interrater difference. Continuous line represents overall mean difference (0.8°). Dashed lines represent 95% confidence intervals.

Table 2. Comparison between the two readers regarding CSA and TDPF.

	Reader 1		Reader 2		mean difference	range of differencesr	sig
	mean	std dev	mean	std dev			
CSA [°]	81.0	8.2	80.0	8.4	1.0	0–8.2	0.95	<.001
TDPF [mm]	38.1	8.5	38.1	8.7	0.0	0–6.4	0.95	<.001

Std dev = standard deviation, sig = level of significance.

Discussion

In this study, a comparably large number of normal fetuses and fetuses with ONTDs and CNTDs were evaluated with regard to their CSA and TDPF in order to be able to differentiate between the two entities based on posterior fossa morphometry.

In contrast to d'Addario et al. [10], we were able to prove that, based on the results of the present and a recent study by Grant et al. [17], there is a low but significant correlation of the CSA with gestational age both in fetuses with NTDs and in fetuses with a normal CNS. Thus, our data represent the most extensive analysis of the CSA and TDPF to date, as Grant et al. [17] included a smaller number of fetuses. Increasing values of both the CSA and TDPF during gestation imply that normal values (mean, standard deviation, and 10th and 90th percentiles) have to be established for each gestational week based on a sufficient number of measurements.

In both our study and the study by Grant et al., measurements of the CSA were performed on MR images [17], whereas the measurements that remained constant during gestation obtained by d'Addario et al. were based on ultrasound examinations [10]. The difference between the ultrasound data and the present data may be related to methodological differences. T2-weighted SSFSE and SSFP MR-sequences are free of sonographic shadowing by osseous structures, and offer a very high contrast between the hypointense bony structures (clivus, supraocciput) and the CSF spaces of the posterior fossa. The lines by which the CSA is measured are positioned at the interfaces between these high and low signal intensities. Therefore, MRI might serve as a better tool than ultrasound to precisely identify these structures.

Aside from these differences, the mean values obtained by d'Addario et al. and Grant et al. are comparable to our findings. D'Addario et al. reported the mean value of the CSA in normal fetuses to be 79.3° which is within the 10th and 90th percentile of our measurements in the majority of fetuses (GW 21 and 24–32) [10]. Grant et al. measured a mean CSA of 75.4° in normally developing fetuses [17], while, in our study, the mean CSA of all fetuses with a normal CNS was 82.4°. Grant et al. reported that, in fetuses with Chiari II malformations, between 19 and 25 GW the mean CSA was 57.8°, which is comparable to our mean CSA in fetuses with ONTDs of 53.4°.

A group-wise comparison of fetuses with ONTDs and CNTDs revealed a significant difference with regard to the CSA but not the TDPF. Differentiation between ONTDs and CNTDs is limited, based on the TDPF, as standard deviations of the TDPF overlap in all three comparisons (ONTDs versus controls, CNTDs

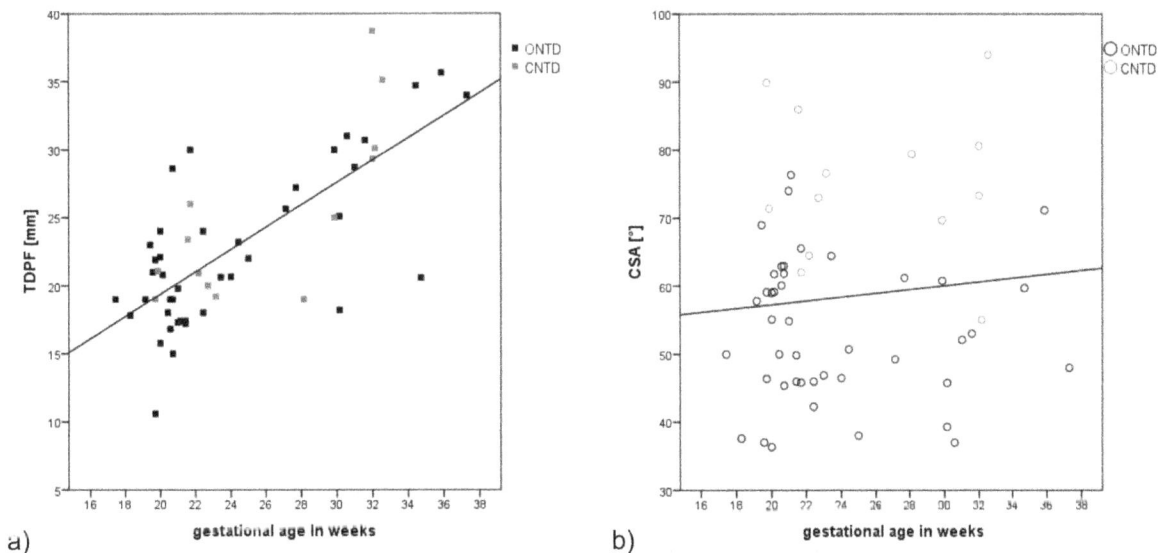

a)

b)

Figure 4. The TDPF and CSA in fetuses with ONTDs and CNTDs plotted against gestational age. a) Correlation of the TDPF with gestational age was significant (r = .943, p<.000) (see correlation line). b) The CSA in fetuses with ONTDs and CNTDs plotted against gestational age. Correlation was low and insignificant (r = .103, p = .452).

Table 3. Descriptive statistics of fetuses with normal CNS development, ONTDs and CNTDs.

GW	TDPF [mm] normal mean	std dev	0.1	0.9	ONTDs mean	max	min	CNTDs mean	max	min	CSA [°] normal mean	std dev	0.1	0.9	ONTDs mean	max	min	CNTDs mean	max	min	GW
21	26.9	2.6	23.6	30.2	18.0	22.0	16.0				74.2	5.1	67.7	80.8	54.7	63.0	36.3				21
22	28.4	1.7	26.2	30.6	18.0	20.0	17.0	26.0	29.0	23.0	70.2	6.5	61.9	78.4	54.1	74.0	45.9	76.4	79.4	73.3	22
23	30.0	2.3	27.0	32.9	21.0	21.0	21.0	21.0	21.0	21.0	69.6	5.9	62.0	77.3	44.3	44.3	44.3	71.4	71.4	71.4	23
24	31.7	1.2	30.1	33.2	22.0	22.0	21.0	19.0	19.0	19.0	74.6	8.8	63.3	85.8	54.7	64.5	46.9	59.0	59.0	59.0	24
25	32.9	1.7	30.7	35.1	22.0	23.0	21.0				74.4	4.2	68.9	79.8	48.6	50.7	46.5				25
26	36.0	2.0	33.4	38.5							76.8	5.1	70.3	83.3							26
27	37.3	2.3	34.4	40.2							81.5	5.1	74.9	88.0							27
28	39.7	2.2	36.8	42.5	26.0	27.0	26.0				82.0	4.9	75.7	88.3	51.1	50.7	49.3				28
29	42.1	2.8	38.5	45.7	30.0	30.0	30.0	19.0	19.0	19.0	84.3	6.9	75.5	93.2	60.8	60.8	60.8	86.0	86.0	86.0	29
30	42.6	3.0	38.8	46.4	25.0	30.0	18.0				86.0	8.6	75.1	97.0	47.8	57.4	39.3	89.9	89.9	89.9	30
31	45.6	2.6	42.3	49.0	30.0	31.0	29.0				88.8	10.4	75.4	102.1	52.6	53.0	52.1				31
32	47.0	4.3	41.5	52.6	34.0	34.0	34.0				88.8	8.3	78.2	99.5	65.1	65.1	65.1				32
33	49.6	3.5	45.1	54.0				33.0	39.0	29.0	87.3	4.6	81.4	93.2				65.6	94.0	45.1	33
34	49.4	3.4	45.0	53.8							91.2	8.2	80.7	101.7							34
35	51.2	2.1	48.5	53.9	28.0	35.0	21.0				89.4	4.1	84.3	94.7	63.6	67.4	59.7				35
36	53.9	2.8	50.3	57.5	36.0	36.0	36.0				91.7	7.6	81.9	101.4	71.2	71.2	71.2				36
37	54.4	1.9	52.0	56.9							90.3	3.6	85.7	94.9							37
all	41.1	9.1									82.4	7.6									all

GW = gestational week, TDPF = maximum transverse diameter of the posterior fossa, CSA = clivus-supraocciput angle, ONTD = open neural tube defect, CNTD = closed neural tube defect, std dev = standard deviation, 0.1 = 10th percentile, 0.9 = 90th percentile; max = maximum, min = minimum.

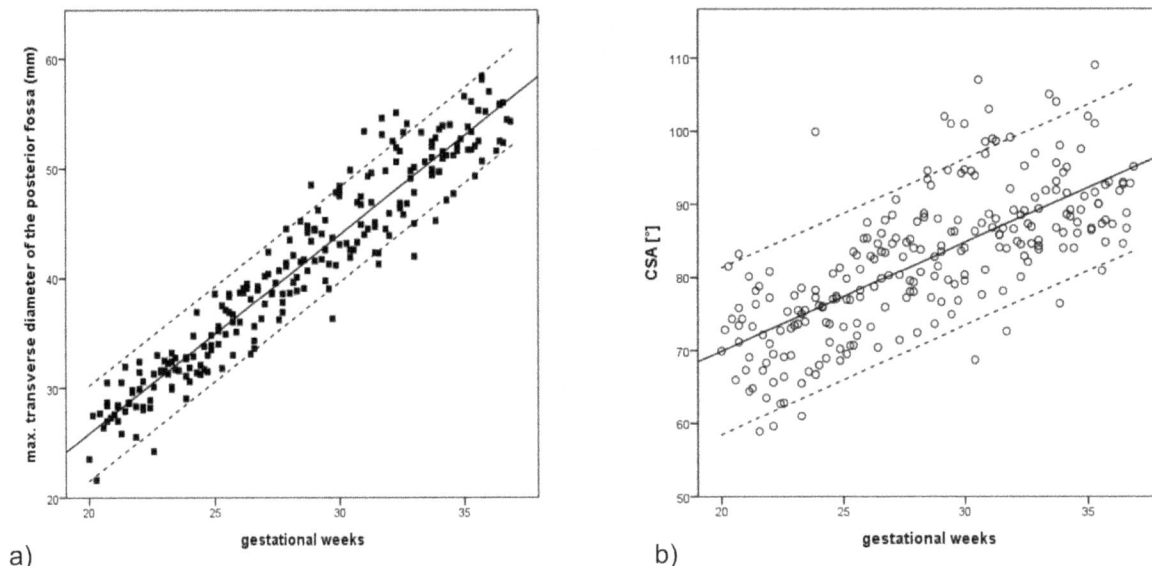

Figure 5. Correlations of the TDPF and CSA with gestational age. a) Correlation between the TDPF and gestational age in 238 fetuses with normal CNS development. Squares show TDPF values. The regression line is continuous (r = .956; p<.001). Dashed lines show calculated 10th and 90th percentiles. b) Correlation between the CSA and gestational age. Circles show CSA values of 238 fetuses with normal CNS development. The regression line is continuous (r = .714; p<.001). Dashed lines show 10th and 90th percentiles.

versus controls, and ONTDS versus CNTDs), with the highest overlap in the comparison of ONTDs to CNTDs. In contrast, the standard deviations calculated for the CSA in ONTDs and controls do not overlap. Comparisons of the CSA in CNTDs versus age-matched controls, or CNTDs versus ONTDs, revealed overlapping standard deviations. With regard to CNTDs versus ONTDs, in particular, this overlap is small and could, theoretically, be overcome with a higher number of measurements. Supported by our data we believe the CSA to be a sensitive tool to distinguish between ONTDS and CNTDs on fetal MRI.

Our findings reveal a smaller TDPF in fetuses with CNTDs than with a normal CNS development, implying that, in CNTDs, the posterior fossa also undergoes malformation, but apparently to a lesser extent than in ONTDs. The hydrodynamic theory [18–20] cannot explain this observation. More probably, a genetic background might be the missing link between the pathogenesis of ONTDs and CNTDs and might explain the different development of the posterior fossa.

It has been shown that members of the HOX gene family play important roles both in the formation of the neural tube [21] and in the growth of the enchondral bones of the skull base [22], eventually contributing to the formation of NTDs and Chiari malformations [23]. Most studies on the genetic background of NTDs focus on ONTDs or evaluate pooled data from NTDs without classifying according to ONTDs and CNTDs, mostly due to the small numbers of patients and the lack of patients with CNTDs. Therefore, a study aimed at the distinction of genetic factors that contribute to the formation of ONTDs and CNTDs should be undertaken. A multicentric approach appears to be necessary to be able to include large enough numbers of patients with ONTDs or CNTDs.

The limitations of our study are, firstly, that the evaluation of fetuses was limited to fetuses aged 17–37 GW. Secondly in those fetuses with NTDs that were lost to follow up differentiation between ONTDs and CNTDs was based on imaging findings alone. Furthermore, as this was a single center study, the number of fetuses with NTDs was limited to those patients referred to our MRI unit for diagnostic work-up.

This study shows that the skull base morphology in fetuses with ONTDs differs significantly from cases with CNTDs and normal controls. We show for the first time that the CSA is a reliable imaging biomarker to distinguish between ONTDs and CNTDs in early pregnancy, regardless of the morphology of the spinal defect. Furthermore, our work raises questions concerning the pathogen-

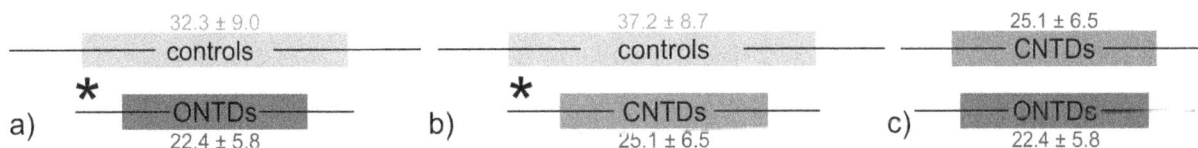

Figure 6. Comparisons of the TDPF in ONTDs, CNTDs and the respective control groups. Bars represent mean values and lines represent standard deviations of the TDPF in fetuses with ONTDs (a, c), in fetuses with CNTDs (b, c) and their respective age matched control fetuses with normal CNS development (a, b). Asterisks indicate significant differences between ONTDs and control fetuses with normal CNS and between CNTDs and control fetuses with normal CNS development (p<.001).

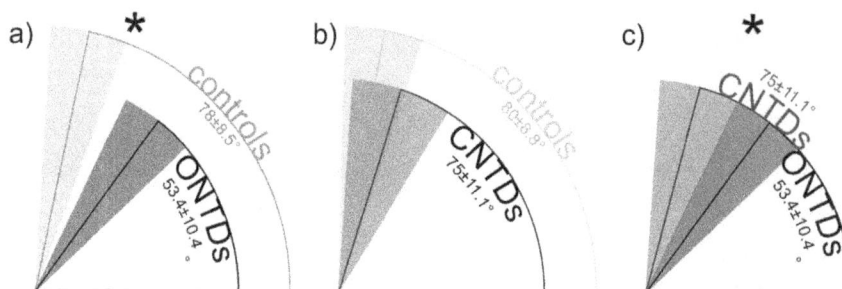

Figure 7. Comparisons of the CSA in ONTDs, CNTDs and the respective control groups. Sector outlines represent mean values and gray sectors represent standard deviations of the CSA in fetuses with ONTDs (a, c), with CNTDs (b, c) and their respective age matched control fetuses with normal CNS development (a, b). Asterisks indicate significant differences between ONTDs and control fetuses with normal CNS and between ONTDs and CNTDs (p<.001).

esis of Chiari II malformations in relation to ONTDs, and also, CNTDs, possibly initiating future studies that could focus on a genetic basis as a link between these two entities.

Author Contributions

Conceived and designed the experiments: RW AD JF UA RS DB GK DP. Performed the experiments: RW AD JF UA GA. Analyzed the data: RW AD MW. Contributed reagents/materials/analysis tools: MW GA PCB. Contributed to the writing of the manuscript: RW AD MW RS DB VS GA PCB JF UA DP GK.

References

1. Tortori-Donati P, Rossi AMD, Biancheri R (2005) Pediatric neuroradiology; Springer, editor. Berlin [Great Britain]: Springer.
2. Stevenson KL (2004) Chiari Type II malformation: past, present, and future. Neurosurg Focus 16: E5.
3. Nishino A, Shirane R, So K, Arai H, Suzuki H, et al. (1998) Cervical myelocystocele with Chiari II malformation: magnetic resonance imaging and surgical treatment. Surg Neurol 49: 269–273.
4. Naidich TP, Pudlowski RM, Naidich JB (1980) Computed tomographic signs of the Chiari II malformation. III: Ventricles and cisterns. Radiology 134: 657–663.
5. Naidich TP, Pudlowski RM, Naidich JB (1980) Computed tomographic signs of Chiari II malformation. II: Midbrain and cerebellum. Radiology 134: 391–398.
6. Naidich TP, Pudlowski RM, Naidich JB, Gornish M, Rodriguez FJ (1980) Computed tomographic signs of the Chiari II malformation. Part I: Skull and dural partitions. Radiology 134: 65–71.
7. Van den Hof MC, Nicolaides KH, Campbell J, Campbell S (1990) Evaluation of the lemon and banana signs in one hundred thirty fetuses with open spina bifida. Am J Obstet Gynecol 162: 322–327.
8. Campbell J, Gilbert WM, Nicolaides KH, Campbell S (1987) Ultrasound screening for spina bifida: cranial and cerebellar signs in a high-risk population. Obstet Gynecol 70: 247–250.
9. Thomas M (2003) The lemon sign. Radiology 228: 206–207.
10. D'Addario V, Pinto V, Del Bianco A, Di Naro E, Tartagni M, et al. (2001) The clivus-supraocciput angle: a useful measurement to evaluate the shape and size of the fetal posterior fossa and to diagnose Chiari II malformation. Ultrasound Obstet Gynecol 18: 146–149.
11. Fujisawa H, Kitawaki J, Iwasa K, Honjo H (2006) New ultrasonographic criteria for the prenatal diagnosis of Chiari type 2 malformation. Acta Obstet Gynecol Scand 85: 1426–1429.
12. Chaoui R, Benoit B, Mitkowska-Wozniak H, Heling KS, Nicolaides KH (2009) Assessment of intracranial translucency (IT) in the detection of spina bifida at the 11–13-week scan. Ultrasound Obstet Gynecol 34: 249–252.
13. D'Addario V, Rossi AC, Pinto V, Pintucci A, Di Cagno L (2008) Comparison of six sonographic signs in the prenatal diagnosis of spina bifida. J Perinat Med 36: 330–334.
14. Chen SC, Simon EM, Haselgrove JC, Bilaniuk LT, Sutton LN, et al. (2006) Fetal posterior fossa volume: assessment with MR imaging. Radiology 238: 997–1003.
15. Lachmann R, Chaoui R, Moratalla J, Picciarelli G, Nicolaides KH (2011) Posterior brain in fetuses with open spina bifida at 11 to 13 weeks. Prenat Diagn 31: 103–106.
16. Prayer D, Brugger PC, Prayer L (2004) Fetal MRI: techniques and protocols. Pediatr Radiol 34: 685–693.
17. Grant RA, Heuer GG, Carrion GM, Adzick NS, Schwartz ES, et al. (2011) Morphometric analysis of posterior fossa after in utero myelomeningocele repair. J Neurosurg Pediatr 7: 362–368.
18. McLone DG, Dias MS (2003) The Chiari II malformation: cause and impact. Childs Nerv Syst 19: 540–550.
19. McLone DG, Knepper PA (1989) The cause of Chiari II malformation: a unified theory. Pediatr Neurosci 15: 1–12.
20. Naidich TP, McLone DG, Fulling KH (1983) The Chiari II malformation: Part IV. The hindbrain deformity. Neuroradiology 25: 179–197.
21. Safra N, Bassuk AG, Ferguson PJ, Aguilar M, Coulson RL, et al. (2013) Genome-wide association mapping in dogs enables identification of the homeobox gene, NKX2-8, as a genetic component of neural tube defects in humans. PLoS Genet 9: e1003646.
22. Sarnat HB (2008) Disorders of segmentation of the neural tube: Chiari malformations. Handb Clin Neurol 87: 89–103.
23. Sarnat HB (2004) Regional ependymal upregulation of vimentin in Chiari II malformation, aqueductal stenosis, and hydromyelia. Pediatr Dev Pathol 7: 48–60.

4

Maximizing Negative Correlations in Resting-State Functional Connectivity MRI by Time-Lag

Gadi Goelman[1]*, **Noam Gordon**[1], **Omer Bonne**[2]

1 MRI/MRS Lab, The Human Biology Research Center, Department of Medical Biophysics, Hadassah Hebrew University Medical Center, Jerusalem, Israel, **2** Department of Psychiatry, Hadassah Hebrew University Medical Center, Jerusalem, Israel

Abstract

This paper aims to better understand the physiological meaning of negative correlations in resting state functional connectivity MRI (*r-fcMRI*). The correlations between anatomy-based brain regions of 18 healthy humans were calculated and analyzed with and without a correction for global signal and with and without spatial smoothing. In addition, correlations between anatomy-based brain regions of 18 naïve anesthetized rats were calculated and compared to the human data. T-statistics were used to differentiate between positive and negative connections. The application of spatial smoothing and global signal correction increased the number of significant positive connections but their effect on negative connections was complex. Positive connections were mainly observed between cortical structures while most negative connections were observed between cortical and non-cortical structures with almost no negative connections between non-cortical structures. In both human and rats, negative connections were never observed between bilateral homologous regions. The main difference between positive and negative connections in both the human and rat data was that positive connections became less significant with time-lags, while negative connections became more significant with time-lag. This effect was evident in all four types of analyses (with and without global signal correction and spatial smoothing) but was most significant in the analysis with no correction for the global signal. We hypothesize that the valence *of r-fcMRI* connectivity reflects the relative contributions of cerebral blood volume (CBV) and flow (CBF) to the BOLD signal and that these relative contributions are location-specific. If cerebral circulation is primarily regulated by CBF in one region and by CBV in another, a functional connection between these regions can manifest as an *r-fcMRI* negative and time-delayed correlation. Similarly, negative correlations could result from spatially inhomogeneous responses of rCBV or rCBF alone. Consequently, neuronal regulation of brain circulation may be deduced from the valence of *r-fcMRI* connectivity.

Editor: Alessandro Gozzi, Italian Institute of Technology, Italy

Funding: Funding was provided by Israel Ministry of Health grant number 8430 under the Era-Net-Neuron program and the Israeli Ministry of Science grant number 3-9814. The funders had no role in study design, data collection and analysis, decision to publish, or preparation of the manuscript.

Competing Interests: The authors have declared that no competing interests exist.

* Email: gadig@hadassah.org.il

Introduction

Coherent low frequency fluctuations of the blood oxygenation level-dependent (BOLD) signal in the resting-state were shown to contain functional neuronal network information [1,2]. Such information is derived from correlations between the temporal fluctuations of the BOLD signal in various brain regions in the absence of external stimuli [3–5]. Multiple resting-state networks (RSN) were defined [3,6,7] in this manner, and their reliability and robustness were established [8–10]. RSNs were also shown in anesthetized animals [11,12]. Most RSN sets show positive correlations between the brain regions comprising these networks. However, several RSNs were shown to be inversely correlated. For example, it was shown that the default mode network is negatively correlated with the dorsal attention system [4,5]. Alterations in such anti-correlated networks between healthy subjects and patients with, for example, schizophrenia [13], ADHD [14], bipolar disorder [15] and Alzheimer's disease [16] were observed.

The physiological mechanisms underlying resting-state functional brain connectivity MRI (r-fcMRI) are however, not clear. Positive correlations between regions comprising such networks are assumed to reflect synchronized activity between these regions, but the nature of negative correlations is debatable. A distinction should be made between *physiological* sources of negative correlations, such as negative BOLD signals [17–26], and possible data analysis biases [27–31]. Several studies have demonstrated negative correlations using methodologies that are free of such biases [32,33], thereby strengthening the assumption that both negative and positive correlations reflect genuine physiological processes. Potential physiological sources for negative correlations within resting state networks are neuronal inhibition [26,34] and pure non-neuronal hemodynamic processes [31].

In this study we aim to better understand the physiological mechanisms underlying negative correlations in *r-fcMRI*. Since the distinction between positive and negative correlations may be

Table 1. Regions of interest (ROIs) in the human brain, their mean MNI coordinates and number of voxels.

#	Name	X	Y	Z	Volume
0	R amygdala	25.1	−0.2	−18.5	34
1	L amygdala	−21.4	−0.3	−18.8	30
2	R dmPFC	19.9	37.3	34.3	115
3	L dmPFC	−22.6	37.2	32.9	119
4	R dorsolateral PFC	34.1	50.1	29.4	27
5	L dorsolateral PFC	−30.8	49.6	29.3	30
6	R dmPFC -b	19.5	61.3	24.8	41
7	L dmPFC -b	−16.4	61.3	24.6	41
8	R habenula	7.6	−20.0	4.9	43
9	L habenula	−4.5	−20.2	4.8	43
10	R medial BA8-b	23.6	17.4	50.8	415
11	L medial BA8-b	−20.3	17.6	50.8	419
12	R medial BA8	13.6	39.5	48.9	208
13	L medial BA8	−10.4	39.5	48.7	215
14	R Caudate	12.4	10.8	9.8	137
15	L Caudate	−9.4	10.4	9.7	140
16	R medial BA9	37.3	21.4	36.6	335
17	L medial BA9	−34.6	21.6	36.7	328
18	R GP	20.6	−1.4	−0.6	75
19	L GP	−16.1	−1.0	−0.3	72
20	R hippocampus	31.6	−17.1	−14.3	23
21	L hippocampus	−27.7	−17.9	−14.1	29
22	R medial PFC	5.5	67.6	−3.3	56
23	L medial PFC	−2.2	67.8	−3.0	62
24	R NAc	11.6	13.3	−7.7	121
25	L NAc	−8.8	13.2	−7.8	122
26	R posterior Cingulate-b	9.4	−48.5	14.6	416
27	L posterior Cingulate-b	−6.5	−48.7	14.7	423
28	R pregenual ACC	11.6	31.5	22.7	85
29	L pregenual ACC	−8.6	31.5	22.7	86
30	R insula	41.2	−3.9	10.1	492
31	L insula	−36.9	−3.6	10.1	494
32	R mammillary	9.0	−12.5	−4.4	2
33	L mammillary	−6.5	−14.5	−1.9	3
34	R STN	11.3	−11.0	−5.3	4
35	L STN	−8.3	−11.0	−5.3	4
36	R subgenual ACC	7.6	33.4	0.5	281
37	L subgenual ACC	−4.5	33.6	0.5	279
38	R subgenual cingulate	3.2	27.7	−19.3	124
39	L subgenual cingulate	−0.2	27.5	−19.3	123
40	R ventral striatum	21.9	15.3	−1.3	43
41	L ventral striatum	−14.6	11.4	−5.4	42
42	R ParaHippocampal	26.7	−13.0	−21.1	246
43	L ParaHippocampal	−19.9	−13.5	−21.2	231
44	R Posterior Cingulate	7.4	−40.7	40.7	281
45	L Posterior Cingulate	−4.4	−40.5	40.6	283
46	R putamen	25.5	3.5	3.0	198
47	L putamen	−21.6	3.2	3.1	196
48	R SN	12.0	−13.5	−11.3	6
49	L SN	−7.5	−13.3	−11.9	4

Table 1. Cont.

#	Name	X	Y	Z	Volume
50	R visual BA19	5.7	−72.4	30.3	109
51	L visual BA19	−2.6	−72.9	30.7	111
52	R supp motor	9.9	2.2	61.2	541
53	L supp motor	−4.0	6.6	60.6	523
54	Medial BA9	3.7	51.5	22.5	37
55	Superior precuneus	3.3	−56.6	38.6	320
56	DRN	1.5	29.4	−17.3	340

Abbreviations: dmPFC, dorsal medial prefrontal cortex; PFC, prefrontal cortex; BA, Brodman area; GP, globus pallidus; NAc, nucleus accumbens; M1, primary motor; M2, secondary motor; SIJ, primary sensory cortex (jaw region); CPu, caudate putamen; GP, globus pallidus; STN, subthalamic nucleus; ACC, anterior cingulate cortex; DRN, dorsal raphe nucleus.

made difficult by the presence of a global effect that biases all correlations toward positive values (for example see [30]), we analyzed our r-fcMRI data with and without correction for the global signal. We also tested the effect of spatial smoothing by analyzing the data with and without smoothing. We then compared human and rat r-fcMRI data, trying to account for both similarities (brain organization and functionality) and differences (hemodynamic functions) in cerebral function among the species. Based on our findings we conclude that negative and positive correlations have distinct physiological properties and propose a mechanism for negative correlations in r-fcMRI that accounts for all our findings.

Methods

Human data

Eighteen human data-sets of healthy subjects (age 29.2 ± 7.4; 8 males and 10 females) were downloaded from the NITRC site (http://www.nitrc.org/projects/fcon_1000/). Data was generated by professors Milham, M.P. and Castellanos, F.X. groups' and generously posted in this site for public use (data taken from NewYork_a_part1 and part2). Data sets were chosen randomly without any exclusion criteria. To allow reproduction of the results, analysis was performed in the 'Data Processing Assistant for Resting-State fMRI (DPARSF) Advanced Edition' (Release = V2.3_130615, http://www.restfmri.net) [35] which is based on Statistical Parametric Mapping (SPM8, Welcome Department, London UK) and Resting-State fMRI Data Analysis Toolkit [36], thus available to the public. Images were realigned, co-registered to T1 anatomy, segmented, normalized, either smoothed by a [4×4×4] voxel kernel or not smoothed, de-trended, filtered ($0.01<>0.08$ Hz), covaried by the 6 rigid body functions and either with or without the global signal and then scrubbed (FD> 0.5 with 'bad' data points removed [37]). Using a WFU PickAtlas toolbox [38,39], 57 ROIs (36 cortical and 21 non-cortical) were selected in the MNI space (Table 1) covering the extended limbic system. ROIs were implemented in the DPARSFA toolbox, functional connectivity between them was calculated and their time courses were extracted. The analyses yielded four connectivity analysis sets. (1) Without spatial smoothing and without global regression (marked hereafter as '-S –G'). (2) With spatial smoothing and without global regression ('+S –G'). (3) Without

smoothing but with global regression ('-S +G') and (4) with smoothing and with regression ('+S +G'). All further analysis was performed in custom-made IDL software.

Rat data

The study was approved by the *Animal Care and Use Committee of the Hebrew University*. Experiments were carried out in accordance with the NIH Guidelines regarding the care and use of animals for experimental procedures (NIH approval number: OPRR-A01-5011).18 male Sprague-Dawley (380–450 g, age 19 ± 2 weeks supplied by Harlan, Rehovot Israel) rats were included in the study.

Data were collected with a 4.7T Bruker BioSpec scanner (Bruker Biospin Ettlington, Germany) using a Dotty quadrature rat head coil. Rats were anesthetized with isoflurane (1.5% +30:70 $O_2:N_2O$). Respiration rates were continuously monitored and were held between 55–65 min^{-1} by small adjustments of the isoflurane concentration. Body temperature was kept stable (37°C ±1) using a water heating bed. 2D T2-weighted coronal images were acquired for anatomy. Functional BOLD contrast MRI was collected with EPI-FID (TR = 2, TE = 20 ms, 300 repetitions, matrix = 128×64×15, FOV = 3×3 cm^2, 1mm slice width and three sequential sets). Functional data was first processed in SPM8 using standard spatial preprocessing steps. Images were slice-time corrected, realigned and resliced. At a second step, analysis was performed using custom-made IDL and Matlab software. It included regression-out the six functions related to motion, alignment of the MRI images to the rat brain atlas[40], data smoothing by a 3-point-Gaussian kernel, and band-pass filtering ($0.01<>0.1$ Hz). 69 ROIs (24 cortical and 45 non-cortical) were pre-selected in the atlas (Table 2) covering the extended limbic system. Correlations between predefined ROIs were obtained by calculating Pearson correlations between all possible pairs and applying Fischer's z transformation.

Statistics

A one group t-statistic random effect analysis on the Fisher transformed values between subjects was performed. To correct for multiple comparisons, False Discovery Rate (FDR) correction with a threshold of $\alpha = 0.001$ for humans and $\alpha = 0.01$ for rats was used (the difference was due to the weaker effect in rats that is expected due to the anesthesia). To define significant connections,

Table 2. Regions of interest (ROIs) in the rat brain, their mean coordinates and volume in ml.

#	Name	X	Y	Z	Volume
0	R M1 (rostral)	3.4	2.6	3.7	7.00
1	L M1 (rostral)	−3.5	2.6	3.7	6.96
2	R M2 (rostral)	1.3	1.6	3.7	2.39
3	L M2 (rostral)	−1.4	1.6	3.7	2.38
4	R cingulate area 1	0.6	2.1	1.9	5.36
5	L cingulate area 1	−0.7	2.1	1.9	5.28
6	R pre-limbic	0.6	3.7	3.3	4.07
7	L pre-limbic	−0.7	3.7	3.3	4.10
8	R infra-limbic	0.4	5.0	3.2	1.20
9	L infra-limbic	−0.5	5.0	3.1	1.23
10	R frontal area 3	4.2	4.2	3.7	1.34
11	L frontal area 3	−4.2	4.2	3.7	1.35
12	R insular	3.8	5.1	3.7	2.62
13	L insular	−3.9	5.1	3.7	2.62
14	R NAc core	1.5	6.6	2.7	1.27
15	L NAc core	−1.5	6.6	2.7	1.29
16	R NAc shell	1.2	7.4	2.7	1.02
17	L NAc shell	−1.2	7.4	2.7	1.06
18	R sensory SIJ	5.0	4.5	2.3	8.57
19	L sensory SIJ	−5.0	4.5	2.3	8.71
20	R CPu rostral	2.8	5.5	1.2	17.92
21	L CPu rostral	−2.9	5.5	1.2	18.00
22	R cingulate area 2	0.5	3.1	0.9	3.73
23	L cingulate area 2	−0.6	3.1	0.9	3.60
24	R CPU caudal	3.8	5.8	−0.6	12.77
25	L CPU caudal	−3.8	5.7	−0.6	13.14
26	R basal nucleus	3.2	8.0	−1.3	0.15
27	L basal nucleus	−3.2	7.9	−1.3	0.18
28	R GP,	3.5	7.0	−1.6	2.80
29	L GP	−3.6	6.9	−1.6	2.91
30	R VPL	2.8	6.4	−2.3	1.35
31	L VPL	−3.0	6.4	−2.3	1.21
32	R VA+VL	1.9	6.1	−2.3	2.20
33	L VA+VL	−2.0	6.2	−2.3	2.20
34	R EP	2.8	7.9	−2.3	0.33
35	L EP	−2.9	7.9	−2.3	0.22
36	R S1BF	5.3	3.0	−2.3	5.77
37	L S1BF	−5.4	3.0	−2.3	5.76
38	R amygdala	4.2	9.2	−2.6	9.88
39	L amygdala	−4.4	9.2	−2.5	8.78
40	R Hab	0.7	5.0	−3.3	0.48
41	L Hab	−0.7	5.0	−3.3	0.48
42	R Po (thalamus)	2.2	5.9	−3.3	2.03
43	L Po (thalamus)	−2.3	5.8	−3.3	1.84
44	R hippocampus	2.2	3.3	−3.3	5.55
45	L hippocampus	−2.5	3.3	−3.3	6.31
46	R granular cortex	0.6	1.7	−4.7	7.47
47	R granular cortex	−0.7	1.7	−4.8	7.89
48	R hypothalamus	0.9	9.0	−3.3	2.96
49	L hypothalamus	−0.9	9.0	−3.3	2.64

Table 2. Cont.

#	Name	X	Y	Z	Volume
50	R zona inserta	2.6	7.5	−4.3	0.99
51	L zona inserta	−2.8	7.5	−4.3	0.95
52	Mammillary	−0.1	9.3	−4.3	2.70
53	R SNr	2.3	8.4	−5.3	1.52
54	L SNr	−2.4	8.4	−5.3	1.40
55	R Red nucleus	1.0	7.5	−5.3	0.52
56	L Red nucleus	−1.1	7.5	−5.3	0.50
57	R VTA	0.6	8.2	−6.3	0.58
58	L VTA	−0.8	8.1	−6.3	0.53
59	R sup colliculus	1.3	4.1	−6.8	9.49
60	L sup colliculus	−1.4	4.2	−6.8	9.67
61	R DG	4.2	5.8	−6.3	5.89
62	L DG	−4.3	5.9	−6.3	6.03
63	IP	−0.1	9.0	−6.3	0.84
64	R pontine	0.8	10.1	−7.3	1.33
65	L pontine nuc	−0.9	10.1	−7.3	1.36
66	DRN	0.0	6.4	−7.3	1.16
67	R STN	2.6	8.1	−3.3	0.30
68	L STN	−2.7	8.1	−3.3	0.30

Abbreviations: M1, primary motor cortex; M2, secondary motor cortex; NAC, nucleus accumbens; SIJ, primary sensory cortex (jaw region); CPu, caudate-putamen; GP, globus pallidus; VPL, ventral posterolateral thalamic nucleus; VA, ventral anterior thalamic nucleus; VL, ventrolateral thalamic nucleus; EP, entopeduncular nucleus; S1BF, primary sensory cortex (barrel field); Hab, habenula; Po, post thalamic nucleus; SNr, substantia nigra; VTA, ventral tegmental area; DG, dentate gyrus; IP, interpeduncular nucleus; DRN, dorsal raphe nucleus; STN, subthalamic nucleus.

we used the lowest threshold amongst the four analyses (the threshold corresponding to '+S –G'). Each of the four analyses (-S-G; +S-G; -S+G; +S+G) had a FDR cutoff corresponding to $\alpha = 0.001$. To minimize differences due to thresholds, the same cutoff was used in all groups. Connections whose p-values were lower than the threshold are termed hereafter 'significant connections'. Categorizing connections as 'positive' or 'negative' was done based on their t-values. Significant connections with positive t-values were named 'positive-connections' and significant connections with negative t-values were named 'negative connections'. For the definition of the t-values we subtracted the global mean correlation (all Fisher transformed values from the entire group) from all correlations and then divided it by the standard error (similarly to [41]). This resulted in distributions that were centered at zero.

Effect of time lags

To test the effect of time-lags on the correlations, we calculated the correlation values for each significant connection introducing a time-lag ranging from −26 to 26 seconds. This time range was chosen based on reported BOLD signal post-stimulus length in humans [42] and in rats [43]. Specifically, we counted the number of positive connections whose correlations became more positive and the number of negative connections whose correlations became more negative as a function of the time-lag values.

Results

Figure 1 presents the distributions of the Fisher-transformed values and of the group t-values for all ROI pairs for the four different analyses of the human data. As expected [30], the distribution of the Fisher-transformed values of the uncorrected data centered on positive values and was shifted approximately to zero by removing the global signal. The distributions of t-values were, as expected, centered on zero but had different widths. The distribution of the Fisher-transformed values of the rat data was centered approximately on zero. For that reason no global signal removal was applied on the rat data.

Figures 2–5 show the significant positive (A & B) and significant negative (C & D) connections in the human data, each for a different analysis. In figure 6 we show the numbers of significant positive and significant negative connections that were obtained by these analyses in the human data. Whereas spatial smoothing and correction for the global signal increased the number of positive connections, the effect on the negative connections was more complex. To better quantify the differences between the analyses, we calculated the percentage of common connections (positive and negative separately) between the analyses. Table 3 shows that whereas most of the positive connections were common regardless of the analysis used, different negative connections were obtained when a correction for global signal was applied.

Careful inspection of Figures 2–5 suggests that negative and positive connections differ with respect to the structures they

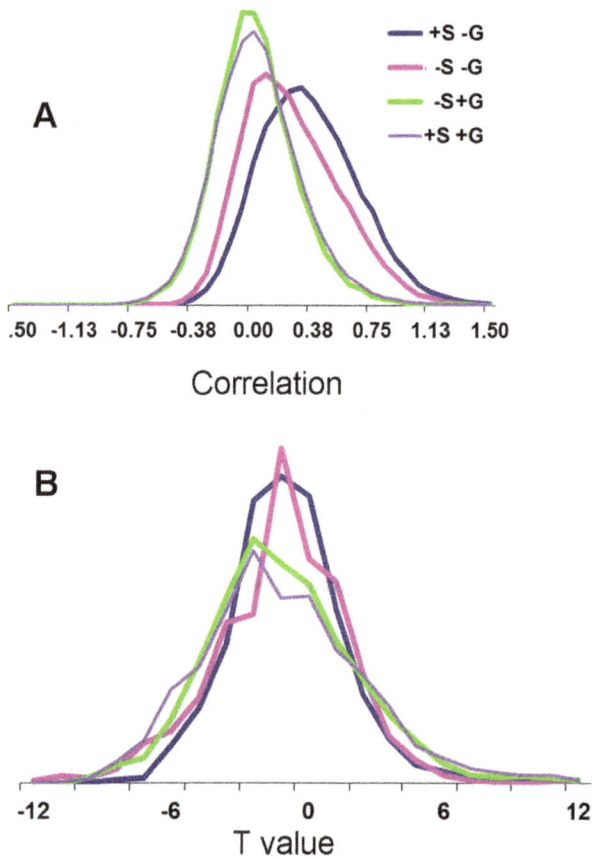

Figure 1. Distributions of Fisher transformed and of t-values for the four different analyses of the human data. *(A)* Distributions of Fisher transformed values. *(B)* Distributions of t-values. The analyses differed in either applying or not applying spatial smoothing and correction for global signal. '–S -G' – analysis without smoothing and without global regression, '+S -G' – analysis with smoothing and without global regression, '–S +G' – analysis without smoothing and with global regression and '–S -G' – analysis with smoothing and with global regression.

connect. To quantify this point, we categorized all negative and positive significant connections into three types: those connecting between two cortical ROIs ("Intra-Cx"), those connecting between two non-cortical ROIs ("Extra-Cx"), and those connecting a

cortical with a non-cortical ROI ("Between"). The percentages of these categories are shown in Figure 7 for the four different analyses of the human data. There was a clear distinction between positive and negative connections with almost no negative connections linking non-cortical regions and only few positive connections linking cortical and non-cortical regions. As seen in Figure 7, the effect of the different analyses on the distribution of positive connections was small while it was greater on the negative connections. Spatial smoothing had a relatively minor effect compared to the significant effect of global regression.

Figure 8 shows the 171 positive (Figure 8 A & B) and 158 negative (Figure 8 C & D) significant connections observed in the rat data where no correction for global signal was used (as it was not needed since the distribution of the correlation values was centered approximately at zero). Each connection is shown as a colored line connecting two ROIs on coronal and axial rat-brain figures derived from the rat atlas [40] with ROIs numbers corresponding to the brain regions presented in Table 2.

Several common features across both species are evident from Figures 2 and 8. First, while many homologous bilateral regions (e.g. right and left anterior cingulate) have positive connections between each other, not even a single negative connection exists between homologous right and left hemispheric structures. Second, both negative and positive connections express a relatively high level of inter-hemispheric (non-homologous) symmetry. Note that in both the human and rat data, several regions had multiple positive connections, several had multiple negative connections and several had both multiple positive and negative connections (e.g., the right and left insula (#30, 31) in humans and the amygdala (#38 and 39) in rats), emphasizing the fact that Fisher-transformed values between regions reflect connection-specific rather than region-specific properties.

Positive correlations between ROI pairs are obtained if ROI time courses express similar periodical behaviors without a time-lag. Negative correlations between ROI pairs can theoretically be obtained if both ROIs express similar periodical behaviors but with a time-lag between them. The effect of time–lags on the positive and the negative connections is presented in Figure 9 for humans and in Figure 10 for rats. The figures show the percentage of significant positive and negative connections that time-lags made them even more significant (higher Fisher-transformed values for positive connections and lower for negative connections). Since the calculations were performed on the data of each subject separately, a statistical comparison is possible. Table 4 gives the p-values for that comparison for each time-lag and each type of analysis. As seen in these Figures and in Table 4, time-lags of more than a few seconds reduced positive correlations while making negative correlations more negative. Specifically we note

Table 3. Percentage of overlap between the significant connections obtained by the four types of analyses of the human data.

	-S-G	+S-G	-S+G	+S+G
-S-G		78(+)	75(+)	89(+)
+S-G	81(−)		78(+)	86(+)
-S+G	30(−)	14(−)		97(+)
+S+G	42(−)	16(−)	88(−)	

Percentage of overlap between positive connections is shown by (+) and between negative connections by (−). –S-G: analysis without spatial smoothing and without global signal regression; +S-G: analysis with spatial smoothing and without global signal regression; -S+G: analysis without spatial smoothing and with global signal regression; +S+G: analysis with spatial smoothing and with global signal regression;

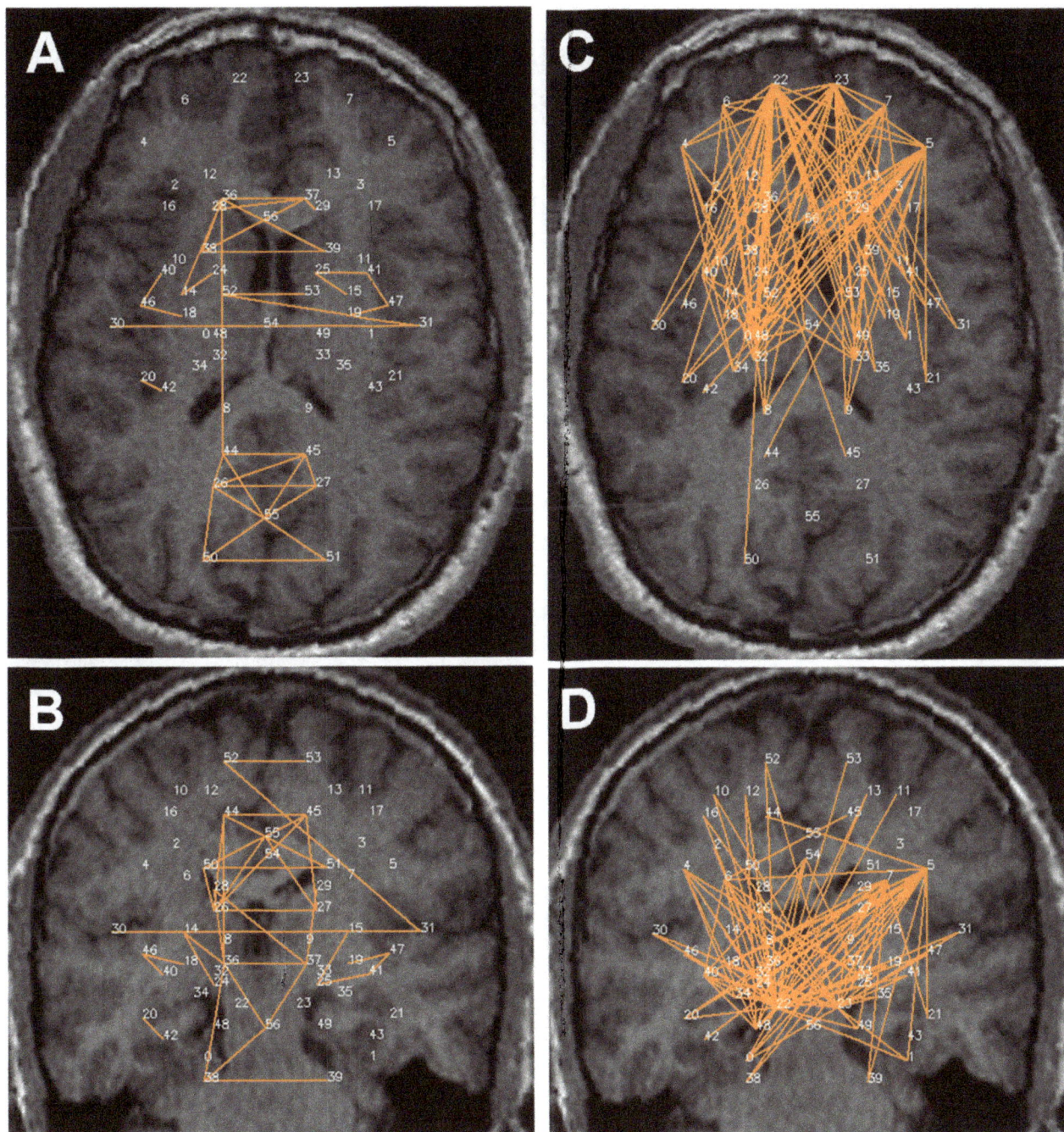

Figure 2. Significant connections within the 57 predefined human regions for the –S-G analysis. Significant connections are presented as 2D projections on top of T1-weighted coronal and axial MRI images. ROIs are annotated using numbers provided in Table 1. *A & B.* Positive connections. *C & D.* Negative connections.

the following: (i) most positive connections were more significant with a zero time-lag, (ii) most negative connections were more significant with a non-zero time-lag, (iii) the time-lags that improve negative connections were of a wide range, (iv) the division between positive and negative connections was sharper when no

correction for global signal was used, (v) the transition points from which any increase of the time-lag resulted in more negative than positive connections becoming more significant were at 4 sec in the human data and at 6 sec in the rat data, (vi) the use of global signal corrections increased the number of negative connections

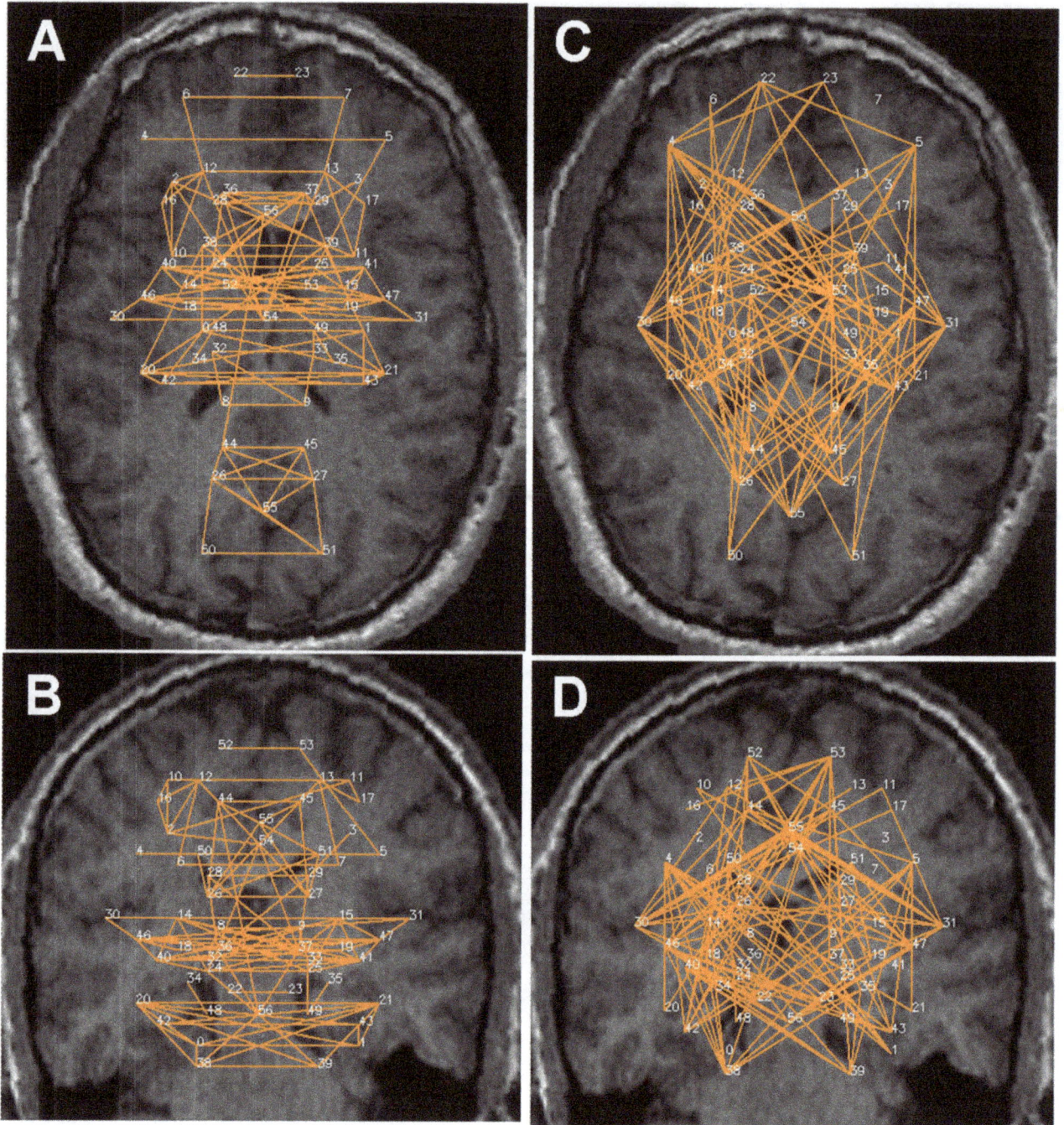

Figure 3. Significant connections within the 57 predefined human regions for the +S+G analysis. Significant connections are presented as 2D projections on top of T1-weighted coronal and axial MRI images. ROIs are annotated using numbers provided in Table 1. *A & B.* Positive connections. *C & D.* Negative connections.

Discussion

for which the most significant correlation was obtained using a zero time-lag (thus being similar to the positive connections). In contrast, the number of such 'zero time-lag' negative connections was negligible when no global signal correction was used. (vii) The rat data was qualitatively similar to human data.

This study aimed to better understand the mechanisms underlying negative correlations in resting-state functional connectivity MRI. Analysis was performed on BOLD contrast

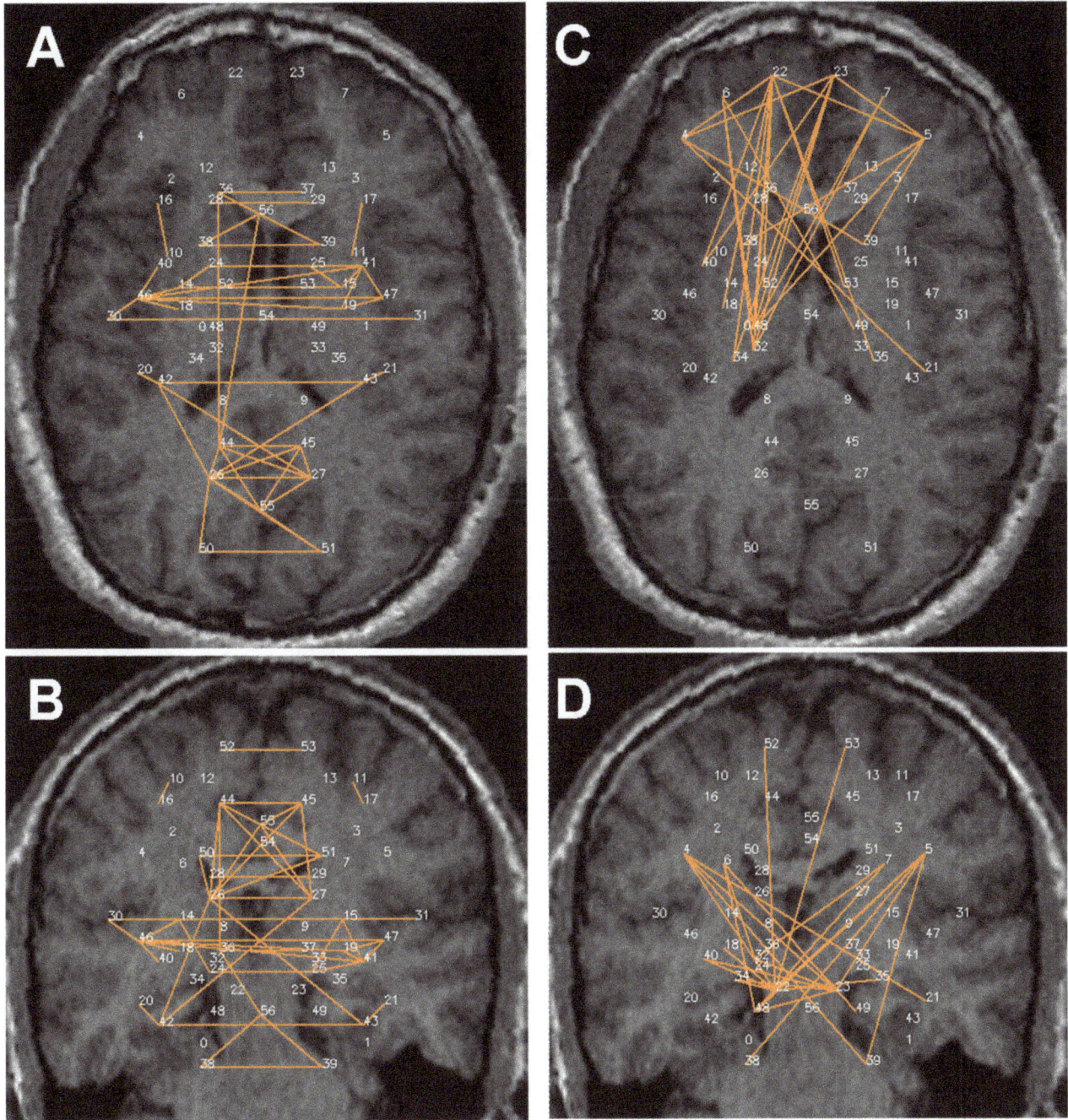

Figure 4. Significant connections within the 57 predefined human regions for the +S-G analysis. Significant connections are presented as 2D projections on top of T1-weighted coronal and axial MRI images. ROIs are annotated using numbers provided in Table 1. *A & B.* Positive connections. *C & D.* Negative connections.

temporal signals obtained from predefined anatomical ROIs. This type of analysis has several advantages, including a more robust signal-to-noise ratio (the average ROI signal was used), being less sensitive to registration and realignments errors, making the examination of symmetry between hemispheres possible and

visualizing the functional connectivity organization on a broad and global level.

By comparing the positive and negative connections obtained through four different analysis methods applied on the human data, we demonstrated critical differences between positive and negative connections that were evident in all types of analysis. The

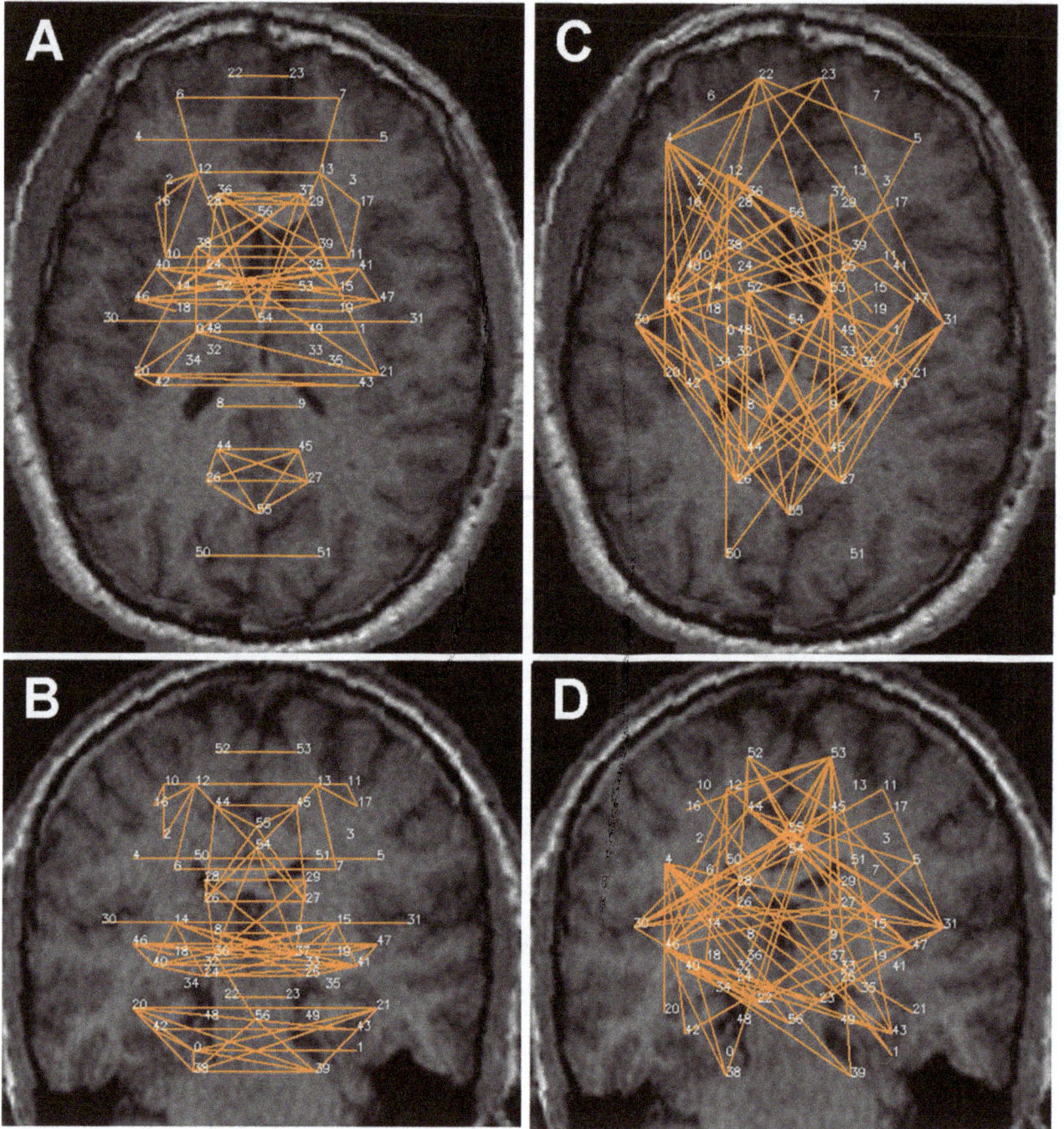

Figure 5. Significant connections within the 57 predefined human regions for the -S+G analysis. Significant connections are presented as 2D projections on top of T1-weighted coronal and axial MRI images. ROIs are annotated using numbers provided in Table 1. *A & B.* Positive connections. *C & D.* Negative connections.

major difference was that introducing non-zero time-lags between ROIs reduced the significance of the positive connections, while increasing the significance of the negative connections. In addition, positive and negative connections typically linked between different regional categories. For example, no negative

connections were found linking two non-cortical structures. When comparing the different analyses, the following differences were observed: (i) spatial smoothing and correction for the global signal increased the number of significant positive connections while its effect on the negative connections was more complex (Figure 6),

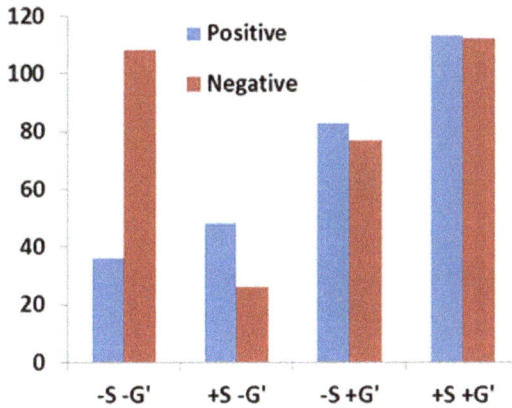

Figure 6. Number of significant positive and negative connections for the different human analyses.

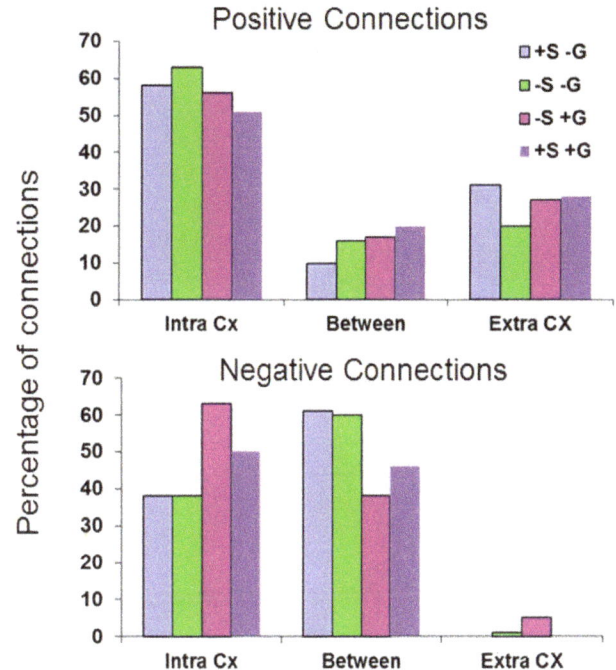

Figure 7. Categorization of positive and negative human connections. Percentages of significant connections into the 'Intra Cx' (between two cortical ROIs), the 'Extra-Cx' (between two non-cortical ROIs) and the 'Between' (between cortical and non-cortical ROIs) categories. *Top.* Positive connections. *Bottom.* Negative connections.

(ii) spatial smoothing and global signal correction had a small effect on positive connections with respect to their regional categorization and to the degree of their overlap, while the global signal correction had a major effect on negative connections, resulting in almost no overlap between connections that were significant with and without global signal correction (Figure 7 and Table 3), and (iii) the differential effect that time-lags had on positive and negative connections was the strongest when no global signal correction was applied.

When comparing the results from the human and the rat data, the patterns of inter-hemispheric symmetry and the prevalence of positive bilateral homologous connections were found to be similar. More importantly, negative connections in both species generally became more negative by introducing time-lags, while positive connections did not. It must however be emphasized that, in rodents, sedation was shown to yield superior *r-fcMRI* results compared to general anesthesia [44], suggesting that our rat data should be considered with caution. Additionally, no attempt was done to regress for cardiac and respiration pulsation although such filtering might have improved the results. We avoided doing this in order for the human and rat data processing to be as similar as possible. Nevertheless, we recently have shown significant *r-fcMRI* results using isoflurane anesthesia [45–47] and without cardiac and respiration regression, which strengthens our confidence in our rat data.

All these results support the assumption that the different forms of *r*-fcMRI correlations reflect different underlying physiological mechanism. We suggest a hypothesis that integrates the above findings into an inclusive model for understanding the mechanism of negative and positive connections. We are aware however, that the current evidence supporting this hypothesis is only circumstantial. The BOLD signal is affected by changes in both rCBF and rCBV. The coupling between CBF, CBV and the BOLD signal is complex, nonlinear, spatially inhomogeneous and even layer dependent [48]. The positive phase of the hemodynamic response function in response to stimulus is assumed to be dominated by rCBF changes, while the post stimulus undershoot is assumed to be affected by a *delayed* rCBV response [43,49,50]. An increase in rCBF presumably results in a decrease in blood deoxy-hemoglobin levels, causing an increase in the BOLD signal. In contrast, an increase in rCBV causes a total increase in deoxy-hemoglobin, resulting in a decrease of the BOLD signal. The balance between rCBF and rCBV could therefore determine the overall resulting BOLD signal (i.e., if the signal at any specific time point is above or below the baseline). We hypothesis that if the activity of two groups of neurons in two separate regions is highly synchronized, and if the hemodynamic response of one is rCBF dominated while that of the other is rCBV dominated, the temporal correlation between the BOLD signal in these regions will be negative. Moreover, since rCBV increases are delayed compared to rCBF increases, there will be a time-lag until the negative correlation reaches its maximal value. This view is based on the assumption that changes in BOLD signals during rest and following stimuli are comparable in magnitude [51] and mechanism. The long time-lags observed in the data (Figure 7) are in line with the reported post-stimulus length in humans [42] and in rats [43]. We further hypothesis that if the rCBV and/or the rCBF responses are spatially dependent (for example, synchronized neuronal activity resulting in an increase of rCBV in one region and a decrease in rCBV in another) one can also expect to find negative correlations with no time lags between such regions. Overall, we suggest that negative connections are the results of complex spatially inhomogeneous hemodynamic responses that are mediated by neuronal activity.

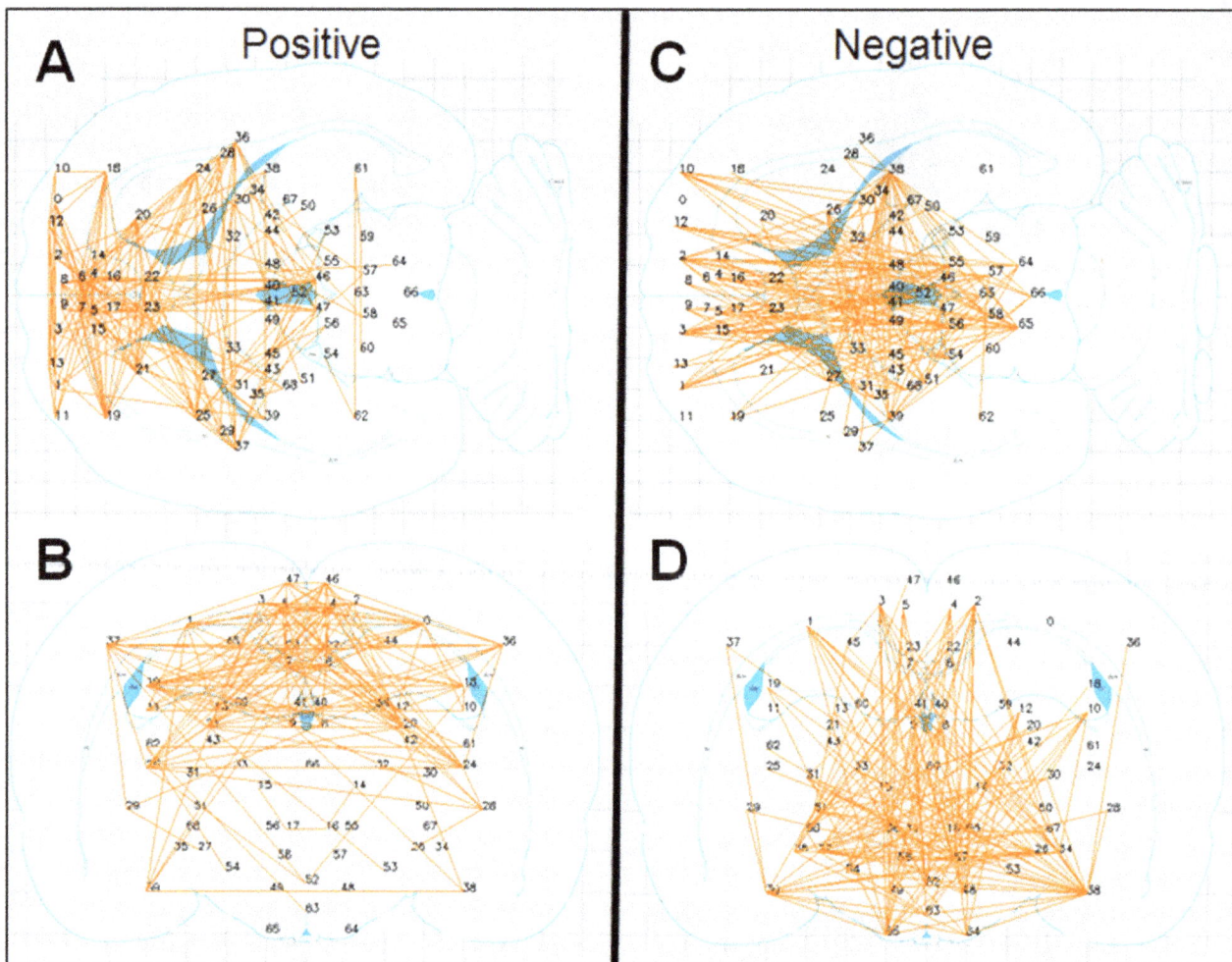

Figure 8. Significant connections within the 69 predefined rat regions. Significant connections are presented as 2D projections on top of coronal and axial Figures from the rat brain atlas. ROIs are annotated using numbers provided in Table 2. *A & B*. Positive connections. *C & D*. Negative connections.

Table 4. T-values for the comparison between the numbers of positive and negative connections that time-lag made more significance.

	-S-G	+S+G	+S-G	-S+G	rats
0	2.90369E-26	2.99046E-13	1.57702E-26	1.69953E-11	1.66596E-10
2	8.40016E-06	0.800385948	7.38712E-07	0.450100779	3.91086E-11
4	0.000407685	2.44899E-06	0.012682339	0.004888566	0.001371955
6	4.73828E-08	9.33376E-07	7.36576E-05	0.000790463	0.811502824
8	2.60049E-07	6.57005E-06	0.001934496	4.07728E-05	0.002860986
10	3.48352E-09	8.16819E-05	0.000272562	0.003190054	0.000538446
12	3.2188E-08	0.000238064	1.03808E-05	0.001122026	0.001629137
14	9.87039E-09	0.000522939	0.000942835	0.000260738	1.8236E-06
16	1.95238E-12	1.99754E-05	7.12566E-06	0.017933245	0.001564497
18	3.14229E-08	1.52653E-05	4.45951E-05	0.006811102	1.2003E-05
20	1.38689E-08	9.0614E-05	0.001227115	0.004817849	0.000457931
22	5.55054E-08	5.0776E-07	3.7641E-05	0.000158922	0.000431086
24	3.93325E-07	1.33919E-06	0.000267121	0.000903292	9.5524E-05
26	1.12124E-06	0.001065601	0.000725739	0.000401245	9.63E-06

More significance positive/negative connections were defined as connections with higher/lower Fisher transform values. Comparison was done for each time-lag and for the four human analyses as well as for the rat data. The rows are for different time-lags that are given is sec.

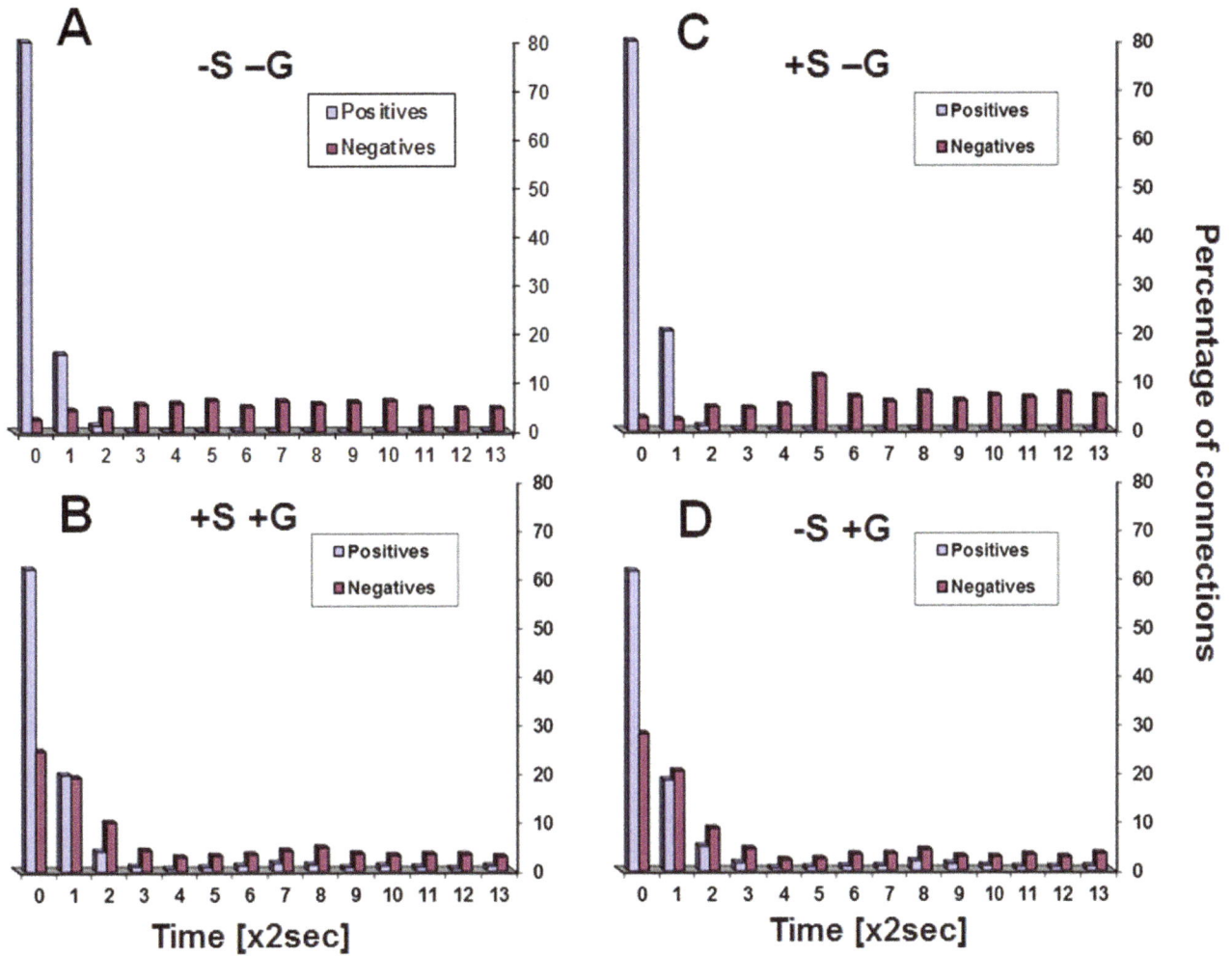

Figure 9. Effect of time-lags on correlation strengths in the human data. Percentage of connections that time-lags made more significant (more positive for positive connections and more negative for negative connections) at each time-lag value. A. Results for the analysis without smoothing and without global regression ('–S -G'), B. Results for the analysis with smoothing and with global regression ('+S +G'), C. Results for the analysis with smoothing and without global regression ('+S -G', D. Results for the analysis without smoothing and with global regression ('–S +G').

Our hypothesis is supported by several published findings suggesting that monoamines, mainly dopamine and serotonin, differentially affect CBV and CBF in different brain regions [52–57]. For example, it was shown that administration of agonists for the excitatory D_1-like dopamine receptors causes an increase in CBV in certain regions, while agonists for the inhibitory D_2-like receptors cause a decrease in CBV in other regions [57]. Such a relationship fits in well with the proposed CBV-based mechanism of negative connections, in which a positive synchronization between the activities of neurons within two regions that are differentially influenced by CBV will result in a negative correlation between their BOLD signals. Similarly, Shin et al. [56] demonstrated that in response to noxious electrical stimulation of the rat forepaw (known to induce endogenous dopaminergic neurotransmission), CBV was increased in the sensory cortex and at the same time was decreased in the caudate-putamen (CPu), although immunohistochemistry and electrophysiological recording demonstrated increased neuronal activity in the CPu.

The following findings lend further support to the hypothesis that differential neurovascular mechanisms are responsible for the positive and negative correlations between brain regions observed in r-fcMRI connectivity measurements: (i) All homologous bilateral connections were positive. Hemodynamic responses in homologous bilateral regions are expected to be similar (similar weightings of CBF and CBV). Consequently, the correlation between their BOLD signals is expected to be positive. (ii) Most of the negative connections became more significant when adding time-lags of a few seconds. Since rCBV changes were shown to be delayed compared to rCBF changes [43,49,50], BOLD signals that are affected by CBV are expected to be more time-delayed compared to BOLD signals affected by CBF. The observed range of 'significance-optimizing' time-lags matches the post-stimulus delays found in humans and rats. (iii) Similar findings were obtained for both human and rat data. Human and rat data were acquired by two different protocols, with different field strengths, at different arousal states, with different resolutions and were analyzed by different software algorithms. Their anatomy,

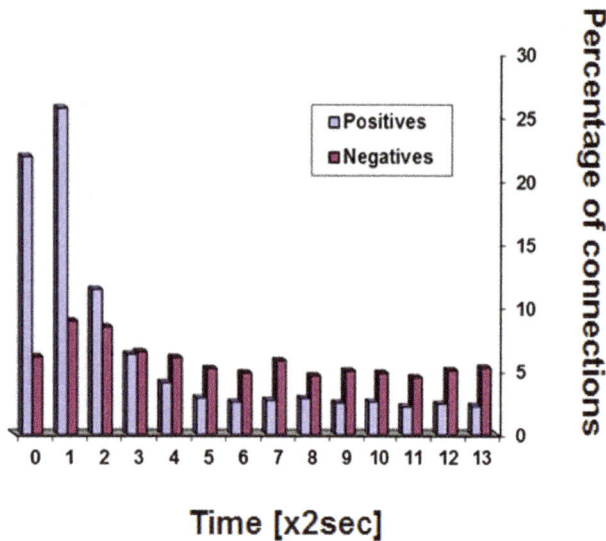

Figure 10. Effect of time-lags on correlation strengths in the rat data. Percentage of connections that time-lags made more significant (more positive for positive connections and more negative for negative connections) at each time-lag value.

We recall that the definition of negative correlations is critical and the use of different definitions makes the comparison between studies difficult. For example, in a recent publication [58] mice *r-fcMRI* of BOLD and CBV weighed data, were compared. Similar independent component analysis (ICA) anti-correlated networks were observed with BOLD and with CBV data, opposing our hypothesis. However, it is likely that not finding significant negative connections in their ROI-based analysis results from the different definition of negative connection. Here we used a t-statistic distribution centered at zero to define positive and negative connections. As described above, the significant differences observed between positive and negative connections, as per this definition, strengthens our belief in its relevance.

In conclusion, we propose that positive and negative connections in *r-fcMRI* result from neuronal-mediated hemodynamic mechanisms leading to temporal and spatial heterogeneity in *r-fcMRI* BOLD responses. We suggest that positive connections are expected to be found between regions with synchronized neuronal activity and homogeneous hemodynamic responses while negative connections are expected to be found between regions with synchronized neuronal activity, yet with heterogeneous hemodynamic responses.

Author Contributions

Conceived and designed the experiments: GG. Performed the experiments: NG. Analyzed the data: GG. Contributed reagents/materials/analysis tools: GG NG. Wrote the paper: GG OB NG.

hemodynamic responses and brain organization are different. In spite of all these, remarkable similarities between human and rat results were observed.

References

1. Buckner RL, Andrews-Hanna JR, Schacter DL (2008) The brain's default network: anatomy, function, and relevance to disease. Ann N Y Acad Sci 1124: 1–38.
2. Fox MD, Raichle ME (2007) Spontaneous fluctuations in brain activity observed with functional magnetic resonance imaging. Nat Rev Neurosci 8: 700–711.
3. Biswal B, Yetkin FZ, Haughton VM, Hyde JS (1995) Functional connectivity in the motor cortex of resting human brain using echo-planar MRI. Magn Reson Med 34(4): 537–541.
4. Fox MD, Snyder AZ, Vincent JL, Corbetta M, Van Essen DC, et al. (2005) The human brain is intrinsically organized into dynamic, anticorrelated functional networks. Proc Natl Acad Sci U S A 102: 9673–9678.
5. Greicius MD, Krasnow B, Reiss AL, Menon V (2003) Functional connectivity in the resting brain: a network analysis of the default mode hypothesis. Proc Natl Acad Sci U S A 100: 253–258.
6. Raichle ME, MacLeod AM, Snyder AZ, Powers WJ, Gusnard DA, et al. (2001) A default mode of brain function. Proc Natl Acad Sci U S A 98: 676–682.
7. Deco G, Jirsa VK, McIntosh AR (2011) Emerging concepts for the dynamical organization of resting-state activity in the brain. Nat Rev Neurosci 12: 43-56.
8. Damoiseaux JS, Rombouts SA, Barkhof F, Scheltens P, Stam CJ, et al. (2006) Consistent resting-state networks across healthy subjects. Proc Natl Acad Sci U S A 103: 13848–13853.
9. Shehzad Z, Kelly AM, Reiss PT, Gee DG, Gotimer K, et al. (2009) The resting brain: unconstrained yet reliable. Cereb Cortex 19: 2209–2229.
10. Zuo XN, Kelly C, Adelstein JS, Klein DF, Castellanos FX, et al. (2010) Reliable intrinsic connectivity networks: test-retest evaluation using ICA and dual regression approach. Neuroimage 49: 2163–2177.
11. Wang K, van Meer MP, van der Marel K, van der Toorn A, Xu L, et al. (2011) Temporal scaling properties and spatial synchronization of spontaneous blood oxygenation level-dependent (BOLD) signal fluctuations in rat sensorimotor network at different levels of isoflurane anesthesia. NMR Biomed 24: 61–67.
12. Liu X, Zhu XH, Zhang Y, Chen W (2011) Neural origin of spontaneous hemodynamic fluctuations in rats under burst-suppression anesthesia condition. Cereb Cortex 21: 374–384.
13. Whitfield-Gabrieli S, Thermenos HW, Milanovic S, Tsuang MT, Faraone SV, et al. (2009) Hyperactivity and hyperconnectivity of the default network in schizophrenia and in first-degree relatives of persons with schizophrenia. Proc Natl Acad Sci U S A 106: 1279–1284.
14. Castellanos FX, Margulies DS, Kelly C, Uddin LQ, Ghaffari M, et al. (2008) Cingulate-precuneus interactions: a new locus of dysfunction in adult attention-deficit/hyperactivity disorder. Biol Psychiatry 63: 332–337.
15. Chai XJ, Whitfield-Gabrieli S, Shinn AK, Gabrieli JD, Nieto Castanon A, et al. (2011) Abnormal medial prefrontal cortex resting-state connectivity in bipolar disorder and schizophrenia. Neuropsychopharmacology 36: 2009–2017.
16. Wang K, Liang M, Wang L, Tian L, Zhang X, et al. (2007) Altered functional connectivity in early Alzheimer's disease: a resting-state fMRI study. Hum Brain Mapp28: 967–978.
17. Grimm S, Boesiger P, Beck J, Schuepbach D, Bermpohl F, et al. (2009) Altered negative BOLD responses in the default-mode network during emotion processing in depressed subjects. Neuropsychopharmacology 34: 932–943.
18. Kastrup A, Baudewig J, Schnaudigel S, Huonker R, Becker L, et al. (2008) Behavioral correlates of negative BOLD signal changes in the primary somatosensory cortex. Neuroimage 41: 1364–1371.
19. Kobayashi E, Bagshaw AP, Grova C, Dubeau F, Gotman J (2006) Negative BOLD responses to epileptic spikes. Hum Brain Mapp27: 488–497.
20. Nakata H, Sakamoto K, Ferretti A, Gianni Perrucci M, Del Gratta C, et al. (2009) Negative BOLD effect on somato-motor inhibitory processing: an fMRI study. Neurosci Lett 462: 101–104.
21. Northoff G, Walter M, Schulte RF, Beck J, Dydak U, et al. (2007) GABA concentrations in the human anterior cingulate cortex predict negative BOLD responses in fMRI. Nat Neurosci 10: 1515–1517.
22. Pasley BN, Inglis BA, Freeman RD (2007) Analysis of oxygen metabolism implies a neural origin for the negative BOLD response in human visual cortex. Neuroimage 36: 269–276.
23. Schridde U, Khubchandani M, Motelow JE, Sanganahalli BG, Hyder F, et al. (2008) Negative BOLD with large increases in neuronal activity. Cereb Cortex 18: 1814–1827.
24. Shmuel A, Yacoub E, Pfeuffer J, Van de Moortele PF, Adriany G, et al. (2002) Sustained negative BOLD, blood flow and oxygen consumption response and its coupling to the positive response in the human brain. Neuron 36: 1195–1210.
25. Smith AT, Williams AL, Singh KD (2004) Negative BOLD in the visual cortex: evidence against blood stealing. Hum Brain Mapp21: 213–220.
26. Shmuel A, Augath M, Oeltermann A, Logothetis NK (2006) Negative functional MRI response correlates with decreases in neuronal activity in monkey visual area V1. Nat Neurosci 9: 569–577.
27. Fox MD, Zhang D, Snyder AZ, Raichle ME (2009) The global signal and observed anticorrelated resting state brain networks. J Neurophysiol 101: 3270–3283.
28. Murphy K, Birn RM, Handwerker DA, Jones TB, Bandettini PA (2009) The impact of global signal regression on resting state correlations: are anti-correlated networks introduced? Neuroimage 44: 893–905.
29. Weissenbacher A, Kasess C, Gerstl F, Lanzenberger R, Moser E, et al. (2009) Correlations and anticorrelations in resting-state functional connectivity MRI: a

quantitative comparison of preprocessing strategies. Neuroimage 47: 1408–1416.

30. Chai XJ, Castanon AN, Ongur D, Whitfield-Gabrieli S (2011) Anticorrelations in resting state networks without global signal regression. Neuroimage 59: 1420–1428.

31. Bianciardi M, Fukunaga M, van Gelderen P, de Zwart JA, Duyn JH (2011) Negative BOLD-fMRI signals in large cerebral veins. J Cereb Blood Flow Metab 31: 401–412.

32. Chang C, Glover GH (2010) Time-frequency dynamics of resting-state brain connectivity measured with fMRI. Neuroimage 50: 81–98.

33. Carbonell F, Bellec P, Shmuel A (2011) Global and system-specific resting-state FMRI fluctuations are uncorrelated: principal component analysis reveals anti-correlated networks. Brain Connect 1: 496–510.

34. Devor A, Tian P, Nishimura N, Teng IC, Hillman EM, et al. (2007) Suppressed neuronal activity and concurrent arteriolar vasoconstriction may explain negative blood oxygenation level-dependent signal. J Neurosci 27: 4452–4459.

35. Chao-Gan Y, Yu-Feng Z (2010) DPARSF: A MATLAB Toolbox for "Pipeline" Data Analysis of Resting-State fMRI. Front Syst Neurosci 4: 13.

36. Song XW, Dong ZY, Long XY, Li SF, Zuo XN, et al. (2011) REST: a toolkit for resting-state functional magnetic resonance imaging data processing. PLoS One 6: e25031.

37. Power JD, Barnes KA, Snyder AZ, Schlaggar BL, Petersen SE (2012) Spurious but systematic correlations in functional connectivity MRI networks arise from subject motion. Neuroimage 59: 2142–2154.

38. Maldjian JA, Laurienti PJ, Kraft RA, Burdette JH (2003) An automated method for neuroanatomic and cytoarchitectonic atlas-based interrogation of fMRI data sets. Neuroimage 19: 1233–1239.

39. Maldjian JA, Laurienti PJ, Burdette JH (2004) Precentral gyrus discrepancy in electronic versions of the Talairach atlas. Neuroimage 21: 450–455.

40. Paxinos G, Watson C (2007) The Rat Brain in Stereotactic Coordinates 6th edition: Academic Press.

41. Lowe MJ, mock BJ, Sorenson JA (1998) Functonal Connectivity in Single and multislice Echoplanar Imaging Using Resting-State Fluctuations. Neuroimage 7: 119–132.

42. Arichi T, Fagiolo G, Varela M, Melendez-Calderon A, Allievi A, et al. (2012) Development of BOLD signal hemodynamic responses in the human brain. Neuroimage 63: 663–673.

43. Zong X, Kim T, Kim SG (2012) Contributions of dynamic venous blood volume versus oxygenation level changes to BOLD fMRI. Neuroimage 60: 2238–2246.

44. Kalthoff D, Po C, Wiedermann D, Hoehn M (2013) Reliability and spatial specificity of rat brain sensorimotor functional connectivity networks are superior under sedation compared with general anesthesia. NMR Biomed 26: 638–650.

45. Lotan A, Lifschytz T, Lory O, Goelman G, Lerer B (2014) Amygdalar disconnectivity could underlie stress resilience in the Ahi1 knockout mouse: conclusions from a resting-state functional MRI study. Mol Psychiatry 19: 144.

46. Lotan A, Lifschytz T, Slonimsky A, Broner EC, Greenbaum L, et al. (2014) Neural mechanisms underlying stress resilience in Ahi1 knockout mice: relevance to neuropsychiatric disorders. Mol Psychiatry 19: 243–252.

47. Goelman G, Ilinca R, Zohar I, Weinstock M (2014) Functional connectivity in prenatally stressed rats with and without maternal treatment with ladostigil, a brain-selective monoamine oxidase inhibitor. Eur J Neurosci.

48. Goense J, Merkle H, Logothetis NK (2012) High-resolution fMRI reveals laminar differences in neurovascular coupling between positive and negative BOLD responses. Neuron 76: 629–639.

49. Buxton RB, Wong EC, Frank LR (1998) Dynamics of blood flow and oxygenation changes during brain activation: the balloon model. Magn Reson Med 39: 855–864.

50. Buxton RB, Uludag K, Dubowitz DJ, Liu TT (2004) Modeling the hemodynamic response to brain activation. Neuroimage 23 Suppl 1: S220–233.

51. Kenet T, Bibitchkov D, Tsodyks M, Grinvald A, Arieli A (2003) Spontaneously emerging cortical representations of visual attributes. Nature 425: 954–956.

52. Chen YI, Choi JK, Xu H, Ren J, Andersen SL, et al. (2010) Pharmacologic neuroimaging of the ontogeny of dopamine receptor function. Dev Neurosci 32: 125–138.

53. Choi JK, Mandeville JB, Chen YI, Grundt P, Sarkar SK, et al. (2010) Imaging brain regional and cortical laminar effects of selective D3 agonists and antagonists. Psychopharmacology (Berl) 212: 59–72.

54. Mueggler T, Razoux F, Russig H, Buehler A, Franklin TB, et al. (2011) Mapping of CBV changes in 5-HT(1A) terminal fields by functional MRI in the mouse brain. Eur Neuropsychopharmacol 21: 344–353.

55. Easton N, Marshall FH, Marsden CA, Fone KC (2009) Mapping the central effects of methylphenidate in the rat using pharmacological MRI BOLD contrast. Neuropharmacology 57: 653–664.

56. Shih YY, Chen CC, Shyu BC, Lin ZJ, Chiang YC, et al. (2009) A new scenario for negative functional magnetic resonance imaging signals: endogenous neurotransmission. J Neurosci 29: 3036–3044.

57. Choi JK, Chen YI, Hamel E, Jenkins BG (2006) Brain hemodynamic changes mediated by dopamine receptors: Role of the cerebral microvasculature in dopamine-mediated neurovascular coupling. Neuroimage 30: 700–712.

58. Sforazzini F, Schwarz AJ, Galbusera A, Bifone A, Gozzi A (2014) Distributed BOLD and CBV-weighted resting-state networks in the mouse brain. Neuroimage 87: 403–415.

5

Prospective Randomized Trial of Enoxaparin, Pentoxifylline and Ursodeoxycholic Acid for Prevention of Radiation-Induced Liver Toxicity

Max Seidensticker[1,2]*, **Ricarda Seidensticker**[1,2], **Robert Damm**[1,2], **Konrad Mohnike**[1,2], **Maciej Pech**[1,2,7], **Bruno Sangro**[3], **Peter Hass**[4], **Peter Wust**[5], **Siegfried Kropf**[6], **Günther Gademann**[4], **Jens Ricke**[1,2]

1 Universitätsklinik Magdeburg, Klinik für Radiologie und Nuklearmedizin, Magdeburg, Germany, **2** International School of Image-Guided Interventions, Deutsche Akademie für Mikrotherapie, Magdeburg, Germany, **3** Clinica Universidad de Navarra, Liver Unit, Department of Internal Medicine, Pamplona, Spain, **4** Universitätsklinik Magdeburg, Klinik für Strahlentherapie, Magdeburg, Germany, **5** Charité Universitätsmedizin Berlin, Klinik für Radioonkologie und Strahlentherapie, Berlin, Germany, **6** Universitätsklinik Magdeburg, Institut für Biometrie und Medizinische Informatik, Magdeburg, Germany, **7** Medical University of Gdansk, 2nd Department of Radiology, Gdansk, Poland

Abstract

Background/Aim: Targeted radiotherapy of liver malignancies has found to be effective in selected patients. A key limiting factor of these therapies is the relatively low tolerance of the liver parenchyma to radiation. We sought to assess the preventive effects of a combined regimen of pentoxifylline (PTX), ursodeoxycholic acid (UDCA) and low-dose low molecular weight heparin (LMWH) on focal radiation-induced liver injury (fRILI).

Methods and Materials: Patients with liver metastases from colorectal carcinoma who were scheduled for local ablation by radiotherapy (image-guided high-dose-rate interstitial brachytherapy) were prospectively randomized to receive PTX, UDCA and LMWH for 8 weeks (treatment) or no medication (control). Focal RILI at follow-up was assessed using functional hepatobiliary magnetic resonance imaging (MRI). A minimal threshold dose, i.e. the dose to which the outer rim of the fRILI was formerly exposed to, was quantified by merging MRI and dosimetry data.

Results: Results from an intended interim-analysis made a premature termination necessary. Twenty-two patients were included in the per-protocol analysis. Minimal mean hepatic threshold dose 6 weeks after radiotherapy (primary endpoint) was significantly higher in the study treatment-group compared with the control (19.1 Gy versus 14.6 Gy, p = 0.011). Qualitative evidence of fRILI by MRI at 6 weeks was observed in 45.5% of patients in the treatment versus 90.9% of the control group. No significant differences between the groups were observed at the 12-week follow-up.

Conclusions: The post-therapeutic application of PTX, UDCA and low-dose LMWH significantly reduced the extent and incidence fRILI at 6 weeks after radiotherapy. The development of subsequent fRILI at 12 weeks (4 weeks after cessation of PTX, UDCA and LMWH during weeks 1–8) in the treatment group was comparable to the control group thus supporting the observation that the agents mitigated fRILI.

Trial Registration: EU clinical trials register 2008-002985-70 ClinicalTrials.gov NCT01149304

Editor: Vincent Wong, The Chinese University of Hong Kong, Hong Kong

Funding: This study was funded in full by Sirtex medical (http://www.sirtex.com.au/eu/), funding received by university hospital of Magdeburg. The writing of this paper was funded in part by Sirtex medical. Writing support was provided by Rae Hobbs and was funded by Sirtex medical. Apart from that, the funders had no role in study design, data collection and analysis, decision to publish, or preparation of the manuscript.

Competing Interests: M. Seidensticker has served as a speaker for Bayer Healthcare and Sirtex medical, and has received research funding from Sirtex medical. R. Seidensticker has served as a speaker for Bayer Healthcare and Sirtex medical, and has received research funding from Sirtex medical. J. Ricke has served as a speaker for Bayer Healthcare and Sirtex medical, and has received research funding from Sirtex medical, Bayer Healthcare and Siemens. M. Pech has served as a speaker for Sirtex medical. B. Sangro has served as a speaker and an advisory board member for Sirtex medical.

* Email: max.seidensticker@med.ovgu.de

Introduction

Highly targeted radiotherapy of liver malignancies has found to be effective in selected patients. Stereotactic radiotherapy, radioembolization using yttrium-90 (^{90}Y) microspheres as well as image-guided brachytherapy (BT) have been described in the literature with promising results [1,2,3]. A key limiting factor of these therapies is the relatively low tolerance of the liver parenchyma to radiation leading to either subclinical focal or generalized injury of the liver parenchyma. When the intensity or the extent of radiation-induced liver injury (RILI) exceeds the functional reserve, clinical complications appear in the form of radiation (radioembolization) induced liver disease (RILD or REILD) [4,5,6,7]. Prior exposure or concomitant chemotherapy is thought to increase the risk of RILD (or REILD), and as a consequence is a relatively common complication, for example, after conditioning therapy prior to bone marrow transplantation (BMT) [5,8,9,10]. Liver damage whether associated with whole body irradiation or liver-directed radiotherapy have the same pathology, i.e. veno-occlusive disease (VOD) [5,11,12,13].

Medication designed to reduce RILI could improve the safety as well as enable more aggressive radiotherapy. Clinical studies have shown with varying strength of evidence that VOD/RILD after BMT can be ameliorated by pentoxifylline (PTX), ursodeoxycholic acid (UDCA) and low molecular weight heparin (LMWH) [14,15,16,17,18,19,20,21,22] (see Table 1). However, the equivocal nature of the results from most studies probably reflect the heterogeneous study populations (including patients who have received prior chemotherapy or had underlying liver disease) [23]. Thus, a more standardized clinical model is needed to evaluate the protective effects of prophylactic regimens against VOD/RILD.

Image-guided, single-fractioned, high-dose-rate BT of liver malignancies is associated with a well-characterized focal RILI (fRILI), which can be visualized and quantified using functional hepatobiliary magnetic resonance imaging (MRI) (see Figure 1) [6,7]. Importantly, the histopathological evidence of fRILI (i.e. sinusoidal congestion with hepatocyte atrophy and increased reticulin deposits) correlates well with the absence of the hepatocyte uptake of hepatolbiliary MRI contrast media [24]. We have previously found that development of areas of fRILI were maximal at 6–8 weeks post-BT which correlates to the peak incidence of RILD/REILD after conditioning therapy/radio-embolization throughout the first 2 months post-intervention [5,6,7,25]. We conducted a prospective study to quantify fRILI in patients who were randomized to BT with and without prophylactic PTX, UDCA and low-dose LMWH. To minimize the confounding effects of prior chemotherapy on radiation tolerability, only patients with liver metastases from colorectal cancer (mCRC) were included because these patients tend to have a more consistent pattern of prior exposition to chemotherapy. The cumulative effect of three drugs over a period of 8 weeks [26,27,28] was assessed and patients followed-up at 6 and 12 weeks.

Materials and Methods

The protocol for this trial and supporting CONSORT checklist are available as supporting information; see Checklist S1 and Protocol S1.

Study design

This was a prospective, randomised phase II, parallel-group, open-label study conducted at a single centre. The study was approved by the competent authorities (Federal Institute for Drugs and Medical Devices (in german: Bundesinstitut für Arzneimittel und Medizinprodukte - BfArM)) and the local ethics committee (Ethikkommission der Otto-von-Guericke-Universität der Medizinischen Fakultät). Trial registration: Eudra-CT: 2008-002985 70; ClinicalTrials.gov-identifier NCT01149304. Written informed consent was obtained from all patients prior to study entry. Group allocation approach was unrestricted randomization.

Patient characteristics

Consecutive patients (18–80 years) with liver metastases from mCRC, who were scheduled for local ablation with computed-tomography (CT)/MRI-guided BT between 2009 and 2012, were screened (Figure 2). (BT is the local standard ablative treatment in patients ineligible for surgical or all other appropriate intervention).

Women who were pregnant, lactating or of childbearing potential were excluded as were patients with liver cirrhosis, hepatitis B or C, severe coronary artery disease, autoimmune diseases, acute bacterial endocarditis, active major bleedings or high-risk of uncontrolled hemorrhage; severe or moderate renal impairment (GFR <60 mL/min), or known contraindication or hypersensitivity to any of the study treatments or procedures.

Treatment and follow-up

Patients received a single-fraction, CT- or MRI-guided BT of CRC liver metastases (see details below). In those randomized to prophylaxis, the following treatment was initiated during the evening of the day of BT: sc injection of 40 mg q.d. enoxaparin (Clexane, Sanofi Aventis, Paris, France) [20], oral 400 mg t.i.d. PTX (Trental, Sanofi Aventis) [16] and oral 250 mg t.i.d. UDCA (Ursofalk, Falk Pharma, Freiburg, Germany) [17,19]. Patients were discharged usually on the third day post-BT and continued to take study medication at home for 8 weeks. All patients were followed-up on day 3, week 6 and 12 with an optional follow-up at week 24. Within 24 hours of the procedure and at each subsequent visit, blood samples were taken for liver-specific and inflammatory/hemostatic laboratory parameters, and patients were assessed for ECOG-performance status and health-related quality-of-life (using the EQ5D-questionnaire). All adverse reactions related to the study medication or BT were recorded.

Compliance to the prophylactic regimen was evaluated during a dialogue at each visit and the evaluation of anti-Xa-activity at 6 weeks. Insufficient compliance was determined by: either anti-Xa-activity <0.1 IU/mL measured up to 4 hours after last enoxaparin injection, or two dose interruptions of the prophylactic regimen for more than 1 day/week. Non-compliant patients were withdrawn from the per-protocol analysis and study-specific medication stopped.

Image-guided interstitial brachytherapy

The technique of image-guided BT has been described previously [2]. Briefly, the placement of the introducer sheaths (6F Radiofocus, Terumo, Tokyo, Japan) with the BT applicators (Lumencath, Nucletron/Elekta, Veenendaal, The Netherlands) was performed using CT or MRI fluoroscopy. For treatment planning purposes, a spiral CT or T1-weighted MRI of the liver (reconstructed slice thickness: 3 mm) enhanced by intravenous application of iodine contrast media (CT) or Gd-EOB-DTPA (MRI) was acquired.

The high-dose-rate afterloading system (Microselectron, Nucletron/Elekta, Veenendaal, The Netherlands) employed an iridium-192 source with a nominal activity of 10Ci (i.e. 370GBq); decay correction was performed daily. Relative coordinates (x, y, z) of the catheters were determined in the CT/MRI-data set and transferred to the treatment planning system (Oncentra, Nucletron/Elekta). Using these coordinates, the clinical target volume and the predefined minimum dose (20 Gy, delivered as a single fraction [2]), the software calculated a dosimetry and the duration of the iridium-192 source inside the BT catheters. A planning CT with dosimetry is displayed in Figure 1B and F.

Table 1. Summary of published studies on drug treatments for the prevention of VOD/RILD.

Reference	Study design	N	Treatment regimen	Incidence of VOD	p-value*	Bilirubin (µmol/L)	p-value*
Attal et al. 1993 [14]	Prospective RCT	70	**Pentoxifylline** 1,600 mg/d day −8 to day+100 post-BMT	4%	NS	26.4 (mean max)	NS
		70	Control	3%		24.4 (mean max)	
Clift et al. 1993 [22]	Prospective RCT	44	**Pentoxifylline** 2,400 mg/d day −3 to day+70 post-allogeneic BMT	-		26.6 (mean max)	0.62
		44	Control	-		23.47 (mean max)	
Bianco et al. 1991 [16]	Phase 1–2	30	**Pentoxifylline** 1,200, 1,600, and 2,000 mg/d; day −10 to day+100 post-BMT	10%	0.001	-	-
		20	Control (retrospective)	65%		-	
Attal et al 1992 [15]	Prospective RCT	81	**Unfractionated heparin** 100 U/kg/d cont. infusion; day −8 to day+30 post-BMT	2.5%	0.01	7.4% exceeding 34	<0.05
		80	Control	14%		18.7% exceeding 34	
Forrest et al. 2003 (18)	Prospective single-arm	40	**LMWH:** dalteparin 2500 anti-Xa i.u; day −1 to day +30 post-BMT or hospital discharge	22.5%, 2.5% severe			
Or et al. 1996 [20]	Prospective RCT, pilot	61	**LMWH:** enoxaparin 40 mg/day; day+1 to day+40 post-BMT or hospital discharge		0.01	(duration of elevated levels)	0.01
		33	Control				
Essel et al. 1998 [17]	Prospective RCT	34	**UDCA** 600–1200 mg/d; day at least −1 to day +80 post-BMT	15%	0.03	102.6 (mean max)	0.13
		32	Control	40%		188.1 (mean max)	
Ohashi et al. 2000 [19]	Prospective RCT	67	**UDCA** 600 mg/d; day −21 to day+80 post-BMT	3%	0.004	Not reported in detail	NS
		65	Control	18.5%		Not reported in detail	

Table 1. Cont.

Reference	Study design	N	Treatment regimen	Incidence of VOD	p-value*	Bilirubin (μmol/L)	p-value*
Park et al. 2002 [28]	Prospective RCT	82	**UDCA** 600 mg/d + **unfractionated heparin** 5–50 U/kg/d adjusted aPTT of 50 s; day +1 to day +30 post-BMT or hospital discharge (but a minimum of 15d)	16%	0.348	148.8 (mean max)	0.725
		83	**Unfractionated heparin** 5–50 U/kg/d adjusted aPTT of 50 s; day +1 to day +30 post-BMT or hospital discharge (but a minimum of 15d)	19%		173.6 (mean max)	

*Group comparison; LMWH: Low molecular weight heparin; BMT: Bone marrow transplantation; Max: Maximum; NS: Not significant; VOD: Veno-occlusive disease; RCT: Randomized controlled trial; UDCA: ursodeoxycholic acid (ursodiol); aPTT: activated Partial Thromboplastin Time.

Magnetic resonance imaging

MRI (Achieva 1.5T, Philips, Best, The Netherlands) using the hepatobiliary contrast medium Gd-EOB-DTPA (Primovist, Bayer Healthcare, Leverkusen, Germany) was performed 1 day before and 6 and 12 weeks post-BT. MR-sequence of events was as follows: axial 3D T1-weighted (T1-w) gradient echo THRIVE (T1-High-Resolution-Isotropic-Volume-Excitation) (Time-to-Echo/Time-to-Repetition 4/10 ms, flip-angle 10°) with fat-suppression pre-contrast, at 20 s, 60 s and 120 s and 20 minutes after iv 0.1 mL/kg bodyweight Gd-EOB-DTPA. The slice thickness was 3 mm. For the study-specific MRI volumetry, dynamic THRIVE at 60 s (for the exclusion of tumor progression/local recurrence) and hepatobiliary phase THRIVE 20 min after application of Gd-EOB-DTPA (for the determination of area of fRILI) were mandatory.

Identification of the radiation isodose (minimal hepatic threshold dose) that demarcated the border between the fRILI and functioning liver tissue (as defined by non-uptake and uptake of Gd-EOB-DTPA enhanced MRI, respectively) was performed as follows in a blinded matter.

The hepatobiliary phase THRIVE was transferred to the BT-planning software. Image registration of the hepatobiliary phase THRIVE to the contrast-enhanced planning CT/MRI (including the dosimetry) was performed by an isoscalar local semi-automated point-based 3D-3D image registration using predefined match points (3 or 4 corresponding landmarks restricted to liver structures). Registration was only accepted if the target area merged perfectly by visual assessment. As a result of this procedure, the software simultaneously displayed the treatment dosimetry and anatomical structures/fRILI of the hepatobiliary phase THRIVE. The volume of the liver parenchyma with radiation-induced impaired uptake of Gd-EOB-DTPA (i.e. fRILI) was determined. The isodose of the dosimetry encircling this volume was determined at five different axial levels and the mean of these values recorded. This dose resembles the dose which was formerly applied at the now demarcated rim of the fRILI, corresponding to the assumed minimal hepatic tolerance dose. To ensure a negligible registration error, the volume of fRILI was inserted into the dose-volume-histogram of the dosimetry. The corresponding isodose was stored. Results of the two methods showed a high correlation of 0.899 and 0.562 (p<0.001 and p = 0.006) for 6 and 12 weeks, respectively. To minimize methodological errors, the mean isodose value of the two methods was taken. In case of more than one treated lesion, the mean of the determined isodoses was used. If no detectable fRILI was seen in follow-up, the minimal mean hepatic threshold dose was defined as the dose which was previously administered at the tumor margin (since an effect on the liver parenchyma above this dose level cannot be excluded). Figure 1 illustrates the development and appearance of the fRILI in hepatobiliary phase THRIVE.

Endpoints and statistical analyses

The aim of the study was to assess if a combination regimen of PTX, UDCA and low-dose LMWH for 8 weeks provided a preventive effect regarding irradiation damage to liver parenchyma (as resembled by the minimal mean threshold dose of the fRILI volume) at 6 weeks (primary endpoint) and at 12 weeks (secondary endpoint) after BT.

As additional descriptor, detectable fRILI in Gd-EOB-DTPA MRI (yes/no) was recorded at each follow-up. Further secondary objectives included the safety of the study treatment after BT including changes in bilirubin and albumin which were graded according to Common Terminology Criteria for Adverse Events version 3 (CTCAE3.0).

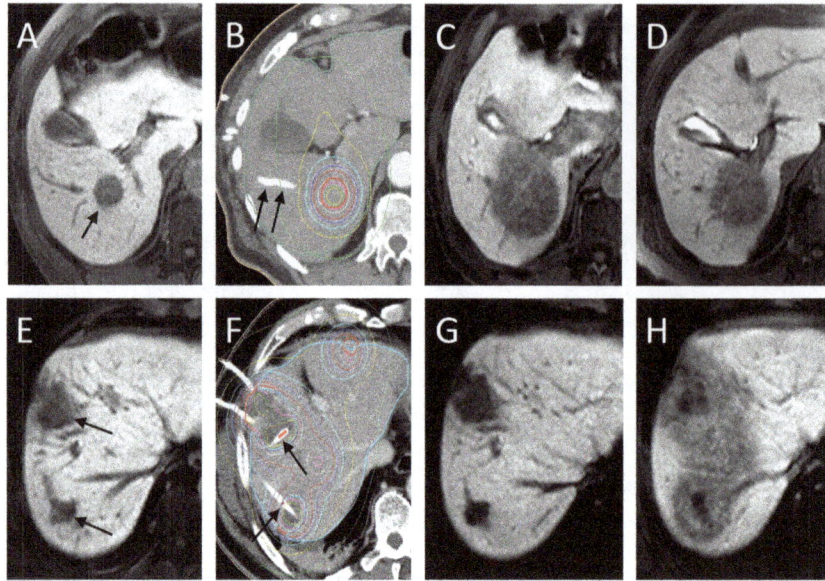

Figure 1. T1w-axial THRIVE 20 min after application of Gd-EOB-DTPA (A, C–E and G, H) and BT planning CT with dosimetry (B and F). A–D, control group. A: pre-treatment MRI displaying a metastasis scheduled for BT treatment (black arrow). B: Planning-CT after introduction of the brachytherapy catheters (black arrows). Clinical target volume (CTV) represented by bold red circle and dosimetry by coloured lines (red: 20 Gy-, blue: 12 Gy-isodose). C: MRI at 6 weeks showing substantial reduction in Gd-EOB-DTPA uptake by liver parenchyma adjacent to treated metastases (i.e. focal radiation-induced liver injury, fRILI). Note: The area of fRILI matches the geometry of the dosimetry (B). Determined threshold dose: 9.75 Gy. D: MRI at 3 months showing shrinkage of the fRILI. Determined threshold dose: 11.9 Gy. E–H, treatment group. E: pre-treatment MRI displaying two metastases (black arrow); two more treated lesions are not displayed in the plane. F: Planning-CT (annotations: see B). G: MRI at 6 weeks showing no fRILI. H: MRI at 3 months after radiotherapy (and 1 month after finishing study treatment) showing a substantial region of fRILI. Determined threshold dose: 15.8 Gy.

The relation between hepatocyte dysfunction and changes in the following liver-specific and inflammatory/hemostatic laboratory values were analysed: fibrinogen, factor-VIII-activity, interleukin-6, protein-C-activity, protein-S-activity, von-Willebrand-factor-activity and antithrombin-III-activity [29].

Determination of sample size was based on the expected minimum between-group difference of 2.1 Gy (SD 2.3 Gy) for minimal mean hepatic threshold dose at 6 weeks after BT (from 9.9 Gy to 12 Gy) [7]. A sequential test with 2 stages according to the Pocock-design was used which yielded a total of 22 observations per group with a scheduled interim analysis after 11 observations per group when a = 0.025 and power 1-b = 0.8. Interim-analysis showed a significant difference between the groups regarding the primary variable with a one-sided p-value of 0.011. A one-sided p of <0.0148 was necessary to terminate the study prematurely.

Statistical analysis was performed using SPSS (SPSS21, IBM, Chicago, Il, USA). Descriptive analysis of patient characteristics and laboratory findings was performed. The primary analysis was evaluated in the per protocol cohort and repeated in the intention-to-treat population as sensitivity analysis. Between-group differences in minimal mean hepatic threshold after BT at 6 and 12 weeks were compared using a two-sample t-tests, and evidence of detectable fRILI were compared using the Fisher's-exact-test. Possible confounding factors were evaluated using the Mann-Whitney-U-test for metric variables and the Fisher's-exact-test for categorical variables, and then between-group differences for the primary endpoint were evaluated with inclusion of the covariables (ANOVA and ANCOVA). The relationship between the minimal mean hepatic threshold dose and laboratory values was tested by Pearson's correlation and ANCOVA. Group comparison regarding ECOG and EQ5D was made by Mann-Whitney-U-test.

Median overall survival was estimated by Kaplan-Meier (group comparison by log-rank test). A p-value of <0.05 was statistically significant.

Results

Of 129 patients screened with liver metastases from colorectal cancer scheduled for BT, 30 patients were included in the study and 22 patients (11 per group) in the primary analyses of the per-protocol group (see CONSORT diagram, Figure 2). Demographic characteristics of randomized patients at screening are summarized in Table 2 and the baseline liver function and other laboratory parameters are presented in Table 3. Group comparison revealed a similar distribution of possible confounders. A tendency towards a larger volume of significantly radiation exposed liver parenchyma (>10 Gy) in the study treatment group (Table 2) may have potentially lowered the hepatic tolerance dose in this group instead of increase it [25].

The minimal mean hepatic threshold dose at 6 weeks after BT (primary endpoint) was significantly higher in the study treatment group than the control (19.1 Gy versus 14.6 Gy, p = 0.011, Table 4) with comparable results with the intention-to-treat analysis (Table 4). Correspondingly, fewer patients in the study treatment group than the control had evidence of fRILI at 6 weeks (45.5% versus 90.9%); this difference was also significant in the intention-to-treat analysis (Table 4). However at 12 weeks after BT (and 4 weeks after cessation of study treatment), these between-group differences were not observed (in neither the per-protocol nor intention-to-treat analyses) for the minimal mean hepatic threshold dose and the proportion of patients with fRILI (Table 4). Results from the optional follow-up at 24 weeks after BT continually showed no between-group differences for the minimal

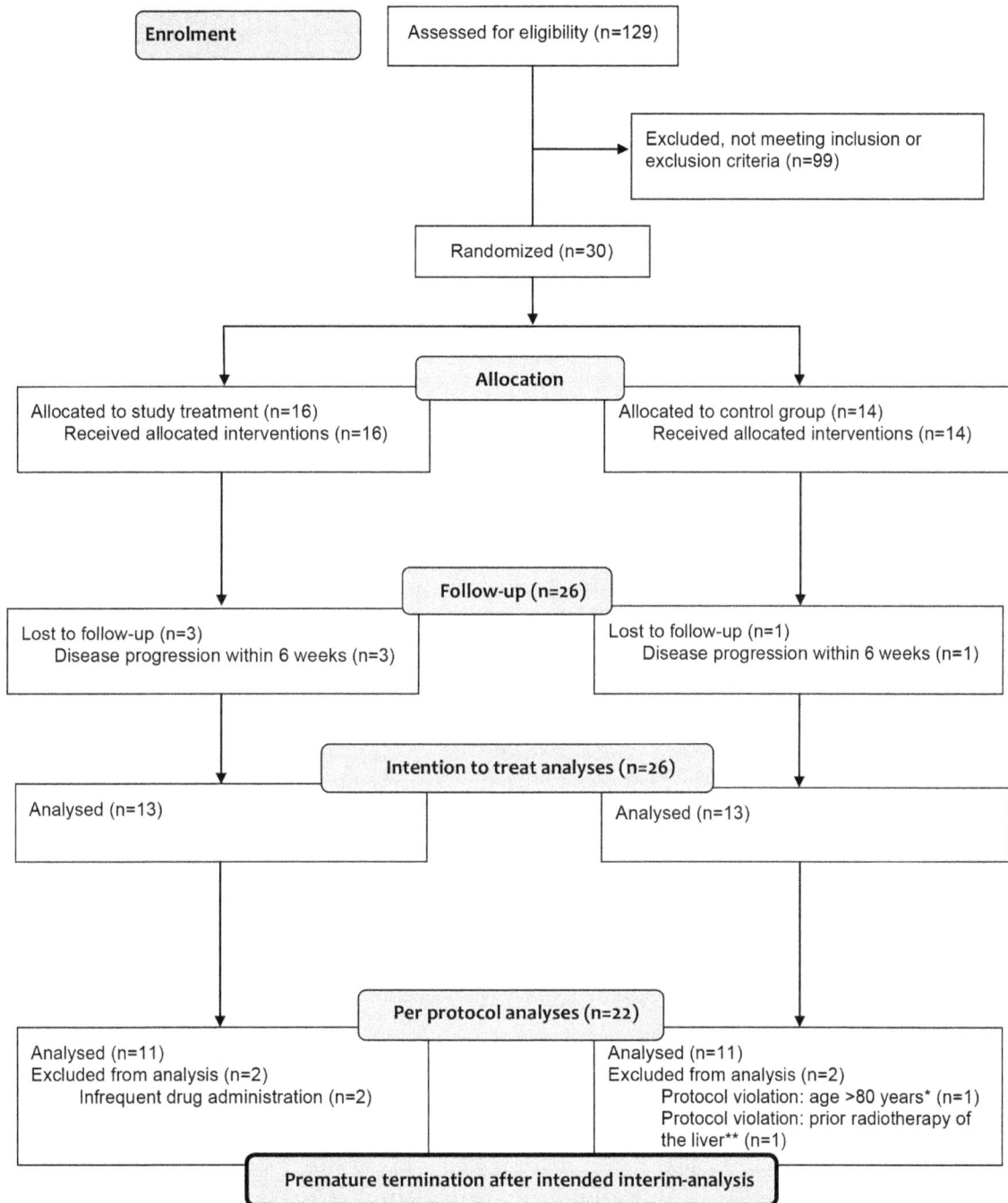

Figure 2. CONSORT-diagram. *Exclusion criterion age was initially disregarded by error in this patient (aged 82). **Exclusion criterion prior radiotherapy was initially disregarded by error in this patient (prior radiotherapy was performed 2 years earlier with location in the contralateral liver lobe).

mean hepatic threshold dose and the proportion of patients with fRILI (no change of the proportion of patients with fRILI as compared to 12 weeks follow-up; the minimal mean hepatic threshold dose for treatment group was 20.1 Gy (1 patient missing) and for the control group 21.0 Gy; p>0.05, per-protocol analysis (with comparable results with the intention-to-treat analysis)).

Covariate analyses also showed no influence of recorded covariables on the primary endpoint; only group allocation was significant (Table 5).

EQ5D (as a descriptor of quality of life) and distribution of ECOG performance status were not significantly different at baseline (Table 2) or at any follow-up visit (Table S1). Median overall survival from time of BT on was not different between the groups with 30.0 months (95%CI: 8.7–51.3) in the treatment group and 39.5 months (27.5–51.5) in the control group (p = 0.430).

Safety analyses were conducted in all 30 patients who received BT. The following mild-to-moderate adverse events CTCAEv3 grade 1–2 were reported (in the treatment/control groups) on day

Table 2. Patient characteristics (per protocol analysis).

Variable	Treatment group (n = 11)	Control (n = 11)	p-value (between group)*
Sex (m/f)	9/2	8/3	1.000
Age (years)	71.09±5.47	65.09±12.55	0.408
Weight (kg)	84.64±11.68	83.91±12.89	0.592
Height (cm)	174.09±6.79	172.64±6.90	0.834
ECOG at baseline (0/1/2)	6/4/1	4/5/2	0.370
EQ5D visual analogue score	72.36±14.56	76.36±13.02	0.446
History of liver surgery	45.5%	45.5%	1.000
Steatosis hepatis	36.4%	18.2%	0.635
Diabetes mellitus	18.2%	27.3%	1.000
Chemotherapy pretreatment			
Applied lines	1.00±0.63	1.00±0.45	1.000
no chemotherapy	18.2%	9.1%	NA
1 line	63.6%	81.8%	0.672
2 lines	18.2%	9.1%	NA
Prior chemotherapy			
Oxaliplatin	63.6%	63.6%	1.000
Irinotecan	36.4%	36.4%	1.000
Biologicals	54.5%	54.5%	1.000
Number of treated metastases	1.91±1.04	1.45±0.52	0.382
Maximum diameter of metastases (mm)	37.18±12.91	29.45±11.79	0.146
Clinical target volume (cm³)	42.82±29.26	31.36±37.14	0.156
Number of used brachytherapy catheters	3.18±1.78	2.27±1.74	0.079
Liver volume (cm³)	1296.1±226.6	1451.3±278.6	0.401
Interval between BT and 6 weeks FU (days)	43.91±4.76	45.09±4.68	0.757
Interval between BT and 3 months FU (days)	87.34±4.52	89.55±6.15	0.505
Liver volume with a dose exposure >10 Gy (%)	22.55±14.45	11.95±10.43	0.056
Chemotherapy during follow-up	18.2%	9.1%	1.000

Continuous data: mean ± standard deviation, frequencies: counts or percent.
*Group comparison, continuous data compared by Mann-Whitney U test, frequency data compared by Pearson's chi square test.

3 after BT: pain (1 patient/1 patient) and fatigue (0/1); at week 6: pain (2/0), fatigue (0/1), nausea (1/0) and diarrhea (2/0); nausea and diarrhea was probably related to PTX or UDCA. One grade 3 subacute bleeding episode from the bile duct, related to BT, occurred in the study treatment group which was successfully managed by endoscopic coagulation.

Analysis of the laboratory data revealed no grade 3/4 changes in bilirubin or albumin. One grade 1 reduction of albumin in the treatment group at 6 weeks was unchanged at week 12. One patient in control group with elevated (grade 1) bilirubin at baseline remained stable throughout follow-up. RILD was not observed on either group.

Laboratory analysis regarding liver-specific and inflammatory/hemostatic parameters found no relevant findings at baseline (Table 3). At week 6, slightly higher gamma-glutamyl-transferase levels and protein-S-activity were recorded in the control group compared with the treatment group. At 6 and 12 weeks, there was slight but significant mean decrease from baseline in cholinesterase in the treatment group. Additionally, mean fibrinogen and von-Willebrand-factor-activity increased significantly from baseline in the treatment group at 6 and 12 weeks; while significant increases

from baseline were recorded with mean fibrinogen, factor-VIII-activity and aspartate-transaminase in the control group at 6 weeks.

No correlation between the minimal mean hepatic threshold and liver-specific and inflammatory/hemostatic laboratory values was found at either week 6 or 12 (data not shown).

Discussion

In this prospective study, we were able to show a significant reduction in fRILI (as measured by hepatobiliary MRI) at 6 weeks after BT of colorectal liver metastases in patients who received low-dose LMWH, PTX and UDCA. Re-assessment of patients at 12 weeks (4 weeks after cessation of study treatment) found that the extent and incidence of fRILI was comparable to the control group, thereby supporting the reliability of our findings. This is further authenticated by the results of the (optional) 24 weeks follow-up. According to our results we believe that we were able to mitigate rather than delay the fRILI by the prophylactic regimen. The finding that the positive effect of the medication to the liver parenchyma as seen at the 6 weeks follow-up vanished after discontinuation of the medication (after 8 weeks) in the 3 months

Table 3. Laboratory parameters at baseline and follow-up (per protocol analysis).

Variable (normal range)		Treatment group (n = 11)	Control (n = 11)	p-value (between group)*	p-value (baseline vs. follow-up)**
Bilirubin	baseline	8.27±2.92	8.39±5.61	0.594	
(<21.0 µmol/L)	6 weeks	9.58±9.94	9.56±7.18	0.641	0.182 (0.350)
	12 weeks	8.71±4.27	8.75±5.95	0.735	0.594 (0.505)
Albumin	baseline	44.21±3.46	44.05±2.45	0.833	
(35.0–52.0 g/L)	6 weeks	42.49±5.16	42.67±3.17	0.743	0.197 (0.060)
	12 weeks	42.84±4.94	43.66±2.31	0.743	0.212 (0.332)
Cholinesterase	baseline	149.26±47.97	144.73±21.73	0.718	
(88–215 µmol/s.L)	6 weeks	136.27±51.65	143.82±29.10	0.433	**0.023** (0.929)
	12 weeks	132.94±49.22	153.36±30.96	0.088	**0.010** (0.423)
Aspartate transaminase	baseline	0.56±0.18	0.46±0.17	0.211	
(0.17–0.83 µmol/s.L)	6 weeks	0.59±0.17	0.55±0.23	0.533	0.373 (**0.016**)
	12 weeks	0.63±0.47	0.54±0.17	0.974	0.563 (0.056)
Alanine transaminase	baseline	0.44±0.20	0.51±0.36	1,000	
(0.17–0.83 µmol/s.L)	6 weeks	0.50±0.18	0.62±0.45	0.742	0.443 (0.109)
	12 weeks	0.53±0.43	0.52±0.27	0.718	0.508 (0.722)
Gamma glutamyltransferase	baseline	1.61±2.62	1.49±1.21	0.189	
(0.17–1.19 µmol/s.L)	6 weeks	0.82±0.83	2.21±1.71	**0.011**	0.100 (0.050)
	12 weeks	1.25±1.17	1.97±1.49	0.139	0.722 (0.306)
Glutamate dehydrogenase	baseline	104.36±91.47	108.82±94.84	0.844	
(<120 nmol/s.L)	6 weeks	67.55±31.43	123.27±105.88	0.490	0.328 (0.308)
	12 weeks	128.11±108.79	126.09±95.19	0.849	0.674 (0.374)
International normalized	baseline	93.9±3.03	95.55±2.98	0.053	
ratio (0.85–1.27)	6 weeks	94.11±2.71	94.8±2.44	0.399	0.438 (0.502)
	12 weeks	94.63±2.50	95.33±3.61	0.732	0.334 (0.498
Interleukin 6	baseline	4.54±3.31	3.71±3.09	0.245	
(<7.0 pg/mL)	6 weeks	8.44±8.53	7.62±4.41	0.809	0.266 (0.038)
	12 weeks	10.50±9.24	4.06±2.42	0.229	0.139 (0.515)
Fibrinogen	baseline	3.72±0.53	3.99±0.46	0.377	
(1.50–4.00 g/L)	6 weeks	4.50±1.17	4.77±0.84	0.365	**0.014 (0.017)**
	12 weeks	4.65±1.04	4.23±0.49	0.416	**0.037** (0.214)
Factor VIII activity	baseline	169.09±41.51	160.60±42.12	0.756	
(70–150%)	6 weeks	195.45±61.02	218.91±60.77	0.490	0.130 (0.093)
	12 weeks	199.7±67.26	257.09±150.23	0.360	0.169 (**0.017**)
Protein C activity	baseline	107.36±33.99	109.70±12.46	0.145	
(>70%)	6 weeks	108±32.68	106.55±18.67	0.767	0.799 (0.475)
	12 weeks	101.5±27.26	114±19.76	0.084	0.113 (0.540)
Protein S activity	baseline	85.36±12.26	86.80±12.55	0.848	
(>60%)	6 weeks	82.18±15.16	104.36±27.09	**0.036**	0.266 (0.086)
	12 weeks	87.3±14.54	91±10.6	0.549	0.799 (0.507)
von Willebrand factor	baseline	164.09±42.81	174.90±71.14	0.973	
activity (70–130%)	6 weeks	222.27±59.75	201.73±71.76	0.554	**0.013** (0.075)
	12 weeks	209.5±77.35	215.27±75.31	0.883	**0.013** (0.333)
Antithrombin III activity	baseline	92.73±13.72	98.90±11.50	0.191	
(>80%)	6 weeks	96.73±15.31	98.2±9.78	0.944	0.082 (0.779)
	12 weeks	96.4±12.08	96.73±9.51	0.751	0.407 (0.681)

*Between group comparison, Mann-Whitney U test;
**Comparison versus baseline (in brackets p-value of control group), Wilcoxon test.

Table 4. Minimal mean hepatic tolerance dose (Gy) and evidence of detectable focal radiation-induced liver injury (fRILI) after BT, group comparison.

Variable	Group			p-value (between groups)
Minimal mean hepatic tolerance dose (primary endpoint)		**Dose (Gy)**	**SD**	
At 6 weeks	Control	14.64 [14.15]	4.01 [3.93]	
	Treatment	19.06 [18.46]	3.35 [3.59]	**0.011 [0.007]**
At 12 weeks	Control	16.38 [16.10]	3.57 [3.60]	
	Treatment	19.04 [18.50]	2.88 [3.11]	0.069 [0.082]
Detectable fRILI		**Counts**	**Frequency**	
At 6 weeks	Control	10 [12]	90.9% [92.3%]	
	Treatment	5 [7]	45.5% [53.8%]	**0.022 [0.027]**
At 12 weeks	Control	10 [12]	90.9% [92.3%]	
	Treatment	10 [12]	90.9% [92.3%]	1.000 [1.000]

Per protocol analysis (n = 22); Intention-to-treat analysis (n = 26) in square brackets.

follow-up, make us believe that the fRILI was in fact mitigated in that period. Further on, the extent of the fRILI at 6 weeks in the treatment group and at 3 months (and 6 months) in both groups was less in size compared to the fRILI in the control group at 6 weeks (the peak of the fRILI in our study). Thus, the maximum extent of the fRILI at 6 weeks was skipped in the treatment group as compared to the control group. However, the radiation damage could not be suppressed completely by the prophylactic regimen with a rebound after cessation of the treatment to the level of the control group in later follow-ups. Thus, it is possibly right to assume additionally a delay on the development of the fRILI by the prophylactic regimen. This delay is considered to be advantageous as well since a rapid formation of the fRILI can be delayed (and mitigated) allowing the liver remnant to compensate for the fRILI. However, although appropriately powered, the study should be understood as a pilot due to the small sample size. To compensate for the rebound of the fRILI after cessation of the prophylactic regimen and for a better understanding of the dynamics of the fRILI, a study concept with a prolonged course for the prophylactic regimen is planned.

RILI remains a challenge in the treatment of liver malignancies by radiotherapy (whether percutaneous, interstitial or by radio-embolization) because it may eventually translate into RILD or REILD. Further on, life-threatening VOD associated with combined-modality induced liver disease occurs in 5–60% of patients undergoing BMT [18,23,26]. For this reason, the potentially protective effects of a number of treatments including low-dose LMWH, PTX and UDCA have been evaluated. Although the efficacy appears equivocal in some studies [14,15,16,17,18,19,20,21,28] (Table 1), we determined that the combination of low-dose LMWH, PTX and UDCA appeared to be the most promising option for further evaluation with BT. We believe that our success in showing a benefit in ameliorating fRILI with this combination is based on the following factors: a highly homogeneous patient cohort; attention to patient compliance to the prophylactic regimen; and direct measurement of damage to the liver parenchyma rather than clinical endpoints.

The treatment course of 8 weeks for the medication was determined on the assumption that occurrence of RILD and fRILI

peaks around 2 months after radiation-exposure [5,6,7,25]. However, our findings suggest that the radiation-induced injury to the liver structures and cell endothelial continues beyond 8 weeks and that discontinuation of the medication at this time allows the development of a veno-occlusive state/liver cell dysfunction. Endothelial cell damage, which triggers local thrombotic mechanisms, leading to microvascular flow insufficiency, production of cytotoxic substances, and ultimately hepatocellular necrosis, has been thought to be an early event in the development of RILD/VOD [5,10,11,30,31]. The current evidence indicates that PTX, low-dose LMWH and UDCA may act through a variety of mechanisms to alleviate these effects. PTX, for example, down regulates tumor-necrosis factor-α (TNF-α), a prime suspect in either the initiation or amplification of tissue injury following radiation. PTX also stimulates vascular endothelial production of non-inflammatory prostaglandins of the E- and I-series, enhancing loco-regional blood flow and promoting thrombolysis [16].

LMWHs are assumed to prevent subsequent thrombosis of hepatic venules after endothelial damage and therefore decrease the risk of VOD/RILD [18].

By oral administration of UDCA the concentration of potentially liver toxic hydrophobic bile acids can be reduced [32]. Several *in vitro* studies suggest that potential attenuating effects of UDCA on the pathogenesis of VOD is achieved through the down-regulation of inflammatory cytokine such as TNF-α and interleukin-1 [33]. These cytokines not only induce and amplify liver damage but are also associated with apoptosis in endothelial cells [34] and the development of VOD. UDCA also appears to have a direct effect on programmed-cell death, inhibiting apoptosis and protecting against the membrane damaging effects associated with hydrophobic bile acids in both hepatocytes and non-liver cells [35].

The rationale for this combined treatment approach is based on the assumption that LMWH, PTX and UDCA, which act through a variety of different mechanisms, may act synergistically or in a complimentary fashion to protect the liver [26,27,28]; although further study is needed to fully evaluate this hypothesis. However, based on the low toxicity profile of these medications, we believe

Table 5. Covariate analysis of minimal mean hepatic tolerance dose 6 weeks after BT (per protocol, n = 22).

Covariate*	p-value (group influence)	p-value (co-variate influence)
Sex (m/f)	0.015	0.458
Age (y)	0.016	0.864
Weight (kg)	0.010	0.117
Height (cm)	0.011	0.485
ECOG at baseline (0 and 1 vs 2)	0.008	0.310
EQ5D visual analogue score	0.015	0.868
History of liver surgery	0.007	0.064
Steatosis hepatis	0.014	0.845
Diabetes mellitus	0.015	0.627
Chemotherapy pre treatment	0.012	0.373
Used chemotherapeutic agents		
Oxaliplatin	0.013	0.991
Irinotecan	0.011	0.327
Biologicals	0.012	0.459
Number of treated metastases	0.013	0.681
Maximum diamter of metastases (mm)	0.023	0.669
Clinical target volume (cm^3)	0.013	0.815
Liver volume (cm^3)	0.018	0.937
Interval from BT to 6 weeks FU (days)	0.008	0.258
Liver volume with a dose exposure >10 Gy (%)	0.013	0.598
Chemotherapy during follow-up	0.015	0.191
Bilirubin baseline	0.030	0.401
Albumin baseline	0.020	0.784
Aspartate transaminase baseline	0.025	0.263
Alanine transaminase baseline	0.006	0.092
Cholinesterase baseline	0.013	0.425
Gamma glutamyltransferase baseline	0.012	0.317
Glutamate dehydrogenase baseline	0.011	0.352
International normalized ratio baseline	0.008	0.783
Interleukin 6 baseline	0.030	0.401
Fibrinogen baseline	0.002	0.232
Factor VIII activity baseline	0.005	0.615
Protein C activity baseline	0.004	0.868
Protein S activity baseline	0.004	0.831
von Willebrand factor activity baseline	0.004	0.763
Antithrombin III activity baseline	0.008	0.261

*Two-way ANOVA for categorical factors, ANCOVA for metric covariables.

that this initial approach can be justified. Although the patient numbers are small, the absence of severe toxicities accords with experience of other published data [15,16,17,19,20,21,28].

Regarding changes of laboratory values, no clinically relevant (grade 3/4) toxicities were observed. The observed slight increases (varying over time and group) of fibrinogen, factor-VIII-activity, protein-S-activity and von-Willebrand-factor-activity correspond most likely to an unspecific increase in acute-phase proteins after radiotherapy or/and to a consequence of radiation-induced endothelial damage of the hepatic veins and sinuses with subsequent platelet aggregation. Regarding the course of liver specific laboratory paramters after BT, it might be argued that the

induced fRILI was possibly too small to induce a significant overall increase of these parameters. However, the slight but significant increase of aspartate transaminase in the control group indicates a parenchymal damage. Interestingly, this increase was not seen in the treatment group, indicating a decreased parenchymal damage under preventive medication.

The primary endpoint in our analysis is based on a surrogate i.e. fRILI visualized and quantified using hepatobiliary contrast agent (Gd-EOB-DTPA)-enhanced MRI. Hepatobiliary contrast agents differ from other gadolinium chelates in that they are selectively taken up by functioning hepatocytes through an organic-anion-transporter-polypeptide (mainly OATP1B1 and 3) and excreted into the bile by the multidrug-resistance-protein-2. For Gd-EOB-DTPA, the biliary excretion rate is approximately 50% in humans [36,37]. Regardless of the mechanism of damage to liver, the hepatobiliary contrast media in functionally altered liver parenchyma is significantly reduced [38]. This is also true for fRILI since a loss of uptake of hepatobiliary contrast media is clearly evident in the liver parenchyma adjacent to the clinical target volume after local radiotherapy (Figure 2) [6,7]. Importantly, an agreement has been found between the histopathological evidence of fRILI/VOD and loss of hepatocellular uptake of hepatobiliary contrast agent [24].

Unlike the reduced uptake of hepatobiliary contrast agents in sinusoidal-obstruction-syndrome observed after platinum-containing chemotherapy (which is reticular in geometry and generalized all over the liver) [39], the reduced uptake of hepatobiliary contrast media after BT is focal, homogenous and circumferential around the clinical target volume (Figure 1) [6,7]. Thus, we believe that we can exclude underlying sinusoidal-obstruction-syndrome as a confounder of our results. Additionally, the history of platinum-containing chemotherapy was equal between the groups and without influence on the endpoint.

We suggest that our study results can be transferred to other established radiation treatment methods of liver malignancies such as ^{90}Y-radioembolization. According to conversion calculations, the dose ranges in the liver parenchyma associated with ^{90}Y-radioembolization and BT are comparable, if re-calculated with respect to the standard fractionation. We therefore hypothesize that preventive treatment approaches against RILD/REILD should be equally effective for both ^{90}Y-radioembolization and BT.

Conclusions

In summary, our results show a highly significant reduction in fRILI after BT of colorectal liver metastases in patients who received low-dose LMWH, PTX and UDCA. Further on, we believe that these findings can be adopted for the prevention of radiation-induced liver damage after other radiotherapeutic approaches as ^{90}Y-radioembolization and that further clinical studies in this area are warranted.

Supporting Information

Table S1 ECOG, EQ5D dimensions and EQ5D VAS, baseline and follow-up; group comparison (per-protocol only).

Checklist S1 Consort Checklist regarding the present study.

Protocol S1 Study protocol as submitted to the competent authorities.

Author Contributions

Contributed to the writing of the manuscript: MS PW JR. Statistical planning and analysis: SK RD MS. Conceived and designed the experiments: MS RS RD BS JR. Performed the experiments: MS RS RD PH GG JR. Analyzed the data: MS RD KM MP RS SK. Contributed reagents/materials/analysis tools: PH GG SK.

References

1. Boda-Heggemann J, Dinter D, Weiss C, Frauenfeld A, Siebenlist K, et al. (2012) Hypofractionated image-guided breath-hold SABR (stereotactic ablative body radiotherapy) of liver metastases–clinical results. Radiation oncology 7: 92.
2. Ricke J, Mohnike K, Pech M, Seidensticker M, Ruhl R, et al. (2010) Local response and impact on survival after local ablation of liver metastases from colorectal carcinoma by computed tomography-guided high-dose-rate brachytherapy. International journal of radiation oncology, biology, physics 78: 479–485.
3. Seidensticker R, Denecke T, Kraus P, Seidensticker M, Mohnike K, et al. (2012) Matched-pair comparison of radioembolization plus best supportive care versus best supportive care alone for chemotherapy refractory liver-dominant colorectal metastases. Cardiovascular and interventional radiology 35: 1066–1073.
4. Emami B, Lyman J, Brown A, Coia L, Goitein M, et al. (1991) Tolerance of normal tissue to therapeutic irradiation. International journal of radiation oncology, biology, physics 21: 109–122.
5. Lawrence TS, Robertson JM, Anscher MS, Jirtle RL, Ensminger WD, et al. (1995) Hepatic toxicity resulting from cancer treatment. International journal of radiation oncology, biology, physics 31: 1237–1248.
6. Ricke J, Seidensticker M, Ludemann L, Pech M, Wieners G, et al. (2005) In vivo assessment of the tolerance dose of small liver volumes after single-fraction HDR irradiation. International journal of radiation oncology, biology, physics 62: 776–784.
7. Seidensticker M, Seidensticker R, Mohnike K, Wybranski C, Kalinski T, et al. (2011) Quantitative in vivo assessment of radiation injury of the liver using Gd-EOB-DTPA enhanced MRI: tolerance dose of small liver volumes. Radiation oncology 6: 40.
8. McDonald GB, Sharma P, Matthews DE, Shulman HM, Thomas ED (1985) The clinical course of 53 patients with venocclusive disease of the liver after marrow transplantation. Transplantation 39: 603–608.
9. Sangro B, Gil-Alzugaray B, Rodriguez J, Sola I, Martinez-Cuesta A, et al. (2008) Liver disease induced by radioembolization of liver tumors: description and possible risk factors. Cancer 112: 1538–1546.
10. Farthing MJ, Clark ML, Sloane JP, Powles RL, McElwain TJ (1982) Liver disease after bone marrow transplantation. Gut 23: 465–474.
11. Fajardo LF, Colby TV (1980) Pathogenesis of veno-occlusive liver disease after radiation. Archives of pathology & laboratory medicine 104: 584–588.
12. Reed GB, Jr., Cox AJ, Jr (1966) The human liver after radiation injury. A form of veno-occlusive disease. The American journal of pathology 48: 597–611.
13. Shulman HM, Gown AM, Nugent DJ (1987) Hepatic veno-occlusive disease after bone marrow transplantation. Immunohistochemical identification of the material within occluded central venules. The American journal of pathology 127: 549–558.
14. Attal M, Huguet F, Rubie H, Charlet JP, Schlaifer D, et al. (1993) Prevention of regimen-related toxicities after bone marrow transplantation by pentoxifylline: a prospective, randomized trial. Blood 82: 732–736.
15. Attal M, Huguet F, Rubie H, Huynh A, Charlet JP, et al. (1992) Prevention of hepatic veno-occlusive disease after bone marrow transplantation by continuous infusion of low-dose heparin: a prospective, randomized trial. Blood 79: 2834–2840.
16. Bianco JA, Appelbaum FR, Nemunaitis J, Almgren J, Andrews F, et al. (1991) Phase I-II trial of pentoxifylline for the prevention of transplant-related toxicities following bone marrow transplantation. Blood 78: 1205–1211.
17. Essell JH, Schroeder MT, Harman GS, Halvorson R, Lew V, et al. (1998) Ursodiol prophylaxis against hepatic complications of allogeneic bone marrow transplantation. A randomized, double-blind, placebo-controlled trial. Annals of internal medicine 128: 975–981.
18. Forrest DL, Thompson K, Dorcas VG, Couban SH, Pierce R (2003) Low molecular weight heparin for the prevention of hepatic veno-occlusive disease (VOD) after hematopoietic stem cell transplantation: a prospective phase II study. Bone marrow transplantation 31: 1143–1149.
19. Ohashi K, Tanabe J, Watanabe R, Tanaka T, Sakamaki H, et al. (2000) The Japanese multicenter open randomized trial of ursodeoxycholic acid prophylaxis for hepatic veno-occlusive disease after stem cell transplantation. American journal of hematology 64: 32–38.
20. Or R, Nagler A, Shpilberg O, Elad S, Naparstek E, et al. (1996) Low molecular weight heparin for the prevention of veno-occlusive disease of the liver in bone marrow transplantation patients. Transplantation 61: 1067–1071.
21. Ruutu T, Eriksson B, Remes K, Juvonen E, Volin L, et al. (2002) Ursodeoxycholic acid for the prevention of hepatic complications in allogeneic stem cell transplantation. Blood 100: 1977–1983.
22. Clift RA, Bianco JA, Appelbaum FR, Buckner CD, Singer JW, et al. (1993) A randomized controlled trial of pentoxifylline for the prevention of regimen-related toxicities in patients undergoing allogeneic marrow transplantation. Blood 82: 2025–2030.
23. McDonald GB, Sharma P, Matthews DE, Shulman HM, Thomas ED (1984) Venocclusive disease of the liver after bone marrow transplantation: diagnosis, incidence, and predisposing factors. Hepatology 4: 116–122.
24. Seidensticker M, Burak M, Kalinski T, Garlipp B, Koelble K, et al. (2014) Radiation-Induced Liver Damage: Correlation of Histopathology with Hepatobiliary Magnetic Resonance Imaging, a Feasibility Study. Cardiovascular and interventional radiology.

25. Wybranski C, Seidensticker M, Mohnike K, Kropf S, Wust P, et al. (2009) In vivo assessment of dose volume and dose gradient effects on the tolerance dose of small liver volumes after single-fraction high-dose-rate 192Ir irradiation. Radiation research 172: 598–606.

26. Shulman HM, Hinterberger W (1992) Hepatic veno-occlusive disease–liver toxicity syndrome after bone marrow transplantation. Bone marrow transplantation 10: 197–214.

27. Lakshminarayanan S, Sahdev I, Goyal M, Vlachos A, Atlas M, et al. (2010) Low incidence of hepatic veno-occlusive disease in pediatric patients undergoing hematopoietic stem cell transplantation attributed to a combination of intravenous heparin, oral glutamine, and ursodiol at a single transplant institution. Pediatric transplantation 14: 618–621.

28. Park SH, Lee MH, Lee H, Kim HS, Kim K, et al. (2002) A randomized trial of heparin plus ursodiol vs. heparin alone to prevent hepatic veno-occlusive disease after hematopoietic stem cell transplantation. Bone marrow transplantation 29: 137–143.

29. Lee JH, Lee KH, Kim S, Lee JS, Kim WK, et al. (1998) Relevance of proteins C and S, antithrombin III, von Willebrand factor, and factor VIII for the development of hepatic veno-occlusive disease in patients undergoing allogeneic bone marrow transplantation: a prospective study. Bone marrow transplantation 22: 883–888.

30. Catani L, Gugliotta L, Vianelli N, Nocentini F, Baravelli S, et al. (1996) Endothelium and bone marrow transplantation. Bone marrow transplantation 17: 277–280.

31. Geraci JP, Mariano MS (1993) Radiation hepatology of the rat: parenchymal and nonparenchymal cell injury. Radiation research 136: 205–213.

32. Kowdley KV (2000) Ursodeoxycholic acid therapy in hepatobiliary disease. The American journal of medicine 108: 481–486.

33. Neuman MG, Shear NH, Bellentani S, Tiribelli C (1998) Role of cytokines in ethanol-induced cytotoxicity in vitro in Hep G2 cells. Gastroenterology 115: 157–166.

34. Lindner H, Holler E, Ertl B, Multhoff G, Schreglmann M, et al. (1997) Peripheral blood mononuclear cells induce programmed cell death in human endothelial cells and may prevent repair: role of cytokines. Blood 89: 1931–1938.

35. Rodrigues CM, Fan G, Ma X, Kren BT, Steer CJ (1998) A novel role for ursodeoxycholic acid in inhibiting apoptosis by modulating mitochondrial membrane perturbation. The Journal of clinical investigation 101: 2790–2799.

36. Pascolo L, Cupelli F, Anelli PL, Lorusso V, Visigalli M, et al. (1999) Molecular mechanisms for the hepatic uptake of magnetic resonance imaging contrast agents. Biochemical and biophysical research communications 257: 746–752.

37. Schuhmann-Giampieri G, Schmitt-Willich H, Press WR, Negishi C, Weinmann HJ, et al. (1992) Preclinical evaluation of Gd-EOB-DTPA as a contrast agent in MR imaging of the hepatobiliary system. Radiology 183: 59–64.

38. Watanabe H, Kanematsu M, Goshima S, Kondo H, Onozuka M, et al. (2011) Staging hepatic fibrosis: comparison of gadoxetate disodium-enhanced and diffusion-weighted MR imaging–preliminary observations. Radiology 259: 142–150.

39. Shin NY, Kim MJ, Lim JS, Park MS, Chung YE, et al. (2012) Accuracy of gadoxetic acid-enhanced magnetic resonance imaging for the diagnosis of sinusoidal obstruction syndrome in patients with chemotherapy-treated colorectal liver metastases. European radiology 22: 864–871.

6

Grey and White Matter Correlates of Recent and Remote Autobiographical Memory Retrieval – Insights from the Dementias

Muireann Irish[1,2,4]*, **Michael Hornberger**[2,3,7], **Shadi El Wahsh**[2,3,4], **Bonnie Y. K. Lam**[2,3], **Suncica Lah**[4,5], **Laurie Miller**[4,6], **Sharpley Hsieh**[2,3,4], **John R. Hodges**[2,3,4], **Olivier Piguet**[2,3,4]

1 School of Psychology, the University of New South Wales, Sydney, Australia, **2** Neuroscience Research Australia, Randwick, Sydney, Australia, **3** School of Medical Sciences, the University of New South Wales, Sydney, Australia, **4** Australian Research Council Centre of Excellence in Cognition and its Disorders, Sydney, Australia, **5** School of Psychology, the University of Sydney, Sydney, Australia, **6** Neuropsychology Unit, Royal Prince Alfred Hospital, and Central Clinical School, University of Sydney, Sydney, Australia, **7** Department of Clinical Neuroscience, University of Cambridge, Cambridge, United Kingdom

Abstract

The capacity to remember self-referential past events relies on the integrity of a distributed neural network. Controversy exists, however, regarding the involvement of specific brain structures for the retrieval of recently experienced versus more distant events. Here, we explored how characteristic patterns of atrophy in neurodegenerative disorders differentially disrupt remote versus recent autobiographical memory. Eleven behavioural-variant frontotemporal dementia, 10 semantic dementia, 15 Alzheimer's disease patients and 14 healthy older Controls completed the Autobiographical Interview. All patient groups displayed significant remote memory impairments relative to Controls. Similarly, recent period retrieval was significantly compromised in behavioural-variant frontotemporal dementia and Alzheimer's disease, yet semantic dementia patients scored in line with Controls. Voxel-based morphometry and diffusion tensor imaging analyses, for all participants combined, were conducted to investigate grey and white matter correlates of remote and recent autobiographical memory retrieval. Neural correlates common to both recent and remote time periods were identified, including the hippocampus, medial prefrontal, and frontopolar cortices, and the forceps minor and left hippocampal portion of the cingulum bundle. Regions exclusively implicated in each time period were also identified. The integrity of the anterior temporal cortices was related to the retrieval of remote memories, whereas the posterior cingulate cortex emerged as a structure significantly associated with recent autobiographical memory retrieval. This study represents the first investigation of the grey and white matter correlates of remote and recent autobiographical memory retrieval in neurodegenerative disorders. Our findings demonstrate the importance of core brain structures, including the medial prefrontal cortex and hippocampus, irrespective of time period, and point towards the contribution of discrete regions in mediating successful retrieval of distant versus recently experienced events.

Editor: Ramon Trullas, IIBB/CSIC/IDIBAPS, Spain

Funding: This work was supported by a National Health and Medical Research Council (NHMRC) of Australia Project Grant [510106], the Australian Research Council (ARC) Centre of Excellence in Cognition and its Disorders [CE110001021], and an ARC Discovery Project [DP10933279]. MI is supported by an ARC Discovery Early Career Research Award [DE130100463]. SL is, in part, supported by the University of Sydney Thompson Fellowship. OP is supported by an NHMRC Career Development Fellowship [1022684]. The funders had no role in study design, data collection and analysis, decision to publish, or preparation of the manuscript.

Competing Interests: The authors have declared that no competing interests exist.

* Email: m.irish@neura.edu.au

Introduction

The ability to reminisce on events from the past represents a unique expression of the episodic memory system, and one that is essential for a sense of identity and continuity across subjective time [1]. Autobiographical memory (ABM) refers to the complex ability to retrieve personally experienced events from the past imbued with a sense of recollection and situated within a coherent spatiotemporal context [2,3]. The recollection of ABMs relies upon the episodic memory system, permitting us to retrieve events from the past that are bound within a unique time and place, for example "My first holiday abroad with my family." While self-referential in nature, ABMs also contain general conceptual knowledge or semantic memory, derived from the abstraction of content from experiences, for example "Paris is the capital of France." ABMs therefore necessarily contain episodic and semantic elements [4,5], as well as rich contextual sensory perceptual details and emotional salience, which facilitate the mental reliving of the original event [6–8].

Given the multifaceted nature of these memories, it is not surprising that a widespread neural network is implicated in the retrieval of autobiographical episodes from the past [9]. Functional neuroimaging studies in healthy individuals converge to reveal a distributed network of regions subtending successful ABM retrieval. Importantly, this core network includes medial temporal lobe (MTL) structures such as the hippocampus and surrounding parahippocampal cortices, lateral temporal lobe cortices, posterior parietal regions including the posterior cingulate cortex and precuneus, as well as frontal regions such as the medial prefrontal cortex (PFC) [9–11]. Crucially, these studies confirm that co-activation of multiple brain regions must occur to support successful ABM retrieval.

One outstanding issue in the literature concerns the extent to which specific brain regions within the ABM core network are differentially recruited during the retrieval of recent versus distant memories. This issue is of central relevance for elucidating how memories are consolidated over time. The standard consolidation theory [12] holds that the hippocampus plays a time-limited role in the storage and retrieval of ABMs, with memories becoming increasingly independent from the MTL and relying on neocortical areas following consolidation. In contrast, the multiple trace theory [13,14] proposes that the hippocampus plays a permanent role in the retrieval of detailed and vivid episodic memories irrespective of remoteness of the memory. The evidence to date largely favours the multiple trace theory, with most neuroimaging studies demonstrating hippocampal activation during ABM retrieval from both recent and remote time periods [15–20].

While the hippocampus has tended to be the focus of most ABM neuroimaging studies, other brain regions within the ABM core network are likely to be sensitive to the age of the memories recalled [11]. For example, midline posterior regions, including the retrosplenial and posterior cingulate cortex, have consistently been shown to exhibit greater activation for retrieval of recent compared with remote ABMs [8,15,19,21]. Several factors have been proposed to account for this preferential recruitment during recent recall, including the retrieval of self-referential information, generation of visual imagery, as well as increased emotional processing and recollection for more recent events [11]. Similarly, frontal cortical regions, including the medial PFC, have been found to preferentially activate with increasing recency of ABMs [10,22] although this finding has not been consistently replicated [16,21]. Finally, it has been suggested that, over time, a process of semanticisation occurs whereby episodic ABMs are transformed into less detailed, schematic memories more akin to semantic representations [23]. By this view, recent memories are more likely to encompass sensory-perceptual elements [24], whereas remote ABMs represent an abstracted or semanticised gist of the formerly evocative event [25]. Accordingly, these remote ABM schematic accounts are posited to draw heavily upon regions specialised for semantic processing in the brain [4]. Differential involvement of the lateral temporal cortices for remote memories, however, has not been consistently reported [3,9,19]. Thus, while functional neuroimaging studies have clarified the overall neuroanatomy of the core network required to support ABM retrieval, it remains unclear which components of this network are differentially involved in recent versus remote retrieval.

One approach to identify the key structures required for recent versus remote memory retrieval, is to study the disruption of ABM in neurodegenerative disorders [26]. It is well established that ABM is severely compromised in Alzheimer's disease (AD) with temporal gradients typically observed whereby remote memories are recalled in significantly better detail compared with more recent time periods [7,27,28] although flat profiles have also been reported [29,30]. Studies incorporating neuroimaging analyses have pointed to the pivotal role of hippocampal and surrounding medial temporal lobe degeneration in the origin of ABM dysfunction in AD [31–33]. In contrast, the syndrome of semantic

dementia (SD) is associated with the converse profile of ABM retrieval, whereby retrieval of recent events is typically disproportionally better compared with distant epochs [28,29,34] although flat profiles have also been noted [35,36]. The loss of remote memories in SD has been ascribed to the progressive deterioration of the lateral temporal cortices, disrupting semantic information that comprises, or is required to access, the memory trace [4,37]. Finally, in the behavioural variant of frontotemporal dementia (bvFTD), the majority of studies have revealed a flat profile, indicating global deficits in ABM irrespective of time period [28,29,38]. These impairments are attributable predominantly to medial prefrontal and lateral temporal dysfunction [39], with recent evidence pointing towards significant medial temporal lobe involvement in the genesis of episodic memory impairments in bvFTD [40].

The objective of the present study was to explicate the neural substrates of recent and remote ABM retrieval on the Autobiographical Interview (AI) [41] using the disease syndromes of AD, SD, and bvFTD as lesion models for this process. By incorporating structural neuroimaging analyses, we sought to clarify how changes in grey matter density, assessed using voxel-based morphometry, and alterations in white matter connectivity, as indicated by fractional anisotropy values extracted from diffusion tensor imaging, differentially associate with the retrieval of recent versus remote ABM retrieval. Based on previous studies, we predicted frontal and medial temporal lobe involvement irrespective of epoch. Integrity of the lateral temporal cortices was predicted to be strongly associated with remote ABM retrieval, suggestive of a crucial role for semantic processing in the retrieval of old memories. In contrast, we expected that integrity of midline posterior parietal structures, important for self-referential processing and visual imagery, would correlate with the retrieval of recent events.

Methods

Participants

Thirty-six dementia patients (bvFTD = 11; SD = 10; AD = 15) and 14 education-matched healthy controls were recruited through FRONTIER at Neuroscience Research Australia, Sydney. All dementia patients met the relevant clinical diagnostic criteria for bvFTD [42], SD (also known as semantic variant Primary Progressive Aphasia) [43] or AD [44]. Clinical diagnoses were established by multidisciplinary consensus among a senior neurologist, clinical neuropsychologist, and occupational therapist based on extensive clinical investigations, cognitive assessment, report of activities of daily living, and structural neuroimaging. Briefly, bvFTD patients presented with decline in behaviour and interpersonal functioning accompanied by loss of insight, increased apathy, and emotional blunting. To exclude potential phenocopy cases in the bvFTD group [45], only those cases showing evidence of progression over time, as reported by their caregivers, and with atrophy on structural MRI scans, were included. SD patients exhibited progressive loss of word meaning with significant naming and comprehension impairments, as well as prosopagnosia and/or associative agnosia, with relatively intact everyday memory. Finally, AD patients displayed significant episodic memory loss, in the context of preserved personality and behaviour.

Healthy controls were recruited from the FRONTIER research volunteer panel and local community clubs. All controls scored 0 on the Clinical Dementia Rating scale (CDR) [46], and 88 or above on the Addenbrooke's Cognitive Examination-Revised (ACE-R) [47].

Exclusion criteria for all participants included prior history of mental illness, significant head injury, movement disorders, cerebrovascular disease, alcohol and other drug abuse, and limited English proficiency.

Ethics Statement

This study was conducted in accordance with the Declaration of Helsinki. Ethical approval was obtained from the Human Research Ethics Committee of the South Eastern Sydney and Illawarra Area Health Service (HREC 10/126) and the University of New South Wales Human Research Ethics Advisory panel D (Biomedical, ref. # 10035). All participants, or their person responsible, provided written informed consent. Capacity to provide informed consent was established by asking participants to signify that they understood the purpose of the research visit by explaining the proposed research in their own words. In the event that patients lacked the capacity to provide informed consent, written informed consent was obtained from the patient's next of kin or legally authorised representative. Withdrawal from the study was permitted at any time if either the patient or the family member elected to discontinue. Participants volunteered their time and were reimbursed for travel costs.

Behavioural testing

General cognitive screening. Participants were assessed across the following neuropsychological tests: ACE-R as a general measure of global cognitive functioning, delayed recall on the Rey Auditory Verbal Learning Test (RAVLT) [48] to measure verbal episodic recall; delayed recall of the Rey Complex Figure (RCF) [49] as an index of non-verbal episodic memory, and the Trail Making Test (Parts B-A) [50] as an index of executive function. Verbal semantic processing was assessed using verbal letter fluency (F, A, S) [51], and the Naming and Comprehension subtests from the Sydney Language Battery (SydBat) [52]. The functional status of patients was determined using the Frontotemporal Dementia Functional Rating Scale (FRS) [53], which is a dementia staging tool sensitive to changes in functional abilities and presence of neuropsychiatric symptomatology.

Assessment of Autobiographical Memory

The procedure for this study has been described in detail elsewhere [29]. Briefly, a shortened version of the Autobiographical Interview (AI) [41] was used to examine episodic autobiographical memory retrieval from across four life epochs; Teenage Years (11–17 years), Early Adulthood (18–35 years), Middle Adulthood (35–55 years), and Recent period (within the last year). The Early Childhood epoch (up to age 11) of the original AI test was omitted to shorten the overall test session and reduce the burden of testing on patient groups.

The AI was administered according to the standardised protocol. Briefly, participants were instructed to provide a detailed description of a personally experienced event that occurred at a specific time and place from each of the four life periods. In the case of participants who were unable to spontaneously retrieve a suitable event, a list of typical events for each time period was presented. In keeping with the original protocol, the level of retrieval structure was manipulated across three conditions; Free Recall, General Probe, and Specific Probe [41]. Participants first spoke extemporaneously about the event in question (free recall), following which general probes were used to encourage greater retrieval of detail. Finally, specific probes targeting five contextual details categories were provided (Event, Time, Place, Perceptual, Emotion/Thoughts). To avoid the contamination of subsequent memories, the specific probe condition was administered after all

events had been retrieved via the free recall and general probe conditions. All interviews were digitally recorded for subsequent transcription and scoring.

Scoring of autobiographical memories. Following the original AI protocol, retrieved events were first segmented into informational bits or details, classified as a unique occurrence, observation or thought, typically expressed as a grammatical clause [41]. Each detail was then categorised as "internal" or "external", representing episodic and semantic memory, respectively. Here, we focused on the retrieval of internal (i.e., episodic) details as an index of overall autobiographical event recollection Internal details were those details relating directly to the main episode, located within a specific spatiotemporal context, and reflected episodic re-experiencing [41]. We constrained our focus to the high retrieval support condition (Probed recall) to reduce the demands on generative search processes in the patient groups and to ensure that specific contextual details were elicited for each retrieved event.

To investigate potential differences across time periods, we averaged internal details retrieved across Teenage Years, Early Adulthood, and Middle Adulthood to create a Remote period composite score, which was then compared with Recent memory performance. The scores of interest in the present context were therefore: (i) Remote Total Retrieval and (ii) Recent Total Retrieval.

Statistical analyses. Cognitive data were analysed using IBM SPSS Statistics (Version 21.0). Multivariate analyses of variance (MANOVA) with Sidak post hoc tests were used to explore main effects of Group (Controls, bvFTD, SD, AD) for all general cognitive tests. The rationale for using the Sidak modification of the traditional Bonferroni post hoc test is that the statistical power of the analyses is not affected [54]. Performance on the Autobiographical Interview was analysed using one overall repeated measures MANCOVA, with age as a covariate, in which main effects of Epoch (Recent, Remote), and Group, as well as relevant interactions were explored. Chi-squared tests (X^2), based on the frequency patterns of dichotomous variables (e.g., sex), were also used.

Imaging acquisition

All participants underwent whole-brain T1- and diffusion-weighted images using a 3T Philips MRI scanner with standard quadrature head coil (8 channels).

The 3D T1-weighted images were acquired using the following sequences: coronal orientation, matrix 256×256, 200 slices, 1×1 mm^2 in-plane resolution, slice thickness 1 mm, echo time/repetition time = 2.6/5.8 ms, flip angle $\alpha = 19°$.

The diffusion-weighted sequences were acquired as follows: 32 gradient direction diffusion-weighted sequence (repetition time/echo time/inversion time: 8400/68/90 ms; b-value = 100 s/mm^2; 55 2.5 mm horizontal slices, end resolution: $2.5 \times 2.5 \times 2.5$ mm^3; field of view 240×240 mm, 96×96 matrix; repeated twice). Two diffusion tensor imaging sequences were acquired for each participant, which were subsequently averaged. All scans were then visually inspected for field inhomogeneity distortions and corrected for eddy current distortions. Diffusion tensor models were fitted at each voxel via FMRIB's software library (http://fsl.fmrib.ox.ac.uk/fsl/fslwiki/FDT) which resulted in the creation of maps of three eigenvalues ($\lambda 1$, $\lambda 2$, $\lambda 3$) allowing the calculation of fractional anisotropy for each participant.

Voxel-based morphometry analysis

Three-dimensional T1-weighted sequences were analysed with FSL-VBM, a voxel-based morphometry analysis [55,56] using the

FSL-VBM toolbox from the FMRIB software package (http://fsl.fmrib.ox.ac.uk/fsl/fslwiki/FSLVBM/UserGuide) [57]. The VBM technique was used to identify grey matter density changes across groups on a voxel-by-voxel basis. Briefly, the brain extraction tool (BET) [58] was used to extract structural MR images, following which, tissue segmentation was carried out on the brain extracted images using FMRIB's Automatic Segmentation Tool (FAST) [59]. The FMRIB non-linear registration approach (FNIRT) [60,61] was then used to align the resulting grey matter partial volumes to the Montreal Neurological Institute standard space (MNI152), using a b-spline representation of the registration warp field [62]. A study-specific template was created using the resulting images, to which the native grey matter images were re-registered nonlinearly. To correct for local expansion or contraction, the registered partial volume maps were then modulated by dividing by the Jacobian of the warp field. Finally, the modulated segmented images were smoothed with an isotropic Gaussian kernel with a sigma of 3 mm.

A voxel-wise general linear model was employed to investigate grey matter intensity differences via permutation-based non-parametric testing [63] with 5000 permutations per contrast. Differences in cortical grey matter intensities between patients (bvFTD, SD, and AD) and Controls were assessed using regression models with separate directional contrasts (i.e., t-tests). Clusters were extracted using the threshold-free cluster enhancement method and corrected for multiple comparisons using Family-Wise Error at $p<.001$. An overlap analysis was conducted to identify spatial overlap between regions of grey matter intensity commonly affected across the patient groups. The statistical maps generated from the atrophy analyses were scaled using a threshold of $p<.001$, following which, the scaled contrasts were multiplied to create an inclusive, or overlap, mask across groups.

Next, correlations between performance on the Autobiographical Interview and grey matter intensity were investigated using the "randomise" permutation-based inference tool in FSL for all participant images combined. This procedure was adopted to increase the study's statistical power to detect brain-behaviour relationships across the entire brain by achieving greater variance in behavioural scores [64,65]. For additional statistical power, a covariate only general linear statistical model was employed in which group effects were not taken into account. Two separate GLMs were run; (i) Remote ABM performance with age included as a nuisance variable (1,0) and (ii) Recent ABM performance with age included as a nuisance variable (1,0). A positive t-contrast was used in the covariate model, providing an index of positive association between grey matter density and ABM scores. An unbiased voxel-wise whole-brain approach was used across all atrophy and covariate VBM analyses. Anatomical locations of significant results were overlaid on the MNI standard brain, with maximum coordinates provided in MNI stereotaxic space. Anatomical labels were determined with reference to the Harvard-Oxford probabilistic cortical atlas. For all covariate analyses, a threshold of 300 contiguous voxels was used, uncorrected at the $p<.001$ threshold. Similar to the atrophy analyses, an overlap analysis was conducted using the statistical maps generated from the recent and remote ABM contrasts to identify common grey matter regions implicated in recent and remote ABM retrieval. In addition, an exclusive masking procedure was employed to identify regions uniquely associated with retrieval in the recent and remote time periods. The scaled images were subsequently divided by each other to create an exclusive mask for each ABM time period.

Diffusion tensor imaging analysis

Tract-based Spatial Statistics [66] from the FMRIB software library were used to perform a skeleton-based analysis of white matter fractional anisotropy. Fractional anisotropy maps for each participant were eddy current corrected and co-registered using non-linear registration (FNIRT) [60,61] to the MNI standard space using the FMRIB58 fractional anisotropy template. Due to the coarse resolution of diffusion tensor imaging data (i.e., 2.5 mm^3) the template was subsampled at 2 mm^3. Following image registration, the fractional anisotropy maps were averaged to produce a group mean fractional anisotropy image. Then, a skeletonization algorithm [66] was applied to define a group template of the lines of maximum fractional anisotropy, corresponding to the centres of white matter tracts. Fractional anisotropy values for each participant were projected onto this group template skeleton, and extracted for use in subsequent correlation analyses with the ABM variables. Clusters were tested using permutation-based non-parametric testing as outlined for the voxel-based morphometry analyses. Age was included as a nuisance variable in these analyses. Clusters are reported using the threshold-free cluster enhancement method and corrected for Family-Wise Error at $p<.05$. Anatomical labels were determined with reference to the John Hopkins University white matter atlas and the ICBM-DTI-WM atlas labels integrated into FSLview [67,68].

Results

Demographics

An overall group difference was evident for age $(F(3, 50) = 4.410, \ p = .008)$, reflecting the fact that Controls were on average 9 years older than the bvFTD group $(p = .011)$. The patient groups were matched for age (all p values >.05). All participant groups were matched for total years of education $(F(3, 50) = .438, p = .727)$. A significant difference was evident for sex distribution $(\chi^2 \ (3) = 9.326, \ p = .025)$, driven by the fact that significantly more females were present in the Control sample. Importantly, the patient groups were matched for disease duration (i.e., months elapsed since symptom onset, $p = .109$; AD versus bvFTD, $p = .909$; AD versus SD, $p = .113$; SD versus bvFTD, $p = .381$). The patients were further matched for functional status (FRS: $F(2, 35) = 3.024, p = .063$) although the suggestion of a greater functional impairment in bvFTD relative to SD $(p = .059)$ was noted.

General cognitive functioning

Neuropsychological testing revealed profiles characteristic of each patient group (Table 1). Briefly, all patient groups were significantly impaired on the ACE-R screening measure $(F(3, 50) = 18.575, p<.0001)$ relative to Controls (bvFTD, $p = .002$; SD, $p<.0001$; AD, $p<.0001$). SD patients exhibited disproportionate deficits on the ACE-R in comparison with the bvFTD $(p = .013)$ and AD $(p = .056)$ groups, reflecting the verbal loading of this task. No differences were evident between the bvFTD and AD groups on the ACE-R $(p = .968)$.

Looking at each patient group separately, bvFTD patients showed significant impairments in verbal letter fluency $(p = .030)$, delayed verbal and non-verbal episodic memory retrieval (RAVLT, $p<.0001$; RCF, $p = .001$) in the context of relatively spared Naming $(p = .066)$ and Comprehension $(p = .113)$ performance in comparison with Controls. No significant differences between bvFTD and Control participants were observed on the Trail Making Task (Part B-A) $(p = .308)$.

Table 1. Demographic and clinical characteristics of study cohort.

Demographics and cognitive tests	bvFTD (n = 11)	SD (n = 10)	AD (n = 15)	Controls (n = 14)	Group effect	Post hoc test
Sex (M/F)	9:2	8:2	12:3	5:9	*	
Age (years)	62.4 (7.3)	64.0 (8.9)	68.3 (8.8)	72.2 (3.9)	**	Controls>bvFTD
Education (years)	11.9 (3.0)	12.8 (3.0)	12.8 (2.9)	11.9 (2.4)	n/s	n/s
Disease duration (months)	44.2 (30.2)	61.8 (23.5)	37.6 (27.1)	n/a	n/s	n/s
FRS	−0.01 (1.5)	1.6 (1.4)	0.9 (1.6)	n/a	n/s	n/s
ACE-R (100)	76.5 (7.6)	61.3 (14.0)	73.2 (14.1)	93.4 (4.0)	***	Controls>Patients bvFTD, AD>SD
RAVLT delayed recall (15)	2.1 (3.2)	n/a	2.2 (2.7)	10.7 (2.3)	***	Controls>AD, bvFTD
RCF 3 min recall (36)	6.9 (5.6)	13.8 (8.4)	3.4 (4.4)	16.5 (4.3)	***	Controls>AD, bvFTD SD = Controls
Naming (30)	20.0 (7.5)	5.6 (4.5)	21.0 (5.3)	25.6 (2.3)	***	Controls>SD
Comprehension (30)	23.7 (8.0)	21.9 (5.2)	25.7 (3.9)	28.7 (1.6)	*	Controls>SD
Letter Fluency	23.9 (12.3)	26.6 (12.3)	31.5 (14.5)	38.9 (10.9)	*	Controls>bvFTD
Trail Making Test Part B-A (s)	102.4 (68.8)	79.2 (81.2)	93.1 (57.1)	54.0 (32.1)	n/s	n/s

Maximum score for each test in brackets where applicable.
*$p < .05$;
**$p < .005$;
***$p < .0001$;
n/s = not significant; n/a = not applicable; bvFTD = behavioural-variant frontotemporal dementia; SD = semantic dementia; AD = Alzheimer's disease; FRS = Frontotemporal Dementia Functional Rating Scale; ACE-R = Addenbrooke's Cognitive Examination Revised; RAVLT = Rey Auditory Verbal Learning Test; RCF = Rey Complex Figure. FRS data not available for 1 AD patient; Trails data available for 9 AD, 10 bvFTD patients, and 13 Controls; Naming data available for 13 Controls; Comprehension data available for 9 bvFTD patients and 13 Controls; RAVLT not administered in SD patients due to the high verbal loading of the task; RCF recall data available for 10 bvFTD and 9 SD patients; Letter fluency data available for 14 AD patients.

The SD group was characterised by significant impairments in semantic Naming ($p < .0001$), and Comprehension ($p = .014$) with relatively preserved delayed non-verbal episodic memory (RCF, $p = .850$), executive functioning ($p = .900$), and letter fluency ($p = .129$) when compared with Controls.

Finally, AD patients demonstrated significant episodic memory impairments across verbal (RAVLT, $p < .0001$) and non-verbal (RCF, $p < .0001$) domains in the context of relatively preserved Naming ($p = .132$), Comprehension ($p = .531$), executive functioning ($p = .586$), and letter fluency ($p = .556$) in comparison with Controls.

Autobiographical Memory Performance

Figure 1 illustrates overall performance under high retrieval support (Probed Recall) across recent and remote time periods on the Autobiographical Interview for all participant groups. A repeated measures MANCOVA revealed that for overall internal details, a significant main effect of Group was evident ($F(3, 45) = 8.794$, $p < .0001$). This group effect reflected the fact that Controls recalled significantly more internal details than all patient groups irrespective of epoch, (AD, $p < .0001$; bvFTD, $p = .001$; SD, $p = .007$).

The repeated measures MANCOVA further revealed a significant Epoch×Group interaction ($F(1, 45) = 3.746$, $p = .017$). A main effect on the threshold of significance was found for Epoch ($F(1, 45) = 3.858$, $p = .056$), indicating that while all patients showed significant impairments for remote retrieval (AD, $p = .001$; bvFTD, $p = .001$; SD, $p = .001$), SD patients scored in line with Control performance for recent retrieval (SD, $p = .279$; AD, $p = .001$; bvFTD, $p = .007$). Further, within-group comparisons revealed that SD patients recalled significantly more internal details in the recent relative to remote periods ($p = .005$), while all other participant groups demonstrated equivalent ABM perfor-

mance across time periods (AD, $p = .155$; bvFTD, $p = .548$; Control, $p = .288$). No significant differences were evident between patient groups for remote or recent retrieval (all p values $> .4$).

Voxel-based morphometry analyses

Grey matter density profiles in patient groups. Figure 2 displays the patterns of grey matter density displayed by each patient group relative to Controls using the threshold free cluster enhancement method (tfce) and corrected for Family-Wise Error

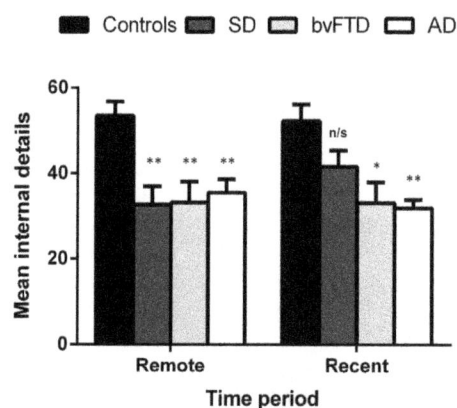

Figure 1. Total internal (episodic) details retrieved across remote and recent periods on the Autobiographical Interview. Error bars represent the standard error of the mean. * $p < .05$; ** $p = .001$; n/s = non-significant. Group differences refer to contrasts between patient groups and Controls. No significant differences were evident between the patient groups for remote or recent retrieval.

(FWE) at $p<.001$. All results reported indicate a decrease in grey matter intensity in patient groups relative to Controls. Briefly, bvFTD patients showed pronounced changes in the medial PFC, frontal poles, orbitofrontal, and insular cortices bilaterally, extending into the left anterior cingulate cortex and left superior frontal gyrus. Medial temporal regions of the brain were also affected including the bilateral inferior and middle temporal gyri, temporal poles, parahippocampal cortices, hippocampi, and amygdalae. Further grey matter density reduction was evident in the cerebellum bilaterally.

The SD group demonstrated characteristic grey matter intensity decrease in bilateral anterior temporal regions, extending into the temporal poles, amygdalae, hippocampi, insular and orbitofrontal cortices bilaterally, and including the left frontal pole.

Finally, AD patients showed widespread grey matter intensity decrease relative to Controls, most pronounced on the left hand side, involving medial temporal regions including the amygdala, and hippocampus bilaterally, the bilateral lateral temporal cortices, and extending to frontal regions, including the orbito-frontal cortex and frontal poles bilaterally. Posterior regions of the brain were also found to harbour significant grey matter density reduction including the right angular gyrus, bilateral supramar-ginal gyrus, as well as the left superior parietal lobule, left precuneus, and left lateral occipital cortices. These patterns of changes are consistent with previous reports in the literature for bvFTD [69], SD [70] and AD [71] (Table 2).

An overlap analysis identified regions of grey matter intensity decrease common to all patient groups, including bilateral lateral and medial temporal regions, notably the temporal poles, amygdalae, hippocampi, as well as the bilateral insular and

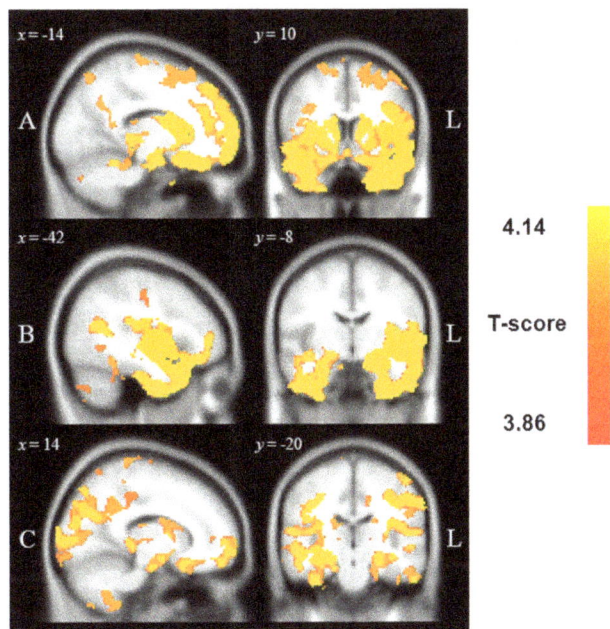

Figure 2. Regions of significant grey matter intensity decrease in patient groups versus Controls. (A) BvFTD (MNI coordinates: $x=-14$, $y=10$, $z=-22$), (B) SD ($x=-42$, $y=-8$, $z=-38$), and (C) AD ($x=14$, $y=-20$, $z=-24$). Coloured voxels show regions that were significant in the voxel-based morphometry analyses at $p<.001$ corrected for Family-Wise Error using the threshold free cluster enhancement method (tfce). Clusters are overlaid on the Montreal Neurological Institute standard brain. Age is included as a covariate in the analyses.

orbitofrontal cortices. The left superior temporal gyrus, left angular gyrus, left lateral occipital cortex, and left postcentral and precentral gyrus were also significantly affected across all of the patient groups (Table S1).

Grey matter correlates of autobiographical memory performance. Data from all participants (n = 50) were com-bined into a single general linear model to examine the neural correlates of recent versus remote ABM retrieval, irrespective of group membership, using a voxel-wise approach, with $p<.001$ uncorrected and a cluster extent threshold of 300 contiguous voxels.

Table 3 displays the neural correlates of successful internal ABM retrieval for remote and recent time periods, indicating a positive association between regions of grey matter intensity and memory performance. Retrieval of remote period internal details was found to correlate positively with grey matter intensity in the following regions bilaterally: temporal pole, orbitofrontal cortex, hippocampus, thalamus, and occipital pole. Further regions implicated in successful remote period retrieval included the left frontal pole and left medial prefrontal cortex, and the left postcentral gyrus (Table 3).

In contrast, recall of recent internal details was positively associated with the integrity of the medial PFC, the frontal pole, and the inferior temporal gyrus bilaterally. Further regions implicated in recent retrieval included the right hippocampus, the left posterior cingulate cortex, left lateral occipital cortices, and the left caudate (Table 3).

To identify the regions significantly associated with retrieval of both remote and recent ABM, we conducted an overlap analysis (Table 4). This analysis revealed the regions commonly implicated irrespective of epoch, namely the left medial PFC, left frontal pole, and the right posterior hippocampus (Figure 3A). Exclusive masking was used to identify the regions that uniquely contributed to ABM retrieval in each time period (Table 4). Integrity of bilateral temporal cortices including the temporal poles, left medial temporal structures including the left hippocampus and amygdala, and the left frontal pole correlated exclusively with remote ABM retrieval (Figure 3B). In contrast, recent ABM retrieval was positively associated with integrity of left frontal cortices including the orbitofrontal cortex and frontal pole, left lateral occipital and posterior parietal regions including the left posterior cingulate cortex and precuneus, bilateral posterior inferior temporal gyrus, right superior frontal gyrus, and the right posterior hippocampus (Figure 3C).

Diffusion tensor imaging

Group differences in fractional anisotropy. Table 5 displays the patterns of fractional anisotropy decrease for each of the patient groups relative to Controls. Diffusion tensor imaging data were not available for 1 bvFTD patient. Analysis of whole-brain fractional anisotropy across groups, controlling for age, revealed the following patterns. Compared to Controls, bvFTD patients showed reduced fractional anisotropy bilaterally in the inferior frontooccipital, uncinate, inferior and superior longitudi-nal fasciculi, as well as the anterior thalamic radiation, forceps minor, forceps major, and cingulum (cingulate gyrus and hippocampal parts). SD patients, by contrast, showed reduced fractional anisotropy predominantly in the left inferior longitudinal fasciculus, and left uncinate fasciculus. Finally AD patients displayed bilateral reduced fractional anisotropy involving the forceps major, forceps minor, the inferior frontooccipital, inferior longitudinal, and uncinate fasciculi, as well as the cingulum (cingulate gyrus) (Table 5). These patterns of fractional anisotropy

Table 2. Voxel-based morphometry results showing regions of significant grey matter intensity decrease for contrasts across patient samples (bvFTD, SD, AD) in comparison with Controls.

Contrast	Regions	Side	Number of voxels	MNI coordinates			T value
				x	y	z	
BvFTD vs. Controls	Right cerebellum, right inferior temporal gyrus, right temporal pole, right parahippocampal gyrus, right hippocampus, right amygdala, right thalamus, right insular cortex, right orbitofrontal cortex, right medial PFC, right frontal pole, extending into left frontal pole, left medial PFC, left orbitofrontal cortex, left anterior cingulate, left insular cortex, left parahippocampal cortex, left amygdala, left hippocampus, left temporal pole, left inferior temporal gyrus	B	67,718	18	-62	-64	4.11
SD vs. Controls	Cerebellum	L	2,707	-26	-84	-52	4.11
	Temporal fusiform cortex, temporal pole, parahippocampal gyrus, amygdala, hippocampus, insular cortex, orbitofrontal cortex, frontal pole	L	20,159	-24	-6	-52	4.14
	Temporal fusiform cortex, temporal pole, parahippocampal gyrus, amygdala, hippocampus, insular cortex, orbitofrontal cortex	R	6,885	34	-8	-52	4.14
	Cerebellum	L	1,250	-26	-82	-54	3.86
AD vs. Controls	Right temporal fusiform cortex, right parahippocampal gyrus, right amygdala, right hippocampus, right supramarginal gyrus, right orbitofrontal cortex, right frontal pole, extending into left frontal pole, left inferior temporal gyrus, left parahippocampal gyrus, left hippocampus, left supramarginal gyrus, left superior parietal lobule, left lateral occipital cortex, left precuneus	B	68,010	30	-2	-54	4.02

All clusters reported using threshold free cluster enhancement technique (tfce) and corrected for Family-Wise Error (FWE) at $p < .001$. For brevity only those clusters above 1,000 contiguous voxels are reported here.
BvFTD = behavioural-variant frontotemporal dementia; SD = semantic dementia; AD = Alzheimer's disease; L = Left; R = Right; B = Bilateral; MNI = Montreal Neurological Institute.

Table 3. Voxel-based morphometry results showing regions of grey matter intensity that covary with remote and recent autobiographical memory (ABM) retrieval in all participants combined (n = 50).

Contrast	Regions	Side	Number of voxels	MNI coordinates		
				x	y	z
Remote	Temporal pole, orbitofrontal cortex	L	1476	−18	4	−50
	Frontal pole, medial PFC	L	1408	−12	50	−28
	Parahippocampal gyrus, hippocampus (posterior), amygdala	L	1082	−14	0	−22
	Hippocampus (posterior), thalamus	R	1066	34	−20	−10
	Postcentral gyrus	L	745	−44	−12	28
	Occipital pole	L	502	−8	−102	−10
	Temporal pole, orbitofrontal cortex	R	378	38	20	−28
	Caudate, thalamus	L	331	−12	4	4
	Occipital fusiform gyrus	R	300	26	−86	−8
Recent	Medial PFC, frontal poles	B	1384	−2	42	−30
	Orbitofrontal cortex, caudate	L	825	−24	24	−8
	Temporal occipital fusiform cortex, hippocampus (posterior)	R	793	34	−40	−14
	Lateral occipital cortex	L	566	−34	−66	16
	Superior frontal gyrus	R	413	22	12	42
	Posterior cingulate cortex	L	397	−4	−30	26
	Inferior temporal gyrus	L	364	−62	−6	−38
	Inferior temporal gyrus	R	313	60	−30	−30
	Occipital pole	L	310	−26	−100	−8

All clusters reported using voxel-wise contrasts and uncorrected at $p<.001$. Age is included as a covariate in all contrasts. All clusters reported at $t>3.80$ with a cluster threshold of 300 contiguous voxels. L = Left; R = Right; B = Bilateral; MNI = Montreal Neurological Institute.

changes are in keeping with previous reports in the literature for bvFTD and SD [72] and AD [73] patients.

Fractional anisotropy correlations with autobiographical memory performance. Fractional anisotropy values of white matter tracts connecting grey matter regions found to correlate positively with ABM retrieval in the voxel-based morphometry analyses were investigated. Masks for the following white matter tracts, taken from the Johns Hopkins probabilistic white matter atlas [74] were created; uncinate fasciculus (connecting medial prefrontal and anterior temporal brain regions), cingulum (running along the surface of the corpus callosum and hippocampal parts), inferior longitudinal fasciculus (connecting the temporal lobes and occipital lobes), superior longitudinal fasciculus (connecting the frontal, temporal, parietal and occipital lobes), and the forceps minor (connecting medial and lateral prefrontal regions). Fractional anisotropy values for each white matter tract were extracted and exported into SPSS. Pearson R correlations, corrected for multiple comparisons at $p<.01$, were then run to investigate positive associations between fractional anisotropy values and recent and remote ABM performance.

Fractional anisotropy values in the left uncinate fasciculus ($r = .449$, $p = .001$), left cingulum (corpus callosum part: $r = .340$, $p = .008$; hippocampal part: $r = .399$, $p = .002$), and the forceps minor ($r = .440$, $p = .001$) were found to correlate significantly with remote ABM retrieval (Figure 4). In contrast, only fractional anisotropy values in the forceps minor ($r = .417$, $p = .001$) and the left cingulum (hippocampal part; $r = .330$, $p = .010$) were significantly associated with recent ABM performance (Figure 5).

Discussion

This study is the first to contrast the neural substrates of recent and remote ABM using a combination of whole-brain voxel-based morphometry analyses and tract-based spatial statistics in neurodegenerative disorders. Distinct grey matter correlates common to both recent and remote time periods were found, including the right posterior hippocampus, left medial prefrontal and frontopolar cortices. Notably, however, discrete regions potentially specialised for the retrieval of information specific to each time period were identified. Remote ABM performance was associated with integrity of the bilateral anterior temporal cortices including the temporal poles, whereas retrieval of recent ABMs was associated with the integrity of left posterior parietal regions including the posterior cingulate cortex. Associations with white matter tract integrity were also found: the forceps minor and left hippocampal portion of the cingulum bundle were significantly associated with both recent and remote retrieval, while a distributed set of predominantly left-lateralised white matter tracts were implicated for remote retrieval. Our findings point towards commonalities and differences between the grey and white matter regions implicated in remote and recent recall and shed further light on the neurocognitive mechanisms supporting ABM retrieval.

Using neurodegenerative disorders as lesion models for declarative memory processes, we have confirmed that ABM retrieval depends upon the integrity of a distributed neural network. Notably, this network comprises not only medial temporal, but also lateral temporal, medial prefrontal and frontopolar structures, as well as posterior regions in the parietal and occipital lobes. Our

Table 4. Voxel-based morphometry results showing regions of significant grey matter intensity that correlate with ABM retrieval irrespective of time period, and regions that correlate exclusively with Remote and Recent time periods in all participants combined (n = 50).

Contrast	Regions	Side	Number of voxels	MNI coordinates		
				x	y	z
Overlap	Medial PFC, frontal pole	L	636	−6	46	−26
	Hippocampus (posterior)	R	472	40	−22	−12
Remote	Temporal pole, inferior temporal gyrus (anterior)	L	1290	−16	2	−46
	Hippocampus, amygdala, putamen	L	947	−14	−14	−24
	Postcentral gyrus, precentral gyrus	L	661	−46	−14	28
	Frontal pole	L	588	−14	44	−28
	Temporal pole, middle temporal gyrus	R	378	48	6	−28
	Superior temporal gyrus, supramarginal gyrus	R	376	44	−32	4
Recent	Orbitofrontal cortex, caudate, putamen	L	540	−26	22	−10
	Lateral occipital cortex, precuneus	L	507	−36	−64	14
	Frontal pole	L	396	−14	58	−16
	Posterior cingulate cortex	L	346	−6	−36	26
	Superior frontal gyrus	R	331	20	20	44
	Inferior temporal gyrus (posterior)	L	331	−62	−6	−40
	Inferior temporal gyrus (posterior)	R	309	60	−30	−30
	Hippocampus (posterior), lingual gyrus	R	306	34	−36	−16

All results reported using voxel-wise contrasts and uncorrected at $p<.001$. Age is included as a covariate in all contrasts. All clusters reported at $t>3.80$ with a cluster threshold of 300 contiguous voxels. L = Left; R = Right; MNI = Montreal Neurological Institute.

findings converge with a large body of literature from functional neuroimaging studies in healthy individuals revealing a core memory network which subtends successful retrieval of events from the past [9,11]. Importantly, our study points to the hippocampus, medial prefrontal, and frontopolar cortices, as pivotal structures for successful ABM retrieval irrespective of time period [19–21,75].

The temporal duration of hippocampal involvement in the retrieval of ABMs from across the lifespan represents a heavily debated issue within the literature. Here, we demonstrate hippocampal involvement in ABM retrieval regardless of the age of the memory, with contributions evident for recent events (i.e., less than 1 year old), as well as for considerably older episodes, stretching back over 40 years prior. Notably, our diffusion tensor imaging analyses reveal that integrity of the hippocampal portion of the left cingulum bundle, projecting from the posterior cingulate gyrus to the entorhinal cortex, also correlates with ABM retrieval irrespective of time period, providing converging grey and white matter evidence in support of a time-invariant role of medial temporal regions for ABM retrieval. These findings resonate with the multiple trace theory [13,14] which delineates a permanent role for the hippocampus in supporting the rich recollection of previously experienced events. Subregions of the hippocampus have been differentially implicated across ABM studies with recent memories shown to activate the anterior hippocampus [19], whereas remote memories appear to be represented more evenly across the hippocampal formation [15]. Recently, both recent and remote memories have been shown to be represented within the anterior and posterior hippocampus, however, the posterior hippocampus appears more sensitive to the retrieval of remote memories [16]. In this study, we found evidence only for posterior

hippocampal involvement in ABM, however, this finding may in part reflect methodological differences in the sampling of ABMs and demarcation of recent versus remote time periods, as well as the use of a post hoc correlation approach in neurodegenerative disorders. Finally, some hippocampal lateralisation effects were observed, with the right hippocampus implicated irrespective of time period, whereas the left hippocampus correlated exclusively with remote memory retrieval. Interestingly, however, only the left hippocampal portion of the cingulum bundle was found to correlate with ABM retrieval irrespective of epoch. Considerable variation exists within the literature regarding the response of the hippocampii according to the age of the retrieved memory, with some studies reporting bilateral hippocampal recruitment irrespective of time period [21], whereas others have demonstrated a time invariant role for the left hippocampus and increasing activation of the right hippocampus according to the recency of the memory [76]. While our overall findings mesh well with existing reports in the literature emphasising a permanent role for the hippocampus in ABM retrieval, our divergent lateralisation effects caution against a simple mapping of results from lesion studies to functional activation studies conducted in healthy individuals. We suggest that functional activation studies in the disease groups in question will serve to considerably strengthen our understanding of the specific neural regions implicated in ABM dysfunction across the lifespan, as has been conducted in semantic dementia [36].

Despite appreciable overlap in the neural substrates of recent and remote ABM retrieval, we further identified discrete neural correlates for each epoch. For remote retrieval, in which memories stretching back over 40 years were sampled, the largest grey matter cluster to correlate exclusively with remote memory resided

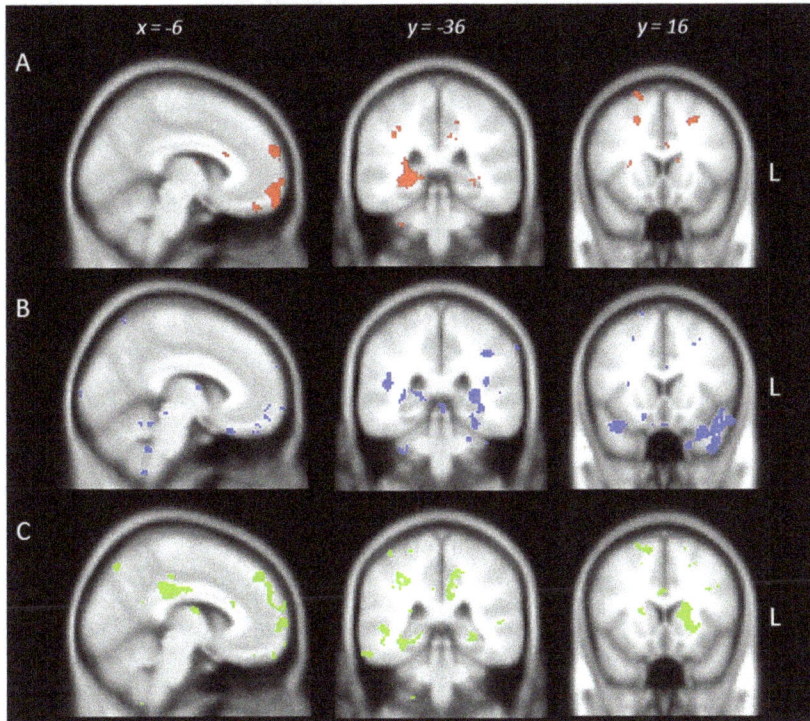

Figure 3. Overlap and exclusive masking results showing brain regions in which grey matter intensity correlates significantly with autobiographical memory retrieval. (A) Overlap in regions irrespective of time period; (B) Regions exclusively implicated in remote memory; (C) Regions exclusively implicated in recent memory. Coloured voxels show regions that were significant in the voxel-based morphometry covariate analyses with $p<.001$ uncorrected with a cluster threshold of 300 contiguous voxels. All clusters reported $t>3.80$ and depict a positive association between grey matter integrity and memory performance. Clusters are overlaid on the Montreal Neurological Institute standard brain. Age is included as a covariate in the analyses.

in the left temporal pole and left anterior inferior temporal gyrus, regions specialised for semantic memory [5,77]. This finding is consistent with the proposal that old memories undergo a process of semanticisation [78]. Over time, repeated recollection and rehearsal of remote memories facilitates abstraction of the gist of the episode, divested of its accompanying sensory-perceptual details [25]. This process of abstraction therefore produces a largely schematic or overgeneral account of the formerly evocative event [4,7]. The sizeable contribution of semantic processing regions to remote memory retrieval found here suggests that, over time, episodic ABMs lose much of their autonoetic flavour, leading to a reliance on predominantly semantic or gist-based representations which represent the most accessible and efficient route of access [79]. Our tract-based spatial statistics results revealed that fractional anisotropy values from predominantly left-lateralised white matter tracts connecting frontal, temporal, and occipital regions (uncinate fasciculus, cingulum, forceps minor) were significantly related to remote ABM retrieval, suggesting the importance of connectivity between a distributed network of regions in supporting recollection of events from the distant past [9].

For retrieval of recent memories (i.e., events that had occurred within the previous year), our voxel-based morphometry analyses revealed the involvement of the right posterior hippocampus, left orbitofrontal, left occipital and bilateral posterior inferior temporal cortices. Most striking, however, was the emergence of the left posterior cingulate cortex as a crucial structure for recent retrieval. Our finding of posterior cingulate cortex involvement exclusively in the recent period is in keeping with prior reports of its

preferential activation in healthy individuals for recent ABMs [8,19]. This midline posterior structure represents a site of particular interest as its functional specialisation in the context of ABM retrieval remains poorly understood. In contrast with the widespread involvement of multiple white matter tracts for remote retrieval, our diffusion tensor imaging analyses revealed that only the forceps minor and the left cingulum bundle (hippocampal portion) were significantly related to recent ABM retrieval. Again, these findings converge to suggest the involvement of frontal and posterior hippocampal/cingulate regions in the successful recollection of recent events. The posterior cingulate has been proposed to facilitate rich contextual re-experiencing [15], and the generation of visuospatial imagery [80], with further studies pointing to its role in the coding of personally familiar places [81] and self-referential processing [82]. With increasing recency, it is likely that the ABMs retrieved by participants are imbued with a sense of recollection, vivid visual imagery, and self-referential connotations [83]. Indeed, recency of events has previously been associated with increased instances of rich autonoetic re-experiencing [3,83]. Accordingly, the preferential involvement of the posterior cingulate cortex for recent period retrieval suggests that this region may be particularly well suited to support the recollective endeavour.

A number of methodological issues warrant consideration in the current context. Our grey matter voxel-based morphometry covariate results did not survive conservative correction for multiple comparisons (i.e., Family-Wise Error) and were therefore reported uncorrected at $p<.001$. To guard against the potential for false positive results, however, we applied strict cluster extent

Table 5. Tract-based spatial statistics results showing regions of white matter integrity decrease in each of the patient groups compared with Controls[a]

Contrast	Tracts	Side	Number of voxels	MNI coordinates			T value
				x	y	z	
BvFTD versus Controls	Inferior longitudinal fasciculus, uncinate fasciculus, inferior fronto-occipital fasciculus, superior longitudinal fasciculus, anterior thalamic radiation, forceps minor, forceps major, cingulum (cingulate gyrus), cingulum (hippocampal part), superior longitudinal fasciculus (temporal part)	B	64,986	−28	0	−36	4.14
SD versus Controls	Inferior longitudinal fasciculus, uncinate fasciculus	L	2,096	−34	−3	−34	2.53
AD versus Controls	Forceps major, forceps minor, inferior fronto-occipital fasciculus, inferior longitudinal fasciculus, uncinate fasciculus, cingulum (cingulate gyrus)	B	31,691	−24	−56	11	3.49

[a]Diffusion tensor imaging data not available for 1 bvFTD patient. Age is included as a covariate in all contrasts. All clusters reported using threshold-free cluster enhancement method and corrected for Family-Wise Error (FWE) at p<.05. BvFTD = behavioural-variant frontotemporal dementia; SD = semantic dementia; AD = Alzheimer's disease; L = Left; B = Bilateral; MNI = Montreal Neurological Institute.

thresholds of 300 contiguous voxels in the covariate analyses. Given our sample size, the application of stringent cluster extent thresholds, and our *a priori* hypotheses, we are confident that our results do not represent false positive findings. The use of dementia syndromes as lesion models for ABM processes presents a number of challenges, one of which concerns the possibility of confabulation in the bvFTD patient group, particularly with the use of structured probing in the high retrieval condition. While this could not be definitively ruled out, details were cross-checked with carers where the veracity of memories was in doubt. It is also important to note that some of the regions to emerge in our voxel-based morphometry analyses for ABM processes have been implicated in behavioural disruption in neurodegenerative disorders [84]. In general, however, the neural correlates of ABM dysfunction identified here correspond remarkably well with the key regions of the core ABM network expounded in healthy individuals [9].

The classification of what constitutes a "recent" memory varies considerably in the literature, ranging from relatively extended periods of time (e.g., within the past 5 years) to more discrete snapshots (e.g., within the past month). It remains unclear whether the differential dissection of time periods impacts the neural correlates of ABM retrieval and this represents an interesting avenue for future investigation. A further caveat concerns the differential statistical thresholds used in the grey and white matter neuroimaging analyses. Future studies with larger sample sizes will permit the use of one statistical threshold across all levels of analyses. One further issue of relevance to the hippocampal contributions to ABM recall concerns the recollective quality of the events retrieved. Previous studies have pointed to the modulating effect of specific recollective aspects of retrieval, with comparable patterns of activation reported for recent and remote ABMs that are matched in terms of vividness [20,85]. As we did not collect subjective ratings from our participants, it is not possible to determine how recollective factors, such as vividness, visual imagery, and emotional tone, potentially modulate the specific neural correlates of recent and remote ABM retrieval reported here. We suggest that future investigations incorporating subjective experiential ratings will be important to clarify the functional specialisation of specific brain regions for recent and remote memory retrieval. Finally, we did not have access to functional connectivity data in our participant cohort, however, it will be crucial to incorporate such measures in future studies to elucidate how alterations in functional connectivity between specific regions disrupt the capacity for ABM retrieval in neurodegenerative disorders.

Conclusions

Using neurodegenerative disorders as lesion models for declarative memory processes, we have demonstrated that recent and remote ABM retrieval is associated with the integrity of common and unique grey and white matter structures. Our findings suggest that regions specialised for semantic memory play an important role in the retrieval of distant memories, whereas midline posterior parietal structures may be preferentially involved for more recent events. Irrespective of time period, however, ABM retrieval appears to be significantly associated with the integrity of the hippocampus, resonating with current theories emphasising a time-invariant role for the medial temporal lobes in retrieving events from the past.

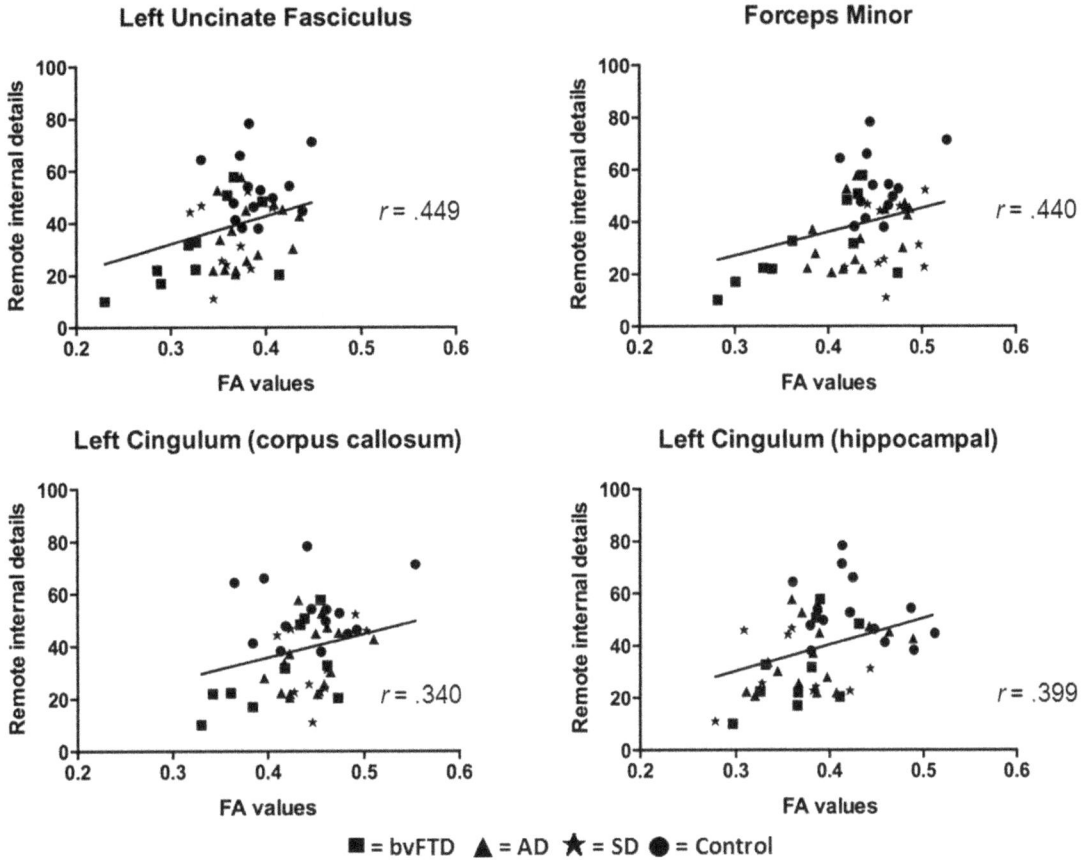

Figure 4. Relationship between fractional anisotropy (FA) values in white matter tracts of interest and remote memory. All participants included in the analyses (n = 49). Age is included as a covariate in the analyses. Plotted data depict a positive association between fractional anisotropy values and memory performance, with the magnitude of this relationship calculated using Pearson's R correlations (r).

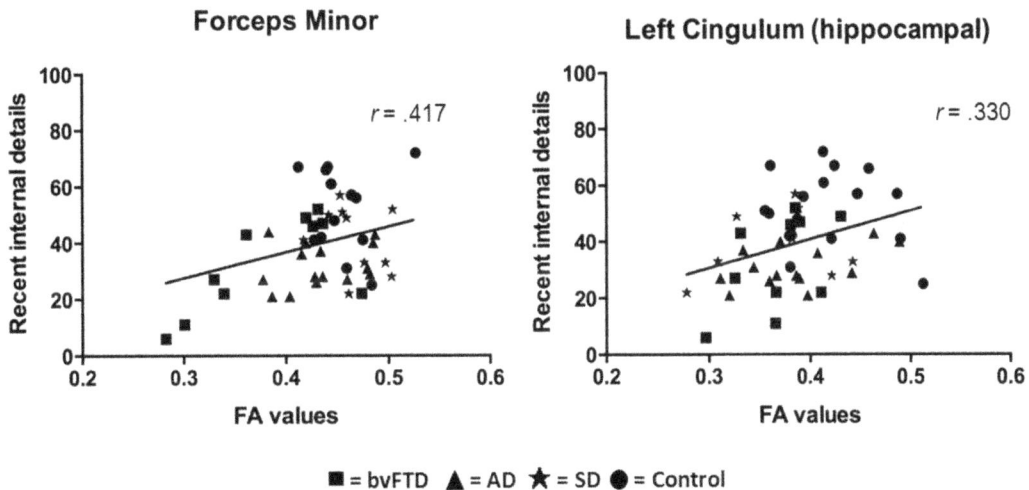

Figure 5. Relationship between fractional anisotropy (FA) values in white matter tracts of interest and recent memory. All participants included in the analyses (n = 49). Age is included as a covariate in the analyses. Plotted data depict a positive association between fractional anisotropy values and memory performance, with the magnitude of this relationship calculated using Pearson's R correlations (r).

Acknowledgments

The authors are grateful to the patients and their families for their continued support of our research.

Author Contributions

Conceived and designed the experiments: MI MH SL LM JRH OP. Performed the experiments: MI MH SEW SH. Analyzed the data: MI SEW OP. Contributed reagents/materials/analysis tools: MH BYKL. Wrote the paper: MI SEW JRH OP. Critically revised the manuscript: MI MH SEW BYKL SL LM SH JRH OP.

References

1. Conway MA, Singer JA, Tagini A (2004) The self and autobiographical memory: Correspondence and coherence. Soc Cogn 22: 491–529.

2. Greenberg DL, Rubin DC (2003) The neuropsychology of autobiographical memory. Cortex 39: 687–728.

3. Piolino P, Desgranges B, Eustache F (2009) Episodic autobiographical memories over the course of time: Cognitive, neuropsychological and neuroimaging findings. Neuropsychologia 47: 2314–2329.

4. Irish M, Piguet O (2013) The pivotal role of semantic memory in remembering the past and imagining the future. Front Behav Neurosci 7: 27.

5. Binder JR, Desai RH, Graves WW, Conant LL (2009) Where is the semantic system? A critical review and meta-analysis of 120 functional neuroimaging studies. Cereb Cortex 19: 2767–2796.

6. Conway MA (2001) Sensory–perceptual episodic memory and its context: Autobiographical memory. Philos Trans R Soc B Biol Sci 356: 1375–1384.

7. Irish M, Lawlor BA, O'Mara SM, Coen RF (2011) Impaired capacity for autonoetic reliving during autobiographical event recall in mild Alzheimer's disease. Cortex 47: 236–249.

8. Piefke M, Weiss P, Zilles K, Markowitsch H, Fink G (2003) Differential remoteness and emotional tone modulate the neural correlates of autobiographical memory. Brain 126: 650–668.

9. Svoboda E, McKinnon MC, Levine B (2006) The functional neuroanatomy of autobiographical memory: a meta-analysis. Neuropsychologia 44: 2189–2208.

10. Maguire EA (2001) Neuroimaging studies of autobiographical event memory. Philos Trans R Soc B Biol Sci 356: 1441–1451.

11. Cabeza R, St Jacques P (2007) Functional neuroimaging of autobiographical memory. Trends Cogn Sci 11: 219–227.

12. Squire L, Alvarez P (1995) Retrograde amnesia and memory consolidation: a neurobiological perspective. Curr Opin Neurobiol 5: 169–177.

13. Moscovitch M, Rosenbaum R, Gilboa A, Addis DR, Westmacott R, et al. (2005) Functional neuroanatomy of remote episodic, semantic and spatial memory: a unified account based on multiple trace theory. J Anat 207: 35–66.

14. Nadel L, Moscovitch M (1997) Memory consolidation, retrograde amnesia and the hippocampal complex. Curr Opin Neurobiol 7: 217–227.

15. Gilboa A, Winocur G, Grady CL, Hevenor SJ, Moscovitch M (2004) Remembering our past: functional neuroanatomy of recollection of recent and very remote personal events. Cereb Cortex 14: 1214–1225.

16. Bonnici HM, Chadwick MJ, Lutti A, Hassabis D, Weiskopf N, et al. (2012) Detecting representations of recent and remote autobiographical memories in vmPFC and hippocampus. J Neurosci 32: 16982–16991.

17. Piolino P, Giffard-Quillon G, Desgranges B, Chetelat G, Baron JC, et al. (2004) Re-experiencing old memories via hippocampus: a PET study of autobiographical memory. NeuroImage 22: 1371–1383.

18. Viard A, Piolino P, Desgranges B, Chetelat G, Lebreton K, et al. (2007) Hippocampal activation for autobiographical memories over the entire lifetime in healthy aged subjects: an fMRI study. Cereb Cortex 17: 2453–2467.

19. Söderlund H, Moscovitch M, Kumar N, Mandic M, Levine B (2012) As time goes by: hippocampal connectivity changes with remoteness of autobiographical memory retrieval. Hippocampus 22: 670–679.

20. Addis DR, Moscovitch M, Crawley AP, McAndrews MP (2004) Recollective qualities modulate hippocampal activation during autobiographical memory retrieval. Hippocampus 14: 752–762.

21. Steinvorth S, Corkin S, Halgren E (2006) Ecphory of autobiographical memories: An fMRI study of recent and remote memory retrieval. NeuroImage 30: 285–298.

22. Oddo S, Lux S, Weiss PH, Schwab A, Welzer H, et al. (2010) Specific role of medial prefrontal cortex in retrieving recent autobiographical memories: an fMRI study of young female subjects. Cortex 46: 29–39.

23. Winocur G, Moscovitch M (2011) Memory transformation and systems consolidation. J Int Neuropsychol Soc 17: 766–780.

24. Hodges JR, Graham KS (2001) Episodic memory: insights from semantic dementia. Philos Trans R Soc Lond B Biol Sci 356: 1423–1434.

25. Rosenbaum RS, Winocur G, Moscovitch M (2001) New views on old memories: re-evaluating the role of the hippocampal complex. Behav Brain Res 127: 183–197.

26. Irish M, Piguet O, Hodges JR (2012) Self-projection and the default network in frontotemporal dementia. Nat Rev Neurol 8: 152–161.

27. Greene J, Hodges J, Baddeley A (1995) Autobiographical memory and executive function in early dementia of Alzheimer type. Neuropsychologia 33: 1647–1670.

28. Piolino P, Desgranges B, Belliard S, Matuszewski V, Lalevee C, et al. (2003) Autobiographical memory and autonoetic consciousness: triple dissociation in neurodegenerative diseases. Brain 126: 2203–2219.

29. Irish M, Hornberger M, Lah S, Miller L, Pengas G, et al. (2011) Profiles of recent autobiographical memory retrieval in semantic dementia, behavioural-variant frontotemporal dementia, and Alzheimer's disease. Neuropsychologia 49: 2694–2702.

30. Barnabe A, Whitehead V, Pilon R, Arsenault-Lapierre G, Chertkow H (2012) Autobiographical memory in mild cognitive impairment and Alzheimer's disease: A comparison between the Levine and Kopelman interview methodologies. Hippocampus 22: 1809–1825.

31. Philippi N, Noblet V, Botzung A, Despres O, Renard F, et al. (2012) MRI-based volumetry correlates of autobiographical memory in Alzheimer's disease. PLoS One 7: e46200.

32. Gilboa A, Ramirez J, Kohler S, Westmacott R, Black SE, et al. (2005) Retrieval of autobiographical memory in Alzheimer's disease: relation to volumes of medial temporal lobe and other structures. Hippocampus 15: 535–550.

33. Meulenbroek O, Rijpkema M, Kessels RP, Rikkert MG, Fernandez G (2010) Autobiographical memory retrieval in patients with Alzheimer's disease. NeuroImage 53: 331–340.

34. Matuszewski V, Piolino P, Belliard S, de la Sayette V, Laisney M, et al. (2009) Patterns of autobiographical memory impairment according to disease severity in semantic dementia. Cortex 45: 456–472.

35. Moss HE, Kopelman MD, Cappelletti M, Davies Pde M, Jaldow E (2003) Lost for words or loss of memories? Autobiographical memory in semantic dementia. Cogn Neuropsychol 20: 703–732.

36. Maguire EA, Kumaran D, Hassabis D, Kopelman MD (2010) Autobiographical memory in semantic dementia: A longitudinal fMRI study. Neuropsychologia 48: 123–136.

37. Westmacott R, Leach L, Freedman M, Moscovitch M (2001) Different patterns of autobiographical memory loss in semantic dementia and medial temporal lobe amnesia: A challenge to consolidation theory. Neurocase 7: 37–55.

38. McKinnon M, Nica E, Sengdy P, Kovacevic N, Moscovitch M, et al. (2008) Autobiographical memory and patterns of brain atrophy in fronto-temporal lobar degeneration. J Cogn Neurosci 20: 1839–1853.

39. Piolino P, Chételat G, Matuszewski V, Landeau B, Mézenge F, et al. (2007) In search of autobiographical memories: A PET study in the frontal variant of frontotemporal dementia. Neuropsychologia 45: 2730–2743.

40. Irish M, Piguet O, Hodges JR, Hornberger M (2014) Common and unique grey matter correlates of episodic memory dysfunction in frontotemporal dementia and Alzheimer's disease. Hum Brain Mapp 35: 1422–1435.

41. Levine B, Svoboda E, Hay JF, Winocur G, Moscovitch M (2002) Aging and autobiographical memory: Dissociating episodic from semantic retrieval. Psychol Aging 17: 677–689.

42. Rascovsky K, Hodges JR, Knopman D, Mendez MF, Kramer JH, et al. (2011) Sensitivity of revised diagnostic criteria for the behavioural variant of frontotemporal dementia. Brain 134: 2456–2477.

43. Gorno-Tempini ML, Hillis AE, Weintraub S, Kertesz A, Mendez M, et al. (2011) Classification of primary progressive aphasia and its variants. Neurology 76: 1006–1014.

44. McKhann GM, Knopman DS, Chertkow H, Hyman BT, Jack CR Jr, et al. (2011) The diagnosis of dementia due to Alzheimer's disease: recommendations from the National Institute on Aging-Alzheimer's Association workgroups on diagnostic guidelines for Alzheimer's disease. Alzheimers Dement 7: 263–269.

45. Kipps CM, Hodges JR, Hornberger M (2010) Nonprogressive behavioural frontotemporal dementia: recent developments and clinical implications of the 'bvFTD phenocopy syndrome'. Curr Opin Neurol 23: 628–632.

46. Morris J (1997) Clinical dementia rating: a reliable and valid diagnostic and staging measure for dementia of the Alzheimer type. Int Psychogeriatr 9: 173–176.

47. Mioshi E, Dawson K, Mitchell J, Arnold R, Hodges JR (2006) The Addenbrooke's Cognitive Examination Revised (ACE R): a brief cognitive test battery for dementia screening. Int J Geriatr Psychiatry 21: 1078–1085.

48. Schmidt M (1996) Rey Auditory and Verbal Learning Test: A handbook. Los Angeles: Western Psychological Services.

49. Meyers J, Meyers K (1995) The Meyers Scoring System for the Rey Complex Figure and the Recognition Trial: Professional Manual. Odessa, FL: Psychological Assessment Resources.
50. Reitan R (1958) Validity of the Trail Making Test as an indicator of organic brain damage. Percept Mot Skills 8: 271–276.
51. Strauss E, Sherman EMS, Spreen O (2006) A compendium of neuropsychological tests: Administration, norms, and commentary. New York: Oxford University Press, USA.
52. Savage S, Hsieh S, Leslie F, Foxe D, Piguet O, et al. (2013) Distinguishing Subtypes in Primary Progressive Aphasia: Application of the Sydney Language Battery. Dement Geriatr Cogn Disord 35: 208–218.
53. Mioshi E, Hsieh S, Savage S, Hornberger M, Hodges JR (2010) Clinical staging and disease progression in frontotemporal dementia. Neurology 74: 1591–1597.
54. Keppel G, Wickens TD (2004) Design and Analysis: A researcher's handbook. Englewood Cliffs (NJ): Prentice Hall.
55. Ashburner J, Friston KJ (2000) Voxel-based morphometry - the methods. NeuroImage 11: 805–821.
56. Mechelli A, Price CJ, Friston KJ, Ashburner J (2005) Voxel-based morphometry of the human brain: methods and applications. Curr Med Imaging Rev 1: 1–9.
57. Smith SM, Jenkinson M, Woolrich MW, Beckmann CF, Behrens TE, et al. (2004) Advances in functional and structural MR image analysis and implementation as FSL. NeuroImage 23: S208–219.
58. Smith SM (2002) Fast robust automated brain extraction. Hum Brain Mapp 17: 143–155.
59. Zhang Y, Brady M, Smith S (2001) Segmentation of brain MR images through a hidden Markov random field model and the expectation-maximization algorithm. IEEE Trans Med Imaging 20: 45–57.
60. Andersson JLR, Jenkinson M, Smith S (2007a) Non-linear optimisation. FMRIB Technical Report TR07JA1. Oxford: University of Oxford FMRIB Centre. Available: http://www.fmrib.ox.ac.uk/analysis/techrep/tr07ja1/tr07ja1.pdf. Accessed June 2013.
61. Andersson JLR, Jenkinson M, Smith S (2007b) Non-linear registration, aka Spatial normalisation. FMRIB Technical Report TR07JA2. Oxford: University of Oxford FMRIB Centre. Available: http://www.fmrib.ox.ac.uk/analysis/techrep/tr07ja2/tr07ja2.pdf. Accessed June 2013.
62. Rueckert D, Sonoda LI, Hayes C, Hill DL, Leach MO, et al. (1999) Nonrigid registration using free-form deformations: application to breast MR images. IEEE Trans Med Imaging 18: 712–721.
63. Nichols TE, Holmes AP (2002) Nonparametric permutation tests for functional neuroimaging: a primer with examples. Hum Brain Mapp 15: 1–25.
64. Sollberger M, Stanley CM, Wilson SM, Gyurak A, Beckman V, et al. (2009) Neural basis of interpersonal traits in neurodegenerative diseases. Neuropsychologia 47: 2812–2827.
65. Irish M, Addis DR, Hodges JR, Piguet O (2012) Considering the role of semantic memory in episodic future thinking: evidence from semantic dementia. Brain 135: 2178–2191.
66. Smith SM, Jenkinson M, Johansen-Berg H, Rueckert D, Nichols TE, et al. (2006) Tract-based spatial statistics: voxelwise analysis of multi-subject diffusion data. NeuroImage 31: 1487–1505.
67. Mori S, Oishi K, Jiang H, Jiang L, Li X, et al. (2008) Stereotaxic white matter atlas based on diffusion tensor imaging in an ICBM template. NeuroImage 40: 570–582.
68. Oishi K, Zilles K, Amunts K, Faria A, Jiang H, et al. (2008) Human brain white matter atlas: identification and assignment of common anatomical structures in superficial white matter. NeuroImage 43: 447–457.
69. Rosen HJ, Gorno-Tempini ML, Goldman WP, Perry RJ, Schuff N, et al. (2002) Patterns of brain atrophy in frontotemporal dementia and semantic dementia. Neurology 58: 198–208.
70. Mion M, Patterson K, Acosta-Cabronero J, Pengas G, Izquierdo-Garcia D, et al. (2010) What the left and right anterior fusiform gyri tell us about semantic memory. Brain 133: 3256–3268.
71. Karas GB, Scheltens P, Rombouts SA, Visser PJ, van Schijndel RA, et al. (2004) Global and local gray matter loss in mild cognitive impairment and Alzheimer's disease. NeuroImage 23: 708–716.
72. Lam BYK, Halliday G, Irish M, Hodges JR, Piguet O (2014) Longitudinal white matter changes in frontotemporal dementia subtypes. Hum Brain Mapp 35: 3547–3557.
73. Chua TC, Wen W, Slavin MJ, Sachdev PS (2008) Diffusion tensor imaging in mild cognitive impairment and Alzheimer's disease: a review. Curr Opin Neurol 21: 83–92.
74. Mori S, Wakana S, Nagae-Poetscher LM, van Zijl PC (2005) MRI atlas of human white matter. Amsterdam: Elsevier.
75. Viard A, Lebreton K, Chetelat G, Desgranges B, Landeau B, et al. (2010) Patterns of hippocampal-neocortical interactions in the retrieval of episodic autobiographical memories across the entire life-span of aged adults. Hippocampus 20: 153–165.
76. Maguire EA, Frith CD (2003) Lateral asymmetry in the hippocampal response to the remoteness of autobiographical memories. J Neurosci 23: 5302–5307.
77. Visser M, Embleton KV, Jefferies E, Parker GJ, Ralph MA (2010) The inferior, anterior temporal lobes and semantic memory clarified: novel evidence from distortion-corrected fMRI. Neuropsychologia 48: 1689–1696.
78. Cermak L (1984) The episodic-semantic distinction in amnesia; Squire L, Butters N, editors. New York: Guilford Press. 55–62 p.
79. Greenberg DL, Verfaellie M (2010) Interdependence of episodic and semantic memory: evidence from neuropsychology. J Int Neuropsychol Soc 16: 748–753.
80. Cavanna AE, Trimble MR (2006) The precuneus: a review of its functional anatomy and behavioural correlates. Brain 129: 564–583.
81. Sugiura M, Shah NJ, Zilles K, Fink GR (2005) Cortical representations of personally familiar objects and places: functional organization of the human posterior cingulate cortex. J Cogn Neurosci 17: 183–198.
82. Northoff G, Bermpohl F (2004) Cortical midline structures and the self. Trends Cogn Sci 8: 102–107.
83. Irish M, Lawlor BA, O'Mara SM, Coen RF (2010) Exploring the recollective experience during autobiographical memory retrieval in amnestic mild cognitive impairment. J Int Neuropsychol Soc 16: 546–555.
84. Rosen HJ, Allison SC, Schauer GF, Gorno Tempini ML, Weiner MW, et al. (2005) Neuroanatomical correlates of behavioural disorders in dementia. Brain 128: 2612–2625.
85. Sheldon S, Levine B (2013) Same as it ever was: Vividness modulates the similarities and differences between the neural networks that support retrieving remote and recent autobiographical memories. NeuroImage 83: 880–891.

7

Comparison of NOGA Endocardial Mapping and Cardiac Magnetic Resonance Imaging for Determining Infarct Size and Infarct Transmurality for Intramyocardial Injection Therapy Using Experimental Data

Noemi Pavo[1], Andras Jakab[2], Maximilian Y. Emmert[3,4,5], Georg Strebinger[1], Petra Wolint[3,4,5], Matthias Zimmermann[6], Hendrik Jan Ankersmit[6,7], Simon P. Hoerstrup[3,4,5], Gerald Maurer[1], Mariann Gyöngyösi[1]*

1 Department of Cardiology, Medical University of Vienna, Vienna, Austria, 2 Department of Biomedical Imaging and Image-guided Therapy, Medical University of Vienna, Vienna, Austria, 3 Swiss Centre for Regenerative Medicine, University of Zürich, Zürich, Switzerland, 4 Division of Surgical Research, University Hospital of Zürich, Zürich, Switzerland, 5 Clinic for Cardiovascular Surgery, University Hospital of Zürich, Zürich, Switzerland, 6 Department of Thoracic Surgery, Medical University of Vienna, Vienna, Austria, 7 Christian Doppler Laboratory for Cardiac and Thoracic Diagnosis and Regeneration, Vienna, Austria

Abstract

Objectives: We compared the accuracy of NOGA endocardial mapping for delineating transmural and non-transmural infarction to the results of cardiac magnetic resonance imaging (cMRI) with late gadolinium enhancement (LE) for guiding intramyocardial reparative substance delivery using data from experimental myocardial infarction studies.

Methods: Sixty domestic pigs underwent diagnostic NOGA endocardial mapping and cMRI-LE 60 days after induction of closed-chest reperfused myocardial infarction. The infarct size was determined by LE of cMRI and by delineation of the infarct core on the unipolar voltage polar map. The sizes of the transmural and non-transmural infarctions were calculated from the cMRI transmurality map using signal intensity (SI) cut-offs of >75% and >25% and from NOGA bipolar maps using bipolar voltage cut-off values of <0.8 mV and <1.9 mV. Linear regression analysis and Bland-Altman plots were used to determine correlations and systematic differences between the two images. The overlapping ratios of the transmural and non-transmural infarcted areas were calculated.

Results: Infarct size as determined by 2D NOGA unipolar voltage polar mapping correlated with the 3D cMRI-LE findings (r = 0.504, p<0.001) with a mean difference of 2.82% in the left ventricular (LV) surface between the two images. Polar maps of transmural cMRI and bipolar maps of NOGA showed significant association for determining of the extent of transmural infarction (r = 0.727, p<0.001, overlap ratio of 81.6±11.1%) and non-transmural infarction (r = 0.555, p<0.001, overlap ratio of 70.6±18.5%). NOGA overestimated the transmural scar size (6.81% of the LV surface) but slightly underestimated the size of the non-transmural infarction (−3.04% of the LV surface).

Conclusions: By combining unipolar and bipolar voltage maps, NOGA endocardial mapping is useful for accurate delineation of the targeted zone for intramyocardial therapy and is comparable to cMRI-LE. This may be useful in patients with contraindications for cMRI who require targeted intramyocardial regenerative therapy.

Editor: Joshua M. Hare, University of Miami Miller School of Medicine, United States of America

Funding: This study was sponsored by the Christian Doppler Laboratory for Cardiac and Thoracic Diagnosis and Regeneration, Vienna, Austria; by the Ludwig Boltzmann Institute Cluster of Cardiovascular Diseases; and by the Swiss Centre for Regenerative Medicine, University of Zurich, Zurich, Switzerland. The funders had no role in study design, data collection and analysis, decision to publish, or preparation of the manuscript.

Competing Interests: The authors have declared that no competing interests exist.

* Email: mariann.gyongyosi@meduniwien.ac.at

Introduction

The border zone of myocardial infarction (MI) represents myocardial areas with decreased viability and reduced wall motion capacity. Perfusion and transport of cell-death waste products, such as oxygen radicals and other metabolic substances, is impaired due to the close proximity to the non-perfused infarcted area, and this may account for the functional decline. These areas are targeted by cardiac regenerative therapies because regenerative cells delivered to these areas may survive and help restore cardiac function.

Compared to intracoronary or intravenous delivery, intramyocardial delivery of regenerative drugs, genes, or cells into the border zone of chronic myocardial ischemia results in higher retention of the applied substances, which may result in more effective therapy [1–4]. However, accurate real-time localization of this area for application of intramyocardial regenerative therapy remains a challenge. Cardiac magnetic resonance imaging (cMRI) with late gadolinium enhancement (LE) is the gold standard for assessing myocardial infarct size, infarct transmurality, and left ventricular (LV) function and for assessing the efficacy of cardiac therapies [5,6]. Identification of subendocardial or non-transmural infarcted areas using cMRI-LE would be ideal for guiding targeted intramyocardial regenerative therapy. However, cMRI is an off-line imaging modality, and there is a delay between diagnostic imaging and application of the therapy. Further, cMRI is contraindicated for patients with cMRI-non-compatible pacemakers or implantable defibrillators.

Three-dimensional (3D) NOGA endocardial mapping and electromagnetic guided percutaneous intramyocardial therapy is the method that is currently used for real-time (on-table) assessment of myocardial viability and for delineation of the infarct and infarct border zone [7–10]. The accuracy and reproducibility of NOGA maps for evaluating myocardial viability have been established [11–15], and this 3D imaging method has been compared with other 3D imaging methods such as myocardial scintigraphy, positron emission tomography, and cMRI [16–20]. Furthermore, histology, echocardiography, and other methods have confirmed that NOGA mapping can be used to correctly assess the size and severity of myocardial necrosis [21]. In order to assess the accuracy of the point-to-point sampling method of NOGA mapping, several research groups have developed fusion software for constructing hybrid images of cMRI and NOGA CARTO mapping [22–29]. These reports on a limited number of patients confirmed that there is good correlation between the two 3D images regarding the location and size of the infarction. However, the reports noted that NOGA mapping does not show good correlation with cMRI-LE in terms of the delineation of non-transmural areas. Moreover, the aim of these multimodality images was to find a focus for arrhythmogen substrates for ablation therapy to treat reentry tachycardias using unipolar and bipolar voltage electrocardiograms.

Here we focused on the accuracy of NOGA mapping to delineate transmural and non-transmural infarction by comparing it with cMRI-LE imaging. We investigated whether NOGA mapping is suitable for guiding intramyocardial drug or cell delivery using data from experimental myocardial infarction studies. We chose to use an animal model of closed chest reperfused MI. This is very similar to human primary percutaneous coronary intervention in acute MI, which simulates post-infarction left ventricular dysfunction.

We hypothesized that real-time, on-table 3D endocardial mapping using the NOGA system can accurately delineate the zone of decreased viability and non-transmural scars that is the target area for percutaneous intramyocardial therapy. Here we show that there is a significant correlation between the two images in terms of infarct size and the sizes of the transmural and non-transmural infarction, with high degree of overlap between endocardial mapping and cMRI-derived infarcted areas.

Materials and Methods

Experimental chronic left ventricular dysfunction post MI

Closed-chest reperfused acute MI was induced in 60 female farm pigs by percutaneous occlusion of the mid left anterior descending coronary artery. Sixty days later, the pigs underwent cMRI-LE images to confirm chronic myocardial infarction. Additional NOGA endocardial mapping was then performed 2±1 days later, just before the animals were euthanized, aiming to search for correlations between the two images.

Briefly, all pigs were sedated with ketamine hydrochloride (12 mg/kg), xylazine (1 mg/kg), and atropine (0.04 mg/kg) intramuscularly. The pigs were intubated intratracheally and anesthetized with isoflurane (1.5–2.5 vol%), O_2 (1.6–1.8 vol%), and N_2O (0.5 vol%). O_2 saturation, blood pressure, and electrocardiography were monitored continuously. After an arteriotomy of the right femoral artery, a 6F introducer sheath (Terumo Medical Corporation, Somerset, NJ, USA) was inserted. Heparin (200 IU/kg) was administered followed by selective angiography of the left coronary artery tree. A balloon catheter (3.0 mm in diameter, 9 mm long; Maverick, Boston Scientific Corp, Natick, MA, USA) was advanced into the left anterior descending coronary artery (LAD). After the origin of the second major diagonal branch, the mid LAD was occluded by inflation of the balloon at 5 atmospheres for 90 minutes, followed by deflation of the balloon to allow opening of the infarct-related artery and reperfusion of the ischemia-affected myocardium. The pigs were then allowed to recover from the anesthesia.

This study was carried out in strict accordance with the recommendations in the Guide for the Care and Use of Laboratory Animals of the National Institutes of Health. The protocol was approved by the Experimental Animal Care and Use Committee at the Faculty of Animal Science of the University of Kaposvar (Hungary) (Permit Numbers: 246/002/SOM2006/11/11 and 246/002/SOM2006/08/11). All procedures were performed under general anesthesia, and all efforts were made to minimize the suffering of the animals.

NOGA electroanatomical mapping of the LV

The electromechanical maps of the pigs were obtained 62±1 days after induction of acute MI. The principles and procedures of NOGA electroanatomical mapping have been described previously [7–10]. Briefly, the external reference patch, which contains a tip sensor, was taped onto the experimental animal's back below its heart. A 7 F introducer sheath was introduced into the left femoral artery, followed by administration of 5000 IU of unfractionated heparin. To begin the navigation process, a fully deflected NogaStar (Johnson & Johnson, Diamond Bar, CA) mapping catheter was introduced through the femoral sheath and was advanced inside the aorta under fluoroscopic guidance. Before entering the LV chamber, the mapping catheter was bent and then introduced through the aortic valve. As soon as the tail of the catheter was inside the LV, the catheter tip was straightened and orientated towards the apex. The first few endocardial points in different regions of the LV (apical point, outflow tract, and lateral and posterior points) were sampled to initiate a three-dimensional silhouette of the heart, which was then updated in real time with every new mapping point which facilitated further electromagnetic navigation with limited use of fluoroscopy.

At least four points were acquired in each of twelve myocardial segments. During the mapping process, simultaneous unipolar and bipolar electrocardiograms were recorded as well as the 3D location and orientation of the catheter tip of several sites within the LV cavity. The electrophysiological and mechanical data were integrated to create a color-coded 3D reconstruction of the LV chamber to facilitate assessment of the regional viability. The stability of the catheter-to-wall contact was evaluated at every location in real time, and only stable location points were accepted to create the 3D maps [9,10]. When constructing the NOGA maps, care was taken to correctly define the apex and the heart axis.

Using the movement of the catheter tip in the LV cavity, the end-diastolic, end-systolic volumes and global ejection fraction were calculated automatically. The average heart rate was calculated during the electroanatomical mapping procedure.

Evaluation of the NOGA maps

ImageJ for Windows (U.S. National Institutes of Health [NIH], Bethesda, Maryland, USA) was used to determine the relative size of the area of interest. The 3D unipolar (UPV) and bipolar (BiPV) voltages of each measuring point were displayed as two-dimensional polar maps (bull's eye format). The same discriminatory threshold values were used for all NOGA maps: <5 mV for non-viable infarcted area, 5–15 mV for infarct border zone and > 15 mV for normal viability in unipolar maps and <0.8 mV for transmural, 0.8–1.9 mV for non-transmural infarction and > 1.9 mV for normal myocardium in bipolar maps. These cut-off values are represented by the color-coding of the NOGA images and facilitate the identification of areas with reduced UPVs and BiPVs (Table 1, Fig. 1). As a next step, in order to validate the discriminatory threshold values for bipolar NOGA maps, we determined the correlation between MRI-based infarct area measurements and different discriminatory bipolar cut-off values. Specifically, we exported the raw images of the NOGA transmurality data (i.e. the bipolar recordings) into the image processing pipeline of Matlab R2010 for Windows, converted the image RGB (red-green-blue) color values into voltage values, and cropped the image to the cMRI-LE infarct area. Using 100 threshold steps (from 0.5 to 1.5 mV), we iteratively exported the NOGA-based transmurality areas to the cMRI transmurality maps and determined the correlation coefficient between the two images using different thresholds (25, 30, 50, 60, and 75% transmurality) (Fig. 2A).

In order to determine the BiPV cut-off that provides the best fit to the size of transmural and non-transmural cMRI-LE areas, we also tested 0.5–1.5 mV and 1.0–2.0 mV BiPV cut-offs (Fig. 3). The fibrous ring and cardiac valves, represented as red zones at the outer edge of the bull's eye NOGA maps, were excluded from analysis as they contained low UPVs and BiPVs that were indicative of non-contractile collagen structures [9,10].

The relative size of the infarct core, border areas, and normal myocardium was determined from the color-coded unipolar voltage polar map, and the sizes of the transmural and non-transmural infarction were delineated on the bipolar maps (Figs. 4 and 5). The demarcation and measurement of these areas on the NOGA maps was carried out by a researcher who was blinded to the results of the cMRI-LE.

cMRI-LE acquisitions

Cardiac magnetic resonance (cMRI) images were acquired on a 1.5 T Siemens Avanto Syngo B17 clinical scanner (Erlangen, Germany) with a phased-array coil and a vector ECG system. Functional (dynamic) images were acquired using a retrospective ECG-gated (HR: 80–100 beats/minute), steady-state free precession (SSFP - TRUFISP sequence) technique in short-axis and long-axis sections of the heart using 1.2-ms echo time (TE), 40-ms repetition time (TR), 25 phases, 50° flip angle, 360-mm field-of-view, 8-mm slice thickness, and a 256×256 image matrix. For quantitative measurement of infarct extent and transmurality, delayed enhancement diastolic phase short-axis images were obtained after injection of 0.05 mmol/kg of contrast medium using an inversion recovery prepared gradient-echo sequence. LE images were obtained 10 minutes after gadolinium contrast agent injection.

Analysis and visualization of cMRI images

In all cases, care was taken to include the entire heart volume from the apex to the level of the great vessels, and the entire left ventricle was included in the MRI analysis. Analysis was consistently restricted to slices between the apex and the basis on which the left ventricle myocardium is seen in 360 degrees. Image analysis was performed using Segment for Windows software (version 1.9; Medviso AB, Lund, Sweden) [30]. The extent and transmurality of the infarct was semi-automatically quantified on the 10-minute LE images using the "2SD" approach. During this procedure, hyperintense image pixels were tagged as infarcted if their signal intensity (SI) was greater than the mean value plus 2 standard deviations of the normal-appearing LV myocardium. Signal intensity was derived from the absolute value of the voxel intensity data, which were stored in the DICOM files from the cMRI-LE acquisitions.

The 3D infarct volume was determined both in absolute units and as a percentage of the total LV myocardium volume (Fig. 1). The entire LV was imaged by both NOGA and cMRI-LE in order to obtain an accurate volume measurement. The non-contractile mitral valve areas, which are clearly visible in both images, were excluded from the quantitative analysis of infarct size and transmurality.

Polar plots were derived from the infarct segmentations using segmental transmurality data. The corresponding bull's eye maps were processed to achieve the same apex, heart axis, and orientation as for NOGA maps.

For these visualizations, viability data from 8 apico-basal slices and 32 wall sectors per slice were interpolated and smoothed. The linear borders of 17 segments were overlaid on the images

---

Table 1. NOGA endocardial unipolar and bipolar map-derived cut-off values.

Cut-off value	Color on the NOGA map	Definition
Unipolar voltage map		
>15 mV	Blue, violet	Normal tissue
5–15 mV	Yellow, green	Border zone of infarction
<5 mV	Red	Area of myocardial infarction
Bipolar voltage map		
>1.9 mV	Blue, violet	Normal tissue
0.8–1.9 mV	Yellow, green	Non-transmural infarction
<0.8 mV	Red	Transmural infarction

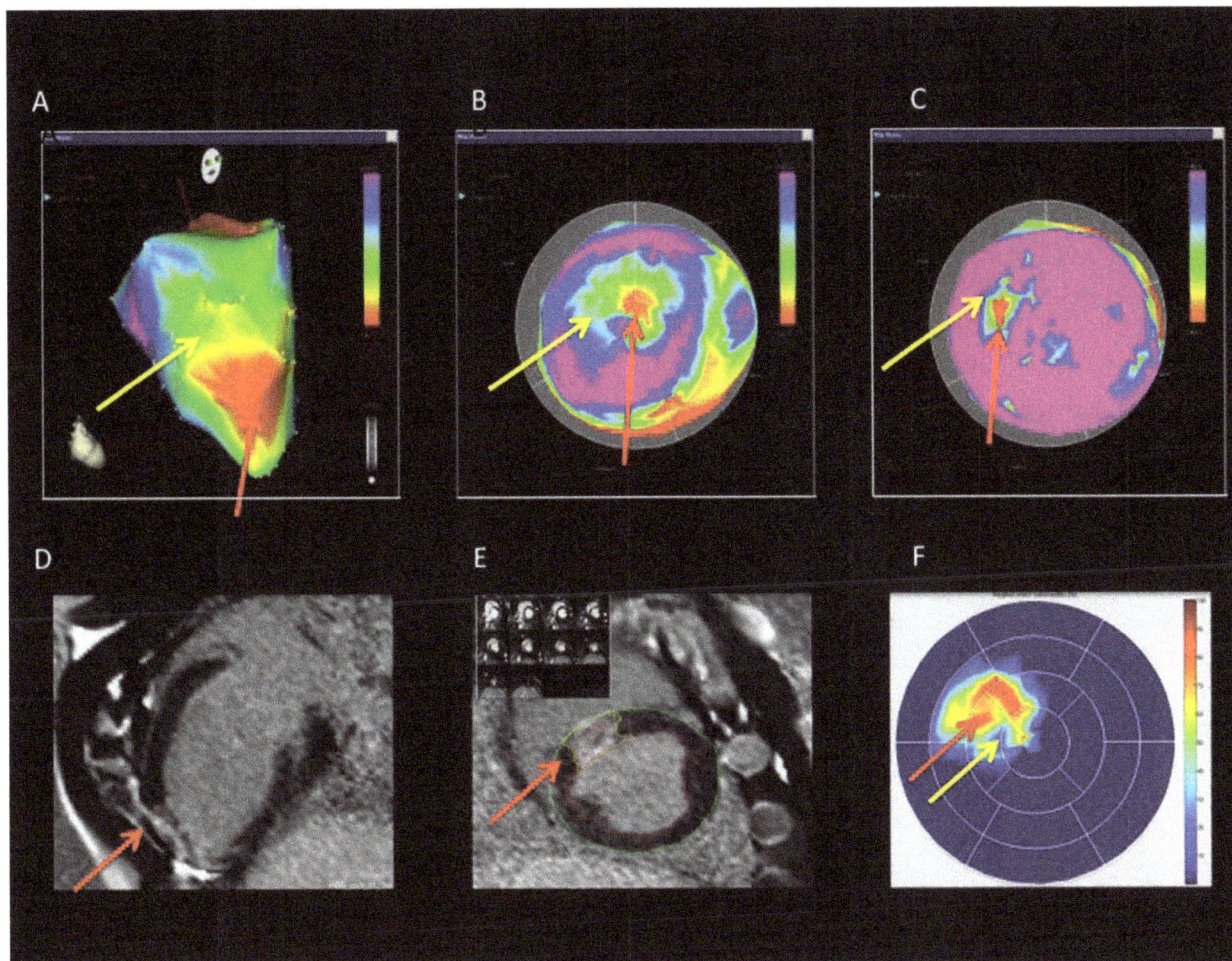

Figure 1. NOGA endocardial mapping and cardiac magnetic resonance imaging (cMRI) of a pig with chronic myocardial ischemia. A. 3D NOGA mapping showing anterior, anteroseptal, and apical myocardial infarction. Red indicates the infarct core (red arrow), the surrounding green-yellow area shows the border zone of infarction (yellow arrow). B. The corresponding unipolar voltage polar map. The color-coding is the same as in A. C. The bipolar voltage polar map of the same pig. Red indicates the transmural infarction (red arrow); yellow-green indicates the non-transmural infarction (yellow arrow), and blue-pink indicates normal myocardium. D. cMRI with late enhancement reveals the myocardial scar (red arrow). Long axis image. E. cMRI late enhancement short axis images with myocardial infarction (red arrow). Quantitative size of infarction was assessed by dividing of the myocardium to 8 slices from heart basis to apex (left upper corner). F. A cMRI transmurality polar map shows the transmural infarction (red arrow) with a surrounding area of non-transmural infarction (yellow arrow).

graphically to help interpret the images using "classical" segmental nomenclature, while the interpolated data originated from 32 sections per slice. The endo- and epicardial borders were segmented, and a segmental model was fitted on the left ventricle model (32 sections per slice). Using the standard transmurality analysis feature of the Segment software (Medviso Inc., Lund, Sweden), the midline was calculated for each section of the LV myocardium. The transmurality of the infarct is given as the radial projection of the segmented scar volume on the midline, summed for each section.

By applying two-dimensional planimetry to the polar plots, we performed two distinct measurements of the transmurality of the infarct. The extents of the transmural or non-transmural infarct and normal areas were defined as the percentage of sectors in which the SI was >75% (infarct core), 51–75% (border zone of infarction), 25–50% (non-transmural infarction), or <25% (normal) [22]. Alternatively, SI>60% was defined as transmural infarct, 31–60% as non-transmural infarct, and <30% as a normal area [21]. To calculate the areas, we used the raw transmurality

data from 32 sections per slice, as noted above. All MRI area measurements are reported as the percentage of segments in the threshold range divided by the total number of segments.

Dynamic MR images were analyzed for myocardial wall movement and functional parameters. We carried out semi-automatic segmentation of the LV endocardial and epicardial borders while the end-diastolic volume (EDV), end-systolic volume (ESV), global LV ejection fraction (EF), and cardiac output (CO) were calculated automatically on short-axis images.

Overlap ratio

The overlap ratio between the cMRI and NOGA bipolar transmurality maps was calculated as follows [28] (Fig. 6):

(NOGA bipolar map overlap area + cMRI transmural map overlap area)/(NOGA bipolar low voltage area + cMRI transmurality area)

For the overlap ratio of the transmural, non-transmural and the combined transmural and non-transmural (not normal) areas the following cut-off values were used:

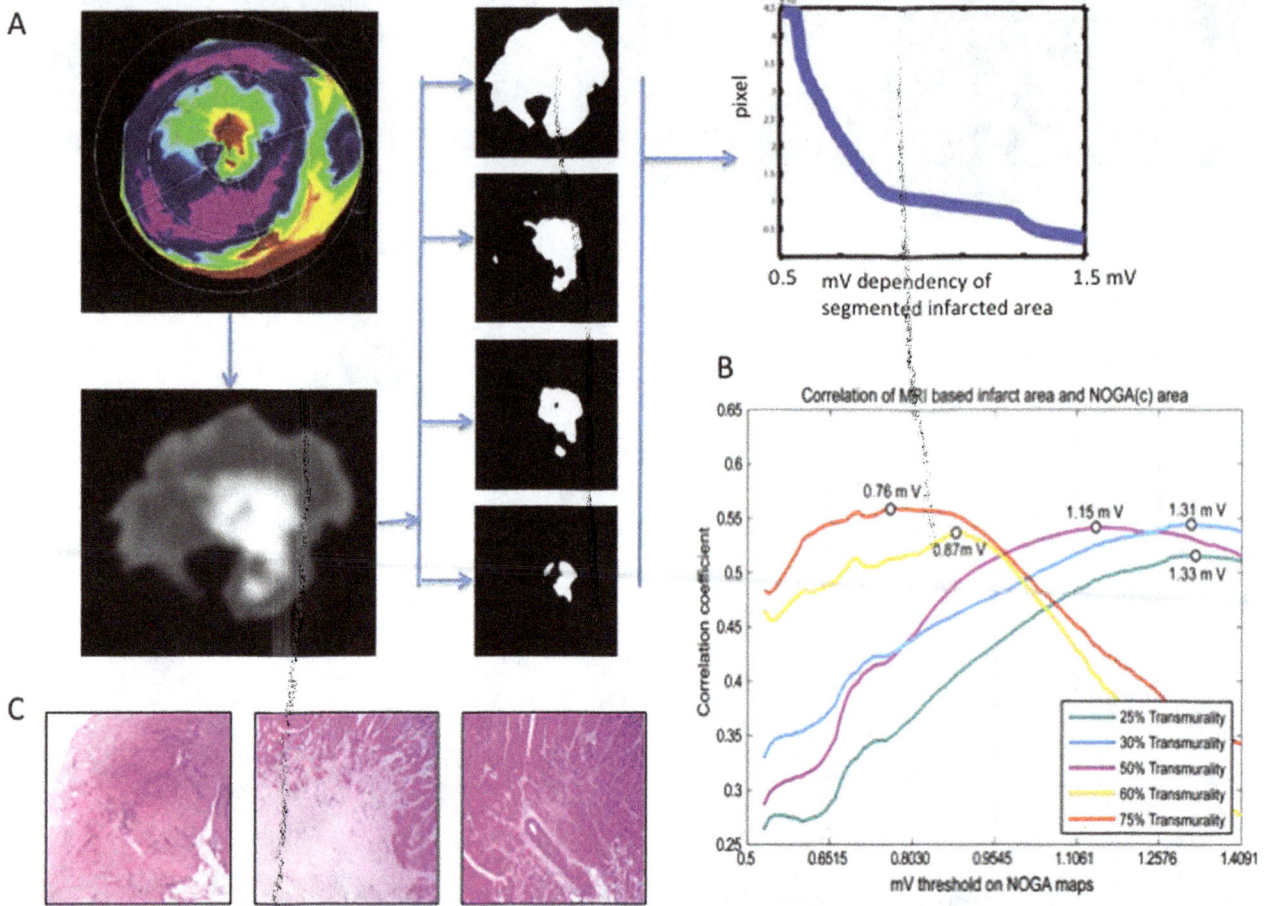

Figure 2. Magnet resonance imaging- (MRI-) derived NOGA bipolar threshold values for infarct transmurality. A. Iterative thresholding of voltage maps (left panel). The original NOGA maps were cropped to infarct areas, converted to a mV scale, then iteratively thresholded using 100 steps from 0.5 to 1.5 mV. The middle panel shows examples of the iterative thresholding process. The right panel shows the association between the area of infarction and the applied mV threshold. B. Voltage-threshold dependence of the correlation between NOGA maps and areas on an MRI. The maximum correlation coefficient is shown for each line plot. C. Histological correlations of transmural (left) and non-transmural (middle) infarctions and normal heart tissue (right). Samples were taken from areas with bipolar voltage values <0.8 mV, between 0.8–1.9 mV, and>1.9 mV with corresponding cMRI-LE transmurality values of>75%, 50%, and <25%, respectively. Magnification: 2x.

– Transmurality overlap ratio: between a NOGA bipolar map area with BipV <0.8 mV and a cMRI transmurality area with SI>75%;

– Non-transmural areas overlap ratio: between a NOGA bipolar map area with BipV 0.8-1.9 mV and a cMRI transmurality area with SI 25–75%;

– Combined transmural and non-transmural (not normal) area overlap ratio: between a NOGA bipolar map area with BipV <1.9 mV and a cMRI transmurality area with SI>25% (Figs. 4 and 5).

Overlap>60% was considered good accuracy [28], and 50–60% overlap was considered moderate accuracy (arbitrary value).

Histology

Myocardial samples were collected from transmural and non-transmural infarctions and from normal heart tissue. These were areas with bipolar voltage values <0.8 mV, from 0.8–1.9 mV, and>1.9 mV with corresponding cMRI-LE transmurality values of>75%, 50%, and <25%, respectively. The samples were stored in 4.5% buffered formalin for at least 24 h and embedded in paraffin. Sections were cut into 4- to 6-μM thick slices and stained with hematoxylin-eosin.

Statistical analysis

Continuous variables are presented as mean values ± standard deviation. The correlation between NOGA- and cMRI-derived parameters (infarct size, transmural and non-transmural infarct size) was calculated by linear regression analysis using Pearson Product Moment Correlation and Bland-Altman plots. Linear regression and Bland-Altman analysis was performed using Matlab R2010 software for Windows. During the iterative fitting of the linear function, a "least absolute residual" robust regression approach was used [31]. For interpretation of the correlations between 2 images the standardized nomenclature was used: if the correlation coefficient is greater than 0.5 is large, 0.5–0.3 is moderate, and 0.3–0.1 is a small correlation [32].

In order to choose the correct BiPV cut-off values for determining the transmural and non-transmural scars, all UPVs were also correlated with the corresponding BiPVs using linear regression analysis. Using a 5 mV UPV value as the cut-off for viability/non-viability, receiver operator curve (ROC) analysis was

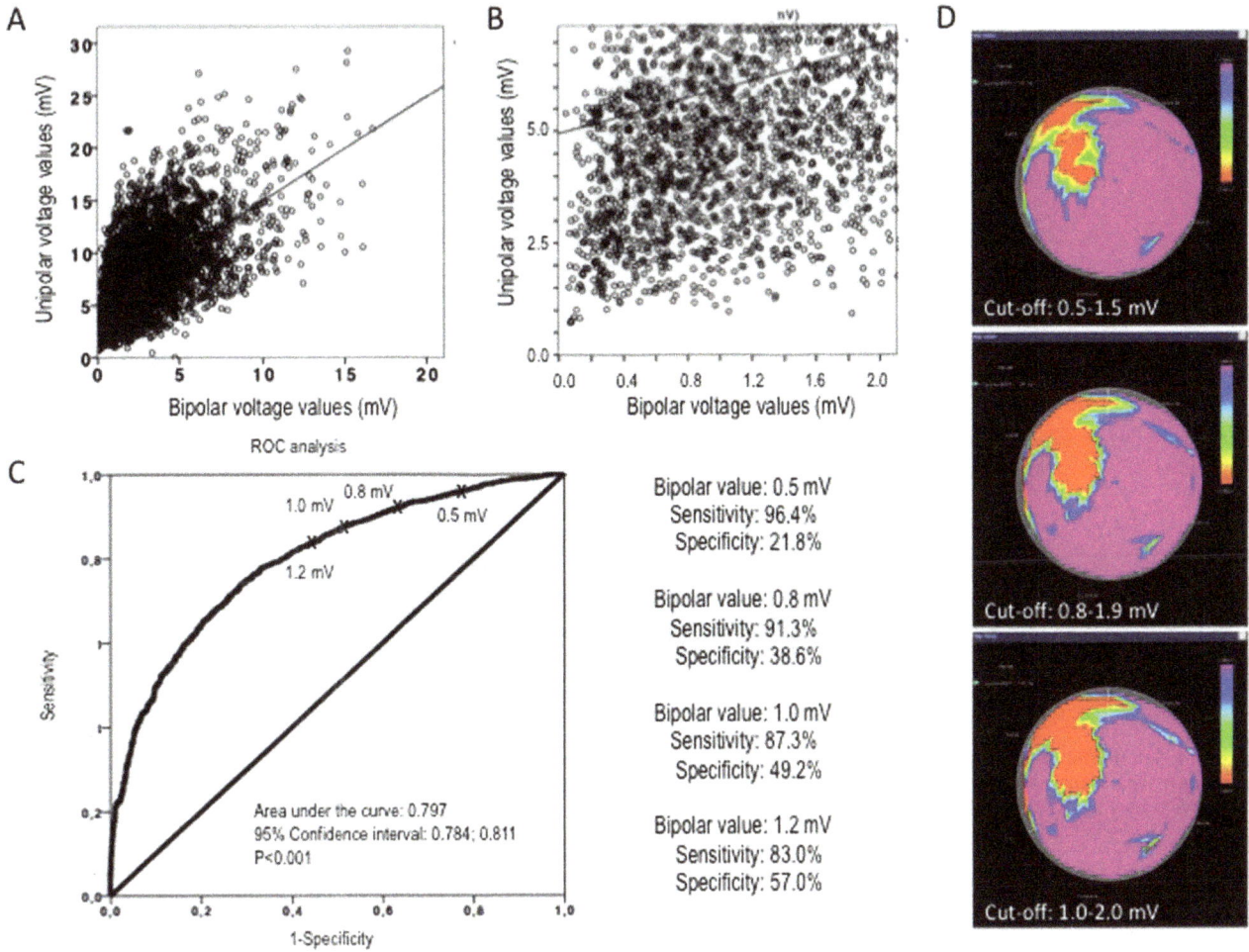

Figure 3. Determination of the bipolar voltage (BiPV) cut-off value for calculating the transmural and non-transmural infarct size using unipolar voltage values. A. Linear correlation between unipolar and bipolar voltage values. B. Part of the correlation showing the non-viable range defined as unipolar voltage values <5 mV. C. Receiver operator characteristics curve for determination of different bipolar voltage cut-off values. D. Display of bipolar maps using different cut-offs.

performed, and the sensitivity, specificity of different BiPV values, and the area under the curve, with 95% confidence intervals, were calculated.

For all statistical analyses, a p-value <0.05 was considered statistically significant.

Results

There were no complications during the NOGA and cMRI-LE procedures that required additional medication or cardiopulmonary resuscitation.

Correlation of NOGA threshold values with MRI-based transmurality

Depending on the threshold values applied to the NOGA bipolar voltage maps, the correlations between the different cut-offs of the two images were r = 0.27–0.57. The 75% MRI transmurality areas showed the best correlation with the NOGA-based areas using a cut-off of 0.76 mV, while the 60% transmurality areas correlated best with NOGA maps using a 0.87 mV threshold. The validation experiment resulted in a cut-off value of 1.3 mV for 25% transmurality. In order to exclude non-

transmural ischemia, we used the usual value of 1.9 mV for normal, non-infarcted areas (Figure 2B). Notably, these cut-offs correlated well with the histological findings (Fig. 2C), confirming the proprietary diagnosis of transmural and non-transmural areas.

cMRI and NOGA mapping results

The cMRI-LE and NOGA endocardial mapping results are summarized in Tables 2 and 3. NOGA mapping and cMRI-LE showed similar results for LV volumes and global EF. Heart rates were slightly higher during the NOGA procedure, probably due to the longer procedure time.

The NOGA endocardial maps contained a mean of 202±31 (range: 152–295) mapping points per animal, with a mapping point distribution of 16.8±5.5 points per segment of the 12-segment view. The mapping points were connected automatically if the distance between points was less than 15 mm. The mean time for the NOGA procedure was 35±9 min.

The BiPV values correlated significantly with the UPV values (Fig. 3). ROC analysis showed that a BiPV value of 0.8 mV as the non-transmural cut-off value had a sensitivity>90% and low but acceptable specificity. Display of the bipolar maps with different cut-offs revealed small differences between the images, with a

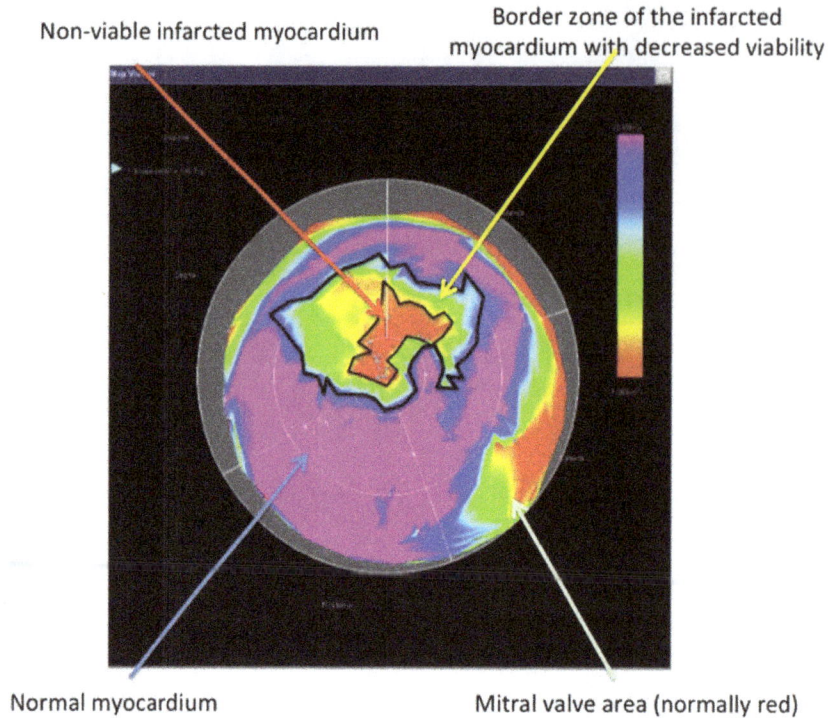

Figure 4. Schematic illustration of the planimetric calculation of the size of the infarct core and the size of the border zone of the infarction with decreased viability in the NOGA endocardial mapping. Red indicates the infarct core, and green-yellow indicates the surrounding area that has decreased viability.

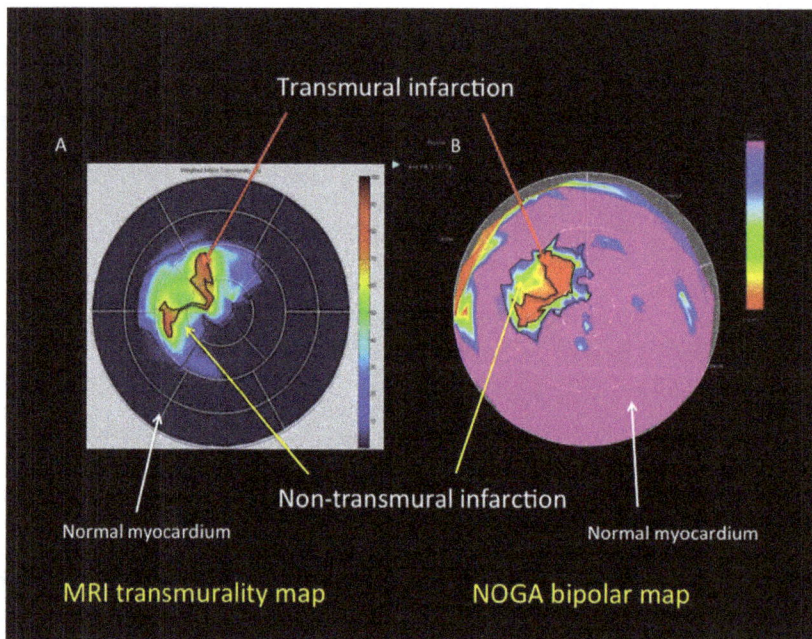

Figure 5. Schematic illustration of the planimetric calculation of the transmural and non-transmural infarct sizes as shown in polar maps from cardiac magnetic resonance imaging (cMRI) and NOGA endocardial mapping. A. Planimetric calculations of the sizes of the transmural and non-transmural infarction by cMRI. B. Planimetric calculations of the sizes of the transmural and non-transmural infarction in a NOGA bipolar voltage map.

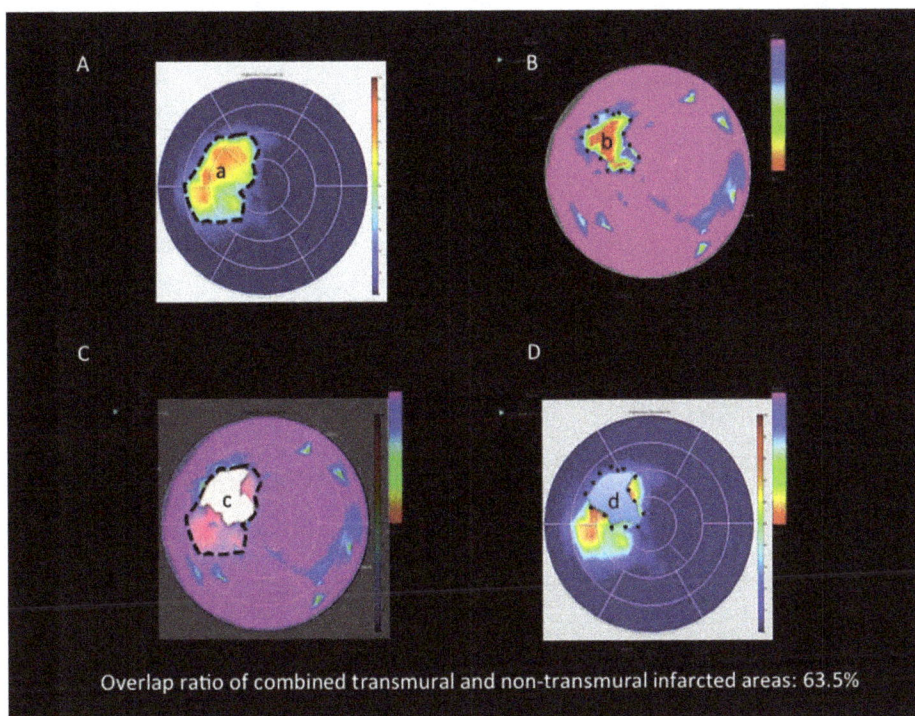

Overlap ratio of combined transmural and non-transmural infarcted areas: 63.5%

Figure 6. Calculation of the overlapping ratio of the transmural plus the non-transmural infarction by cardiac magnetic resonance imaging (cMRI) and NOGA endocardial mapping. A. cMRI transmurality polar map. B. NOGA bipolar polar map. C and D. Overlap of the cMRI and NOGA polar maps. a: The size of the transmural and non-transmural infarction by cMRI; b: the size of transmural and non-transmural infarction by NOGA bipolar mapping; c: overlap of the NOGA bipolar infarct shape on a cMRI polar map; d: overlap of the cMRI infarct shape on a NOGA bipolar map. The overlapping ratio was calculated as follows: (c+d)/(a+b).

transmural infarct size of $12.5 \pm 8.7\%$ using a 0.5-mV cut-off value, $14.1 \pm 6.2\%$ using a 0.8-mV cut-off value, and $16.8 \pm 5.3\%$ using a 1-mV BiPV cut-off value, with no statistically significant differences between the 3 area measurements. Based on the best overlap ratio between the two images, a BiPV cut-off of 0.8–1.9 mV was used for further analysis.

The unipolar voltage map-derived scar size (UPV<5 mV) showed a moderate association with the transmural scar size as determined by bipolar maps (BiPV<0.8 mV) $(r = 0.385,$ $p = 0.002)$. There was better concordance between the border zone of infarction (UPV 5–15 mV) and non-transmural scars (BiPV 0.8–1.9 mV) $(r = 0.457,$ p<0.001). The total size of the

ischemic area showed good correlation between the two maps $(r = 0.575,$ p<0.001).

Correlation of infarct size as determined by cMRI-LE and NOGA mapping

There was a significant correlation $(r = 0.504,$ p<0.001) between the infarct size as determined using the NOGA unipolar voltage polar map and the size determined by cMRI-LE. The Bland-Altman plot showed that NOGA mapping resulted in a systematically higher infarct size compared to cMRI-LE, with a mean difference between the two images of $2.82 \pm 7.43\%$ in the LV surface (Fig. 7).

Table 2. Endocardial NOGA mapping results.

NOGA electromechanical mapping	Value (mean ±SD) (n = 60)
End-diastolic volume	108±12 mL
End-systolic volume	67.1±9.6 mL
Stroke volume	41.3±11.6 mL
Left ventricular ejection fraction	38.7±7.6%
Heart rate	110±7 bpm
Relative size of the infarct core (area of unipolar voltage <5 mV)	19.5±8.1%
Size of the area of border zone of the infarction (area of unipolar voltage 5–10 mV)	20.4±9.7%
Size of the transmural infarction (area of bipolar voltage <0.8 mV)	14.1±6.2%
Size of the non-transmural infarction (area of bipolar voltage 0.8–1.9 mV)	11.6±5.6%

Table 3. Results of cardiac magnetic resonance (cMRI) with late enhancement.

cMRI	Value (mean ±SD) (n = 60)
End-diastolic volume	106±22 mL
End-systolic volume	67.8±22 mL
Stroke volume	38.2±8.4 mL
Left ventricular ejection fraction	37.6±8.9%
Heart rate	102±11 bpm
Cardiac output	4.2±1.1 L/min
Cardiac index	3.7±0.9 L/min/m^2
Left ventricular myocardial mass	108±15 g
Left ventricular myocardial volume	103±14 mL
Relative infarct size of left ventricular myocardial mass	16.9±6.3%
Volume of myocardial infarction	15.7±6.5 mL
0%–30%–60%–100% SI for transmurality	
Size of transmural infarction if SI>60%	10.4±5.1%
Size of non-transmural infarction if SI = 31–60%	8.4±3.9%
Size of non-infarcted tissue if SI<30%	81.2±6.7%
0%–25%–50%–75%–100% SI for transmurality	
Size of transmural infarction if SI>75%	6.4±5.6%
Size of border zone of transmural infarction if SI = 51–75%	7.5±4.3%
Size of non-transmural infarction if SI = 25–50%	6.7±2.9%
Size of non-infarcted tissue if SI<25%	79.4±7.6%

SI: signal intensity.

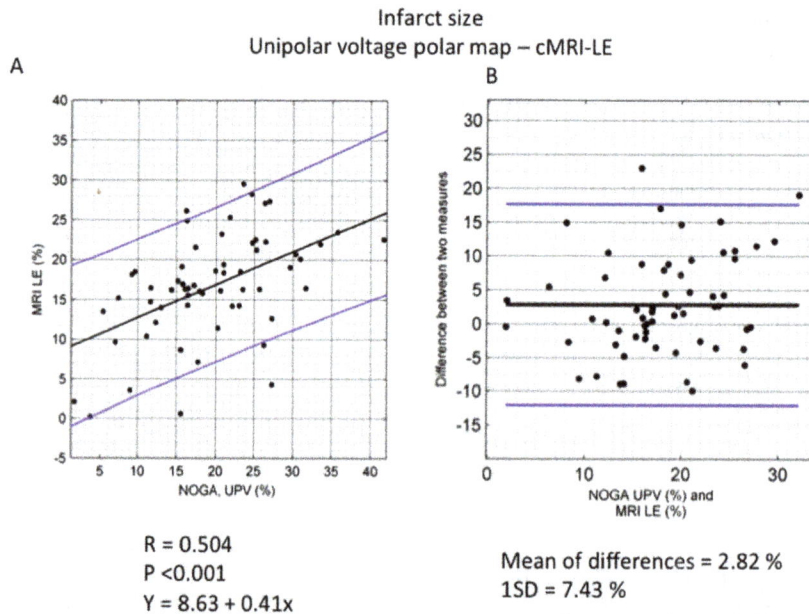

Infarct size
Unipolar voltage polar map – cMRI-LE

A

R = 0.504
P <0.001
Y = 8.63 + 0.41x

B

Mean of differences = 2.82 %
1SD = 7.43 %

Figure 7. Correlation between NOGA endocardial mapping and cardiac magnetic resonance imaging (cMRI) and statistical analysis of the determination of infarct size. A. Regression equation between the size of the infarct core as determined on a unipolar voltage map (UPV) and as determined using late enhancement cMRI. B. Bland-Altman plot of the size of the infarct core as determined on a unipolar voltage map and the size as determined using late enhancement cMRI. Mean (black line) ±2SD (blue line).

Correlation of transmural infarct size as determined by cMRI and NOGA mapping

Using SI>75% and NOGA BipV <0.8 mV, the correlation between the two images was r = 0.727 (p<0.001) for the size of the transmural infarction. NOGA bipolar mapping resulted in a larger transmural infarction size than did cMRI-LE, with a mean difference of 6.81±4.39%) in the LV surface.

Using cut-offs for infarct transmurality of SI>60% and NOGA BipV<0.8 mV, the correlation was slightly lower (r = 0.576, p< 0.001), with a mean difference between the two images of 2.14%±5.62% of LV surface.

Correlation between cMRI and NOGA mapping regarding non-transmural infarct size

Using SI = 51–75% and NOGA BipV 0.8–1.9 mV to define non-transmural infarction, the correlation between the two images was r = 0.555 (p<0.001). NOGA bipolar mapping resulted in a smaller area of non-transmural infarction, with a mean difference of 3.04±5.92% between the two images (Fig. 8).

Using SI = 31–60% and NOGA BipV 0.8–1.9 mV as cut-offs for non-transmural infarction, the correlation was slightly higher

(r = 0.657, p<0.001), with a mean difference between the two images of 3.23±4.56% of LV surface.

Overlap ratio

The overlap ratio was 81.6±11.1% and 70.6±18.5% for delineation of the transmural and non-transmural infarction size on the cMRI and NOGA images, respectively. None of the images showed an overlapping accuracy below 60% regarding transmural infarction. Regarding non-transmurality, two of the 60 animals (3.3%) showed an overlapping ratio between 50% and 60%, which was considered moderate agreement between the two imaging methods.

The overlap ratio of the combined transmural and non-transmural infarction was 70.2±12.2%.

Discussion

Our results indicate that NOGA electroanatomical mapping is accurate enough to guide targeted intramyocardial therapy if both unipolar and bipolar maps are used. The results of NOGA were comparable to those of cMRI-LE, regarding the extent of the transmural and non-transmural scars and viable and reduced viability myocardial areas.

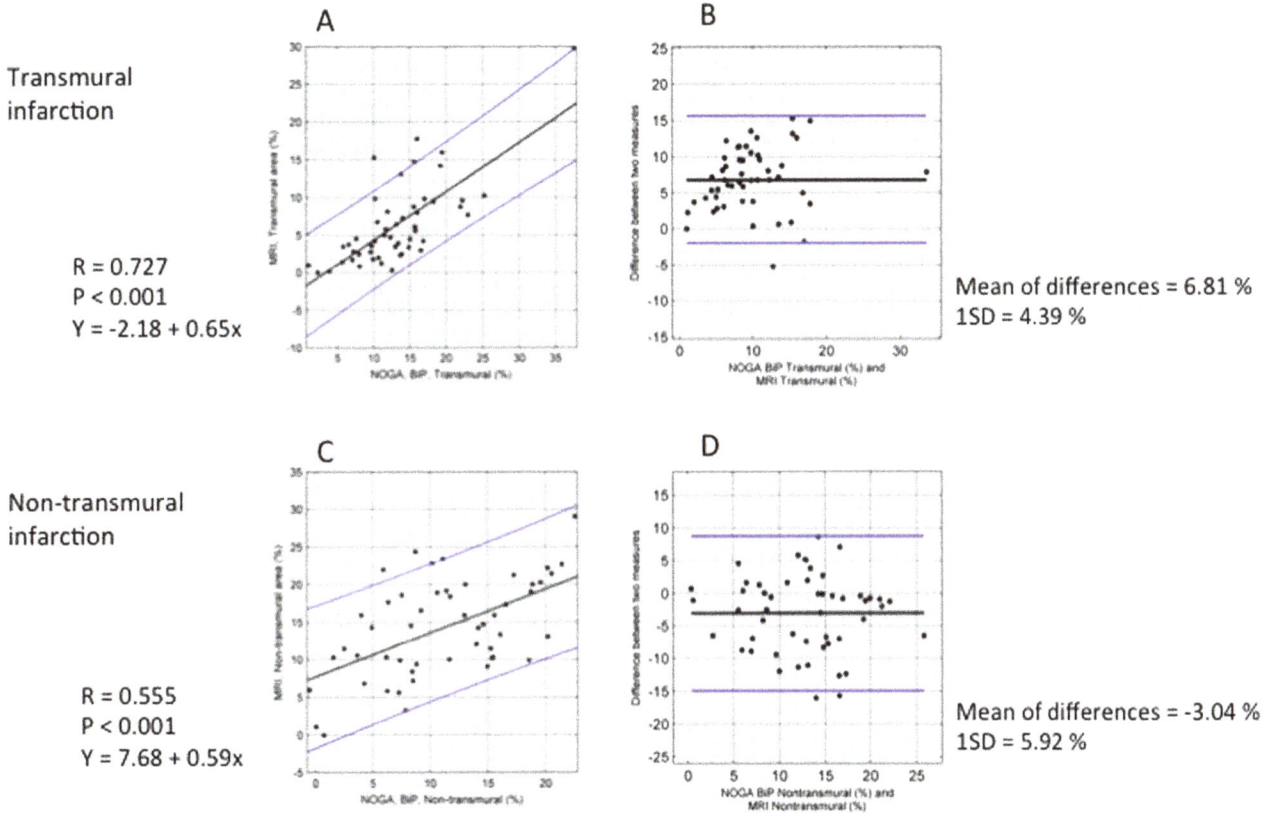

Figure 8. Correlation between NOGA endocardial mapping and cardiac magnetic resonance imaging (cMRI) and statistical analysis of the determinations of transmural and non-transmural infarction. A. Regression equation between the size of the transmural infarction as determined on a bipolar voltage map and the size as determined using cMRI. B. Bland-Altman plot of the size of the transmural infarction as determined on a bipolar voltage map and the size as determined using cMRI. Mean (black line) ±2SD (blue line). C. Regression equation between the size of the non-transmural infarction as determined on a bipolar voltage map and the size as determined using cMRI. D. Bland-Altman plot of the size of the non-transmural infarction as determined on a bipolar voltage map and the size as determined using cMRI. Mean (black line) ±2SD (blue line).

The main difference between the two 3D images is that different sampling methods are used to construct them. The NOGA 3D LV shape is constructed by point-to-point measurements, which is in contrast with the other 3D methods, such as cMRI-LE, which have a spatial resolution of 1.4 mm per voxel. For map construction, a 15-mm point-to-point distance was used by endocardial mapping, while an in-plane resolution of 1–2 mm with an 8-mm slice thickness was utilized for cMRI-LE analysis. Accordingly, the accuracy of the NOGA map depends mainly on the number of gathered and measured points and on the quality of the acquired points used to construct the 3D map. Difficulties in reaching some regions with the mapping catheter due to LV cavity structures such as the papillary muscles or the occurrence of ventricular arrhythmias due to touching vulnerable ischemic areas might lead to insufficient sampling, resulting in incomplete mapping. Nevertheless, unipolar voltage mapping overestimated the infarct size by just 2.82% of the entire LV endocardial surface, and bipolar mapping overestimated the transmural scar by just 6.82% of the LV. These estimates are acceptable for performing intramyocardial procedures safely and accurately. The overestimation of the infarct size and transmural scar as compared to cMRI-LE might result from the quantitative comparison of 2D NOGA polar maps and 3D cMRI-LE and 2D transmurality cMRI-LE images. According to our results, both the unipolar and bipolar voltage maps showed wider zones of interest than on cMRI, which may raise the risk of injecting reparative substances into normal myocardium. The intramyocardial injections are oriented into the non-transmural infarct or into areas with decreased viability. Different cut-offs are suggested for viability and transmurality thresholds in the literature; there are no universally agreed-upon definitions for these terms. Of course, the operators should try to make sure that the intramyocardial injections are made into the correct area, but an injection may be made into the "normal" myocardium if stronger cut-off criteria for non-normal territory are used. However, regenerative cells or other material delivered into the lane neighboring the non-transmural infarction have a good chance of being retained, being functional, and migrating or penetrating into the ischemic area, so a wider zone might result in more effective and safe treatment.

The sizes of the unipolar voltage scar and border zone differed from the sizes of transmural and non-transmural infarction as determined on the bipolar maps. Although the total size of the unhealthy areas on the unipolar and bipolar polar maps showed good correlation, the size of the infarction and border area determined on the unipolar maps was systematically larger than the size of the transmural and non-transmural regions on the bipolar maps. This is not surprising, because an infarct area contains heterogeneously viable myocytes that can be apoptotic or hibernating. Accordingly, the infarct core and the border area (i.e. the extent of infarction) do not necessarily overlap the transmural and non-transmural infarction (i.e. the infarction severity) because the infarct core may include transmural and non-transmural necrotic areas.

The unipolar voltage values represent a summation of the action potentials of the surrounding endocardial surface areas, while the bipolar voltage values represent the amplified difference between the tip of the unipolar electrode and the additional proximal electrode placed within the catheter. Accordingly, a non-transmural infarction with severe endocardial (but not epicardial) necrosis may appear to be an infarct core in the unipolar map. This might explain the differences between the unipolar and bipolar NOGA maps, and between the NOGA maps and other 3D images that measure infarct size. Nevertheless, using both (uni- and bipolar) maps of the NOGA images, information about both the extent and the severity of infarction are available real-time, on-table during a procedure, in contrast to off-line images such as cMRI-LE or myocardial single photon emission computed tomography.

Additionally, to set the correct and right cut-off values of the NOGA maps is of great importance. Several authors used several different cut-off values for definition of viability using the unipolar voltage maps, while the usage of bipolar maps is less common, probably due to the small range of not normal values (0–1.9 mV of interest) suggesting less precise differentiations. We have measured the transmural and non-transmural scars on the cMRI-LE image using two different SI cut-offs, because a SI between 25% and 50% suggests a false positive non-transmural infarction. When the cMRI transmurality threshold is lowered to 60% from 75% and to 31–60% from 51–75%, the size of the transmural and non-transmural infarct areas increase, and the correlations are slightly lower and higher, respectively. The SI of 30% and 60% for cut-off of non-transmural and transmural scars gave a better correlation with slight overestimation of the non-transmural scar by 3.23% of the LV. Since the endocardial injections should target non-transmural infarct areas, higher correlation between the two images in that region is desirable.

Comparison of our results with literature data

The need to localize the arrhythmogenic focus for ablation during catheter-based electrophysiological procedure prompted several research groups to develop hybrid software that analyzes the 3D images of both NOGA maps and cMRI-LE. Fusion of cMRI with electroanatomical mapping of the LV proved to be successful with a registration error of 3.8 ± 0.6 mm [22], with visual mismatches between the NOGA scars and LE in cMRI, particularly in patients with inferior infarction [22]. To enhance the accuracy of the electroanatomical mapping relative to cMRI-LE for the determination of myocardial scars with a presumed arrhythmogenic focus, different cut-off values were tested: 1.5 mV for non-transmural scars and 0.5 mV for dense scars [22]; 1.0 mV [28], 1.3 mV [23], 1.54 mV [24], 1.55 mV [26], and 1.9 mV [27] for bipolar maps; and 5.8 mV [23], 6.52 mV [24], 6.9 mV [18], 6.78 mV [26], 6.7 mV [27], and 5.1 mV [28] for unipolar maps. This reflects the uncertainty of finding the arrhythmogenic focus with electroanatomical mapping alone and emphasizes the visual mismatch between the two images in certain cases. In contrast with these studies, the sample size in our animal study was much larger (n = 60), but we did not use fusion software. Instead, we compared the 2D maps of the NOGA images with the 3D LE and 2D transmurality map of the cMRI. Nevertheless, we did not search for a single focus but rather for an area with reduced viability.

Limitations

We did not use local linear shortening maps of the NOGA for delineating of the hibernating myocardium characterized by preserved viability and decreased segmental wall motion [12], because of the lower accuracy of the local linear shortening map and higher discordance with cMRI [9] regarding the segmental wall motion abnormalities. We overlaid the two images in order to determine the overlapping accuracies, while other research groups used 3D fusion software. Accordingly, our method has several shortcomings in the technique used. The study reports comparisons of 2D transmurality cMRIs and NOGA bipolar maps as well as comparisons of the 2D projection of the NOGA-derived infarct size and the 3D cMRI-LE-derived infarct size. However, both imaging modalities for quantitatively determining infarct size use standardized image processing functions of the software and are widely used.

We are aware that there are ongoing efforts to fuse 3D NOGA endocardial maps and cardiac MRIs to determine the similarities of infarct location and extent. Although numerous percutaneous intramyocardial therapy studies are currently underway with the aim of determining the optimal injection location, currently there is no commercially available 3D MRI-NOGA fusion software. The comparisons of cMRI and NOGA polar maps published previously lack some of the refinements we used, such as comparison of the transmurality map with the bipolar map and calculation of the overlapping ratio.

Unfortunately, we could not perform 3D volumetric co-registration of the compared modalities, as currently we do not have an image-processing tool with which to conduct such a comparison. The spatial correspondence was ensured by (1) similar selection of the basal and apical slice positions and (2) similar orientation of the bull's eye maps. The definition of sector orientation was based on manual selection of the right ventricular insertion point (sector 0) on the most basal MRI slice of the left ventricular myocardium. A real value of the fusion of the off-line cMRI-LE and on-table NOGA endocardial mapping would be the real-time display of the actual catheter position and location of the intramyocardial therapy on the reconstructed hybrid (cMRI and NOGA) image; which software is currently not available.

We have included the NOGA-derived volumetric measurements. The similarities between the NOGA-derived and cMRI-derived end-diastolic and end-systolic volume and calculated stroke volume and ejection fraction (Tables 2 and 3) ensure the acquisition of the entire LV map of the NOGA procedure and also ensure that the two images are comparable.

The use of 2SD method of cMRI-LE might overestimate the infarct size, as compared with the 5SD or "full width at half maximum" (FWHM) method. In our experience, it has not been the case that the 5SD method better reflects the infarct size compared to the 2SD approach, and there are data in the literature that show a higher correlation coefficient for the 2SD approach than the 5SD approach [33]. The FWHM method might correlate better with post-mortem measurements, but this

approach has not yet been implemented into the software we used for our data analysis. Based on the different sampling modes and standardized segmentation of both MRI (17 segments divided into 6 basal, 6 mid and 5 apical segments) and NOGA (9 segments divided into 4 basal, 4 mid and 1 apex segments), direct comparison of segmental mean values to search for a mathematical cut-off for unipolar and bipolar values based on MRI cut-off values would require extensive digital processing and adaptation of both images. However, we correlated the unipolar and bipolar voltage values and calculated different bipolar voltage cut-offs using ROC analysis. Additionally, we have determined the optimal bipolar cut-offs using iterative thresholding and calculated the transmural and non-transmural infarct areas using 3 cut-offs and compared these results with those of the cMRI-LE data. However, we did not search unipolar voltage threshold values based on cMRI-LE images because voltage maps correspond to myocardial viability and cMRI is not the first-choice imaging method for viability assessment. Extensive research has been performed to establish cut-offs for viable, non-viable, and hibernating myocardium using imaging technologies such as myocardial scintigraphy and positron emission tomography [9]. We used these literature-based cut-off values to calculate infarct size.

Conclusions

Our results demonstrate the usefulness of unipolar and bipolar maps generated using real-time electroanatomical mapping for targeted intramyocardial regenerative therapy. NOGA mapping showed good concordance with the off-line gold standard, cMRI-LE imaging. NOGA mapping may be useful in patients with contraindications for cMRI who require targeted intramyocardial regenerative therapy.

Author Contributions

Conceived and designed the experiments: NP AJ ME SH MG. Performed the experiments: NP AJ ME SH MG. Analyzed the data: NP AJ ME GS PW MZ HJA GM MG. Contributed reagents/materials/analysis tools: AJ PW GS MZ. Wrote the paper: NP MG.

References

1. Freyman T, Polin G, Osman H, Crary J, Lu M, et al. (2006) A quantitative, randomized study evaluating three methods of mesenchymal stem cell delivery following myocardial infarction. Eur Heart J 27: 1114–22.

2. Perin EC, Silva GV, Assad JAR, Vela D, Buja LM, et al. (2008) Comparison of intracoronary and transendocardial delivery of allogeneic mesenchymal cells in a canine model of acute myocardial infarction. J Mol Cell Cardiol 44: 486–495.

3. Dib N, Khawaja H, Varner S, McCarthy M, Campbell A (2011) Cell therapy for cardiovascular disease: a comparison of methods of delivery. J Cardiovasc Transl Res. 4: 177–81.

4. Vrtovec B, Poglajen G, Lezaic L, Sever M, Socan A, et al. (2013). Comparison of transendocardial and intracoronary CD34+ cell transplantation in patients with nonischemic dilated cardiomyopathy. Circulation 128(11 Suppl 1): S42–9.

5. Constantine G, Shan K, Flamm SD, Sivananthan MU (2004) Role of MRI in clinical cardiology. Lancet 363: 2162–71.

6. Poon M, Fuster V, Fayad Z (2002) Cardiac magnetic resonance imaging: a "one-stop-shop" evaluation of myocardial dysfunction. Curr Opin Cardiol 17: 663–70.

7. Ben-Haim SA, Osadchy D, Schuster I, Gepstein L, Hayam G, et al. (1996) Nonfluoroscopic, in vivo navigation and mapping technology. Nat Med 2: 1393–5.

8. Gepstein L, Hayam G, Shpun S, Ben-Haim SA (1997) Hemodynamic evaluation of the heart with a nonfluoroscopic electromechanical mapping technique. Circulation 96: 3672–80.

9. Gyöngyösi M, Dib N (2011) Diagnostic and prognostic value of 3D NOGA mapping in ischemic heart disease. Nat Rev Cardiol 8: 393–404.

10. Psaltis PJ Worthley SG (2009) Endoventricular electromechanical mapping—the diagnostic and therapeutic utility of the NOGA XP Cardiac Navigation System. J Cardiovasc Transl Res 2: 48–62.

11. Kornowski R, Hong MK, Leon MB (1998) Comparison between left ventricular electromechanical mapping and radionuclide perfusion imaging for detection of myocardial viability. Circulation 98: 1837–41.

12. Gyöngyösi, M. Khorsand A, Sochor H, Sperker W, Strehblow C, et al. (2005) Characterization of hibernating myocardium with NOGA electroanatomic endocardial mapping. Am J Cardiol 95: 722–8.

13. Gyöngyösi M, Sochor H, Khorsand A, Gepstein L, Glogar D (2001) Online myocardial viability assessment in the catheterization laboratory via NOGA electroanatomic mapping: quantitative comparison with thallium-201 uptake. Circulation 104: 1005–11.

14. Callans DJ, Ren JF, Michele J, Marchlinski FE, Dillon SM (1999) Electroanatomic left ventricular mapping in the porcine model of healed anterior myocardial infarction. Correlation with intracardiac echocardiography and pathological analysis. Circulation 100: 1744–50.

15. Fuchs S, Hendel RC, Baim DS, Moses JW, Pierre A, et al. (2001) Comparison of endocardial electromechanical mapping with radionuclide perfusion imaging to assess myocardial viability and severity of myocardial ischemia in angina pectoris. Am J Cardiol 87: 874–80.

16. Keck A, Hertting K, Schwartz Y, Kitzing R, Weber M, et al. (2002) Electromechanical mapping for determination of myocardial contractility and viability. A comparison with echocardiography, myocardial single-photon emission computed tomography, and positron emission tomography. J Am Coll Cardiol 40: 1067–74.

17. Sheehan FH, Bolson EL, McDonald JA, Reisman M, Koch KC, et al. (2002) Method for three-dimensional data registration from disparate imaging modalities in the NOGA Myocardial Viability Trial. IEEE Trans Med Imaging 21: 1264–70.

18. Perin EC, Silva GV, Sarmento-Leite R, Sousa AL, Howell M, et al. (2002) Assessing myocardial viability and infarct transmurality with left ventricular

electromechanical mapping in patients with stable coronary artery disease: validation by delayed-enhancement magnetic resonance imaging. Circulation 106: 957–61.

19. Wiggers H, Bøtker HE, Søgaard P, Kaltoft A, Hermansen F, et al. (2003) Electromechanical mapping versus positron emission tomography and single photon emission computed tomography for the detection of myocardial viability in patients with ischemic cardiomyopathy. J Am Coll Cardiol 41: 843–8.

20. Graf S, Gyöngyösi M, Khorsand A, Nekolla SG, Pirich C, et al. (2004) Electromechanical properties of the perfusion/metabolism mismatch: comparison of nonfluoroscopic electroanatomic mapping with ^{18}F-FDG PET imaging. J Nucl Med 45: 1611–8.

21. Wolf T, Gepstein L, Dror U, Hayam G, Shofti R, et al. (2001) Detailed endocardial mapping accurately predicts the transmural extent of myocardial infarction. J Am Coll Cardiol 37: 1590–7.

22. Wijnmaalen AP, van der Geest RJ, van Huls van Taxis CF, Siebelink HM, et al. (2011) Head-to-head comparison of contrast-enhanced magnetic resonance imaging and electroanatomical voltage mapping to assess post-infarct scar characteristics in patients with ventricular tachycardias: real-time image integration and reversed registration. Eur Heart J 32: 104–14.

23. Desjardins B, Crawford T, Good E, Oral H, Chugh A, et al. (2009) Infarct architecture and characteristics on delayed enhanced magnetic resonance imaging and electroanatomic mapping in patients with postinfarction ventricular arrhythmia. Heart Rhythm 6: 644–51.

24. Codreanu A, Odille F, Aliot E, Marie PY, Magnin-Poull I, et al. (2008) Electroanatomic characterization of post-infarct scars comparison with 3-dimensional myocardial scar reconstruction based on magnetic resonance imaging. J Am Coll Cardiol 52: 839–842.

25. Gupta S, Desjardins B, Baman T, Ilg K, Good E, et al. (2012) Delayed-enhanced MR scar imaging and intraprocedural registration into an electro-anatomical mapping system in post-infarction patients. JACC Cardiovasc Imaging 5: 207–10.

26. Desjardins B, Yokokawa M, Good E, Crawford T, Latchamsetty R, et al. (2013) Characteristics of intramural scar in patients with nonischemic cardiomyopathy and relation to intramural ventricular arrhythmias. Circ Arrhythm Electrophysiol 6: 891–7.

27. Spears DA, Suszko AM, Dalvi R, Crean AM, Ivanov J, et al. (2012) Relationship of bipolar and unipolar electrogram voltage to scar transmurality and composition derived by magnetic resonance imaging in patients with nonischemic cardiomyopathy undergoing VT ablation. Heart Rhythm 9: 1837–46.

28. Tokuda M, Tedrow UB, Inada K, Reichlin T, Michaud GF, et al. (2013) Direct comparison of adjacent endocardial and epicardial electrograms: implications for substrate mapping. J Am Heart Assoc. 2: e000215.

29. van Slochteren FJ, Teske AJ, van der Spoel TI, Koudstaal S, Doevendans PA, et al. (2012) Advanced measurement techniques of regional myocardial function to assess the effects of cardiac regenerative therapy in different models of ischaemic cardiomyopathy. Eur Heart J Cardiovasc Imaging 13: 808–18.

30. Heiberg E, Sjögren J, Ugander M, Carlsson M, Engblom H, et al. (2010) Design and validation of Segment–freely available software for cardiovascular image analysis. BMC Medical Imaging 10: 1–13.

31. Holland PW, Welsch RE (1977) Robust Regression Using Iteratively Reweighted Least-Squares. Communications in Statistics: Theory and Methods, A6, pp.813–827.

32. Cohen J (1988) Statistical power analysis for the behavioral sciences (2nd ed.). Hillsdale, NJ: Lawrence Earlbaum Associates

33. Amado LC, Gerber BL, Gupta SN, Rettmann DW, Szarf G, et al. (2004) Accurate and objective infarct sizing by contrast-enhanced magnetic resonance imaging in a canine myocardial infarction model. J Am Coll Cardiol 44: 2383–9.

8

Non-Invasive MRI and Spectroscopy of *mdx* Mice Reveal Temporal Changes in Dystrophic Muscle Imaging and in Energy Deficits

Christopher R. Heier[1], **Alfredo D. Guerron**[1], **Alexandru Korotcov**[2], **Stephen Lin**[2], **Heather Gordish-Dressman**[1,3], **Stanley Fricke**[4], **Raymond W. Sze**[5], **Eric P. Hoffman**[1,3], **Paul Wang**[2,6], **Kanneboyina Nagaraju**[1,3]*

1 Center for Genetic Medicine Research, Children's National Medical Center, Washington, D.C., United States of America, **2** Department of Radiology, Howard University College of Medicine, Washington, D.C., United States of America, **3** Department of Integrative Systems Biology, George Washington University School of Medicine and Health Sciences, Washington, D.C., United States of America, **4** Department of Diagnostic Imaging and Radiology, Children's National Medical Center, Washington, D.C., United States of America, **5** Department of Radiology, Children's National Medical Center, Washington, D.C., United States of America, **6** Department of Electrical Engineering, Fu Jen Catholic University, Taipei, Taiwan

Abstract

In Duchenne muscular dystrophy (DMD), a genetic disruption of dystrophin protein expression results in repeated muscle injury and chronic inflammation. Magnetic resonance imaging shows promise as a surrogate outcome measure in both DMD and rehabilitation medicine that is capable of predicting clinical benefit years in advance of functional outcome measures. The *mdx* mouse reproduces the dystrophin deficiency that causes DMD and is routinely used for preclinical drug testing. There is a need to develop sensitive, non-invasive outcome measures in the *mdx* model that can be readily translatable to human clinical trials. Here we report the use of magnetic resonance imaging and spectroscopy techniques for the non-invasive monitoring of muscle damage in *mdx* mice. Using these techniques, we studied dystrophic *mdx* muscle in mice from 6 to 12 weeks of age, examining both the peak disease phase and natural recovery phase of the *mdx* disease course. T2 and fat-suppressed imaging revealed significant levels of tissue with elevated signal intensity in *mdx* hindlimb muscles at all ages; spectroscopy revealed a significant deficiency of energy metabolites in 6-week-old *mdx* mice. As the *mdx* mice progressed from the peak disease stage to the recovery stage of disease, each of these phenotypes was either eliminated or reduced, and the cross-sectional area of the *mdx* muscle was significantly increased when compared to that of wild-type mice. Histology indicates that hyper-intense MRI foci correspond to areas of dystrophic lesions containing inflammation as well as regenerating, degenerating and hypertrophied myofibers. Statistical sample size calculations provide several robust measures with the ability to detect intervention effects using small numbers of animals. These data establish a framework for further imaging or preclinical studies, and they support the development of MRI as a sensitive, non-invasive outcome measure for muscular dystrophy.

Editor: Diego Fraidenraich, Rutgers University -New Jersey Medical School, United States of America

Funding: CRH is supported by the National Institutes of Health's (http://www.nih.gov/) 5T32AR056993 and 5R24HD050846-02 grants. PW and this work were supported in part by the National Institutes of Health's G12MD007597 and United States Army Medical Research and Materiel Command (http://mrmc.amedd.army.mil/) W81XWH 10-1-0767 grants. KN is supported by National Institutes of Health's K26OD011171 and P50AR060836 grants, a Muscular Dystrophy Association (http://mda.org/) translational grant 30000783/4736, and the United States Department of Defense (http://www.defense.gov/) grants W81XWH-05-1-0659, W81XWH-11-1-0782, W81XWH-11-1-0330, and W81XWH-11-1-0782. The funders had no role in study design, data collection and analysis, decision to publish, or preparation of the manuscript.

Competing Interests: The authors have declared that no competing interests exist.

* Email: KNagaraju@childrensnational.org

Introduction

Duchenne muscular dystrophy (DMD) is the most common lethal genetic muscle disease diagnosed in children. Dystrophin-deficient *mdx* mice are a naturally occurring genetic model of DMD and are widely used for preclinical drug testing. Both DMD and *mdx* muscle undergo cycles of degeneration and regeneration, resulting in a chronic inflammatory state in skeletal muscle. Together, a clearly defined genetic cause and animal models establish a logical path for developing therapies for DMD through translational medicine. Several such compounds have now begun to enter clinical trials, including drug classes that target either the skipping of problematic exons [1–3] or inflammation and membrane stability [4].

Two significant problems encountered thus far in the case of DMD and related translational areas are a lack of quantitative surrogate outcome measures [5] and a poor success rate in translating success in preclinical mouse trials into success in human clinical trials [6–8]. Currently, many outcome measures used in early DMD trials consist of measures that can be subjective, could be susceptible to coaching effects or placebo effects, or show high variability [5,9]. In preclinical *mdx* studies, most outcome measures used are unique to mice or must be substantially altered or interpreted to account for species differences.

Magnetic resonance imaging (MRI) is the gold standard for imaging damage to soft-tissue such as muscle. MRI is a non-invasive technique that does not require anesthesia in humans. It provides advantages over microCT, X-ray, and ultrasound imaging techniques in that it does not use ionizing radiation, and provides high-resolution imaging with strong contrast in soft tissues [10,11]. Early MRI and nuclear magnetic resonance (NMR) spectroscopy studies have shown clear differences between DMD and healthy muscle. Adipose tissue replacement of muscle is prominent in standard T2-weighted MRI imaging of advanced-stage DMD patients [12,13]. Fat-suppression MRI techniques allow for enhanced imaging of edema and inflammation [12]. Nuclear magnetic resonance spectroscopy techniques show that DMD muscle is in a state of energy deficiency [14], and detect increased lipid content within muscle [15]. Given these studies establishing dystrophic muscle phenotypes, together with studies comparing clinical groups [16], changes over time [17], and correlation with clinical assessments [18,19], MRI is emerging as a potential key surrogate outcome measure for DMD clinical trials.

Here, we use MRI methodologies to study muscle damage and changes over time in *mdx* mice. One characteristic of the *mdx* disease is the period of peak necrosis and disease severity from 3 to 6 weeks of age; this severe disease is followed by a recovery period that produces mild phenotypes in the mice by 10–12 weeks of age [20–23]. We use a longitudinal strategy in which we image the same mice and muscles repeatedly from 6 to 12 weeks of age. This approach has several advantages: it examines two distinct disease phases, longitudinal measures increase statistical power, it facilitates design of non-invasive studies with technologies that are translatable to human muscle, and by assaying natural recovery periods it provides an idea of what therapeutic efficacy could look like. Here, we show clear MRI and NMR spectroscopy phenotypes in 6-week *mdx* mice in comparison to wild-type. These phenotypes include measures of muscle damage and a deficiency in energy metabolites. Interestingly, many of these differences are eliminated or reduced as *mdx* mice transition into the recovery phase of disease. Taken together, our results support the non-invasive use of MRI surrogate outcome measures for diagnosis, prognosis, and rehabilitation of muscle damage in muscular dystrophy.

Materials and Methods

Ethics Statement

All animal work was conducted according to relevant national and international guidelines. All studies were reviewed and approved by the Institutional Animal Care and Use Committee of Children's National Medical Center, the Washington DC Veterans Affairs Medical Center Institutional Animal Care and Use Committee, and by the Howard University Institutional Animal Care and Use Committee.

Animal care

All experiments were conducted according to protocols approved by the Institutional Animal Care and Use Committees of Children's National Medical Center, the Washington DC Veterans Affairs Medical Center, and Howard University. Animals were maintained in a controlled mouse facility with a 12 h light: 12 h dark photoperiod, fed *ad libitum,* and monitored daily for health. All *mdx* (C57BL/10ScSn-DMD<mdx>/J) and

wild-type (C57BL/10ScSnJ) female mice were obtained from the Jackson Laboratory (Bar Harbor, ME). Groups for the longitudinal study initially consisted of six wild-type and six *mdx* mice each. One wild-type mouse stopped breathing under anesthesia and was removed from the study. Mice were received at 4 weeks of age, allowed to acclimate for 2 weeks, and assayed beginning at 6 weeks of age. MRI and NMR spectroscopy were performed on each mouse every 2 weeks until the mice were 12 weeks of age. To immobilize the animals for MRI and NMR spectroscopy scans, they were anesthetized with 1.5% isoflurane, gently restrained in imaging position upon a plastic plate, and positioned in the center of the MRI scanner. For imaging, mice were placed in a holder that maintained their temperature at 37°C, with monitoring of their body temperature as well as respiratory and heart rates. Hindlimb muscles were examined in two sites per animal, including the leg and the thigh.

MRI and NMR spectroscopy

In vivo monitoring of mouse hindlimbs and muscle damage was performed using a 9.4 T, 89-mm vertical bore NMR spectrometer (Bruker Biospin MRI, Billerica, MA) with a 25-mm inner diameter dual nucleus (^{31}P/^{1}H) birdcage coil. For anatomical positioning, a pilot image set of three orthogonal imaging planes were used. MRI pulse sequences used for data acquisition used T2-weighted imaging (T2) and fat-suppressed T2-weighted imaging (FS) sequences optimized for imaging of muscle inflammation. The imaging sequence used was a rapid acquisition with relaxation enhancement (RARE) sequence: echo time (TE) = 7.4 ms; repetition time (TR) = 3,000 ms; RARE factor 16; flip angle α = 90°; field of view = 2.56 cm×2.56 cm; slice thickness = 1 mm with no gap between slices; matrix size = 256×256; number of averages = 12.

Spectra were processed using TopSpin v1.5 software (Bruker Biospin MRI, Billerica, MA). For ^{31}P spectroscopy studies, un-localized single-pulse spectroscopy was performed with 4k transients and a band width of 50 ppm. Integral areas of spectral peaks corresponding to inorganic phosphorous (Pi), phosphocreatine (PCr), and the three phosphate groups of adenosine triphosphate (α-ATP, β-ATP, and γ-ATP) were measured. Pi peaks were not detectable in several of the mice assayed (3 *mdx* and 5 wild-type); for these mice Pi values were uniformly omitted from the analyses. The presence of phosphomonoester (PME) or phosphodiester (PDE) peaks was also recorded; however, the signal-to-noise ratio of these peaks was not always adequate for accurate quantification. Levels of PCr and Pi were normalized by dividing by either the total ATP present in that spectrum or by the amount of β-ATP present in that spectrum. The results were consistent between both of these normalization methods; data are presented as the ratio of each parameter to total ATP.

For analysis of MRI images, two-dimensional sequential (2dseq) files were converted to digital imaging and communications in medicine (DICOM) files and analyzed using ImageJ v1.48 (NIH) software. To obtain volumetric data and account for possible variability between individual MRI slices, multiple consecutive MRI slices of each leg and thigh were assembled into image stacks encompassing 5- or 3-mm sections of the mouse hindlimb. Each stack was analyzed individually, and values for the two legs or thighs of each mouse were then averaged to obtain a single value for that mouse. For the leg, five consecutive slices along the long axis of the tibia were assayed, beginning 2 mm distal from the tibial plateau as a reference point to ensure mice were assayed at the same anatomical location. For the thigh, three consecutive slices along the long axis of the femur were assayed, beginning 6 mm proximal from the femoral condyles. Within each slice, regions of interest were digitally traced in ImageJ for each leg such that they were defined as the total area internal to the leg or thigh. Within regions of interest in each individual MRI image, we measured the total cross-sectional area, as well as the volumetric area (in voxels, or volume pixels) of bone, of muscle (with bone subtracted), and of tissue exceeding threshold signal intensity. For cross-sectional area, the highest value for each leg or thigh was recorded as the maximal cross-sectional area (CSA_{max}). Bone was measured by digitally tracing the dark outline shape of the tibia or femur in MRI images, and measuring the area outlined. Muscle area was measured by subtracting bone from the combined muscle and bone area making up the full region of interest. Elevated signal intensity was measured using ImageJ software in a semi-automated manner by measuring the volumetric area in voxels that exceeded background threshold within the regions of interest. Percent of tissue with elevated signal intensity was calculated by dividing this measurement by the area in voxels measured for muscle.

Histology

Mice were assayed by T2 imaging of the leg as described above. Immediately after each imaging session, the imaged mouse was sacrificed and the whole leg fixed in formalin. This was performed with 3 *mdx* and 2 wild-type mice at 6 months of age. Paraffin cross-sections of the legs were made at locations of interest corresponding to MRI slices as specified in a sagittal positioning image (Histoserv, Inc.), and sections were stained with H&E. Images were obtained using an Olympus BX61TRF (Olympus, Center Valley, PA) microscope with an Olympus DP71 camera and Olympus DP Controller v3.2.1.276 software. Using ImageJ software, digital tracing and overlap of the tibia structure between H&E and MRI images was used to confirm anatomical location within a corresponding MRI slice. T2 images for specific slices were then compared to corresponding H&E images for qualitative analysis within regions of interest. Multiple images taken with a $4\times$ objective were used to produce full cross-sectional H&E montage images of the leg, and an inset image within a representative area was taken with a $10\times$ objective. Histopathology was assayed qualitatively as reported previously [24].

Statistical Analysis

All statistical analyses were performed by a dedicated biostatistician. Separate regression models were run for each measurement, method, and site. All models were mixed effects linear regression models with the mouse ID as the random coefficient. This approach allowed us to take into account the repeated measures taken at each time point. The main effects of strain and time were tested. All within-strain measurements were approximately normally distributed; therefore, no normalizing transformations were used. All single time-point strain comparisons were done using t-tests without adjustment for multiple testing to facilitate the powered design of trials with single time points. Sample size calculations were performed to determine the number of mice needed to detect a significant change with treatment, to facilitate future preclinical and proof-of-concept studies. Calculations were performed on *mdx* mice only, with the expectation that WT mice would not show the level of changes in inflammation and muscle changes expected in *mdx* mice. For PCr, the percent of voxels with elevated signal, maximum CSA, and volume of tissue with elevated intensity, we performed calculations to show a 20% change in mean value. Power analyses were one-sided in the direction of *mdx* value movement toward wild-type values and assumed a power of 80% and an alpha = 0.05. Throughout the text, all data are presented as means ± standard deviation unless otherwise noted.

Results

NMR spectroscopy shows mdx energetics deficit

To determine the state of energy metabolites in *mdx* versus healthy mice, we assayed the relative levels of phosphate metabolites in mice using un-localized ^{31}P spectroscopy. Here, the levels of phosphocreatine (PCr), inorganic phosphate (Pi), and adenosine triphosphate (ATP, with α-, β- and γ- peaks corresponding to its three phosphate groups) were assayed every 2 weeks beginning at 6 weeks of age (Figure 1A). At 6 weeks of age, PCr levels were significantly lower in *mdx* than in wild-type mice, with PCr:ATP ratios of 0.44±0.05 and 0.58±0.03 ($p\leq0.001$), respectively (Figure 1B). The difference in PCr levels between *mdx* and wild-type mice was reduced by 8 weeks of age, as the *mdx* mice entered the recovery stage of their disease, with *mdx* levels resembling wild-type and no significant difference present from 8 weeks to 12 weeks of age. In contrast to PCr, the levels of Pi:ATP were significantly increased ($p<0.05$) in *mdx* mice compared to wild-type at both 6 weeks and 8 weeks of age, after which they resembled wild-type (Figure 1C). These findings indicate that at 6 weeks of age, during the peak stage of *mdx* weakness and necrosis [20,22,23], the *mdx* mice experience an energy metabolism deficiency that subsequently improves during the recovery phase.

Longitudinal MRI of mdx muscle detects effects of mdx genotype and age

To image dystrophic muscle in live mice during the peak necrosis and recovery phases of the *mdx* condition, we performed T2-weighted imaging and fat-suppressed imaging of leg and thigh muscles every 2 weeks, from 6 to 12 weeks of age. Heterogeneous areas of elevated intensity were visible in all *mdx* mice and at all time points, in contrast to the more uniform and dark signal for healthy control muscle tissue (Figure 2A). Orientation and relevant anatomy are provided (Figure 2B). By aligning anatomically matched MRI slices using the tibial plateau as a reference point across successive time points, we observed qualitative changes in the sites and patterns of hyperintense foci within *mdx* leg muscles between two-week intervals.

Quantitatively, we detected significant effects of the *mdx* genotype on measures of muscle damage and size by both T2-weighted and fat-suppressed imaging, in both the leg and thigh muscles. No significant differences were observed in volumetric bone area between *mdx* and wild-type, for either the tibia or femur, for any of the imaging methods (Figure S1). In T2 imaging of *mdx* leg muscles, we found a significant increase in the percentage of tissue with elevated intensity ($p<0.001$) that changed over time ($p<0.01$), without a significant interaction effect being present. In T2 images of leg muscle, 6-week-old *mdx* mice had 21±3% tissue with elevated signal, as compared to 4±2% for wild-type mice ($p<0.001$; Figure 2C). As the *mdx* mice entered the recovery phase of disease, they showed a 38% reduction in the levels of affected tissue, to a mean of 13±2% of volume pixels (voxels) with elevated intensity at 8 weeks of age ($p<0.001$). These values then remained fairly steady, with no significant decrease from 8 to 12 weeks of age. These data illustrate the ability of MRI to detect significant levels of affected tissue in dystrophic legs in 6- to 12-week old *mdx* mice.

We also wanted to gain insight into whether affected muscle in *mdx* is either being eliminated or being "diluted" as the muscle grows larger and enters the recovery phase. To do this, we assayed the absolute volume of tissue with elevated intensity in the legs as well as the cross-sectional area of the legs. We detected a significant effect of the *mdx* genotype ($p<0.001$), with increased volume of elevated signal over wild-type at all ages (Figure 2D).

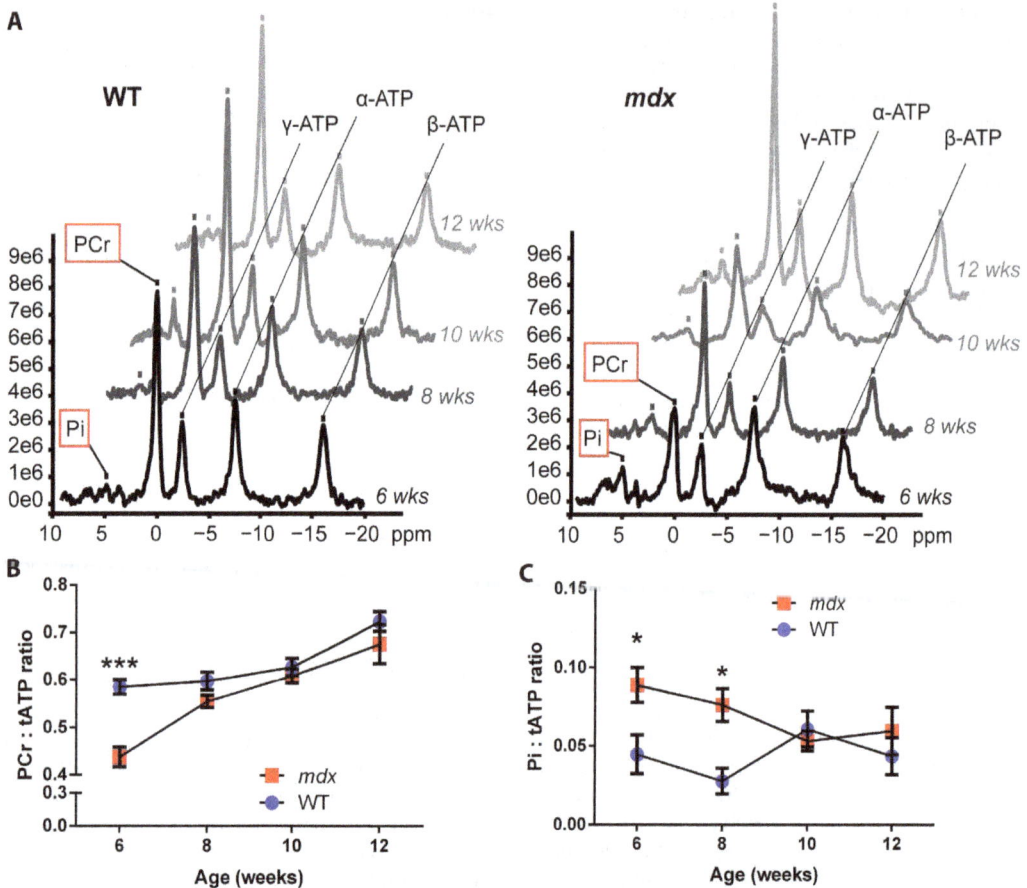

Figure 1. ^{31}P NMR spectroscopy indicates an energy deficit in 6-week-old *mdx* mice. Beginning at 6 weeks of age, *mdx* and wild-type (WT) mice were assayed by ^{31}P spectroscopy every 2 weeks. A) Representative ^{31}P NMR spectra illustrating the peaks of several energy metabolites in one wild-type (left) and one *mdx* (right) mouse, from weeks 6 through 12. The inorganic phosphate, phosphocreatine, and three phosphate group peaks for ATP are labeled and marked by a tick mark. Graphs are aligned by parallel lines connecting the ATP peaks; phosphocreatine and inorganic phosphate showed differences between wild-type and *mdx* mice and are highlighted by a red box. B) Phosphocreatine levels are decreased in 6-week-old *mdx* mice, then change to near wild-type levels during the *mdx* recovery phase. C) Inorganic phosphate levels are elevated at 6 and 8 weeks in *mdx* mice compared to wild-type, then change to near wild-type levels by 10 weeks. Note, peaks for inorganic phosphate were not detectable in several mice of both genotypes (3 *mdx* and 5 wild-type); values for these mice were uniformly omitted from the Pi analysis (Pi, inorganic phosphate; PCr, phosphocreatine; ATP, adenosine triphosphate; tATP, total ATP; n = 3–6 mice per data point; data are means ±SEM; *$p \leq 0.05$, ***$p \leq 0.001$).

We detected no significant effects of time on the volume of elevated signal in *mdx* mice and no significant interaction effect. Examining the sizes of muscles throughout the 6- to 12-week period assayed, we detected significant effects of the *mdx* genotype ($p < 0.001$) and of time ($p < 0.001$) on CSA$_{max}$, without a significant interaction effect. Initially, the *mdx* mice showed a smaller but significant increase over wild-type in CSA$_{max}$ ($p < 0.05$), with values of 27.7 ± 1.3 mm^2 versus 24.7 ± 2.6 mm^2, respectively (Figure 2E). In contrast to the results for elevated signal, as the *mdx* mice progressed into the recovery phase, differences in CSA$_{max}$ between the *mdx* and wild-type mice became larger, with the difference increasing by 113% from week 6 to week 8. At 8 weeks, *mdx* calves had CSA$_{max}$ values of 34.7 ± 2.2 mm^2, versus 28.4 ± 2.5 mm^2 for wild-type ($p < 0.01$), and this difference was maintained through 12 weeks of age, at which point the *mdx* mice had CSA$_{max}$ values of 40.0 ± 3.9 mm^2, versus 33.5 ± 1.3 mm^2 for wild-type ($p < 0.01$). Together, these MRI data show that as *mdx* mice recover from the necrotic phase and assume a milder phenotype [20,22,23], they show a decrease in the percentage of affected tissue driven by an increase in muscle size, without a complete resolution of phenotype.

To enhance the visualization of signal from possible edema and inflammation, given the reduced signal likely from possible fatty infiltration of the muscle, we performed fat-suppressed imaging immediately following the standard T2-weighted imaging (Figure 3). Here again, we saw significant phenotypes in 6-week old *mdx* mice, with an average of $9 \pm 3\%$ tissue with elevated intensity present in *mdx* mice, versus $1 \pm 1\%$ for wild-type mice ($p < 0.001$). Following week 6, *mdx* mice again showed a 40% reduction in affected leg tissue as they entered the recovery phase of disease, to $5 \pm 4\%$ versus $0.6 \pm 0.3\%$ for wild-type ($p < 0.05$) at 8 weeks. Values for both genotypes were then maintained at similar levels through 12 weeks of age. These data are consistent with the T2 imaging results.

For the thigh muscles, results were qualitatively consistent with those found for the leg muscles; we again observed changes in the patterns of affected tissue over time within the same mouse in anatomically aligned MRI slices (Figure 4A). Orientation and relevant anatomy are provided (Figure 4B). In standard T2 images, 6-week old *mdx* mice showed a significant increase in the percentage of tissue with elevated signal, with values of $22 \pm 5\%$ versus $7 \pm 1\%$ for wild-type mice ($p < 0.001$; Figure 4C).

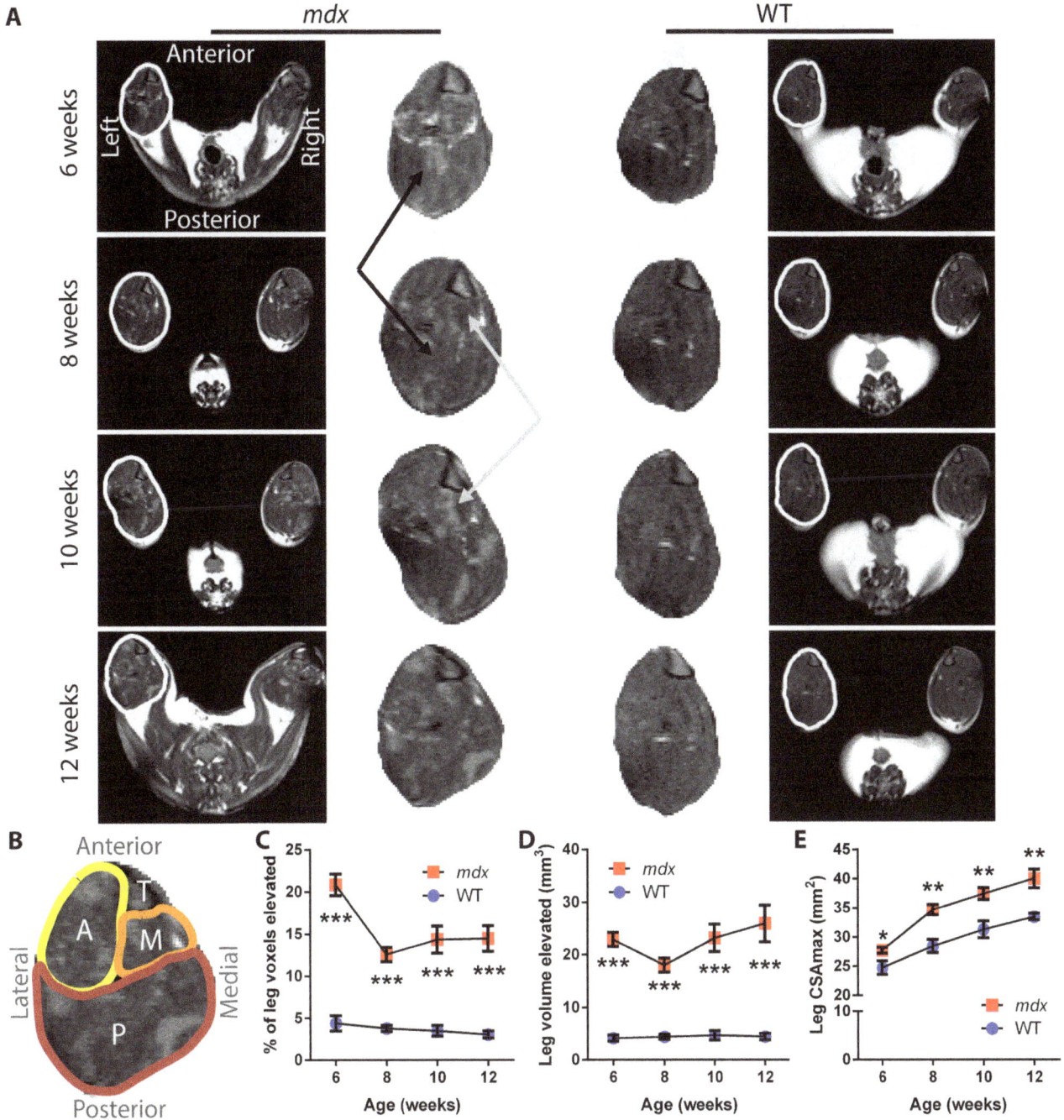

Figure 2. T2 of *mdx* leg shows changes in dystrophic muscle and cross-sectional area over time. A) Representative T2-weighted images from one *mdx* mouse (left) and one wild-type mouse (right) over time, each imaged from 6 to 12 weeks of age. The full MRI image of each mouse is provided on the outside column, with the leg of the left hindlimb for each mouse outlined in white and a magnified version of the leg muscles provided in the center columns. The black arrows mark a region of *mdx* muscle that showed a reduction in intensity between time points, while the gray arrows mark a region that showed an elevation of intensity between time points. The tibia, visible as a triangular structure in the upper right corner of each leg section, was used to orient the muscle slices. B) Orientation and anatomy of the leg cross sections. Anterior muscle groups (A, yellow) include tibialis anterior and extensor digitorum longus. Medial muscle groups (M, orange) include flexor hallucis and flexor digitorum. Posterior muscle groups (P, red) include gastrocnemius, soleus, and plantaris. The tibia bone is also marked (T). C) The percentage of tissue within the leg muscle that showed signal intensity elevated over the threshold that separates healthy muscle from affected tissue illustrates a change between the necrotic (6 week) and recovery phases of *mdx* disease. D) The absolute volume of tissue with elevated signal intensity detected within the leg of mice. E) The CSA$_{max}$ values over time show the growth of muscle, and an increase for the *mdx* mice as compared to wild-type mice (n = 5 wild-type and 6 *mdx* mice; data are means ±SEM; *$p<0.05$, **$p<0.01$, ***$p<0.001$).

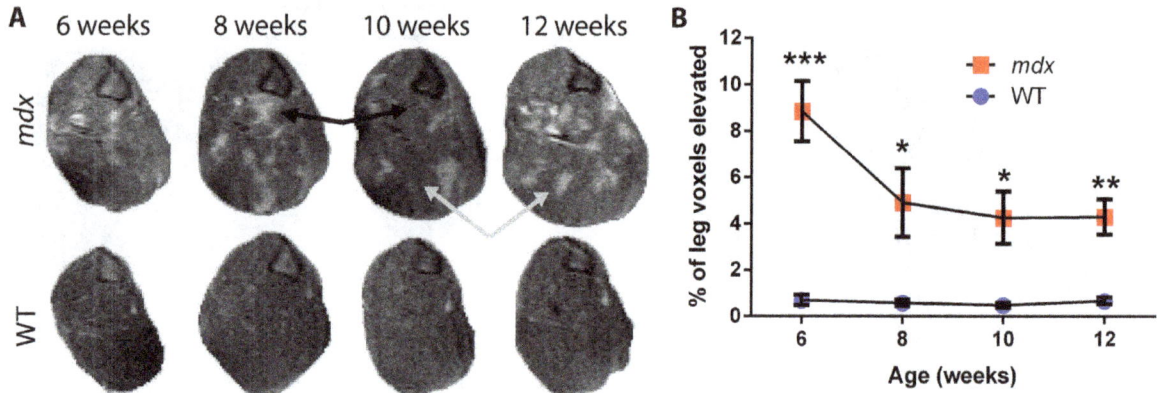

Figure 3. Longitudinal fat-suppressed imaging of dystrophic *mdx* leg muscles. A) Representative fat-suppressed images of leg muscle from the left hindlimb of one *mdx* (top) and one wild-type (bottom) mouse over time, each imaged from 6 to 12 weeks of age. Black arrows mark a region of muscle that showed a reduction in intensity between time points, while gray arrows mark a region that showed an increased intensity between time points. The tibia is present as a triangular structure in the upper right corner of the leg sections. B) The percentage of tissue within the leg that has an elevated signal intensity shows a difference between *mdx* and wild-type mice at all time points and illustrates a change between the peak disease (6 week) and recovery phases of *mdx* disease (n = 5 wild-type and 6 *mdx* mice; data are means ±SEM; *$p < 0.05$, **$p < 0.01$, ***$p < 0.001$).

This parameter decreased steadily over time for the *mdx* thigh, to 14±5% for *mdx* and 5±1% for wild-type mice at 12 weeks ($p < 0.01$). Examining the absolute volume of tissue with increased signal independent of muscle size, we found a significant effect of the *mdx* genotype at all time points ($p < 0.01$), but no significant effect of time over the ages assayed (Figure 4D). The size of the thigh muscle, as measured by CSA_{max}, was not significantly different between genotypes at 6 weeks of age (Figure 4E). However, as with the leg, CSA_{max} increased for the *mdx* thighs when compared to wild-type, beginning at 8 weeks of age with values of 57.9±2.4 mm^2 for *mdx* versus 49.3±6.4 mm^2 for wild-type ($p < 0.05$). This size differential continued to increase through 12 weeks, to 73.0±7.5 mm^2 for *mdx* versus 57.0±3.2 mm^2 for wild-type mice ($p < 0.01$).

In fat-suppressed imaging of the thigh, *mdx* mice again showed a significant increase in the percentage of tissue with elevated signal at 6 weeks, with 17±6% as compared to 2±1% for wild-type ($p < 0.001$; Figure 5). By 10 weeks of age, this decreased to 9±1% for *mdx* and 2±1% for wild-type ($p < 0.001$) as the mice progressed to the recovery stage of disease. Together, thigh data are in agreement with the leg. These data illustrate that *mdx* mice show a substantial decrease in the percentage of affected tissue and an increase in muscle area as they progress from the peak disease phases [20,22,23] to the recovery phase of the disease.

Histopathology present in affected areas of dystrophic mdx leg MRI

To determine pathology present within areas of elevated intensity in MRI of *mdx* hindlimb muscles, we performed an additional experiment comparing H&E histology to matched MRI slices (Figure 6). Here, T2 images of the leg were obtained in 6-month old *mdx* and wild-type mice, with legs collected for histology immediately following MRI. Consistent with younger mice, *mdx* mice but not wild-type mice displayed heterogeneous patterns with foci of elevated signal intensity in their leg muscles (Figure 6A–B). By comparing matched H&E stained sections to MRI slices, we found areas of increased MRI intensity in dystrophic muscle correspond to histology regions containing a mix of inflammation, degenerating fibers, regenerating fibers, and hypertrophic fibers (Figure 6C–D). Inflammation and myofiber degeneration or regeneration were not observed in either of the

wild-type controls. Results were consistent between individual mice with the same genotype. These data indicate areas of elevated intensity in dystrophic *mdx* muscle correspond to dystrophic lesions that include a combination of inflammation with degenerating and regenerating myofibers.

Statistical power calculations suggest assays to use for lowest sample size

To determine the methodology that may be of best utility in preclinical drug or intervention efficacy studies, we performed statistical sample size calculations on MRI and spectroscopy data. Here, we calculated the sample sizes of *mdx* mice needed to detect 20% changes in *mdx* metabolite or imaging measures; in previous studies, we detect up to 40% to 50% effects from drug treatment on measures of muscle pathology and inflammation in similar aged *mdx* mice [4]. Our statistical power analyses indicated that ^{31}P NMR spectroscopy performed along with T2 imaging of leg muscles at 6 weeks of age requires the lowest number of *mdx* mice to detect drug efficacy. At 6 weeks of age significant phenotypes are presented, and 20% intervention effects can be detected with 4 *mdx* mice for ^{31}P phosphocreatine levels, and with 7 or 8 mice for T2 quantification of affected tissue in leg muscle (Table 1). In contrast to the leg, T2 measurements in 6-week-old *mdx* thighs required 13 or more mice for detection of drug effects. Using fat suppression acquisition methods increased the number of 6-week old mice needed for detection of intervention effects to 39 or more mice for both muscle groups. As *mdx* mice grew older, the number of mice needed to detect intervention effects in T2 images also increased to 22 or more at week 12, while ^{31}P phenotypes were absent (Table S1). Together, these data indicate that a protocol of leg T2 MRI combined with ^{31}P spectroscopy in mice that are 6 weeks of age provides several sensitive outcome measures for *mdx* studies.

Discussion

MRI shows promise as a surrogate outcome measure for DMD that is capable of non-invasively detecting muscle damage in patients. Here we use magnetic resonance technologies to identify and longitudinally characterize phenotypes in the *mdx* model of DMD. Since *mdx* mice naturally show a peak of necrosis, weakness

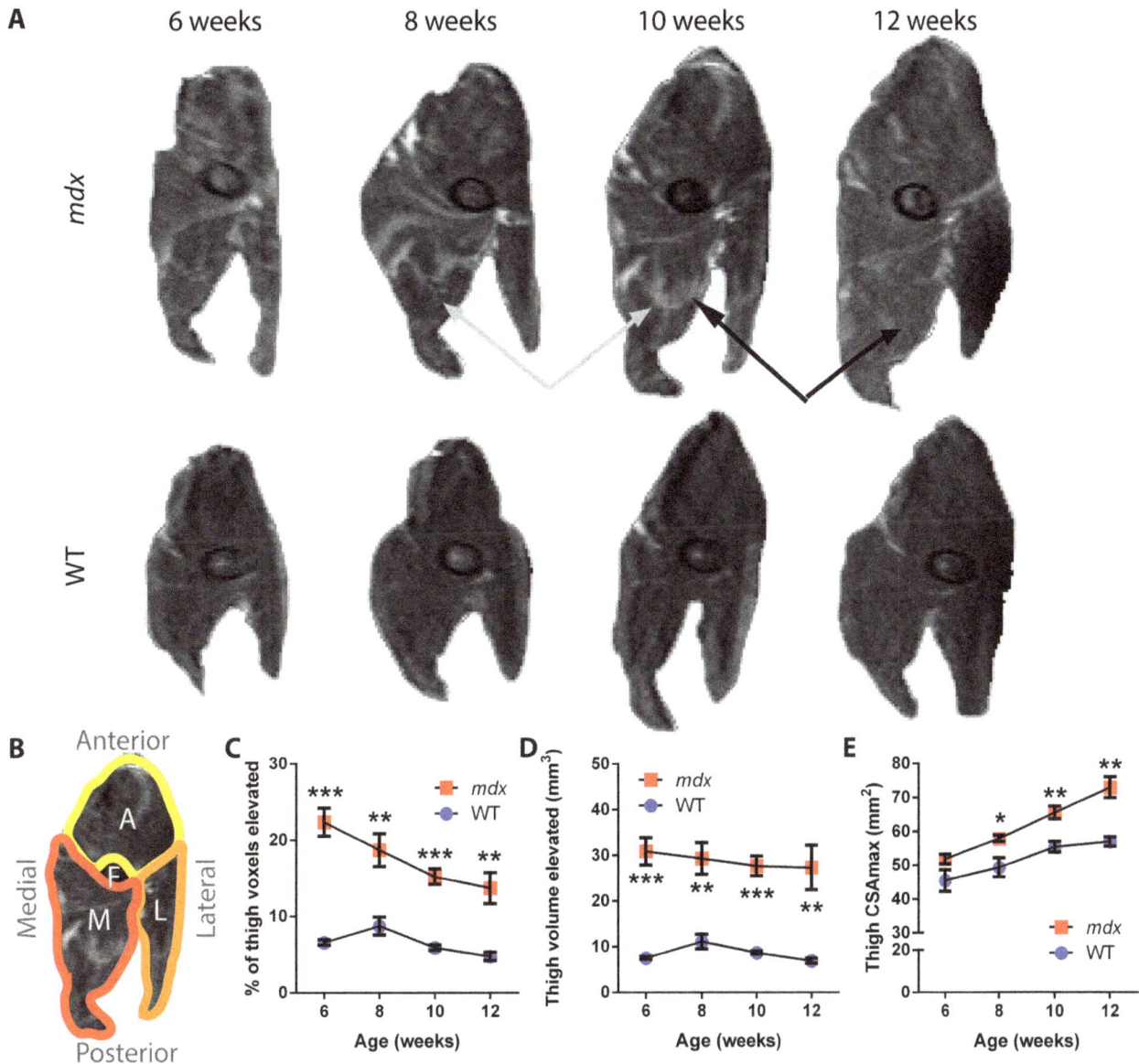

Figure 4. Changes in T2 imaging and cross-sectional area of dystrophic *mdx* thighs over time. A) Representative T2-weighted images of thigh muscle from the right hindlimb of one *mdx* and one wild-type mouse over the study period. The black arrows mark a region of muscle that showed a reduction in intensity over time, while the gray arrows mark a region that showed an increased intensity over time. The femur is visible as an elliptical structure towards the center of the thigh. B) Orientation and anatomy of thigh cross sections. Anterior muscle groups (A, yellow) include vastus intermedius, vastus lateralis, and rectus femoris. Lateral muscle groups (L, orange) include biceps, semitendinosus and semimembranosus muscles. Medial muscle groups (M, red) include gracilis and adductor muscles. The femur bone (F) is also marked. C) The percentage of tissue within the thigh muscle that showed a signal intensity elevated over the threshold that separates healthy muscle from affected tissue shows a difference between *mdx* and wild-type mice at all time points. D) The absolute volume of tissue with an elevated signal within the thigh of *mdx* and wild-type mice. E) CSA$_{max}$ shows growth of the muscle size over time, and an increase in the cross-sectional area of the thigh muscle in *mdx* mice as compared to wild-type mice from 8 weeks onward (n = 5 wild-type and 6 *mdx* mice; data are means ±SEM; *$p < 0.05$, **$p < 0.01$, ***$p < 0.001$).

and disease at 3 to 6 weeks of age [20–23], followed by a natural recovery phase in which they show only mild skeletal muscle disease, the peak disease phase is commonly used to assess preclinical efficacy of therapeutics [4,25]. We find *mdx* mice show significant imaging and spectroscopic alterations during this peak disease phase. Furthermore, these changes decrease as mice progress to the recovery phase. Our findings indicate non-invasive MRI and NMR spectroscopy are sensitive outcome measures that can be used to study disease and evaluate potential therapies in the *mdx* model of muscular dystrophy.

Energy metabolites detected using ^{31}P spectroscopy show a significant deficit of phosphocreatine in 6- to 8-week old *mdx* mice. Significant deficits in phosphocreatine and increased inorganic phosphate are also found in DMD patients [14]. Since energy for muscle contractions comes from phosphocreatine, which is used for generation of ATP through a reversible reaction with creatine phosphokinase, the PCr:ATP ratio is reflective of the energy state of muscle [26–28]. Thus, the decrease in PCr:ATP reflects a muscle bioenergetics deficit in both dystrophic 3- to 12-year-old DMD patients [14] and 6-week-old *mdx* mice. Similar results have

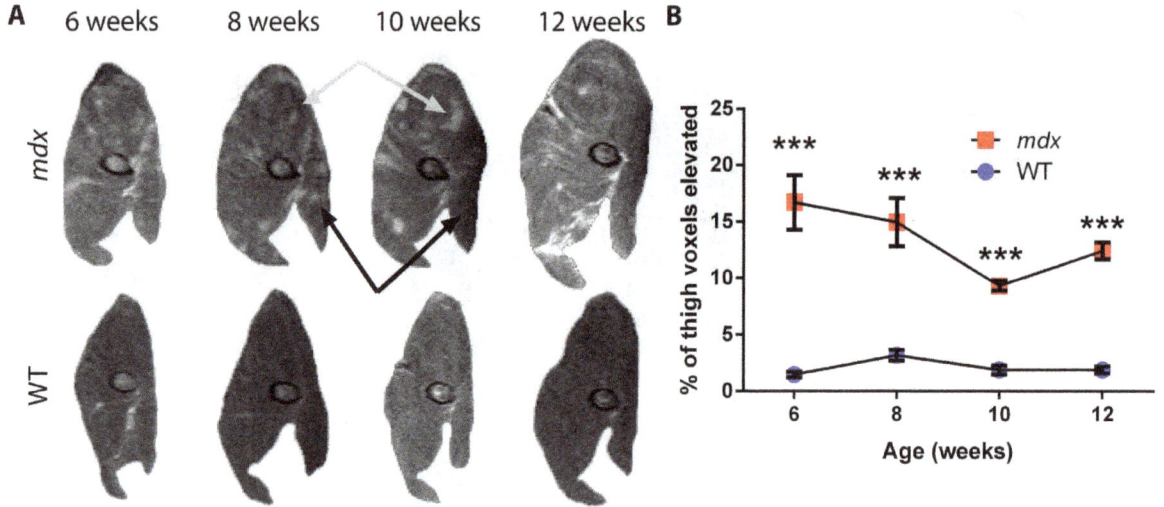

Figure 5. Longitudinal fat-suppressed MRI of dystrophic *mdx* thigh muscles. A) Representative fat-suppressed images of thigh muscle from the right hindlimb of one *mdx* and one wild-type mouse over the course of the study. Black arrows mark a region of muscle that showed a reduction in intensity over time, while gray arrows mark a region that showed an increase in intensity over time. The femur is visible as an elliptical structure in the central area of the thigh. B) The percentage of tissue with an elevated signal intensity within the thigh shows a difference between *mdx* and wild-type mice at all time points (n = 5 wild-type and 6 *mdx* mice; data are means ±SEM; ***$p < 0.001$).

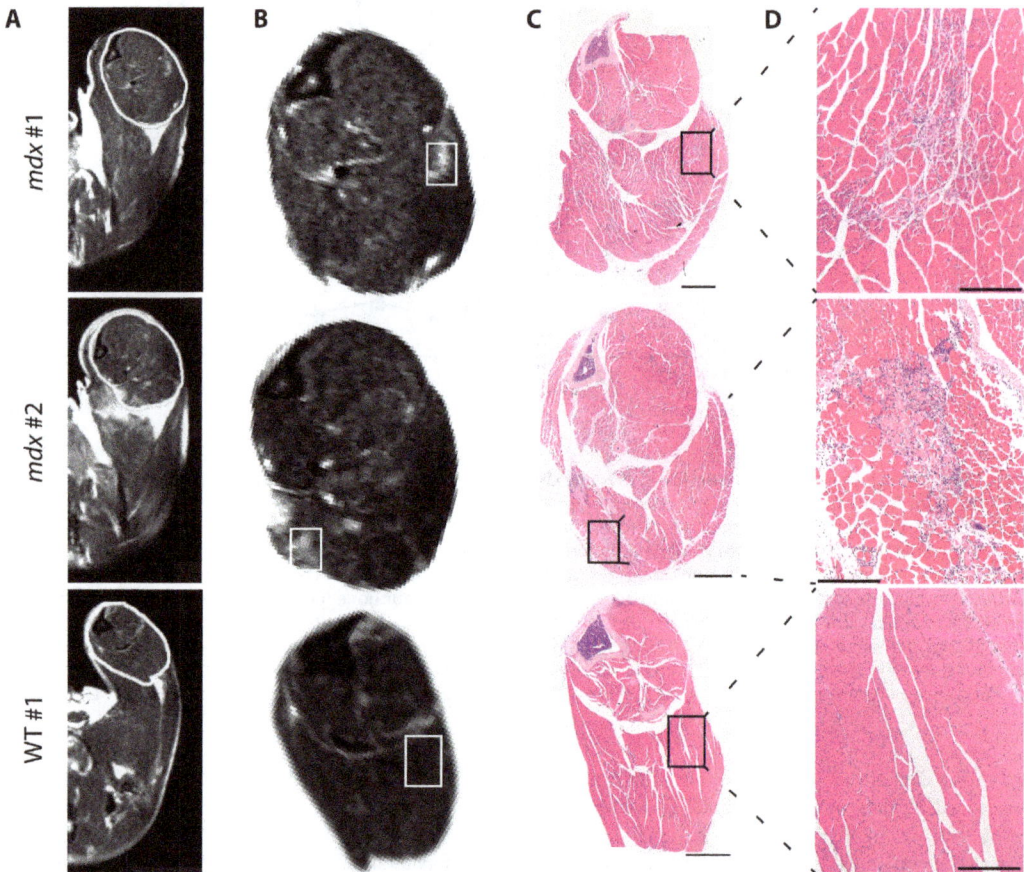

Figure 6. T2 imaging and histology of the *mdx* leg. Additional mice were assayed by T2 imaging at 6 months of age, followed by immediate collection of the whole leg for histology. A) Representative T2 images are provided of *mdx* (top two rows) and wild-type (bottom row) mice. The region of interest outlined in white is shown enlarged in (B). C) H&E stained cross section images corresponding to MRI slices in panels A and B. A montage image of the full leg is provided, with the inset area displayed in (D) at higher magnification (Rectangles in B and C represent the approximate areas presented in higher magnification images in D; Scale bars = 2 mm in C and 0.5 mm in D).

Table 1. Statistical sample size calculations to detect intervention effects in *mdx* mice.

Method	Measure	Site	Values at 6 weeks of age		N per group to detect a 20% change in *mdx*
			WT mean ±SD	*mdx* mean ±SD	
^{31}P NMR Spec	PCr: tATP		0.585±0.030	0.438±0.047	4
T2	% elevated signal	Leg	4±2	21±3	8
	Vol. elevated (mm³)	Leg	4.16±1.36	22.91±3.31	7
	% elevated signal	Thigh	7±1	22±5	13
	Vol. elevated (mm³)	Thigh	7.52±0.75	30.89±7.33	18
Fat Suppression	% elevated signal	Leg	1±1	9±3	41
	Vol. elevated (mm³)	Leg	0.70±0.49	10.00±3.55	39
	% elevated signal	Thigh	1±1	17±6	39
	Vol. elevated (mm³)	Thigh	1.69±0.73	23.34±9.04	58

Abbreviations: NMR Spec, Nuclear Magnetic Resonance spectroscopy; PCr, phosphocreatine; tATP, total adenosine triphosphate; Vol., Volume; WT, wild-type.

been found in *ex vivo* cardiac studies of *mdx* mice, where a decrease in PCr is found in association with a decrease in mitochondrial content of heart tissue [29]. Consistent with heart muscle, we and others find significant mitochondrial deficits in *mdx* skeletal muscle [30]. Other muscle disorders such as mitochondrial myopathies and polio paralysis show a deficit in phosphocreatine levels as well [31,32]. Interestingly, we find the PCr:ATP ratio in *mdx* increases to a level not significantly different from wild-type by 8 to 10 weeks of age. This illustrates an improvement in energetics of dystrophic *mdx* skeletal muscle during the period associated with recovery.

MRI of *mdx* muscle provides significant phenotypes at all ages examined, characterized by hyper-intense foci and a more heterogeneous appearance. Histology shows these imaging phenotypes correspond to dystrophic lesions containing a mix of inflammation with degenerating, regenerating, and hypertrophic myofibers. This is consistent with Walter et al, who find hyperintense regions are consistent with dystrophic lesions and damaged myofibers enhanced by contrast agents, and who use ¹H spectroscopy in *mdx* to show minimal fatty infiltration in comparison to DMD [33]. We see foci of hyper-intense signal change over time, consistent with a dynamic disease process [20] and with time frames established for muscle repair following crush injury [34]. We find cross-sectional area of *mdx* muscle increases over time, while absolute volume of dystrophic lesions in imaging does not. Data in the literature indicate such increases in CSA$_{max}$ are the result of hypertrophy and regeneration [23,35–37].

Comparing spectroscopy and imaging results, there is a discrepancy in *mdx* mice. Spectroscopy shows an initial energetics deficit that is eliminated by 8–10 weeks, while imaging phenotypes improve but persist at all ages examined (including 6 months). Established muscle histology and function data may provide insight into these differences. Through matched histology, we find *mdx* imaging phenotypes are consistent with sites containing inflammation along with myofiber degeneration and regeneration. Previous studies establish this histopathology peaks at 3–6 weeks, then improves but persists throughout the *mdx* lifespan [20–23]. In a longitudinal study we are unable to assay isolated muscles for function, but isometric force data in the literature establish muscle function at stages we examined. Throughout the lifespan of their disease, *mdx* muscles show deficits in normalized strength, where force is measured relative to mass (kN/kg) or cross-sectional area (kN/m²) [4,23,25,37,38]. However, raw absolute force measure-

ments (expressed in kN or mN) behave differently. During peak *mdx* disease (within ages 3–7 weeks), *mdx* muscles show deficits in absolute tetanic forces for extensor digitorum longus (EDL) [23], soleus [23], tibialis anterior (TA) [21], and diaphragm [39]. As *mdx* enter a recovery phase (approximately 2–8 months of age) strength deficits improve [20] and raw measures of isolated EDL [23,37], soleus [37], and TA [38] muscle forces are usually at or above wild-type levels. Comparing these observations and stages, it may be possible that energetics deficits play a role in decreased raw isometric forces during peak *mdx* disease. Consistent with this, creatine treatment targeting energetics deficits in DMD is found to both increase phosphocreatine and preserve muscle function over placebo in a short term study [14]. Alternatively, there may be a threshold of inflammation and muscle damage that manifests as metabolite or force deficits, and mice may cross this during recovery. More investigations will be needed to clarify the relationship of energetics, histopathology, and strength in *mdx* muscle.

Though some measures are consistent between *mdx* and DMD, their disease courses have clear differences. A main difference is that DMD is progressive. As children age they show increasing weakness, fibrosis, and infiltration of muscle with fatty tissue. MRI and NMR studies of DMD (summarized in Table 2) show striking differences from controls as fatty adipose tissue replaces muscle [13,15,40,41]. In DMD, edema is observed within damaged muscle [12]. At advanced ages, *mdx* disease does eventually progress, with injury phenotypes becoming more pronounced after 8 months [38], cardiac deficits around 9 months [42,43], and advanced histopathology with susceptibility to rhabdomyosarcoma around 2 years [44]. However, *mdx* typically do not progress to a point with the degree of muscle wasting and fatty infiltration apparent in DMD. The *mdx* stages we examine here may be most consistent with early DMD, where muscle shows weakness, pathology and inflammation, but patients do not yet exhibit extensive replacement of muscle with fibrotic and fatty tissue. Moving forward, many gene therapy, antisense oligos, and next-generation drug strategies will indeed want to target early DMD stages to prevent muscle loss and to target stages with more myofibers present.

Our power analyses and time course show the period of peak *mdx* disease provides a useful window with more severe phenotypes, ³¹P energetics phenotypes, and increased statistical power for detecting intervention effects. Here we calculate sample

Table 2. MR imaging and spectroscopy phenotypes in dystrophinopathies.

Reference	Study Description	Assay	Study population	Findings in dystrophy	Our findings in *mdx*
Banerjee [57]	DMD vs. controls; effects of creatine	^{31}P NMR Spectroscopy	DMD; 27 patients, 8 controls	**PCr is lower & Pi is higher** in DMD	PCr is lower and Pi higher in 6 week *mdx*
Forbes [58]	Ambulant DMD vs. controls	T2 MR Imaging	DMD; 30 patients, 10 controls	**CSAmax higher** in DMD (MG, Sol, ST)	CSAmax up for *mdx* in all weeks (leg & thigh)
Kinali [13]	Leg muscle of DMD	T2 MR Imaging	DMD; 34 patients	**Non-muscle content** and fat higher in DMD	Non-muscle higher in *mdx* muscle in all weeks
Newman [15]	Forearms of DMD vs. controls	^{1}H NMR Spectroscopy	DMD; 6 patients aged 9–15 years	Fat content higher in DMD	No fatty infiltration visible in *mdx*
Kim [12]	T1 and FS imaging of DMD pelvic muscles	Fat-Suppressed T2 Imaging	DMD; 42 patients	DMD Edema; GMa, VL, GMe most frequent	Inflammation and muscle damage present in *mdx*
Dunn [53]	Quantitative MRI of *mdx* vs. WT	T2 Mapping	*mdx*; 32–48 weeks	T2 decrease, ^{1}H density & water increase	Inflammation and muscle damage present in *mdx*
Zhang [29]	Cardiac function and metabolism in *mdx*	MRI & *ex vivo* ^{31}P NMR Spec	*mdx* and WT; 32 weeks	**Decreased PCr in heart**; RV & LV defects	Decreased PCr in skeletal muscle
McIntosh [34]	Crush injury and *mdx* vs. controls	T2 images	*mdx*; 8–10 weeks	Dystrophic foci seen; **muscle changes over 21 days** post-injury	Changes in natural *mdx* lesions between 2 to 4 week intervals
Stuckey [45]	Cardiac morphology and function in *mdx* vs. controls	Longitudinal cardiac & Gd MRI	*mdx*; 4–52 weeks	RV Dysfunction by 1 & LV by 12 months; fibrosis by 6 months	Heart fibrosis after 6 months; 8 weeks if dosed with prednisone[4]
Pratt [55]	Case study of a single *mdx* leg	MRI	One single *mdx* mouse; 5–80 weeks	Peak in MRI hetero-geneity, recovery after 13 weeks	Peak phenotypes in necrotic phase, damage persists at 8–12 weeks
Straub [46]	Agent-enhanced MRI of *mdx* and *Sgca*$^{-/-}$ mice	MS-325 agent MRI	*mdx* & *Sgca*$^{-/-}$; 8–10 weeks	Enhances dystrophic muscle contrast	
Amthor [47]	Albumin targeting of dystrophic muscle	Gd enhanced MRI	*mdx*; 11–13 weeks	HSA targets to dystrophic muscle	
Odintsov [48]	MRI detection of transplanted stem cells	MRI of labeled stem cells	*mdx* and dKO; 5–30 weeks	MRI tracks Fe-labeled stem cells short-term	
Martins-Bach [51]	Metabolic profiling of *mdx* muscle	*In vitro* ^{1}H NMR Spec	Lysates of *mdx* muscle; 12–24 weeks	Identified metabolites altered in *mdx* lysates	
Xu [52]	Metabolic changes in muscle after injury	^{1}H NMR Spec	Injured WT & *mdx* TAs; 8 weeks	Intramuscular lipids increase post injury	Energetics deficit in necrotic phase
Mathur [54]	Effects of exercise on T2 values in muscle	T2 Mapping	*mdx* and WT; 20–60 weeks	T2, affected area up in *mdx* & after running	Affected area increased in necrotic phase
Walter [33]	Gene therapy effects on dystrophic muscle	T2 Mapping	*mdx* & *γsg*$^{-/-}$ mice; 1 year post-therapy	MRI tracks gene therapy efficacy in *mdx*	6 week *mdx* leg provides best stat power

Abbreviations: CSAmax, maximum cross-sectional area; FS, fat suppressed T2; Gd, gadolinium; GMa, gluteus maximus; GMed, gluteus medius; HSA, human serum albumin; MR, Magnetic Resonance; MG, medial gastrocnemius; PCr, phosphocreatine; RV, right ventricular; Sg, Sarcoglycan; Sgca, Sarcoglycan alpha; Sol, soleus; ST, semitendinosus; tATP, total adenosine triphosphate; VL, vastus lateralis; WT, wild-type.

sizes needed to detect 20% intervention effects. In our experience with prednisone and with VBP15, we observe substantially larger than 20% intervention effects at these ages in *mdx* mice [4]. For example, fluorescent live-imaging shows a 52% decrease in markers of necrosis, and histology a 38% decrease in inflammatory foci with drug treatment [4]. Over the course of only a few weeks, we see elimination of ^{31}P spectroscopy phenotypes and a dramatic reduction in the percentage of muscle affected. These findings will be valuable for design of imaging and pre-clinical therapeutic studies, by providing more phenotypes and larger differences from baseline health in controls.

Other imaging studies provide insight into *mdx* physiology (summarized in Table 2), but most avoid the critical necrotic phase of the *mdx* disease course. Cardiac MRI shows *mdx* mice can exhibit heart dysfunction by one month [45], and decreased cardiac phosphocreatine content at 8 months [29]. Agents can help visualize disrupted muscle integrity [46,47] or detect transplanted stem cells [48–50]. Metabolic profiling shows alterations in injured muscle and lysates of 3- to 6-month old *mdx* mice [51,52]. T2 mapping has been performed in 20- to 60-week-old *mdx* [53,54]. One case study reports a single *mdx* leg assayed longitudinally to 80 weeks [55]. Dunn et al. initially showed dystrophic lesions can be detected via MRI and that crush injuries are repaired over approximately 3 weeks [53], consistent with our findings for naturally occurring *mdx* dystrophic lesions. Mathur and Vohra et al. characterized effects of exercise on *mdx*, finding effects of the *mdx* genotype and of running on muscle T2 and % affected area, with medial muscles particularly affected by running [54]. Gene correction in *mdx* and limb girdle muscular dystrophy mouse models show MRI can be used to detect therapeutic improvement in muscular dystrophy [33,56].

The *mdx* mouse provides researchers with a genetic model of the cause of DMD (dystrophin deficiency), and MRI is emerging as an important surrogate outcome measure for muscle damage.

In the present study we have found NMR phenotypes and provide new information on the dynamic disease process in *mdx* mice. Although *mdx* is typically regarded as a very mild disease model, we find ^{31}P spectroscopy and T2 imaging of the 6-week old *mdx* leg show significant differences from WT mice and could provide robust outcome measures, even with relatively few animals. These findings can improve preclinical trial design by reducing the number of animals required to detect effects, allowing for longitudinal non-invasive quantification of muscle disease, and using measures that are translatable to human clinical studies.

Supporting Information

Figure S1 Measurement of bone sizes within hindlimb sections assayed by MRI. Within the MRI slice stacks encompassing the 5-mm leg and 3-mm thigh regions analyzed, bone volume was assayed for each hindlimb. A) Tibia volume as measured in assayed T2 images of the leg. C) Tibial volume within the fat suppressed sections of leg that were analyzed. B) Femur

volume in assayed T2 sections of the thigh. D) Femur volume as measured within assayed fat suppressed images of the thigh.

Acknowledgments

The authors would like to thank Debbie McClellan for assistance with this manuscript.

Author Contributions

Conceived and designed the experiments: CRH ADG AK SL HGD SF RS EPH PW KN. Performed the experiments: CRH ADG ALK SL HGD. Analyzed the data: CRH ADG AK SL HGD SF PW KN. Contributed reagents/materials/analysis tools: CRH ADG AK HGD SF RS EPH PW KN. Wrote the paper: CRH ADG SL HGD PW KN.

References

1. Alter J, Lou F, Rabinowitz A, Yin H, Rosenfeld J, et al. (2006) Systemic delivery of morpholino oligonucleotide restores dystrophin expression bodywide and improves dystrophic pathology. Nat Med 12: 175–177.
2. Yokota T, Lu QL, Partridge T, Kobayashi M, Nakamura A, et al. (2009) Efficacy of systemic morpholino exon-skipping in Duchenne dystrophy dogs. Ann Neurol 65: 667–676.
3. Mendell JR, Rodino-Klapac LR, Sahenk Z, Roush K, Bird L, et al. (2013) Eteplirsen for the treatment of Duchenne muscular dystrophy. Ann Neurol 74: 637–647.
4. Heier CR, Damsker JM, Yu Q, Dillingham BC, Huynh T, et al. (2013) VBP15, a novel anti-inflammatory and membrane-stabilizer, improves muscular dystrophy without side effects. EMBO Mol Med 5: 1569–1585.
5. Hoffman EP, McNally EM (2014) Exon-skipping therapy: a roadblock, detour, or bump in the road? Sci Transl Med 6: 230fs214.
6. Prinz F, Schlange T, Asadullah K (2011) Believe it or not: how much can we rely on published data on potential drug targets? Nat Rev Drug Discov 10: 712.
7. Perrin S (2014) Preclinical research: Make mouse studies work. Nature 507: 423–425.
8. Scott S, Kranz JE, Cole J, Lincecum JM, Thompson K, et al. (2008) Design, power, and interpretation of studies in the standard murine model of ALS. Amyotroph Lateral Scler 9: 4–15.
9. Lu QL, Cirak S, Partridge T (2014) What Can We Learn From Clinical Trials of Exon Skipping for DMD? Mol Ther Nucleic Acids 3: e152.
10. Huang Y, Majumdar S, Genant HK, Chan WP, Sharma KR, et al. (1994) Quantitative MR relaxometry study of muscle composition and function in Duchenne muscular dystrophy. J Magn Reson Imaging 4: 59–64.
11. Mercuri E, Pichiecchio A, Allsop J, Messina S, Pane M, et al. (2007) Muscle MRI in inherited neuromuscular disorders: past, present, and future. J Magn Reson Imaging 25: 433–440.
12. Kim HK, Merrow AC, Shiraj S, Wong BL, Horn PS, et al. (2013) Analysis of fatty infiltration and inflammation of the pelvic and thigh muscles in boys with Duchenne muscular dystrophy (DMD): grading of disease involvement on MR imaging and correlation with clinical assessments. Pediatr Radiol 43: 1327–1335.
13. Kinali M, Arechavala-Gomeza V, Cirak S, Glover A, Guglieri M, et al. (2011) Muscle histology vs MRI in Duchenne muscular dystrophy. Neurology 76: 346–353.
14. Banerjee B, Sharma U, Balasubramanian K, Kalaivani M, Kalra V, et al. (2010) Effect of creatine monohydrate in improving cellular energetics and muscle strength in ambulatory Duchenne muscular dystrophy patients: a randomized, placebo-controlled 31P MRS study. Magn Reson Imaging 28: 698–707.
15. Newman RJ, Bore PJ, Chan L, Gadian DG, Styles P, et al. (1982) Nuclear magnetic resonance studies of forearm muscle in Duchenne dystrophy. Br Med J (Clin Res Ed) 284: 1072–1074.
16. Forbes SC, Walter GA, Rooney WD, Wang DJ, DeVos S, et al. (2013) Skeletal muscles of ambulant children with Duchenne muscular dystrophy: validation of multicenter study of evaluation with MR imaging and MR spectroscopy. Radiology 269: 198–207.
17. Willcocks RJ, Arpan IA, Forbes SC, Lott DJ, Senesac CR, et al. (2014) Longitudinal measurements of MRI-T2 in boys with Duchenne muscular dystrophy: effects of age and disease progression. Neuromuscul Disord 24: 393–401.
18. Kim HK, Laor T, Horn PS, Racadio JM, Wong B, et al. (2010) T2 mapping in Duchenne muscular dystrophy: distribution of disease activity and correlation with clinical assessments. Radiology 255: 899–908.

19. Arpan I, Forbes SC, Lott DJ, Senesac CR, Daniels MJ, et al. (2013) T(2) mapping provides multiple approaches for the characterization of muscle involvement in neuromuscular diseases: a cross-sectional study of lower leg muscles in 5-15-year-old boys with Duchenne muscular dystrophy. NMR Biomed 26: 320–328.
20. Muntoni F, Mateddu A, Marchei F, Clerk A, Serra G (1993) Muscular weakness in the mdx mouse. J Neurol Sci 120: 71–77.
21. Dangain J, Vrbova G (1984) Muscle development in mdx mutant mice. Muscle Nerve 7: 700–704.
22. Tanabe Y, Esaki K, Nomura T (1986) Skeletal muscle pathology in X chromosome-linked muscular dystrophy (mdx) mouse. Acta Neuropathol 69: 91–95.
23. Anderson JE, Bressler BH, Ovalle WK (1988) Functional regeneration in the hindlimb skeletal muscle of the mdx mouse. J Muscle Res Cell Motil 9: 499–515.
24. Spurney CF, Gordish-Dressman H, Guerron AD, Sali A, Pandey GS, et al. (2009) Preclinical drug trials in the mdx mouse: assessment of reliable and sensitive outcome measures. Muscle Nerve 39: 591–602.
25. Huynh T, Uaesoontrachoon K, Quinn JL, Tatem KS, Heier CR, et al. (2013) Selective modulation through the glucocorticoid receptor ameliorates muscle pathology in mdx mice. J Pathol 231: 223–235.
26. Kushmerick MJ (1985) Patterns in mammalian muscle energetics. J Exp Biol 115: 165–177.
27. Kushmerick MJ (1987) Energetics studies of muscles of different types. Basic Res Cardiol 82 Suppl 2: 17–30.
28. Kushmerick MJ (1995) Skeletal muscle: a paradigm for testing principles of bioenergetics. J Bioenerg Biomembr 27: 555–569.
29. Zhang W, ten Hove M, Schneider JE, Stuckey DJ, Sebag-Montefiore L, et al. (2008) Abnormal cardiac morphology, function and energy metabolism in the dystrophic mdx mouse: an MRI and MRS study. J Mol Cell Cardiol 45: 754–760.
30. Jahnke VE, Van Der Meulen JH, Johnston HK, Ghimbovschi S, Partridge T, et al. (2012) Metabolic remodeling agents show beneficial effects in the dystrophin-deficient mdx mouse model. Skelet Muscle 2: 16.
31. Sharma U, Kumar V, Wadhwa S, Jagannathan NR (2007) In vivo (31)P MRS study of skeletal muscle metabolism in patients with postpolio residual paralysis. Magn Reson Imaging 25: 244–249.
32. Taylor DJ, Kemp GJ, Radda GK (1994) Bioenergetics of skeletal muscle in mitochondrial myopathy. J Neurol Sci 127: 198–206.
33. Walter G, Cordier L, Bloy D, Sweeney HL (2005) Noninvasive monitoring of gene correction in dystrophic muscle. Magn Reson Med 54: 1369–1376.
34. McIntosh LM, Baker RE, Anderson JE (1998) Magnetic resonance imaging of regenerating and dystrophic mouse muscle. Biochem Cell Biol 76: 532–541.
35. Coulton GR, Curtin NA, Morgan JE, Partridge TA (1988) The mdx mouse skeletal muscle myopathy: II. Contractile properties. Neuropathol Appl Neurobiol 14: 299–314.
36. Coulton GR, Morgan JE, Partridge TA, Sloper JC (1988) The mdx mouse skeletal muscle myopathy: I. A histological, morphometric and biochemical investigation. Neuropathol Appl Neurobiol 14: 53–70.
37. Lynch GS, Hinkle RT, Chamberlain JS, Brooks SV, Faulkner JA (2001) Force and power output of fast and slow skeletal muscles from mdx mice 6-28 months old. J Physiol 535: 591–600.
38. Dellorusso C, Crawford RW, Chamberlain JS, Brooks SV (2001) Tibialis anterior muscles in mdx mice are highly susceptible to contraction-induced injury. J Muscle Res Cell Motil 22: 467–475.

39. Kumar A, Bhatnagar S, Kumar A (2010) Matrix metalloproteinase inhibitor batimastat alleviates pathology and improves skeletal muscle function in dystrophin-deficient mdx mice. Am J Pathol 177: 248–260.

40. Lamminen AE (1990) Magnetic resonance imaging of primary skeletal muscle diseases: patterns of distribution and severity of involvement. Br J Radiol 63: 946–950.

41. Phoenix J, Betal D, Roberts N, Helliwell TR, Edwards RH (1996) Objective quantification of muscle and fat in human dystrophic muscle by magnetic resonance image analysis. Muscle Nerve 19: 302–310.

42. Quinlan JG, Hahn HS, Wong BL, Lorenz JN, Wenisch AS, et al. (2004) Evolution of the mdx mouse cardiomyopathy: physiological and morphological findings. Neuromuscul Disord 14: 491–496.

43. Spurney CF, Knoblach S, Pistilli EE, Nagaraju K, Martin GR, et al. (2008) Dystrophin-deficient cardiomyopathy in mouse: expression of Nox4 and Lox are associated with fibrosis and altered functional parameters in the heart. Neuromuscul Disord 18: 371–381.

44. Chamberlain JS, Metzger J, Reyes M, Townsend D, Faulkner JA (2007) Dystrophin-deficient mdx mice display a reduced life span and are susceptible to spontaneous rhabdomyosarcoma. FASEB J 21: 2195–2204.

45. Stuckey DJ, Carr CA, Camelliti P, Tyler DJ, Davies KE, et al. (2012) In vivo MRI characterization of progressive cardiac dysfunction in the mdx mouse model of muscular dystrophy. PLoS One 7: e28569.

46. Straub V, Donahue KM, Allamand V, Davisson RL, Kim YR, et al. (2000) Contrast agent-enhanced magnetic resonance imaging of skeletal muscle damage in animal models of muscular dystrophy. Magn Reson Med 44: 655–659.

47. Amthor H, Egelhof T, McKinnell I, Ladd ME, Janssen I, et al. (2004) Albumin targeting of damaged muscle fibres in the mdx mouse can be monitored by MRI. Neuromuscul Disord 14: 791–796.

48. Odintsov B, Chun JL, Mulligan JA, Berry SE (2011) 14.1 T whole body MRI for detection of mesoangioblast stem cells in a murine model of Duchenne muscular dystrophy. Magn Reson Med 66: 1704–1714.

49. Cahill KS, Gaidosh G, Huard J, Silver X, Byrne BJ, et al. (2004) Noninvasive monitoring and tracking of muscle stem cell transplants. Transplantation 78: 1626–1633.

50. Walter GA, Cahill KS, Huard J, Feng H, Douglas T, et al. (2004) Noninvasive monitoring of stem cell transfer for muscle disorders. Magn Reson Med 51: 273–277.

51. Martins-Bach AB, Bloise AC, Vainzof M, Rahnamaye Rabbani S (2012) Metabolic profile of dystrophic mdx mouse muscles analyzed with in vitro magnetic resonance spectroscopy (MRS). Magn Reson Imaging 30: 1167–1176.

52. Xu S, Pratt SJ, Spangenburg EE, Lovering RM (2012) Early metabolic changes measured by 1H MRS in healthy and dystrophic muscle after injury. J Appl Physiol (1985) 113: 808–816.

53. Dunn JF, Zaim-Wadghiri Y (1999) Quantitative magnetic resonance imaging of the mdx mouse model of Duchenne muscular dystrophy. Muscle Nerve 22: 1367–1371.

54. Mathur S, Vohra RS, Germain SA, Forbes S, Bryant ND, et al. (2011) Changes in muscle T2 and tissue damage after downhill running in mdx mice. Muscle Nerve 43: 878–886.

55. Pratt SJ, Xu S, Mullins RJ, Lovering RM (2013) Temporal changes in magnetic resonance imaging in the mdx mouse. BMC Res Notes 6: 262.

56. Pacak CA, Walter GA, Gaidosh G, Bryant N, Lewis MA, et al. (2007) Long-term skeletal muscle protection after gene transfer in a mouse model of LGMD-2D. Mol Ther 15: 1775–1781.

57. Bach JR (2007) Medical considerations of long-term survival of Werdnig-Hoffmann disease. Am J Phys Med Rehabil 86: 349–355.

58. Roos M, Sarkozy A, Chierchia GB, De Wilde P, Schmedding E, et al. (2009) Malignant ventricular arrhythmia in a case of adult onset of spinal muscular atrophy (Kugelberg-Welander disease). J Cardiovasc Electrophysiol 20: 342–344.

9

Simple and Reliable Determination of Intravoxel Incoherent Motion Parameters for the Differential Diagnosis of Head and Neck Tumors

Miho Sasaki, Misa Sumi, Sato Eida, Ikuo Katayama, Yuka Hotokezaka, Takashi Nakamura*

Department of Radiology and Cancer Biology, Nagasaki University School of Dentistry, Nagasaki, Japan

Abstract

Intravoxel incoherent motion (IVIM) imaging can characterize diffusion and perfusion of normal and diseased tissues, and IVIM parameters are authentically determined by using cumbersome least-squares method. We evaluated a simple technique for the determination of IVIM parameters using geometric analysis of the multiexponential signal decay curve as an alternative to the least-squares method for the diagnosis of head and neck tumors. Pure diffusion coefficients (D), microvascular volume fraction (f), perfusion-related incoherent microcirculation (D*), and perfusion parameter that is heavily weighted towards extravascular space (P) were determined geometrically (Geo D, Geo f, and Geo P) or by least-squares method (Fit D, Fit f, and Fit D*) in normal structures and 105 head and neck tumors. The IVIM parameters were compared for their levels and diagnostic abilities between the 2 techniques. The IVIM parameters were not able to determine in 14 tumors with the least-squares method alone and in 4 tumors with the geometric and least-squares methods. The geometric IVIM values were significantly different ($p < 0.001$) from Fit values ($+2 \pm 4\%$ and $-7 \pm 24\%$ for D and f values, respectively). Geo D and Fit D differentiated between lymphomas and SCCs with similar efficacy (78% and 80% accuracy, respectively). Stepwise approaches using combinations of Geo D and Geo P, Geo D and Geo f, or Fit D and Fit D* differentiated between pleomorphic adenomas, Warthin tumors, and malignant salivary gland tumors with the same efficacy (91% accuracy = 21/23). However, a stepwise differentiation using Fit D and Fit f was less effective (83% accuracy = 19/23). Considering cumbersome procedures with the least squares method compared with the geometric method, we concluded that the geometric determination of IVIM parameters can be an alternative to least-squares method in the diagnosis of head and neck tumors.

Editor: Sune N. Jespersen, Aarhus University, Denmark

Funding: The authors received the funds of this study from the internal source of Nagasaki University. The funders had no role in study design, data collection and analysis, decision to publish, or preparation of the manuscript.

Competing Interests: The authors have declared that no competing interests exist.

* Email: taku@nagasaki-u.ac.jp

Introduction

Diffusion occurs because of the non-ending movement of every single molecule [1]. Brown first observed this phenomenon (although Ingenhousz found the phenomenon earlier than Brown did), and Einstein later gave this phenomenon a sound mathematical description considering a free diffusion process, where the molecules only collide with other molecules in a homogeneous container without boundaries. Diffusion-weighted imaging (DWI) is based on MR signal attenuations caused by the displacement of intracellular and extracellular water molecules for a given time. In biological tissues, however, the environment of water molecules can hardly be called homogeneous: membranes, macromolecules, and fibers hamper the diffusion process [2]. Furthermore, there is other incoherent motion within a voxel that can lead to signal attenuation; in particular, the water molecules in blood capillaries exhibit a pseudorandom motion in the tortuous capillaries.

Le Bihan proposed that intravoxel incoherent motion (IVIM) imaging can distinguish between the pure molecular diffusion and motion of water molecules in the capillary network with a single DWI acquisition technique, provided that high b-values (≥ 200 s/mm^2) and low b-values (< 200 s/mm^2) are used [3]. The IVIM imaging can be characterized by 3 parameters: pure diffusion coefficient (D); microvascular volume fraction (f); and perfusion-related incoherent microcirculation (D*) [4]. To determine the IVIM parameters from a multiexponential signal decay curve, the least-squares method is usually used [4,5]. However, the method is cumbersome, and thus may not be suitable for routine clinical use.

Recently, some researchers have applied simplified methods for determining IVIM parameters to characterize tumors in the liver, prostate, and head and neck region [6–9]. For example, Lewin et al shoed that the perfusion fraction parameter f determined by using a geometric analysis of DW MR images can be a marker of sorafenib treatment of patients with advanced hepatocellular carcinoma [7]. However, they did not indicate how precise the geometric determination of the perfusion parameter compared with the conventional technique. In addition, Mazaheri et al noted that the linear fit of the logarithmic signal using limited numbers of b-value is statistically less appropriate than fitting the signals to exponential functions using a least-squares method [8]. The

Table 1. 105 head and neck tumors.

Tumor	n
Benign	35
Salivary gland tumor	
Pleomorphic adenoma	15
Warthin tumor	8
Odontogenic tumor	
Ameloblastoma	2
Keratocystic odontogenic tumor	2
Odontogenic fibroma	2
Odontogenic myxoma	1
Hemangioma	1
Angiomyoma	1
Myofibroma	1
Papiloma	1
Adenomatous goiter	1
Malignant	70
SCC	25
SCC node	12
Lymphoma	14
Salivary gland tumor	
Carcinoma ex. pleomorphic adenoma	2
Adenoid cystic carcinoma	1
Acinic cell carcinoma	1
Adenocarcinoma	1
Dedifferentiated carcinoma	1
Salivary duct carcinoma	1
Lymph node metastasis from malignant salivary gland tumor	4
Malignant melanoma	1
Nasopharyngeal carcinoma	1
Neuroendocrine carcinoma	1
Papillary thyroid carcinoma	1
Lymph node metastasis from papillary thyroid carcinoma	3
Ameloblastic carcinoma	1
Total	105

SCC, squamous cell carcinoma.
Of 105 tumors, 18 were excluded from the study owing to measurement errors, including 6 pleomorphic adenomas, 2 lymphomas, 2 SCCs (oropharynx and hypopharynx), 1 SCC node, 1 adenocarcinoma, 1 metastatic node from papillary thyroid carcinoma, 1 neuroendocrine carcinoma, 1 ameloblastic carcinoma, 1 hemangioma, 1 keratocystic odontogenic tumor, 1 myxoma.

authors also suggested the importance of b-value selection used for the simplified IVIM analysis. In simplified methods, the IVIM parameters are estimated by using a limited number [3–4] of b-values compared with the authentic IVIM imaging, which uses 9–13 b-values [4,5,10,11]. However, the reliability in measurements and effectiveness in diagnosing tumors with simplified IVIM techniques using limited numbers of b-value has not been fully investigated. Sasaki et al. reported the reproducibility of IVIM parameter measurements in evaluating the technique for functional assessment of the masticator muscles [12]. However, there was no published report that presented the reproducibility of IVIM parameters in diagnosing tumors. In the present study, we directly compared the IVIM parameter values that were

determined by a simplified geometric method with those determined by the conventional least-squares method. We have also compared the diagnostic accuracy for diagnosing head and neck squamous cell carcinomas (SCCs) and lymphomas as well as benign and malignant salivary gland tumors between the 2 methods.

Materials and Methods

Ethics statement

The Ethics Committee of Nagasaki University approved this study. Informed consent was waived due to the retrospective

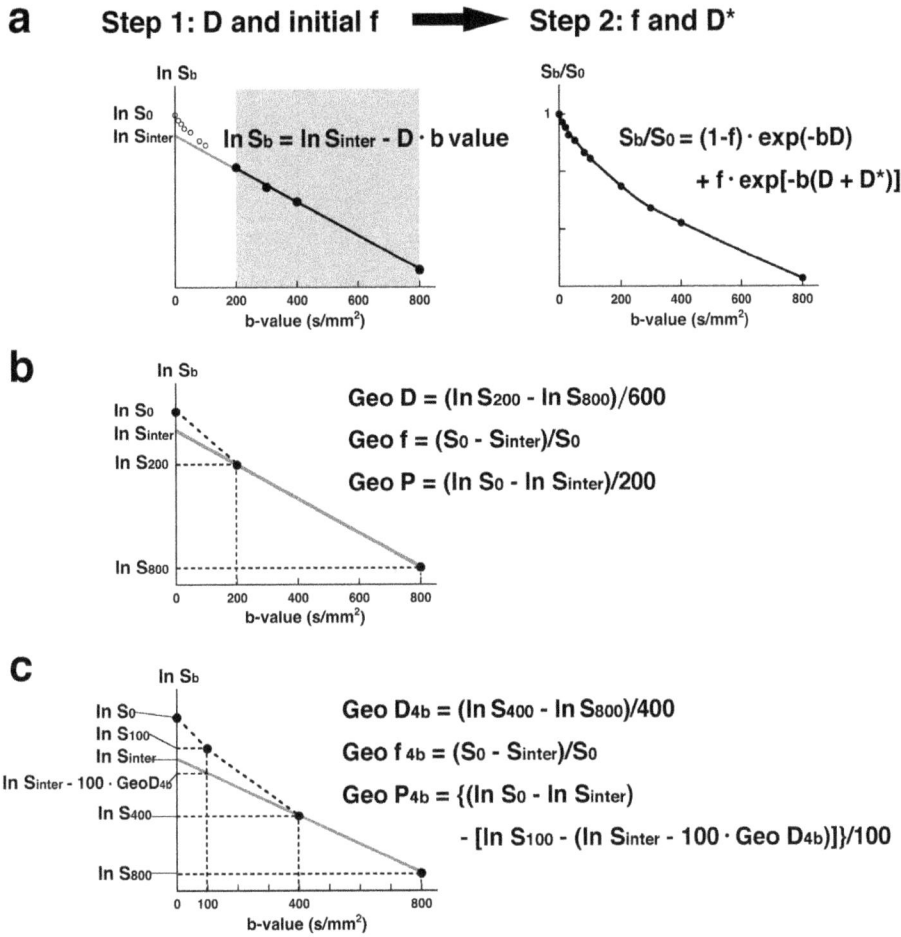

a **Step 1: D and initial f** ➡ **Step 2: f and D***

$$\ln S_b = \ln S_{inter} - D \cdot b\ value$$

$$S_b/S_0 = (1-f) \cdot \exp(-bD)$$
$$+ f \cdot \exp[-b(D + D^*)]$$

b

$$Geo\ D = (\ln S_{200} - \ln S_{800})/600$$
$$Geo\ f = (S_0 - S_{inter})/S_0$$
$$Geo\ P = (\ln S_0 - \ln S_{inter})/200$$

c

$$Geo\ D_{4b} = (\ln S_{400} - \ln S_{800})/400$$
$$Geo\ f_{4b} = (S_0 - S_{inter})/S_0$$
$$Geo\ P_{4b} = \{(\ln S_0 - \ln S_{inter})$$
$$- [\ln S_{100} - (\ln S_{inter} - 100 \cdot Geo\ D_{4b})]\}/100$$

Figure 1. IVIM parameter determination by least-squares or geometric method. a, Least-squares method. Upper panel shows a representative signal decay curve obtained by using 11 b-values (0, 10, 20, 30, 50, 80, 100, 200, 300, 400, 800 s/mm^2). At first step, D (Fit D) can be obtained by least-squares method using $\ln S_{200}$, $\ln S_{300}$, $\ln S_{400}$, and $\ln S_{800}$, and initial f value is calculated as $(S_0 - S_{inter})/S_0$, where S_{inter} is the interception of the logarithmic regression line obtained by using b-values of 200, 300, 400, and 800 s/mm^2 with the y-axis. Right panel shows relationship between S_b/S_0 and varying b-values. Given D and initial f and D* values, f (Fit f) and D* (Fit D*) values can be obtained by least-squares method based on the equation: $S_b/S_0 = (1-f) \cdot \exp(-bD) + f \cdot [-b(D+D^*)]$. **b,** Geometric method. Graph shows geometric determination of IVIM parameters using 3 (0, 200, and 800 s/mm^2) of the 11 b-values. D is calculated by the equation $GeoD = (\ln S_{200} - \ln S_{800})/600$. f is estimated by the equation $Geof = (S_0 - S_{inter})/S_0$, and P is estimated by the equation $GeoP = (\ln S_0 - \ln S_{inter})/200$Geo P = (ln S$_0$–ln S$_{inter}$)/200. **c,** Geometric method based on 4-b-value data. Graph shows geometric determination of IVIM parameters using 4 (0, 100, 400, and 800 s/mm^2) of the 11 b-values. D is calculated by the equation $GeoD_{4b} = (\ln S_{400} - \ln S_{800})/400$, f is estimated by the equation $Geof4b = (S_0 - S_{inter})/S_0$, and P is estimated by the equation $GeoP_{4b} = \{(\ln S_0 - \ln S_{inter}) - [\ln S_{100} - (\ln S_{inter} - 100 \cdot GeoD_{4b})]\}/100$.

Table 2. Inter- and intraobserver errors in measuring Geo and Fit IVIM parameters.

	IVIM parameters	%CV	
		Geo	Fit
Interobserver errors	D	0.5±0.2	0.5±0.3
	f	5.2±0.8	9.7±7.8
	P/D*	5.1±0.8	16.2±11.0
Intraobserver errors	D	0.9±0.9	1.0±0.9
	f	5.4±5.4	11.4±7.9
	P/D*	5.5±5.5[a]	19.7±8.6[a]

%CV, percent coefficient of variation; Geo, geometric measurement; Fit, least-squares method. P/D*, Geo P/Fit D*.
a, significant difference between Geo and Fit values (p=0.0195, Wilcoxon signed-rank test).

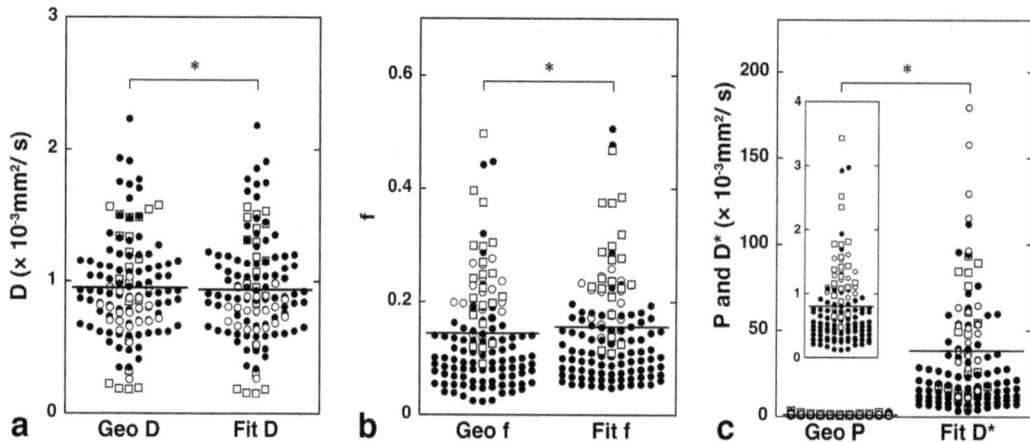

Figure 2. IVIM parameters of normal structures and tumors in the head and neck region. Plot graphs show D (Geo D), f (Geo f), and P (Geo P) values that were determined by geometric method; and D (Fit D), f (Fit f), and D* (Fit D*) values that were determined by least-squares method of normal structures (parotid glands, open circles; and masseter muscles, open squares) and head and neck tumors (closed circles). Broken white contours indicate tumor areas. Parotid gland: Geo D, Geo f and Geo P = $0.76\pm0.17\times10^{-3}$ mm^2/s, 0.20 ± 0.04, and $1.12\pm0.27\times10^{-3}$ mm^2/s, respectively; and Fit D, Fit f, and Fit D* = $0.75\pm0.16\times10^{-3}$ mm^2/s, 0.20 ± 0.05, and $62.96\pm46.78\times10^{-3}$ mm^2/s, respectively. Masseter muscle: Geo D, Geo f, and Geo P = $0.99\pm0.51\times10^{-3}$ mm^2/s, 0.24 ± 0.10, and $1.41\pm0.71\times10^{-3}$ mm^2/s, respectively; and Fit D, Fit f, and Fit D* = $0.96\pm0.51\times10^{-3}$ mm^2/s, 0.25 ± 0.10, and $40.50\pm30.13\times10^{-3}$ mm^2/s, respectively. Tumors: Geo D, Geo f, and Geo P = $1.00\pm0.38\times10^{-3}$ mm^2/s, 0.11 ± 0.08, and $0.61\pm0.48\times10^{-3}$ mm^2/s, respectively; Fit D, Fit f, and Fit D* = $0.99\pm0.37\times10^{-3}$ mm^2/s, 0.12 ± 0.08, and $24.14\pm21.15\times10^{-3}$ mm^2/s, respectively. Insert, Geo P distribution on a small scale. The values are the results of integrated signal intensities within the ROIs. *, p<0.001 (Wilcoxon signed-rank test).

nature of the study. Patient records/information was anonymized and de-identified prior to analysis.

Patients

We retrospectively studied DW MR images of patients with head and neck tumors who underwent preoperative MR examinations between March 2003 to April 2012. We selected head and neck tumors from patients (1) who underwent diffusion-weighted MR imaging as well as conventional contrast-enhanced and non-enhanced T1-weighted and fat-suppressed T2-weighted MR imaging; (2) whose tumors were excised and histologically proven; and (3) whose DW images were good in quality without any severe susceptibility artifacts that would interfere with IVIM analysis. Consequently, the study cohort included 105 head and neck tumors (35 benign and 70 malignant tumors) that arose in 94 patients (56 men and 38 women; average age, 62 ± 15 years; age range, 3–91 years). Detailed tumor pathology is listed in Table 1.

DW MR images of the healthy parotid glands (n = 21) and the masseter muscles (n = 21) of the contralateral sides in patients with parotid tumor were also analyzed for comparing the IVIM parameters determined by using geometric or least-squares methods.

MR imaging

MR imaging was performed using a 1.5-T MR unit (Gyroscan Intera 1.5T Master; Philips Healthcare, Best, The Netherlands). 73 patients were scanned by using a 2-channel 17-cm×14-cm (Synergy-Flex M), 7 patients by using a 2-channel 20-cm (Synergy-Flex L) surface coil, and 14 patients by using a 3-channel head and neck coil (Synergy Head Neck).

T1- and T2-weighted MR imaging

We obtained axial T1- and fat-suppressed (spectral attenuated with inversion recovery, [SPAIR]) T2-weighted MR images (TR/TE/number of signal acquisitions = 500 ms/15 ms/2 and 6385 ms/80 ms/2, respectively) by using a turbo spin-echo

(TSE) sequence (TSE factor = 3 and 15, respectively). We used a 200-mm FOV, 256×204 scan and 512×512 reconstruction matrix sizes, a 4-mm slice thickness and a 0.4-mm slice gap. For contrast-enhanced T1-weighted MR imaging, a gadolinium-based agent (gadopentatate dimeglutimine, Magnevist; Bayer Healthcare, Berlin, Germany) was intravenously injected at a dose of 0.2 mL per kg of body weight and a rate of 1.5 mL/s.

DW MR imaging

Axial DW images (TR/TE = 1625 ms/81 ms) were obtained using single-shot, spin-echo echo planar imaging (SE-EPI). The EPI factor was 47, and Sensitivity Encoding (SENSE) factor was 2. We used a 200-mm FOV, 4-mm slice thickness, 0.4-mm slice gap, and 112×90 matrix size. The measured pixel size was 1.79/2.28/4 mm. We used 11 b-values (0, 10, 20, 30, 50, 80, 100, 200, 300, 400, and 800 s/mm^2). The total acquisition time was 1 min 53 s per 5 slices.

Regions of interest

A region of interest (ROI) was manually placed onto each tumor area such that it encompassed as much of the tumor area as possible. The mean ROI area was 3.4 ± 2.8 cm^2 (0.8–18.1 cm^2). Visually large cystic or necrotic areas were excluded from the present analysis. We used the contrast-enhanced T1-weighted and fat-suppressed T2-weighted MR images as references to determine tumor areas on the corresponding DW images. We compared the IVIM values between geometric and least-squares methods based on the IVIM values calculated from ROI-averaged signal intensities. We used DW image slices including the 1–3 maximal tumor areas, and the IVIM values obtained from each ROIs were averaged. For the healthy parotid glands and masseter muscles, irregular ROIs were placed so that they included as much of the gland or muscle area as possible, but did not include large vessels, such as the retromandibular vein, or intraglandular main ducts. A radiologist with 20-year experience in head and neck radiology placed ROIs and analyzed IVIM images.

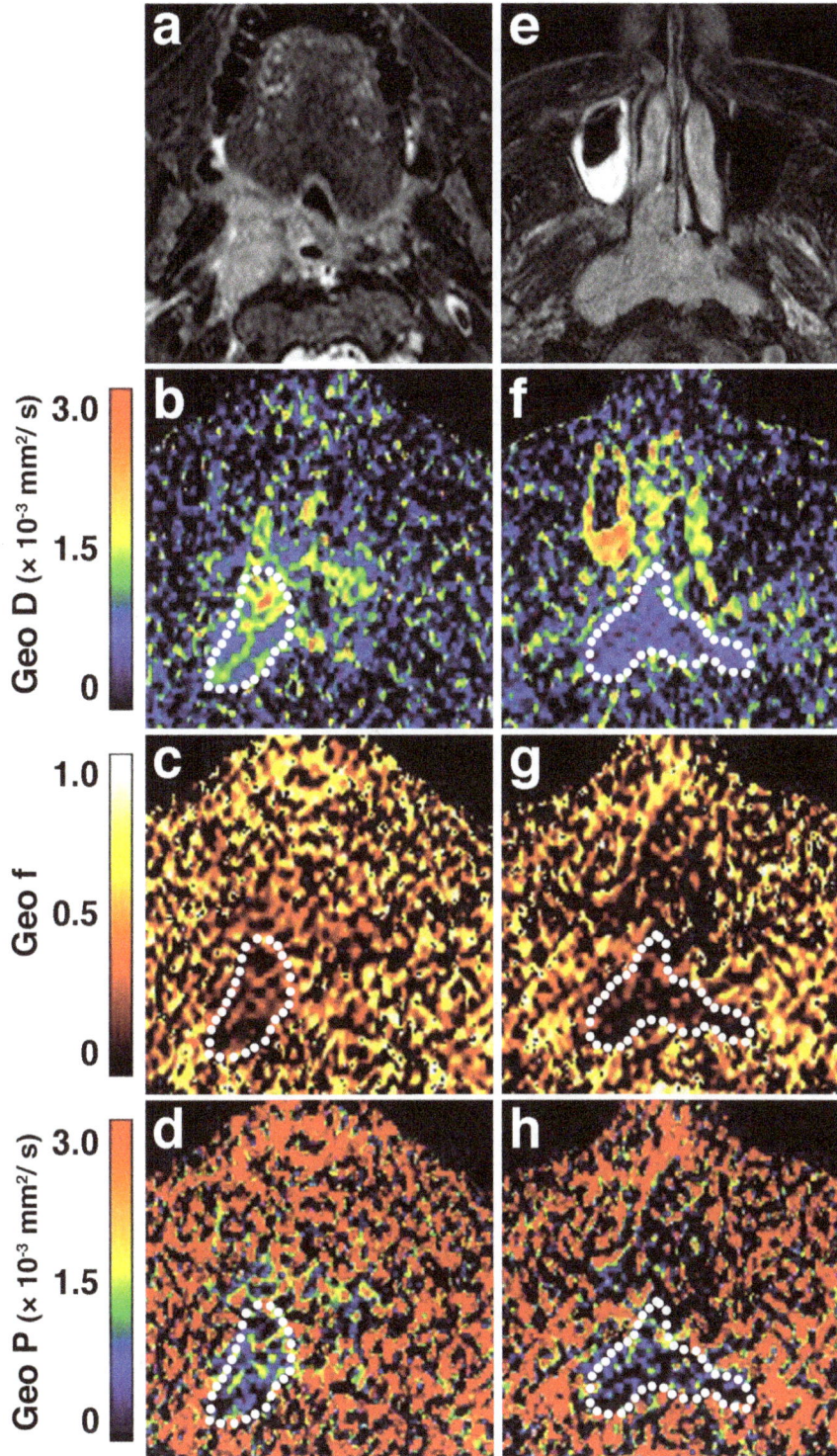

Figure 3. IVIM maps of SCC and lymphoma. a–d, Axial fat-suppressed T2-weighted MR image (**a**), and Geo D (**b**), Geo f (**c**), and Geo P (**d**) maps of 72-year-old man with SCC in oropharynx show tumor with homogeneous T2-signals and IVIM parameter values of Geo D, Geo f, and Geo P = 1.16×10^{-3} mm^2/s, 0.14, and 0.76×10^{-3} mm^2/s, respectively; and Fit D, Fit f, and Fit D* = 1.14×10^{-3} mm^2/s, 0.18, and 8.50×10^{-3} mm^2/s, respectively. **e–h,** Axial fat-suppressed T2-weighted MR image (**e**), and Geo D (**f**), Geo f (**g**), and Geo P (**h**) maps of 79-year-old man with lymphoma In nasopharynx show tumor with homogeneous T2 signals and IVIM parameter values of Geo D, Geo f, and Geo P = 0.59×10^{-3} mm^2/s, 0.08, and 0.41×10^{-3} mm^2/s, respectively; and Fit D, Fit f, and Fit D* = 0.60×10^{-3} mm^2/s, 0.07, and 17.01×10^{-3} mm^2/s, respectively. The values are the results of integrated signal intensities within the ROIs.

Table 3. IVIM parameters of SCCs and lymphomas.

IVIM parameter	SCC (n = 34)	Lymphoma (n = 12)
D ($\times 10^{-3}$ mm^2/s)		
Geo	0.93 ± 0.23^a	0.63 ± 0.16^a
Fit	0.93 ± 0.23^b	0.62 ± 0.15^b
f		
Geo	0.13 ± 0.10	0.09 ± 0.04
Fit	0.14 ± 0.10	0.10 ± 0.03
P/D* ($\times 10^{-3}$ mm^2/s)		
Geo	0.74 ± 0.65	0.49 ± 0.23
Fit	27.11 ± 22.06	28.52 ± 15.01

IVIM, intravoxel incoherent motion; SCC, squamous cell carcinoma; Geo, IVIM parameters determined by geometric method; Fit, IVIM parameters determined by least squares method. P/D*, Geo P/Fit D*.
[a, b]significant differences (p = 0.0002, Mann-Whitney U test).

IVIM analysis based on least squares method

The relationship between signal intensities and b-values based on the IVIM theory can be expressed using the following equation:

$$S_b/S_o = (1-f) \cdot \exp(-bD) + f \cdot \exp[-b(D+D^*)] \quad (1)$$

where f is microvascular volume fraction, D is pure diffusion coefficient, and D* represents perfusion-related incoherent microcirculation [4]; S_0 and S_b are signal intensities at b = 0 and b = 10, 20, 30, 50, 80, 100, 200, 300, 400, or 800 s/mm^2, respectively. Using logarithmic plots (Fig. 1a), D (Fit D) can be obtained with a linear regression algorithm (the least-squares methods using b-values of 200, 300, 400, and 800 s/mm^2). Given a D value, the initial f value was estimated as y-axis intersection of the linear regression (Fig. 1a). Then, the corresponding f (Fit f) and D* (Fit D*) values can be calculated using a nonlinear regression algorithm based on equation (1) (Fig. 1a). Fit f and Fit D* values were obtained after substituting initial f and D* values into the Levenberg-Marquardt algorithm [13], using SPSS software (Version 18.0, IBM incorporation). The initial values used for the least-squares method were as follows: f = −0.06–0.49 (average, 0.11 ± 0.08); D* = 0.01 [5,7]. The convergence criterion was 0.00000001.

IVIM analysis based on geometric method

Separately, we analyzed signal decay curves by using the geometric method as described previously [6,7,9]. By using logarithmic plots, D can be estimated as a decline between b = 200–800 s/mm^2, (ln S_{200}–ln S_{800})/600 (Fig. 1b). Given an estimated D value, we estimated the tissue perfusion by geometrically estimating the f as 1–S_{inter}/S_0 (S_{inter} is the interception of the logarithmic regression line obtained using b-values of 200 and 800 s/mm^2 with the y-axis) (Fig. 1). On the other hand, perfusion property can be geometrically estimated by the formula as (ln S_0–ln S_{inter})/200. Fit D* reflects the vascular space only. However, the geometrically defined perfusion parameter is heavily weighted towards the perfusion in the extravascular space. Therefore, the geometrically perfusion parameter is fundamentally different from Fit D*. We introduced a perfusion parameter Geo P, which reflects and averages the vascular and extravascular spaces.

Separately, we determined IVIM parameters based on 4 b-value (b = 0, 100, 400, and 800 s/mm^2) data according to the followings (Fig. 1c):

$$GeoD_{4b} = (lnS_{400} - \ln S_{800})/400$$

$$Geof_{4b} = (S_0 - S_{inter})/S_0$$

$$GeoP_{4b} =$$

$$\{(\ln S_0 - \ln S_{inter}) - [\ln S_{100} - (\ln S_{inter} - 100 \cdot GeoD_{4b})]\}/100$$

$$= (\ln S_0 - \ln S_{100} - 100 \cdot GeoD_{4b})/100$$

DW images in a DICOM format were converted to 2D color maps of geometrically determined f, D, and D* values by using the ImageJ software (NIH, http://rsweb.nih.gov/ij/index.html). We used an existing fit plug-in for ImageJ software. The color maps were generated purely for qualitative illustration and were not employed in the quantitative performance comparison of the least squares and geometrical methods for calculating IVIM parameters.

Interobserver and intraobserver errors

Separate sets of DW MR images, including conventional T1- and T2-weighted, contrast-enhanced T1-weighted, and DW MR images, from 5 patients with head and neck tumors were analyzed independently by 3 separate radiologists with 17–20-year experience. The radiologists were asked to place an ROI onto each of DW MR images at b-values of 0, 200, and 800 s/mm^2. One day after, the same radiologists were asked to repeat the same procedure with the same sets of DW MR images. Interobserver and intraobserver errors were assessed by calculating percent coefficient of variation (%CV) of IVIM parameters obtained from different ROIs placed on the same DW MR images.

Statistics

Wilcoxon signed-rank test was used for the comparison of the IVIM parameters between the 2 techniques. Steel-Dwass test was used for the comparison of the IVIM parameters between the 3 different types of salivary gland tumors. Mann-Whitney U-test was used for the comparison of the IVIM parameters between lymphomas and SCCs. Cluster analysis was used to determine the best threshold for the IVIM criteria for discriminating between different tumor groups, where the best cutoff IVIM values were determined so that the values differentiated with the highest

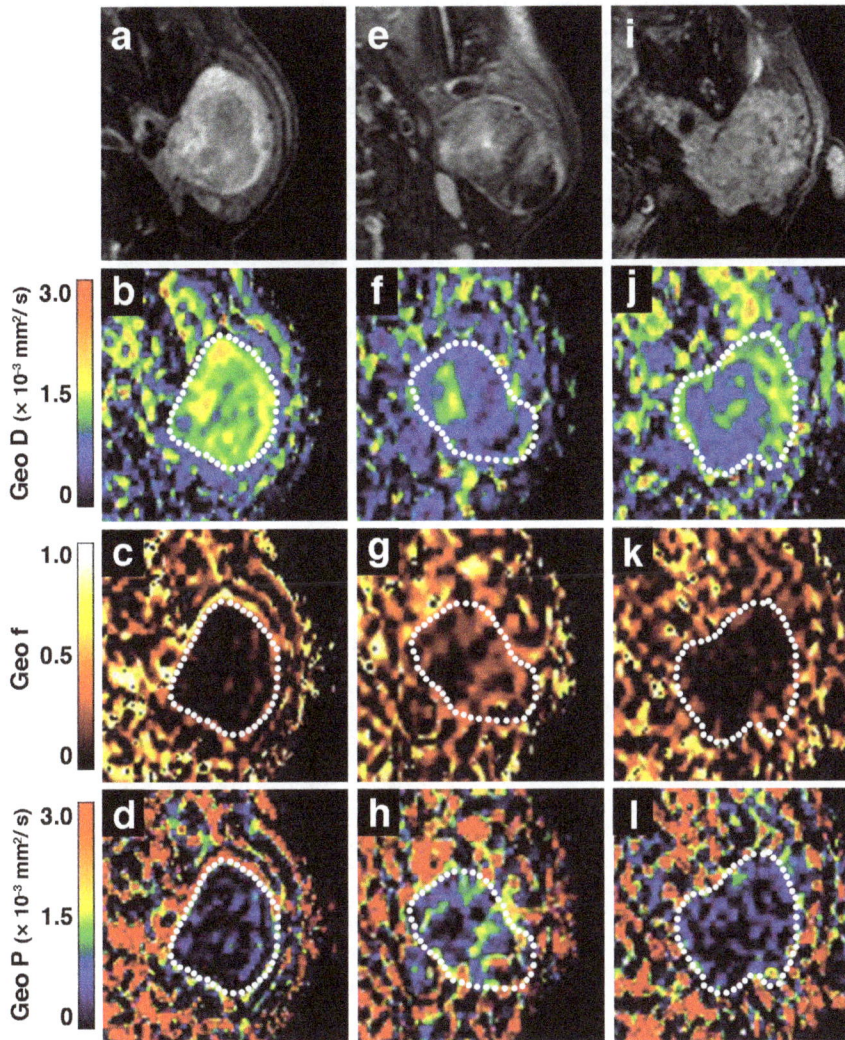

Figure 4. IVIM maps of benign and malignant salivary gland tumors. a–d, Axial fat-suppressed T2-weighted MR image (**a**), and Geo D (**b**), Geo f (**c**), and Geo P (**d**) maps of 67-year-old man with pleomorphic adenoma in left parotid gland show tumor with heterogeneous T2-signals and IVIM parameter values of Geo D, Geo f, and Geo P = 1.37×10^{-3} mm²/s, 0.02, and 0.12×10^{-3} mm²/s, respectively; and Fit D, Fit f, and Fit D* = 1.37×10^{-3} mm²/s, 0.05, and 4.23×10^{-3} mm²/s, respectively. Broken white contours indicate tumor areas. **e–h**, Axial fat-suppressed MR image (**e**), and Geo D (**f**), Geo f (**g**), and Geo P (**h**) maps of 65-year-old woman with Warthin tumor in left parotid gland show tumor with heterogeneous T2-signals and IVIM parameter values of Geo D, Geo f, and Geo P = 0.87×10^{-3} mm²/s, 0.14, and 0.75×10^{-3} mm²/s, respectively; and Fit D, Fit f, and Fit D* = 0.84×10^{-3} mm²/s, 0.16, and 23.32×10^{-3} mm²/s, respectively. Broken white contours indicate tumor areas. **i–l**, Axial fat-suppressed T2-weighted MR image (**i**), and Geo D (**j**), Geo f (**k**), and Geo P (**l**) maps of 59-year-old woman with carcinoma ex. Pleomorphic adenoma in left parotid gland show tumor with heterogeneous T2-signals and IVIM parameter values of Geo D, Geo f, and Geo P = 0.89×10^{-3} mm²/s, 0.04, and 0.20×10^{-3} mm²/s, respectively; and Fit D, Fit f, and Fit D* = 0.88×10^{-3} mm²/s, 0.05, and 10.00×10^{-3} mm²/s, respectively. Broken white contours indicate tumor areas. The values are the results of integrated signal intensities within the ROIs.

accuracy between different tumor groups that were categorized by Ward's method using dendrogram. The statistical analyses were performed using SPSS (Version 18.0, IBM Corporation) and Excel Statistics 2012 (Version 1.00; SSRI).

Results

Errors in ROI placement

Interobserver and intraobserver errors of IVIM parameters were similar between Geo and Fit methods, except for intraobserver errors of D* values (Tables 2, S1, and S3).

Computation-induced invalidity

IVIM imaging of 18 out of the 105 head and neck tumors resulted in invalid IVIM values from the whole ROI, including 4 tumors, in which f values were negative with geometric method; 3 tumors, in which initial f values were negative with least-squares method; and 17 tumors, in which obtained f or D* values were the same as the initial values with least-squares method. Consequently, IVIM parameters were not able to be determined in 14 tumors owing to computation-induced invalidity with the least-squares method alone, and 4 tumors owing to measurement errors with both methods.

Table 4. IVIM parameters of pleomorphic adenomas, Warthin tumors, and malignant SG tumors.

IVIM parameter	Pleomophic adenoma (n = 9)	Warthin tumor (n = 8)	Malignant SG tumor (n = 6)
D ($\times 10^{-3}$ mm²/s)			
Geo	1.41±0.28[a,b]	0.80±0.27[a]	0.93±0.20[b]
Fit	1.40±0.28[a,b]	0.79±0.27[a]	0.94±0.22[b]
f			
Geo	0.07±0.04[c]	0.13±0.04[c]	0.09±0.04
Fit	0.09±0.04	0.13±0.03[d]	0.08±0.03[d]
P/D* ($\times 10^{-3}$ mm²/s)			
Geo	0.35±0.19[e]	0.70±0.20[e]	0.47±0.22
Fit	15.16±17.15[f]	36.23±28.61[f]	18.38±17.84

IVIM, intravoxel incoherent motion; SG, salivary gland; Geo, IVIM parameters determined by geometrical method; Fit, IVIM parameters determined by least squares method. P/D*, Geo P/Fit D*.
[a-f]significant differences (p<0.05, Steel-Dwass test).

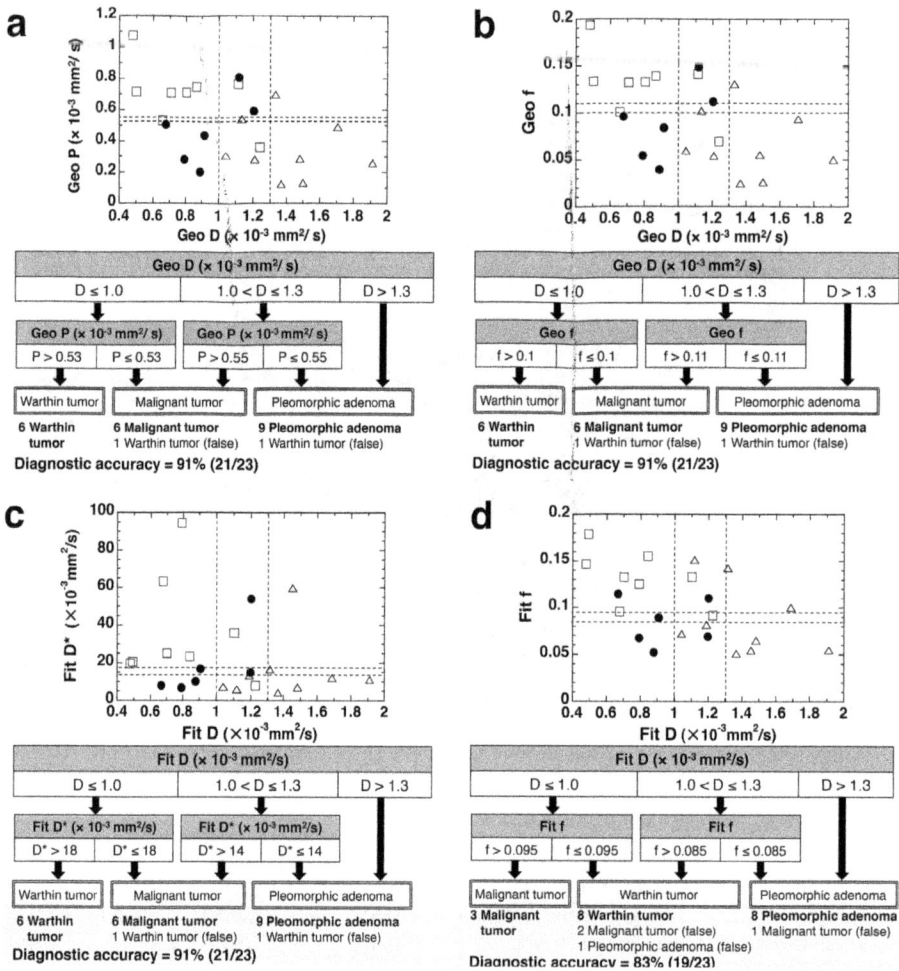

Figure 5. Stepwise differentiation between pleomorphic adenomas, Warthin tumors, and malignant salivary gland tumors using D, f, and D* or P values that were determined by geometric (Geo) or least-squares (Fit) method. Plot graphs show 2D distributions of Geo P and GeoD (**a**), Geo f and Geo D (**b**), Fit D* and Fit D (**C**), or Fit f and Fit D (**d**). Open triangles, open squares, and closed circles indicate pleomorphic adenomas, Warthin tumors, and malignant salivary gland tumors, respectively. In combinations of Geo D and Geo P (a), Geo D and Geo f, or Fit D and Fit D*, stepwise approach diagnosed 21 of 23 salivary gland tumors correctly; in these approaches, the same Warthin tumor was incorrectly diagnosed as a malignant salivary gland tumor owing to having a large Geo D (=1.11×10⁻³ mm²/s) or Fit D values (=1.11×10⁻³ mm²/s); or incorrectly diagnosed as a pleomorphic adenoma owing to having a large Geo D (=1.24×10⁻³ mm²/s) or Fit D (=1.23×10⁻³ mm²/s) and small Geo P (=0.36×10⁻³ mm²/s) or Fit D* (=7.90×10⁻³ mm²/s) values. The diagnostic accuracy with stepwise approach using Fit D and Fit f was lower than that using the corresponding geometric parameters (**b, d**). Diagnostic accuracy was provided for the respective classifications at the bottom of each diagram.

Table 5. IVIM parameters of 23 salivary gland tumors that were determined by least squares, 3b-geometrical, or 4b-geometrical methods.

IVIM parameters	Fit	3b-Geo	4b-Geo
D ($\times 10^{-3}$ mm^2/s)	1.07 ± 0.37	1.07 ± 0.37	1.03 ± 0.38
f	0.10 ± 0.04	0.09 ± 0.04	0.08 ± 0.04
P/D* ($\times 10^{-3}$ mm^2/s)	$23.3 \pm 23.1^{a,b}$	0.50 ± 0.25^a	0.80 ± 0.47^b

IVIM, intravoxel incoherent motion; Fit, least squares method; 3b-Geo, geometric method using 3 b-values; 4b-Geo, geometric method using 4 b-values. P/D*, Geo P/Fit D*.
[a, b]significant differences (p<0.05) (Steel-Dwass test).

Differences in values of IVIM parameters between geometric and least-squares methods

D values determined by the geometric method (Geo D, $0.96 \pm 0.39 \times 10^{-3}$ mm^2/s) were significantly (p<0.001) greater than those determined by the least squares method (Fit D, $0.94 \pm 0.38 \times 10^{-3}$ mm^2/s) (Fig. 2, Tables S1 and S2). Geo f values (0.15 ± 0.09) were significantly (p<0.001) smaller than Fit f valued (0.16 ± 0.09). The differences were very small (2 ± 4% for D values and -7 ± 24% for f values) between 2 techniques.

Differences in diagnostic abilities of IVIM parameters between geometric and least-squares methods

Given the significant differences in values of IVIM parameters between geometric and least squares methods, we next tested whether these differences would affect the diagnostic abilities of IVIM parameters in differentiating SCCs and lymphomas (Fig. 3, Tables 3, S1, and S4). We found that f and P/D* values were ineffective for differentiating the 2 types of malignant tumors, resulting in 59% accuracy with Geo f and Fit f values; and 59% and 50% accuracy with Geo P and Fit D*, respectively. However, D values differentiated between SCCs and lymphomas with diagnostic abilities of 71% sensitivity, 100% specificity, and 78% accuracy with Geo D; and 74% sensitivity, 100% specificity, and 80% accuracy with Fit D.

Although significant differences in the IVIM values were found between the different types of salivary gland tumors (pleomorphic adenomas, Warthin tumors, and malignant salivary gland tumors), any single use of the parameters was ineffective in discriminating between the different tumor types (Fig. 4, Tables 4, S1, and S5). Therefore, we attempted to discriminate between the 3 different tumor types by using a stepwise approach with combined uses of the 3 IVIM parameters that were determined by the geometric or the least-squares methods (Fig. 5. Tables S1 and S5). The stepwise differentiation using Geo D and Geo P (Fig. 5a), Geo D and Geo f (Fig. 5b), or Fit D and Fit D* (Fig. 5c) differentiated 21 (91%) of the 23 salivary gland tumors correctly; consequently, the same 2 Warthin tumors were incorrectly diagnosed as malignant tumor or pleomorphic adenoma. However, a stepwise approach using Fit D and Fit f differentiated the salivary gland tumors less effectively; 3 malignant tumors were incorrectly diagnosed as Warthin tumors or pleomorphic adenoma; and 1 pleomorphic adenoma as Warthin tumor (Fig. 5d).

Lastly, we tested whether the use of 4 b-values (0, 100, 400, and 800 s/mm^2) could significantly influence the IVIM parameter levels and their diagnostic abilities compared with the use of 3 b-values (0, 200, and 800 s/mm^2). We found that Geo D and Geo f values of salivary gland tumors determined by the 3 b- or 4 b-values were not significantly different (Tables 5, S1, and S5). Furthermore, the use of 4 b-values resulted in less effective differentiation of salivary gland tumors compared with the IVIM

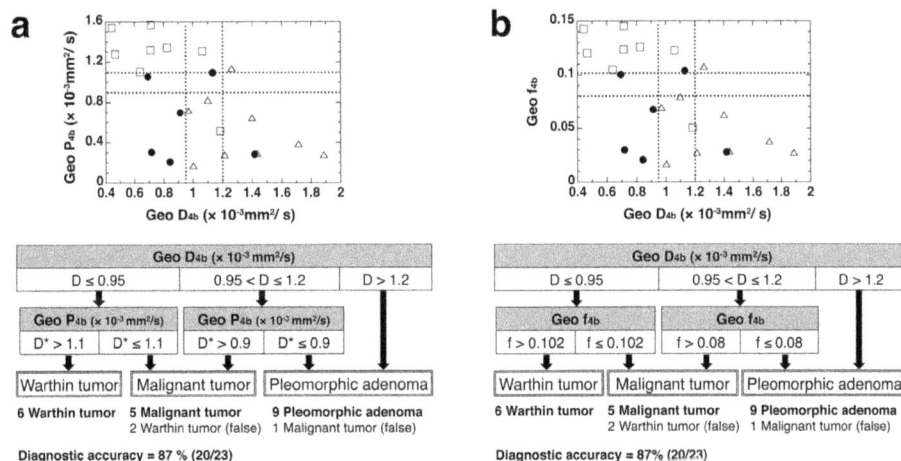

Figure 6. Stepwise differentiation between pleomorphic adenomas, Warthin tumors, and malignant salivary gland tumors using D, f, and D* or P values that were determined by geometric (Geo) method using 4 b-values (0, 100, 400, and 800 s/mm^2). Plot graphs show 2D distributions of Geo P and GeoD (**a**), or Geo f and Geo D (**b**). Open triangles, open squares, and closed circles indicate pleomorphic adenomas, Warthin tumors, and malignant salivary gland tumors, respectively. Diagnostic accuracy was provided for the respective classifications at the bottom of each diagram.

parameters that were determined using 3 b-values, and 3 tumors were incorrectly diagnosed (Fig. 6, Tables S1 and S5).

Discussion

The present results showed that levels of IVIM parameters that were determined by geometric method were significantly different from those determined by least-squares method. However, differences in levels of D and f values were very small between the 2 methods, and diagnostic abilities of geometrically determined IVIM parameters were equivalent to those of IVIM parameters determined by least-squares method in differentiating between lymphomas and SCCs, and between different types of salivary gland tumors (pleomorphic adenomas, Warthin tumors, and malignant salivary gland tumors). Considering cumbersome procedures with least-squares method, the simple geometric IVIM assessment could be an alternative to least-squares method in the clinics.

By using a limited number of b-values, IVIM imaging has the advantage of achieving DW MR images that have better quality and of examining broader areas of head and neck region in a single scan compared with IVIM imaging using more b-values; for example, IVIM imaging using 11 b-values requires 1 min 53 s for obtaining 10 DW image slices per patient; on the other hand, IVIM imaging using 3 b-values requires 26 s for obtaining the same number of DW images per patient. The 3 b-value IVIM technique abandoned the idea of using low b-value (<100 s/mm^2) DWI for a fine analysis of the different vascular compartments with different sizes of vessels [14–16]. Perfusion contributes to signal decays in DWI in a biexponential mode for b-values in very low range (0–200 s/mm^2) [3,14,15]. Indeed, the significant differences in D, f, and D* values between the geometric and least-squares methods may be owing to the use of the upper limit of this b-value range (200 s/mm^2) for assessing the perfusion-related and pure molecular diffusion parameters separately in the present study. However, the use of 4 b-values did not improve the diagnostic abilities in differentiating the different tumor types. These results suggest that the use of 3 b-values (0, 200, and 800 s/mm^2) is clinically feasible for assessing perfusion and diffusion of head and neck tumors in routine examinations.

The present study showed that computation-induced invalidity occurred less frequently with the geometric method compared with the least-squares one. However, these results do not necessarily ensure the better performance of the implied IVIM technique. Basically, the least-squares method has better performance than the geometric method in terms of predicting lesional perfusion and diffusion characteristics with less artifacts and higher signal-to-noise ratios compared with the simplified technique. For example, some perfusion property may be lost during the simplified IVIM parameter calculation with limited numbers of small (<200 s/mm^2) b-values. Furthermore, many of the computation-induced errors with the least-squares technique could be avoided through the use of appropriate scan setting and/or b-values.

The 3 b-value geometric assessment of IVIM parameters was slightly less effective in the diagnosis of salivary gland tumors compared with a previous study, which achieved 100% accuracy [5]. The difference in study cohort may be a possible reason for the difference in diagnostic accuracy. In the present study, stepwise approaches using Fit D and Fit D* or Geo D and Geo P diagnosed 21 of the 23 salivary gland tumors correctly (91% accuracy). In both the combinations of Fit and Geo IVIM parameters, the 2 same Warthin tumors were incorrectly diagnosed as malignant or pleomorphic adenoma (Fig. 5). However, diagnostic accuracy with

stepwise approaches using Fit D and Fit f values was lower than that using Geo D and Geo f values (19/23 = 83% vs 21/23 = 91%), implying advantages of geometric method for the clinical use in diagnosing salivary gland tumors.

A major limitation of this study was the small patient cohort. Different or additional cutoff points might be required for effective discrimination in a larger patient cohort that is comprised of increased numbers of tumors within each tumor type and broader types of head and neck tumors. For example, the present study cohort of salivary gland tumor did not include oncocytoma, which histologically mimics Warthin tumor or malignant salivary gland tumors such as acinic cell carcinoma and clear cell carcinoma [17]. The retrospective nature, including the exclusion of patients with severe susceptibility artifacts from the study cohort, also limit the value of this study. In addition, the benefit of using the simplified IVIM technique may largely depends on disease types. Furthermore, the perfusion-related parameter Geo P defined by the simplified IVIM technique is fundamentally different from the conventional one (Fit D*). For example, in some cases where the diffusion property is important for diagnosing tumors/diseases, the simplified IVIM technique may be beneficial; however, in other cases where the perfusion assessment is essential for diagnosing tumors/disease, the simplified technique will provide perfusion parameters that are greatly different from those obtained with the least squares technique using multiple b-values and may thus mislead the diagnosis.

Another limitation of the present study may reside in ROI placement errors. We found that the interobserver and intraobserver errors were relatively small. However, there were substantial overlaps in IVIM parameters between different tumor types, and thus a small change in the value due to ROI placement may lead to a different result in tumor categorization based on IVIM imaging. In addition, distortion of tumor area due to susceptibility and motion artifacts may be critical factors against precise IVIM parameter measurements.

Conclusion

In this study, we showed that the IVIM parameters determined by geometric method were significantly different from those determined by conventional least-squares method. Nonetheless, both yielded very similar results in terms of differential diagnosis of major types of head and neck tumors, including SCCs, lymphomas, and salivary gland tumors. Therefore, we concluded that geometric determination of IVIM parameters could be an alternative to least-squares methods in the diagnosis of head and neck tumors.

Supporting Information

Table S1 All numerical data for Figs. 2, 5 and 6, and Tables 2, 3, 4 and 5 are summarized. Signal intensities relative to varying b-values (0–800 s/mm^2) are shown for each of benign (n = 26) and malignant (n = 61) head and neck tumors.

Table S2 IVIM parameters (Geo D, Geo f, Geo P, Fit D, Fit f, and Fit D*) are shown for each of benign (n = 26) and malignant (n = 61) head and neck tumors.

Table S3 IVIM parameters (Geo D, Geo f, Geo P, Fit D, Fit f, and Fit D*) determined 5 times (#1–#5) by 3 observers (1–3) are shown for 5 head and neck tumors (Cases 1–5).

Table S4 IVIM parameters (Geo D, Geo f, Geo P, Fit D, Fit f, and Fit D*) for lymphomas (n = 12), primary SCCs (n = 23), and SCC nodes (n = 11) are shown.

Table S5 IVIM parameters determined by least squares method (Fit D, Fit f, and Fit D*), geometrical method using 3 b-values (Geo D3b, Geo f3b, and Geo P3b), or geometrical method using 4 b-values (Geo D4b, Geo f4b, Geo P4b) for benign (n = 17) and malignant (n = 6) salivary gland tumors are shown.

Author Contributions

Conceived and designed the experiments: TN MS MS. Analyzed the data: MS MS SE IK YH. Wrote the paper: TN MS MS.

References

1. Nakamura T, Sumi M, Van Cauteren M (2009) Salivary gland tumors: Preoperative tissue characterization with apparent diffusion coefficient mapping. *In* Methods of Cancer Diagnosis, Therapy, and Prognosis. Hyat MA ed. Vol 7: NY, Springer: 255–269.
2. Le Bihan D (2003) Looking into the functional architecture of the brain with diffusion MRI. Nat Rev Neurosci 4: 469–480.
3. Le Bihan D, Breton E, Lallemand D, Aubin ML, Vignaud J, et al. (1988) Separation of diffusion and perfusion in intravoxel incoherent motion imaging. Radiology 168: 497–505.
4. Luciani A, Vignaud A, Cavet M, Tran Van Nhieu J, Mallat A, et al. (2008) Liver cirrhosis: Intravoxel incoherent motion MR imaging – Pilot study. Radiology 249: 891–899.
5. Sumi M, Van Cauteren M, Sumi T, Obara M, Ichikawa Y, Nakamura T (2012) Salivary gland tumors: use of intravoxel incoherent motion MR imaging for assessment of diffusion and perfusion for the differentiation of benign and malignant tumors. Radiology 263: 770–777.
6. Moteki T, Horikoshi H (2006) Evaluation of hepatic lesions and hepatic parenchyma using diffusion-weighted echo-planar MR with three values of gradient b-factor. J Magn Reson Imaging 24: 637–645.
7. Lewin M, Fartoux L, Vignaud A, Arrivé L, Menu Y, et al. (2011) The diffusion-weighted maging perfusion fraction f is a potential marker of sorafenib treatment in advanced hepatocellular carcinoma: a pilot study. Eur Radiol 21: 281–290.
8. Mazaheri Y, Vargas HA, Akin O, Goldman DA, Hricak H (2012) Reducing the influence of b-value selection on diffusion-weighted imaging of the prostate: Evaluation of a revised monoexponential model within a clinical setting. J Magn Reson Imaging 35: 660–668.
9. Sumi M, Nakamura T (2013) Head and neck tumors: Assessment of perfusion-related parameters and diffusion coefficients based on the intravoxel incoherent motion model. AJNR Am J Neuroradiol 34: 410–416.
10. Patel J, Sigmund EE, Rusinek H, Oei M, Babb JS, Taouli B (2010) Diagnosis of cirrhosis with intravoxel incoherent motion diffusion MRI and dynamic contrast-enhanced MRI alone and in combination: Preliminary experience. J Magn Reson Imaging 31: 589–600.
11. Lai V, Li X, Lee VHF, Lam KO, Chan Q, et al. (2013) Intravoxel incoherent motion MR imaging: Comparison of diffusion and perfusion characteristics between nasopharyngeal carcinoma and post-chemoradiation fibrosis. Eur Radiol 23: 2793–2801.
12. Sasaki M, Sumi M, Van Cauteren M, Obara M, Nakamura T (2013) Intravoxel incoherent motion imaging of masticatory muscles: A pilot study for the assessment of perfusion and diffusion during clenching. AJR AM J Roentgenol 201: 1101–1107.
13. Gao Q, Srinvasan G, Magin RL, Zhou XJ (2011) Anomalous diffusion measured by a twice-refocused spin echo pulse sequence: Analysis using fractional order calculus. J Magn Reson Imaging 33: 1177–1183.
14. Le Bihan D (2008) Intravoxel incoherent motion perfusion MR imaging: A wake-up call. Radiology 249: 748–752.
15. Koh DM, Collins DJ (2007) Diffusion-weighted MRI in the body: Applications and challenges in oncology. AJR Am J Roentgenol 188: 1622–1635.
16. Penner AH, Sprinkart AM, Kukuk GM, Gütgemann I, Gieseke J, et al. (2013) Intravoxel incoherent motion model-based liver lesion characterisation from three b-value diffusion-weighted MRI. Eur Radiol 23: 2773–2783.
17. Barnes L, Everson JW, Reichart P, Sidransky D (2005) Pathology and genetics of head and neck tumours. World Health Organization classification of tumors. IARC Press, Lyon, France.

10

Efficacy of Distortion Correction on Diffusion Imaging: Comparison of FSL Eddy and Eddy_Correct Using 30 and 60 Directions Diffusion Encoding

Haruyasu Yamada[1], Osamu Abe[1]*, Takashi Shizukuishi[1], Junko Kikuta[1], Takahiro Shinozaki[2], Ko Dezawa[2], Akira Nagano[3], Masayuki Matsuda[3], Hiroki Haradome[1], Yoshiki Imamura[2]

1 Department of Radiology, Nihon University School of Medicine, Tokyo, Japan, 2 Department of Oral Diagnostic Sciences, Nihon University School of Dentistry, Tokyo, Japan, 3 Department of Radiological Technology, Nihon University Itabashi Hospital, Tokyo, Japan

Abstract

Diffusion imaging is a unique noninvasive tool to detect brain white matter trajectory and integrity in vivo. However, this technique suffers from spatial distortion and signal pileup or dropout originating from local susceptibility gradients and eddy currents. Although there are several methods to mitigate these problems, most techniques can be applicable either to susceptibility or eddy-current induced distortion alone with a few exceptions. The present study compared the correction efficiency of FSL tools, "eddy_correct" and the combination of "eddy" and "topup" in terms of diffusion-derived fractional anisotropy (FA). The brain diffusion images were acquired from 10 healthy subjects using 30 and 60 directions encoding schemes based on the electrostatic repulsive forces. For the 30 directions encoding, 2 sets of diffusion images were acquired with the same parameters, except for the phase-encode blips which had opposing polarities along the anteroposterior direction. For the 60 directions encoding, non–diffusion-weighted and diffusion-weighted images were obtained with forward phase-encoding blips and non–diffusion-weighted images with the same parameter, except for the phase-encode blips, which had opposing polarities. FA images without and with distortion correction were compared in a voxel-wise manner with tract-based spatial statistics. We showed that images corrected with eddy and topup possessed higher FA values than images uncorrected and corrected with eddy_correct with trilinear (FSL default setting) or spline interpolation in most white matter skeletons, using both encoding schemes. Furthermore, the 60 directions encoding scheme was superior as measured by increased FA values to the 30 directions encoding scheme, despite comparable acquisition time. This study supports the combination of eddy and topup as a superior correction tool in diffusion imaging rather than the eddy_correct tool, especially with trilinear interpolation, using 60 directions encoding scheme.

Editor: Joseph Najbauer, University of Pécs Medical School, Hungary

Funding: This study was supported by a Grant-in-Aid for Scientific Research on Innovative Areas (Comprehensive Brain Science Network) from the Ministry of Education, Science, Sports and Culture of Japan. The funders had no role in study design, data collection and analysis, decision to publish, or preparation of the manuscript.

Competing Interests: The authors have declared that no competing interests exist.

* Email: abe.osamu27@nihon-u.ac.jp

Introduction

Diffusion magnetic resonance imaging (MRI) is a unique and noninvasive tool to detect the white matter trajectory and integrity in vivo [1]. However, this technique suffers from spatial distortion and signal pileup or dropout, originating from local susceptibility-induced field gradient, since ultrafast acquisition techniques, such as echo-planar imaging (EPI), are exclusively employed to measure minute motion of water molecules in the brain tissue without motion-induced artifacts. Furthermore, eddy current resulting from the strong motion-probing gradients (MPG) is another source of geometric distortion, theoretically constrained by scale, shear, and translation deformations. To resolve these problems, several methods have been advocated. Multireference [2], field map with point-spread function mapping [3], and k-space traversal [4–6] can correct for susceptibility-induced distortions. Post-processing registration [7–12], twice-refocused spin echo [13] and character-ization of the 3-D eddy current field with linear response theory [14] can be used to compensate for the eddy current induced distortion. Finally, k-space traversal combined with improvement of the method of Bowtell [15,16] allows for both susceptibility and eddy current correction.

Although these methods are sometimes efficient to unwarp spatial distortion in diffusion imaging, several issues remain [6,14,15]: (a) subject motion during the acquisition of reference and diffusion-weighted images, resulting in misregistration between the two images and unwarping error; (b) prolonged scanning time to acquire reference images which do not contribute to functional or structural analyses of the brain; (c) inefficient correction of signal pileup or dropout; (d) signal intensity difference in areas of high signal intensity on non–diffusion-weighted images and low intensity on diffusion-weighted images (i.e., cerebrospinal fluid), and coherent white matter fascicles with

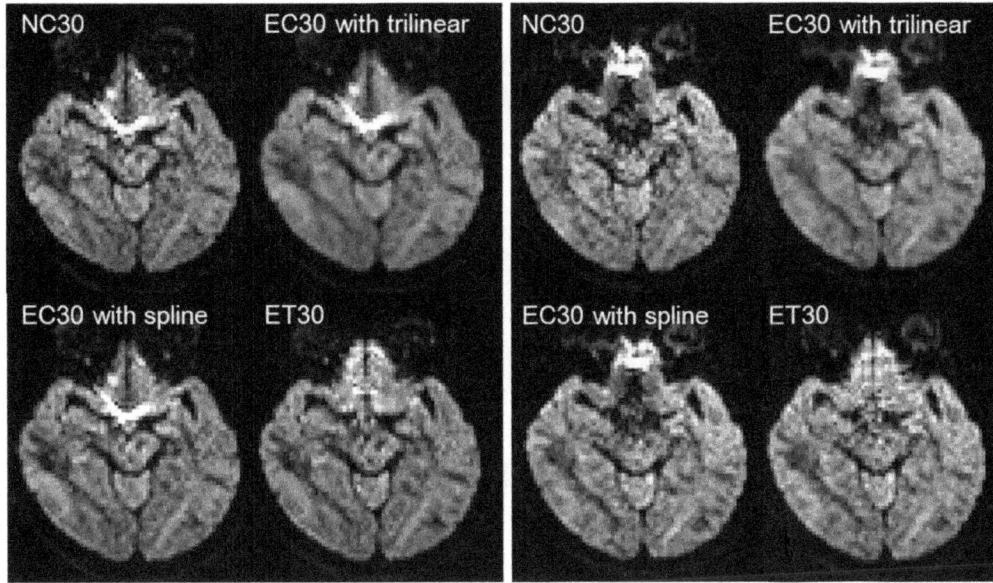

Figure 1. Representative diffusion-weighted images with the 30 directions encoding scheme. The images were from the same subject and slice location, with forward phase-encoding blips (left panel), and with reversed phase-encoding blips (right panel). NC30 had an artifactual signal pileup around the frontal base of the skull, which was corrected not in EC30 with trilinear or spline but in ET30. The EC30 with trilinear interpolation were blurred, compared with EC30 with spline interpolation.

high or low signal intensity, depending on MPG directionality, resulting in inefficient image registration and the erroneous calculation of diffusion properties; and (e) longer echo time, resulting in undesirable signal loss because of T2 decay. Furthermore, most proposed techniques can be applicable either to susceptibility or eddy-current induced distortion alone with a few exceptions [14,15]. More importantly, subject motion and eddy current induced distortion cannot be separated with registration based techniques, which are compensatory operations. Therefore, the efficient distortion correction method in diffusion imaging remains to be an open question.

The Functional Magnetic Resonance Imaging of the Brain Software Library (FSL) offers a comprehensive toolset to analyze neuroimages for functional and structural connectivity, and morphometry (http://fsl.fmrib.ox.ac.uk/fsl/fslwiki) [17]. Initially, FSL provided a tool, named "eddy_correct", to correct eddy current-induced image stretching, shearing, and translation on the basis of a classical affine transformation, but it did not offer the function to mitigate susceptibility-induced distortion and signal pileup. The "topup" and "eddy" FSL tools have been recently developed to estimate susceptibility and eddy current induced distortions, respectively, and correct them simultaneously [4,18–20].

The calculation of diffusion tensor properties (i.e., fractional anisotropy; FA, and mean diffusivity) requires a minimum of 6 diffusion-weighted images with noncollinear MPG directions and 1 non–diffusion-weighted image. However, several diffusion-encoding schemes have been proposed for precise and robust measures, one of which is based on electrostatic repulsive forces. Among them, 30 and 60 noncollinear directions, with a ratio of the total number of diffusion-weighted images over non–diffusion-weighted images equal to 5 [21,22], have been validated in clinical settings [23].

The present study compared the diffusion-derived FA values of non–distortion-corrected images (NC), images corrected with the eddy_correct tool (EC), and images corrected with the eddy and topup tools (ET), in a voxel-wise manner with Tract-Based Spatial Statistics (TBSS) [24]. Furthermore, the diffusion-weighted images were acquired with 2 acquisitions of 30 noncollinear MPG directions and 1 acquisition of 60 noncollinear MPG directions, with equivalent acquisition time. To our knowledge, this is the first report comparing uncorrected diffusion-weighted images to those corrected with the eddy_correct tool or a combination of the eddy and topup tools, using 30 and 60 directions encoding schemes in the human brain.

Materials and Methods

Participants

The subjects were 10 healthy volunteers (7 females; mean age: 34.0 ± 5.5 years; range: 27–43 years). The ethical committee of the Nihon University Itabashi Hospital approved this study (No. RK121109-08). This was part of the ongoing research project investigating brain structural and functional alterations in patients with glossodynia. The exclusion criteria were drug use (antihypertensive, antianxiety, or antidepressant agents) or abuse, previous head trauma and operation, claustrophobia, diabetes, anemia, vitamin deficiency, and infections such as candidiasis. At least one of the trained neuroradiologists (O.A., T.S., or J.K.) evaluated all the anatomical MRI scans, including T1-weighted and T2-weighted images obtained in the same session, and found no gross abnormality in any of the participants. All subjects specifically consented to publication of medical information, including MR images, as well as participation in the study and written informed consents were obtained from them after a complete explanation of the study.

MRI acquisition

The MRI data were obtained using a 1.5-T scanner (Achieva 1.5T; software version 3.2.1, Philips Medical Systems, The Netherlands) at the Nihon University Itabashi Hospital. Spin-echo EPI was used to obtain 60 contiguous axial images (repetition

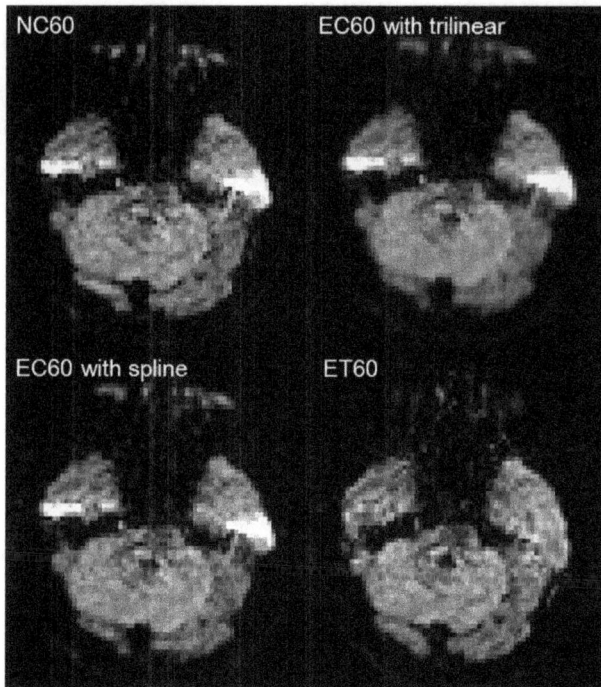

Figure 2. Representative diffusion-weighted images with the 60 directions encoding scheme. The images were from the same subject and slice location. The NC60 with forward phase-encoding blips had an artifactual signal pileup around the temporal base of the skull, which was not corrected in EC60, but corrected in ET60. Again, the EC30 with trilinear were blurred, compared with EC30 with spline interpolation.

time/echo   time = 8100/88.66 ms;   spatial   resolution = 2.5×2.5×2.5 mm) using an 8-channel phased-array head coil with a parallel imaging factor of 2. The MPG directions were conformed to 30 noncollinear directions on the basis of electrostatic repulsive forces (number of excitation = 5 for non–diffusion-weighted image; 1 for diffusion-weighted images), and to 60 noncollinear directions (number of excitation = 10 for non–diffusion-weighted image; 1 for diffusion-weighted images) with a b value of 1000 s/mm^2 [21]. The ratio of the total number of diffusion-weighted over non–diffusion-weighted images was determined on the basis of previous literature [21–23]. The multiple non–diffusion-weighted images were averaged in-line to yield a single non–diffusion-weighted image from the scanner.

For the 30 directions encoding, 2 sets of diffusion images were acquired with the same parameters, except for the phase-encode blips which had opposing polarities along the anteroposterior direction. The acquisition time was 5 min 7 s per session, and the total scan time to encode 30 directions was 10 min 14 s. For the 60 directions encoding, only the non–diffusion-weighted images were acquired with 2 sets of phase encoding blips of opposite polarity (acquisition time: 3 min 14 s) and diffusion-weighted images were obtained with forward phase-encoding blips (acquisition time: 8 min 6 s). The total scan time for the 60 directions encoding protocol was 11 min 20 s, which was comparable with the 30 directions encoding protocol.

Image processing

These digital imaging and communication in medicine (DICOM) images were transferred to a Linux workstation (HP Z820 workstation; Hewlett-Packard Japan, Tokyo) comprised of a

CentOS 6.5 (64-bit version; 48 GBs memory) and dual central processing units (Intel Xeon Processor E5-2630 v2, Santa Clara, CA). The Sun Grid Engine grid computing cluster software system allowed parallel processing on this workstation. All DICOM images were converted into Neuroimaging Informatics Technology Initiative (NIfTI) format using the MRIcron tool named dcm2nii (http://www.mccauslandcenter.sc.edu/mricro/mricron/install.html). Then, the corresponding diffusion images, with opposing polarities of phase-encode blips for 30 and 60 directions encoding, were merged and treated as NC30 and NC60 images, respectively, both of which had 62 imaging volumes. Next the eddy current correction was applied with the eddy_correct tool [17] using the default settings, and these corrected images were processed at later stages as EC30 with trilinear interpolation for 30 directions, and as EC60 with trilinear interpolation for 60 directions encoding. In this step of the image processing, the first non–diffusion-weighted image was set as the target image, into which the remaining 61 volumes were registered. In the default setting of FSL, eddy_correct uses a trilinear function as an interpolation method and does not have the option selecting other interpolation methods. Therefore, we modified the script of eddy_correct and the interpolation function was changed from the default trilinear to spline, and the created images were EC30 and EC60 with spline interpolation. Finally, the topup and eddy tools were applied to the NC30 and NC60 images, which were named ET30 and ET60, respectively. Topup estimates the susceptibility-induced off-resonance field from pairs of images, with reversed phase-encode blips and distortions going in opposite directions (http://fsl.fmrib.ox.ac.uk/fsl/fslwiki/TOPUP) [4]. Two non–diffusion-weighted images with opposed phase encoding polarities were extracted, and susceptibility induced distortion was estimated with topup. The eddy tool corrects image distortions by assuming that diffusion signals obtained from 2 MPG directions with a small angle difference are similar, combining the correction for susceptibility and eddy currents/movements (http://fsl.fmrib.ox.ac.uk/fsl/fslwiki/EDDY). These diffusion images were processed with the FSL tool "dtifit," and FA images were created for NC, EC, and ET. For the analyses with TBSS, FMRIB58_FA was set as the target image used in the registrations [24]. The value that thresholded the mean FA skeleton image was set at 0.2. All FA images were attached as supporting Information (Data S1).

Statistical analyses

Permutation-based tests were conducted using the FSL tool "randomise_parallel," with 50,000 permutations and the threshold-free cluster enhancement option [24]. Age and gender were not treated as covariates because their effects could be cancelled out in a paired analysis.

In the first step, paired t-tests were conducted between NC30 and EC30 with trilinear, and between NC60 and EC60 with trilinear interpolation. Second, tripled paired t-tests were conducted between NC30, EC30 with spline, and ET30, and between NC60, EC60 with spline interpolation, and ET60, separately. Third, a paired t-test was conducted between images derived from 30 and 60 directions encoding with the best performance, on the basis of the results of the tripled paired t-tests. We assumed that misregistration due to spatial distortions would result in lower FA values in tensor calculation. Although both eddy currents and subject movement can cause artificially elevated FA values at the interface between structures with high and low diffusivities, for example, gray matter and cerebrospinal fluid, the white matter skeleton is not the case. Therefore, the image with the best performance should have the highest FA values with TBSS analysis. The significance level was set at a P value of no more

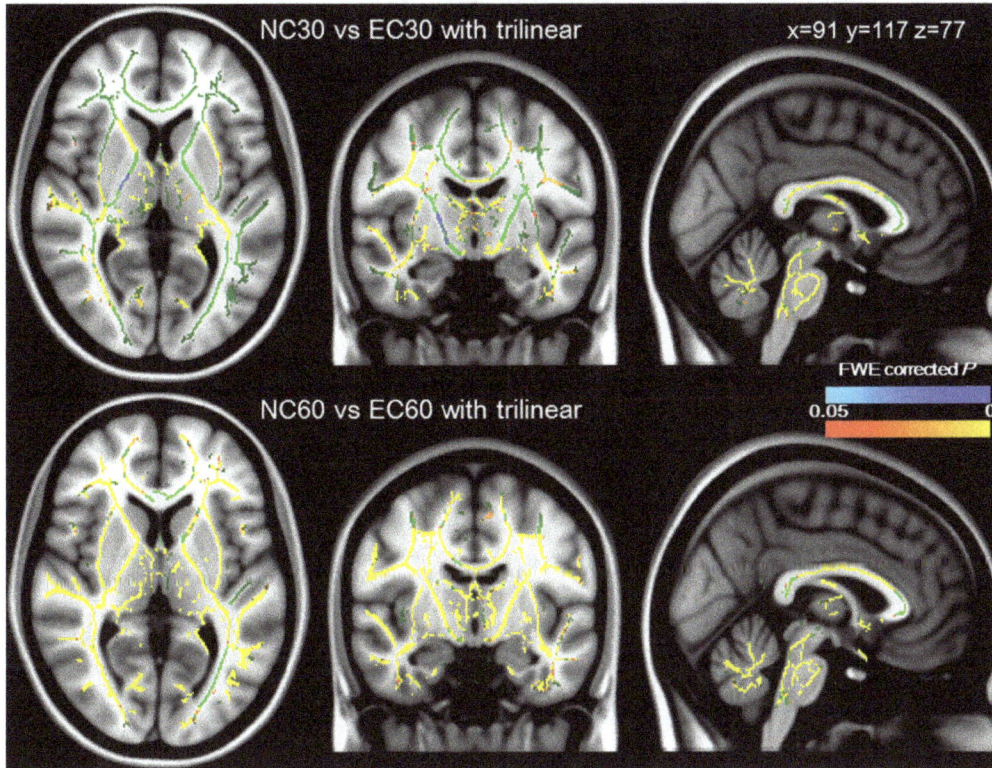

Figure 3. Comparisons between NC and EC images with trilinear interpolation. The white matter skeletons with the higher FA for NC30 or NC60 were shown in red/yellow, and those with higher FA for EC30 or EC60 with trilinear interpolation were shown in blue/lightblue. The upper and lower row showed paired comparisons between NC30 and EC30 with trilinear, NC60 and NC60 with trilinear interpolation, respectively. NC30 and NC60 had higher FA values in most white matter skeletons, compared with EC30 and EC60 with trilinear interpolation, except in the posterior limb of the right internal capsule in the upper row. These data were overlaid onto the MNI152_T1_1 mm template, with the mean FA skeletons shown in green. The significance level was set at a P value of <0.05 with FWE correction.

than 0.05 with family-wise error (FWE) correction for multiple comparisons.

Results

Visual inspections of the correction efficiency

Figure 1 showed representative diffusion-weighted images with the 30 directions encoding scheme. Diffusion images with forward and reverse phase encode blips were shown on the left and right panel, respectively. Before correction, NC30 showed an artifactual signal pileup around the frontal base of the skull with both forward and reversed phase encoding blips. These artifacts were not corrected in EC30 with trilinear or spline interpolation, but were corrected in ET30. With respect to EC30, images blurring occurred with trilinear interpolation (FSL default setting), but not with spline interpolation. Representative movie files of the sagittal, coronal, and axial non–diffusion-weighted and diffusion-weighted images were shown in Fig. S1–S4. Compared with those of NC (Fig. S1), EC with trilinear (Fig. S2) and spline interpolation (Fig. S3), brain surfaces were well-registered among ET images (Fig. S4) by visual inspection. Furthermore, concave or convex distortions were alleviated in ET images.

Figure 2 showed representative diffusion-weighted images acquired with the 60 directions encoding and forward phase encoding blips. Before correction, NC60 showed an artifactual signal pileup around the temporal base of the skull, which was not corrected in EC60, but corrected in ET60. Likewise, image blurring was only detected in EC60 with trilinear interpolation

(FSL default setting). Therefore, both acquisition schemes offered better images with the eddy and topup corrections. Representative movie files of the sagittal, coronal, and axial non–diffusion-weighted and diffusion-weighted images were shown in Fig. S5–S8. Compared with those of NC (Fig. S5), EC with trilinear (Fig. S6) and spline interpolation (Fig. S7), brain surfaces were well-registered among ET images (Fig. S8) by visual inspection. Furthermore, concave or convex distortions were alleviated in ET images.

Comparisons between NC and EC images with trilinear interpolation

Paired t-tests with TBSS were conducted between NC30 and EC30 with trilinear interpolation, and between NC60 and EC60 with trilinear interpolation (Fig. 3). The white matter skeleton with significantly higher FA for NC30 or NC60 were shown in red/yellow, and those with the significantly higher FA for EC30 or EC60 were shown in blue/light blue (FWE corrected P<0.05 for all comparisons). Surprisingly, most of the white matter skeleton showed higher FA values for NC30 and NC60 than those for EC30 and EC60 with trilinear interpolation. The only exception was in the posterior limb of the right internal capsule between NC30 and EC30 with trilinear interpolation. Therefore, we decided not to conduct further analysis of EC30 or EC60 with trilinear interpolation (FSL default setting).

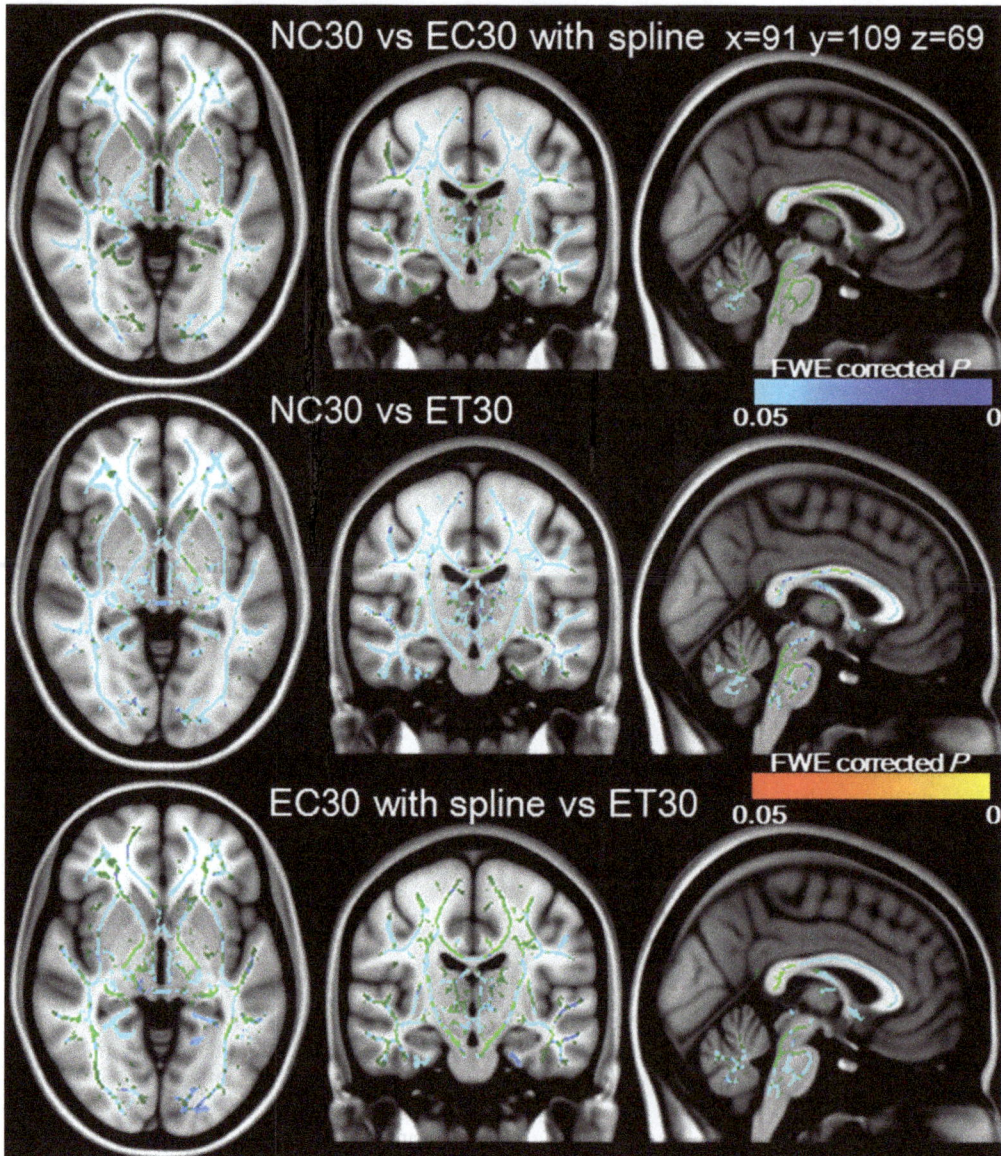

Figure 4. Efficiency of correction schemes acquired with 30 directions diffusion encoding. Tripled paired group comparisons with TBSS were conducted between NC30 and EC30 with spline interpolation in the upper, NC30 and ET30 in the middle, and EC30 with spline interpolation and ET30 in the lower row. The FA values for ET30 were significantly higher than those for NC30 or EC30 in most white matter skeletons (blue/lightblue). The FA values for EC30 with spline interpolation were significantly higher than those for NC30 (blue/lightblue), and lower than those for ET30 in most white matter skeletons. These data were overlaid onto the MNI152_T1_1 mm template, with the mean FA skeletons shown in green. The significance level was set at a P value of <0.05 with FWE correction.

Efficiency of correction schemes acquired with 30 directions diffusion encoding

Figure 4 showed tripled paired t-tests with TBSS between NC30 and EC30 with spline interpolation in the upper, between NC30 and ET30 in the middle, and between EC30 with spline interpolation and ET30 in the lower row, respectively. The FA values for ET30 were significantly higher than those for NC30 or EC30 with spline in most of the white matter skeleton (blue/light blue), and there was no skeleton where FA values for ET30 was significantly lower than those for the others (FWE corrected $P<0.05$ for all comparisons). In addition, the FA values for NC30 were never significantly higher than those for the others in the entire skeleton. Finally, the FA values for EC30 with spline

interpolation were significantly higher than those for NC30 (blue/light blue), and lower than those for ET30 (red/yellow) in most of the white matter skeleton (FWE corrected $P<0.05$ for all comparisons). These data suggested that ET30 provided the most efficient image correction.

Efficiency of correction schemes acquired with 60 directions diffusion encoding

Figure 5 showed tripled paired t-tests with TBSS between NC60 and EC60 with spline interpolation in the upper, between NC60 and ET60 in the middle, and between EC60 with spline interpolation and ET60 in the lower row, respectively. As for the previous scheme, the FA values for ET60 were significantly higher

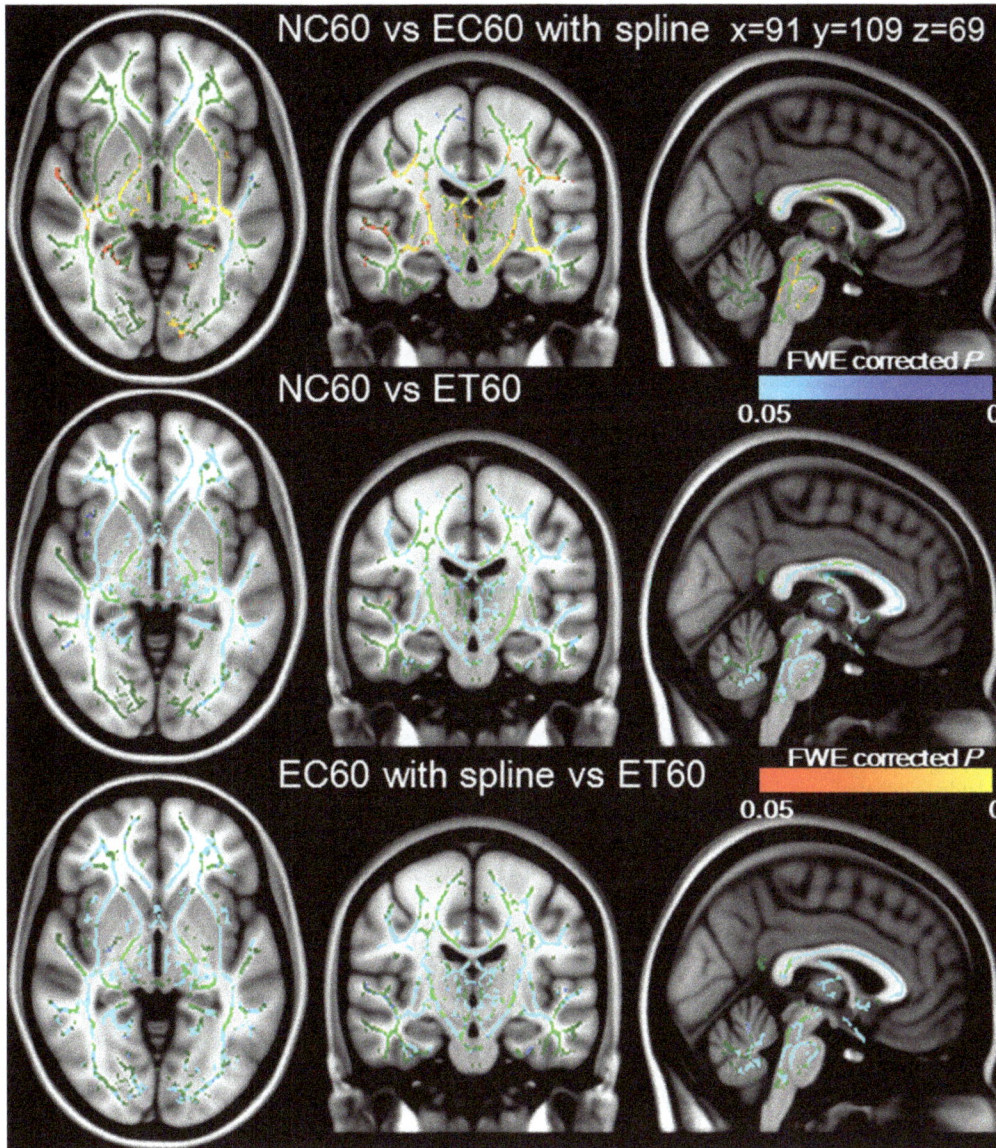

Figure 5. Efficiency of correction schemes acquired with 60 directions diffusion encoding. Tripled paired group comparisons with TBSS were conducted between NC60 and EC60 with spline interpolation in the upper, NC60 and ET60 in the middle, and EC60 with spline and ET60 in the lower row. The FA values for ET60 were significantly higher than those for NC60 or EC60 in most of the white matter skeleton (blue/lightblue). In contrast, white matter skeleton with significantly higher (blue/lightblue) and lower (red/yellow) FA values for EC60 with spline interpolation than those for NC60 were observed in various areas. These data were overlaid onto the MNI152_T1 template, and the mean FA skeleton is shown in green. The significance level was set at a P value of <0.05 with FWE correction.

than those for NC60 or EC60 with spline interpolation in most of the white matter skeleton, and there was no skeleton where FA values for ET60 was significantly lower than those for the others (FWE corrected $P<0.05$ for all comparisons). In contrast, various areas of the white matter skeleton showed significant higher (blue/light blue) or lower (red/yellow) FA values for EC60 with spline interpolation than those for NC60 (FWE corrected $P<0.05$ for all comparisons). Therefore, ET60 exhibited the most efficient image correction.

Comparison of ET30 and ET60 images

The two most efficient correction protocols were compared by paired t-test with TBSS (Fig. 6). The FA values for ET60 were significantly higher than those for ET30 in widespread white

matter, with slight left hemisphere predominance (blue/lightblue; FWE corrected $P<0.05$). On the other hand, there was no skeleton where FA value for ET60 was significantly lower than that for ET30. Altogether, these data suggested that the 60 directions encoding scheme provided more reliable FA measurements than the 30 directions encoding scheme after the eddy and topup corrections.

Discussion

MRI remains the most powerful noninvasive neuroimaging technique to clarify task-related cortical activation, functional connectivity at rest, cerebral perfusion, as well as regional morphology and metabolic activity. Among the recent applica-

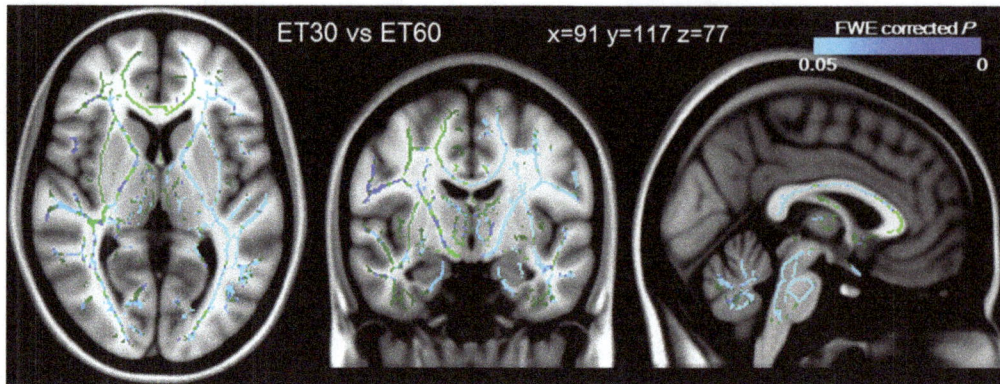

Figure 6. Comparison of ET30 and ET60 images. The FA values for ET60 were significantly higher than those for ET30 in most of the white matter, with slight left hemisphere predominance. These data were overlaid onto the MNI152_T1 template, and the mean FA skeleton is shown in green. The significance level was set at a P value of <0.05 with FWE correction.

tions, diffusion imaging can reveal structural connectivity and white matter integrity. However, structural distortion is a serious problem for these methods since EPI-based acquisition is employed. In terms of diffusion imaging, two major factors contribute to spatial distortion: local susceptibility gradient and eddy current due to the strong MPG application. Without distortion correction, calculations of diffusion properties may be erroneous because of misregistration.

The present study compared the FA values of uncorrected images with those of images corrected with the eddy_correct tool or a combination of the topup and eddy tools. The latter exhibited the highest FA values in most of the white matter skeleton with the 30 directions as well as 60 directions encoding schemes. Furthermore, the FA values of images corrected with the topup and eddy tools were significantly higher in widespread white matter with 60 directions than with 30 directions. Slight residual misregistrations between the two images, especially diffusion-weighted images with opposing phase-encoding directions in the ET30 set, might remain, resulting in the observed reduction in FA. In the current study, however, we did not acquire two imaging sets with the phase encoding blips of the same polarity in terms of 30 directions diffusion encoding, and could not compare them with 60 directions encoded images. In contrast, residual misregistrations between the two images, especially diffusion-weighted images with opposing phase-encoding directions in the ET30 set, can cause artificially elevated FA values at the interface between structures with high and low diffusivities, for example, gray matter and cerebrospinal fluid. Furthermore, at the resolution being probed in this study misregistration of the white matter tracts would have a similar poor correspondence with the gray/white matter boundary and result in abnormally high FA measures on the edge of the white matter tracts. In ET60, however, there was only one data set of diffusion-weighted images. Misregistration between two sets of image data were not applicable and was not a reason for higher FA values in ET60, which might exert a minor effect on the results. Although the exact cause remains unknown, the 60 directions encoding scheme is believed to be superior as measured by increased FA values to the 30 directions encoding scheme because there was no white matter skeleton with FA values for 30 directions higher than those for 60 directions in the entire hemispheres. Furthermore, a higher number of encoding directions increases angular resolution, which might facilitate the analysis of complicated diffusion parameters beyond diffusion tensor, such as high angular resolution diffusion imaging [25].

Previous reports investigating the optimal number of MPG suggested that about or at least 30 directions offered the best performance. However, one report did not evaluate 60 directions [23], and the other study only used a simulation model [21]. Future imaging studies, however, are clearly needed to evaluate the difference between FA values for 30 and 60 directions encoding scheme with the phase encoding blips of the same polarity.

The topup tool uses the reversed direction of phase encoding to estimate the EPI distortion caused by local susceptibility gradient [4]. The estimated distortion field is then advanced into a Gaussian process predictor that uses all the data to estimate the eddy current-induced field inhomogeneities and head motion for each imaging volume [18]. All these distortions are corrected in a single process using the eddy tool [18–20]. In contrast, the eddy_correct tool can register diffusion-weighted images into the reference image, usually a non–diffusion-weighted image which has a different contrast from diffusion-weighted images, with a classical affine transformation-based method. But this tool cannot correct susceptibility-induced distortion, which might explain why images corrected with the eddy_correct tool had significantly lower FA values than those corrected with the topup and eddy tools. Sotiropoulos et al. found that, with measurements of sum of squared differences in signal intensities within the brain, an affine-based correction provided better results than without correction, but clearly performed worse than the Gaussian Process approach, which achieves a better registration between volumes [20]. This study was in good agreement with our current results. Furthermore, the FA values for EC60 even with spline interpolation were significantly lower than those for uncorrected images in some areas of the white matter skeleton. In addition, the FA values for EC30 and EC60 with trilinear interpolation, the default interpolation methods in the eddy_correct tool, were significantly lower than those for NC30 and NC60 in widespread white matter. Therefore, we strongly recommended the topup and eddy tools for distortion correction in diffusion imaging, rather than the eddy_correct tool, especially with the default trilinear interpolation.

The correction method using topup and eddy tools has a few limitations. First, when subjects move between two acquisitions, with different phase encoding polarities, the corrected images would be different from the real shape of the brain because topup attempts to estimate the distortion correction field that will maximize the similarities between the corrected images. If significant movement occurs, another acquisition will be needed.

On the other hand, most image correction methods share this problem. Second, we did not apply MPG reorientation when unwarping images. When a brain is transformed onto another one, such as the standard brain (i.e. spatially normalized template), which is quite different from a subject brain, MPG reorientations would be indispensable according to the rotation matrix around the x, y, and z axes. However, in the current settings, distortion-corrected images have the native shape of the brain, and MPG has been applied to the native shape. Therefore, we believe that MPG reorientation was unnecessary. Finally, we did not use over 60 gradient directions because the amount of acquisition time for diffusion imaging was limited in clinical or even research settings. Because this study investigated brain alterations in subjects diagnosed with glossodynia, other imaging sequences might be required to evaluate functional connectivity and structural deficit. The effect of a hundred or more MPG directions on diffusion imaging is a subject for future studies, especially after multiband technology becomes routinely feasible [19,20].

In conclusion, structural distortions cause misregistration in non–diffusion-weighted and diffusion-weighted images during tensor calculation, resulting in lower FA values. The present study showed that ET images had higher FA values than EC images, which suggested that distortion correction with the topup and eddy tools might be indispensable for accurate measurements of diffusion parameters. Furthermore, the 60 directions encoding scheme was superior as measured by increased FA values to the 30 directions encoding scheme based on electrostatic repulsive forces, despite comparable acquisition time.

Supporting Information

Figure S1 Representative movie files of non–diffusion-weighted and diffusion-weighted images of NC for the 30 directions encoding. Sagittal, coronal, and axial non–diffusion-weighted and diffusion-weighted images of NC were shown.

Figure S2 Representative movie files of non–diffusion-weighted and diffusion-weighted images of EC with trilinear interpolation for the 30 directions encoding. Sagittal, coronal, and axial non–diffusion-weighted and diffusion-weighted images of EC with trilinear interpolation were shown.

Figure S3 Representative movie files of non–diffusion-weighted and diffusion-weighted images of EC with spline interpolation for the 30 directions encoding. Sagittal, coronal, and axial non–diffusion-weighted and diffusion-weighted images of EC with spline interpolation were shown.

Figure S4 Representative movie files of non–diffusion-weighted and diffusion-weighted images of ET for the 30 directions encoding. Sagittal, coronal, and axial non–diffusion-

weighted and diffusion-weighted images of ET were shown. Compared with those of NC (Fig. S1), EC with trilinear (Fig. S2) and spline interpolation (Fig. S3), brain surfaces were well-registered among ET images (Fig. S4) by visual inspection. Furthermore, concave or convex distortions were alleviated in ET images.

Figure S5 Representative movie files of non–diffusion-weighted and diffusion-weighted images of NC for the 60 directions encoding. Sagittal, coronal, and axial non–diffusion-weighted and diffusion-weighted images of NC were shown.

Figure S6 Representative movie files of non–diffusion-weighted and diffusion-weighted images of EC with trilinear interpolation for the 60 directions encoding. Sagittal, coronal, and axial non–diffusion-weighted and diffusion-weighted images of EC with trilinear interpolation were shown.

Figure S7 Representative movie files of non–diffusion-weighted and diffusion-weighted images of EC with spline interpolation for the 60 directions encoding. Sagittal, coronal, and axial non–diffusion-weighted and diffusion-weighted images of EC with spline interpolation were shown.

Figure S8 Representative movie files of non–diffusion-weighted and diffusion-weighted images of ET for the 60 directions encoding. Sagittal, coronal, and axial non–diffusion-weighted and diffusion-weighted images of ET were shown. Compared with those of NC (Fig. S5), EC with trilinear (Fig. S6) and spline interpolation (Fig. S7), brain surfaces were well-registered among ET images (Fig. S8) by visual inspection. Furthermore, concave or convex distortions were alleviated in ET images.

Data S1 Preprocessed fractional anisotropy maps for all subjects. The prefixes NC, EC, and ET indicate reconstructed images with no correction, eddy_correct with spline interpolation, and topup and eddy, respectively. NC30, EC30, and ET30 images were obtained from 30 directions diffusion encoding, and NC60, EC60, and ET60 from 60 directions encoding. The postfix for each filename denote subject number.

Author Contributions

Conceived and designed the experiments: OA YI. Performed the experiments: T. Shizukuishi JK AN MM. Analyzed the data: AN MM HH. Contributed reagents/materials/analysis tools: T. Shinozaki KD YI. Contributed to the writing of the manuscript: HY OA. Designed the diffusion imaging protocol: T. Shizukuishi JK HH.

References

1. Le Bihan D (2003) Looking into the functional architecture of the brain with diffusion MRI. Nat Rev Neurosci 4: 469–480.
2. Wan X, Gullberg GT, Parker DL, Zeng GL (1997) Reduction of geometric and intensity distortions in echo-planar imaging using a multireference scan. Magn Reson Med 37: 932–942.
3. Zeng H, Constable RT (2002) Image distortion correction in EPI: comparison of field mapping with point spread function mapping. Magn Reson Med 48: 137–146.
4. Andersson JL, Skare S, Ashburner J (2003) How to correct susceptibility distortions in spin-echo echo-planar images: application to diffusion tensor imaging. Neuroimage 20: 870–888.
5. Gallichan D, Andersson JL, Jenkinson M, Robson MD, Miller KL (2010) Reducing distortions in diffusion-weighted echo planar imaging with a dual-echo blip-reversed sequence. Magn Reson Med 64: 382–390.
6. Holland D, Kuperman JM, Dale AM (2010) Efficient correction of inhomogeneous static magnetic field-induced distortion in Echo Planar Imaging. Neuroimage 50: 175–183.
7. Andersson JL, Skare S (2002) A model-based method for retrospective correction of geometric distortions in diffusion-weighted EPI. Neuroimage 16: 177–199.
8. Mangin JF, Poupon C, Clark C, Le Bihan D, Bloch I (2002) Distortion correction and robust tensor estimation for MR diffusion imaging. Med Image Anal 6: 191–198.

9. Rohde GK, Barnett AS, Basser PJ, Marenco S, Pierpaoli C (2004) Comprehensive approach for correction of motion and distortion in diffusion-weighted MRI. Magn Reson Med 51: 103–114.

10. Zhuang J, Hrabe J, Kangarlu A, Xu D, Bansal R, et al. (2006) Correction of eddy-current distortions in diffusion tensor images using the known directions and strengths of diffusion gradients. J Magn Reson Imaging 24: 1188–1193.

11. Techavipoo U, Lackey J, Shi J, Guan X, Lai S (2009) Estimation of mutual information objective function based on Fourier shift theorem: an application to eddy current distortion correction in diffusion tensor imaging. Magn Reson Imaging 27: 1281–1292.

12. Mohammadi S, Moller HE, Kugel H, Muller DK, Deppe M (2010) Correcting eddy current and motion effects by affine whole-brain registrations: evaluation of three-dimensional distortions and comparison with slicewise correction. Magn Reson Med 64: 1047–1056.

13. Reese TG, Heid O, Weisskoff RM, Wedeen VJ (2003) Reduction of eddy-current-induced distortion in diffusion MRI using a twice-refocused spin echo. Magn Reson Med 49: 177–182.

14. O'Brien K, Daducci A, Kickler N, Lazeyras F, Gruetter R, et al. (2013) 3-d residual eddy current field characterisation: applied to diffusion weighted magnetic resonance imaging. IEEE Trans Med Imaging 32: 1515–1525.

15. Embleton KV, Haroon HA, Morris DM, Ralph MA, Parker GJ (2010) Distortion correction for diffusion-weighted MRI tractography and fMRI in the temporal lobes. Hum Brain Mapp 31: 1570–1587.

16. Bowtell R, McIntyre DJO, Commandre MJ, Glover PM, Mansfield P (1994) Correction of geometric distortion in echo planar images. Proceedings of 2nd Annual Meeting of the Society for Magnetic Resonance; San Francisco.

17. Smith SM, Jenkinson M, Woolrich MW, Beckmann CF, Behrens TE, et al. (2004) Advances in functional and structural MR image analysis and implementation as FSL. Neuroimage 23 Suppl 1: S208–219.

18. Andersson JLR, Xu J, Yacoub E, Auerbach E, Moeller S, et al. A comprehensive Gaussian process framework for correcting distortions and movements in diffusion images.; 2012, Proceedings of the International Society for Magnetic Resonance in Medicine (ISMRM) 20th Annual Meeting and Exhibition; Melbourne.

19. Glasser MF, Sotiropoulos SN, Wilson JA, Coalson TS, Fischl B, et al. (2013) The minimal preprocessing pipelines for the Human Connectome Project. Neuroimage 80: 105–124.

20. Sotiropoulos SN, Jbabdi S, Xu J, Andersson JL, Moeller S, et al. (2013) Advances in diffusion MRI acquisition and processing in the Human Connectome Project. Neuroimage 80: 125–143.

21. Jones DK (2004) The effect of gradient sampling schemes on measures derived from diffusion tensor MRI: a Monte Carlo study. Magn Reson Med 51: 807–815.

22. Alexander DC, Barker GJ (2005) Optimal imaging parameters for fiber-orientation estimation in diffusion MRI. Neuroimage 27: 357–367.

23. Zhu T, Liu X, Gaugh MD, Connelly PR, Ni H, et al. (2009) Evaluation of measurement uncertainties in human diffusion tensor imaging (DTI)-derived parameters and optimization of clinical DTI protocols with a wild bootstrap analysis. J Magn Reson Imaging 29: 422–435.

24. Smith SM, Jenkinson M, Johansen-Berg H, Rueckert D, Nichols TE, et al. (2006) Tract-based spatial statistics: voxelwise analysis of multi-subject diffusion data. Neuroimage 31: 1487–1505.

25. Tuch DS, Reese TG, Wiegell MR, Makris N, Belliveau JW, et al. (2002) High angular resolution diffusion imaging reveals intravoxel white matter fiber heterogeneity. Magn Reson Med 48: 577–582.

11

Mapping of Autogenous Saphenous Veins as an Imaging Adjunct to Peripheral MR Angiography in Patients with Peripheral Arterial Occlusive Disease and Peripheral Bypass Grafting: Prospective Comparison with Ultrasound and Intraoperative Findings

Ann-Marie Bintu Munda Jah-Kabba[1], Guido Matthias Kukuk[1], Dariusch Reza Hadizadeh[1], Frank Träber[1], Arne Koscielny[2], Mustapha Sundifu Kabba[2], Frauke Verrel[2], Hans Heinz Schild[1], Winfried Albert Willinek[1]*

1 University of Bonn, Dept. of Radiology, Germany, 2 University of Bonn, Dept. of Surgery, Germany

Abstract

Background: Mapping of the great saphenous vein is very important for planning of peripheral and coronary bypass surgery. This study investigated mapping of the great saphenous vein as an adjunct to peripheral MR angiography using a blood pool contrast agent in patients who were referred for evaluation of peripheral arterial occlusive disease and bypass surgery.

Methods: 38 patients with peripheral arterial occlusive disease (21 men; mean age: 71 years, range, 44–88 years) underwent peripheral MR angiography using the blood pool contrast agent Gadofosveset trisodium. Apart from primary arterial assessment images were evaluated in order to determine great saphenous vein diameters at three levels: below the saphenofemoral junction, mid thigh and 10 cm above the knee joint (usability: diameter range: >3 and <10 mm at one level and >3.5 and <10 mm at a neighboring level). Duplex ultrasound was performed by an independent examiner providing diameter measurements at the same levels. Additionally, vessel usability was determined intraoperatively by the vascular surgeon during subsequent bypass surgery.

Results: Mean venous diameters for MR angiography/duplex ultrasound were $5.4\pm2.6/5.5\pm2.8$ mm (level 1), $4.7\pm2.7/4.6\pm2.9$ mm (level 2) and $4.4\pm2.2/4.5\pm2.3$ mm (level 3), respectively, without significant differences between the modalities ($P = 0.207/0.806/0.518$). Subsequent surgery was performed in 27/38 patients. A suitable saphenous vein was diagnosed in 25 and non-usability was diagnosed in 2 of the 27 patients based on MR angiography/duplex ultrasound, respectively. Usability was confirmed by intraoperative assessment in all of the 24 patients that received a venous bypass graft in subsequent bypass surgery. In 1 case, in which the great saphenous vein was assessed as useable by both MR angiography and duplex ultrasound, it was not used during subsequent bypass surgery due to the patients clinical condition and comorbidities.

Conclusion: Simultaneous mapping of the great saphenous vein as an imaging adjunct to peripheral MR angiography with a blood pool contrast agent is an alternative to additive duplex ultrasound in patients undergoing subsequent peripheral bypass grafting.

Editor: Alberto Aliseda, University of Washington, United States of America

Funding: These authors have no support or funding to report.

Competing Interests: The authors have read the journals policy and have the following conflicts: Winfried Willinek has/had speakers bureau appointments with Bracco, Bayer AG, Lantheus Medical Imaging, Koninklijke Philips Electronics and General Electric Company. He is/was on the advisory board of Bayer AG, Lantheus Medical Imaging and General Electric Company.

* Email: Winfried.Willinek@ukb.uni-bonn.de

Introduction

The first bypass surgery with an autologous saphenous vein was carried out by Jean Kunlin in 1948 [1]. Nowadays bypass grafting has been fully established as a standard surgical treatment option in peripheral arterial occlusive disease (PAOD). An autologous saphenous vein is generally regarded as the material of choice for a femorodistal bypass [2]–[4], since it provides the best patency rates [4] and its anatomic position, its length and its wall strength make it suitable to be used as an arterial bypass graft [5]. This is particularly true if it is of good quality i.e. wide enough in diameter

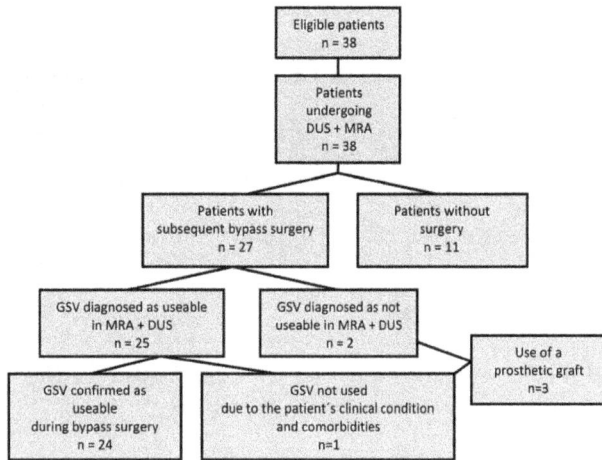

Figure 1. Flowchart portraying the study design.

as well as free of varicosities, thrombotic segments and too many tributaries [6].

Since the 1970 s, the preoperative assessment of the saphenous vein regarding its anatomic configuration, venous abnormalities and pathologic changes has been proven successful in evaluating its suitability as a bypass graft in arterial reconstructions [7], [8]. In the 1980 s, the use of phlebography [9] was challenged by B-mode ultrasound [10], [11] being a procedure which is not invasive, prevents confusion concerning the discrimination of deep and superficial veins and last but not least renders more accurate information about the venous diameters [12], [13].

The advantages of the preoperative saphenous vein mapping, i.e. reduction in morbidity, operation time and hospital stay [13], have been evaluated in several studies on coronary artery grafts [14], [15] as well as peripheral bypass surgery [16], [17].

The major quantitative parameter which has to be determined during venous mapping and has been identified as the predominant technical factor in predicting primary patency, primary assisted patency and secondary patency is the internal venous diameter [4]. In this context the superiority of veins having a larger diameter (>3.5 mm) over narrow ones (<3 mm) is well established [4], [18]. However, Wengerter et al. demonstrated that grafts having a diameter of 3.5 mm as well as grafts which have a diameter of 3.0 mm and are at the same time not longer than 45 mm, present similar patency rates compared to grafts which have a diameter of at least 4.0 mm [19]. This highlights the point that the decisive factor for the short- and long-term success of the bypass surgery is the suitability of the venous conduit, which may be even more important than the quality of the arteries.

B-mode ultrasound has been established as the gold standard in the preoperative mapping of the great saphenous vein (GSV) [20]. However, this noninvasive procedure is highly operator dependent, very time consuming, especially in patients who have already undergone venous surgery, and has technical limitations in patients with edema, obesity and ulcerations.

Contrast-enhanced magnetic resonance angiography (CE-MRA) is considered an alternative to digital subtraction angiography (DSA) in the diagnosis and assessment of patients with peripheral arterial occlusive disease [21], [22] and increasingly replaces DSA in the imaging of the arterial vascular system [23]. However, spatial resolution is limited with standard extracellular Gadolinium chelates during "first pass" imaging. Recently, a contrast agent, with a reversible albumin binding and an extended

intravascular retention and contrast enhancement [24], a "blood pool contrast agent (BPCA)", was approved by the U.S. Food and Drug Administration (FDA). During "first pass" it offers an image quality which, depending on the dose, is at least as good as that of standard extracellular contrast agents [25]–[27]. In addition to first pass MR angiography, blood pool contrast agents allow contrast enhancement during an "equilibrium phase" (i.e. steady state) due to the lack of a relevant extravasation of the contrast agent into the interstitial space. Providing an imaging window of up to 60 minutes [28], the equilibrium phase facilitates the acquisition of much higher spatial resolution images without a significant loss of vessel-to-background contrast [28]–[30]. Steady state MRA with the blood pool contrast agent Gadofosveset trisodium in patients with peripheral arterial occlusive disease was found to render better results than first pass imaging alone [31] and leads – as an add-on – to the simultaneous visualization of the venous system [30]. The additional visualization of veins to that of arteries is inherent to steady state MRA and requires neither a second contrast administration nor any other change of examination parameters. As early as in 1998, Grist et al. indicated the benefits which might be drawn from the simultaneous visualization of arteries and veins in the steady state imaging with Gadofosveset [29]. Today, preliminary data supports the hypothesis that this approach allows for MR-venography as an add-on to the MRA of the arterial system [32]–[34]. Gadofosveset-enhanced MR-imaging has already been proven successful in the detection of thromboembolic processes. Deep venous thrombosis [35] as well as collateral pathways in patients suffering from a massive thromboembolic occlusion of the central veins were reliably detected; the latter could even be achieved in a way better than conventional X-ray-based phlebography [30].

The basis of this work was the hypothesis that peripheral MRA in the steady state using a blood pool contrast agent to image the size and quality of great saphenous veins would be a useful adjunct to arterial phase MRA to improve the performance of peripheral bypass surgery in patients with PAOD. Thus, the purpose of this study was to prospectively determine the accuracy of high-spatial-resolution steady-state MR angiography using the blood pool contrast agent Gadofosveset trisodium in comparison to color-coded duplex ultrasound (DUS) as the standard of reference in order to assess the usability of autologous saphenous veins for subsequent peripheral bypass surgery. Results were correlated with intraoperative findings.

Methods

Ethics Statement

The study protocol was approved by the institutional ethic committee of the University Hospital Bonn, Germany (approval number: 132/07). All patients provided written informed consent.

Patients

This prospective, intraindividual comparative study included 38 consecutive patients (mean age, 71 years; range, 44–88 years) (21 men, 17 women) (table 1) with peripheral arterial occlusive disease who underwent 3D-enhanced MR angiography in preparation for or evaluation of a peripheral (femoropopliteal, popliteocrural or femorocrural) bypass surgery (figure 1).

Clinical inclusion criteria were PAOD stage IIb-IV (Fontaine classification) and indication for MRA. Exclusion criteria were contraindications for 3D contrast-enhanced MR angiography (e.g. allergy, metallic implants that are incompatible with MR imaging including pacemakers). The indication for MRA was defined clinically by the vascular surgeons. Every patient who was enrolled

Table 1. Clinical and demographic characteristics of the study population.

	PAOD stage II b	PAOD stage III	PAOD stage IV
number of patients	13	9	16
age range - years	57–78	45–88	56–85
male sex - no.	7	3	11

All patients were of white ethnicity.

into the study also underwent DUS. 3D contrast-enhanced MR angiographic and ultrasound examinations were carried out in random order. MR-angiographic venous mapping was performed as an adjunct to the BPCA-MRA which was done in order to assess arterial occlusive disease. A possible surgical intervention was not delayed for any patient because of his or her participation in this study.

MR Angiography

MR imaging was performed as previously described [31]: A 1.5-T whole–body imager (Achieva; Philips Healthcare) (maximum gradient amplitude, 33 mT/m; slew rate, 200 T/m/sec) was used to acquire three-dimensional contrast-enhanced MR angiographic sequences of the vasculature. While images of the lower legs were obtained using a commercially available flexible four-channel phased-array coil (Philips Healthcare, Best, the Netherlands), an

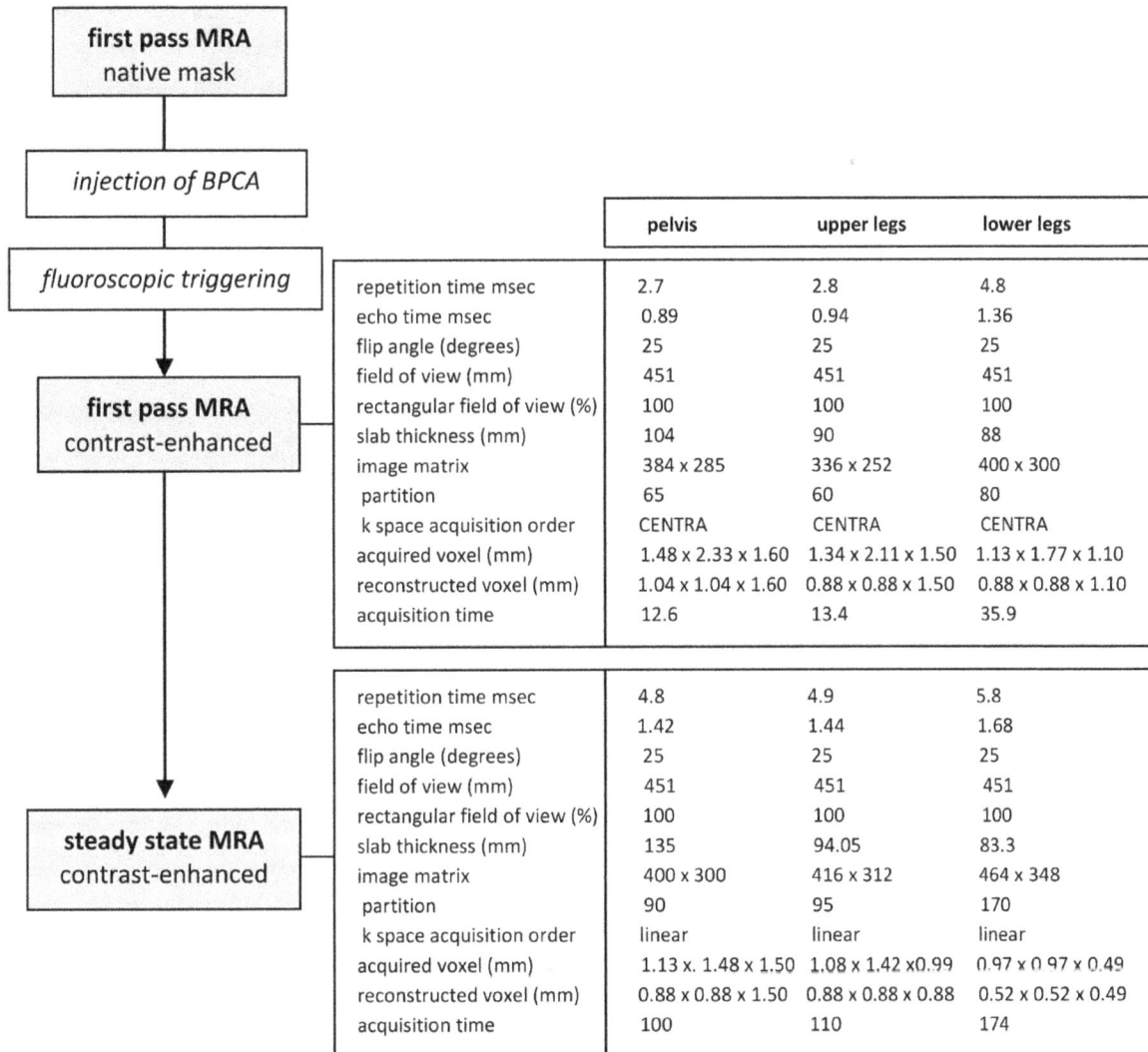

	pelvis	upper legs	lower legs
repetition time msec	2.7	2.8	4.8
echo time msec	0.89	0.94	1.36
flip angle (degrees)	25	25	25
field of view (mm)	451	451	451
rectangular field of view (%)	100	100	100
slab thickness (mm)	104	90	88
image matrix	384 x 285	336 x 252	400 x 300
partition	65	60	80
k space acquisition order	CENTRA	CENTRA	CENTRA
acquired voxel (mm)	1.48 x 2.33 x 1.60	1.34 x 2.11 x 1.50	1.13 x 1.77 x 1.10
reconstructed voxel (mm)	1.04 x 1.04 x 1.60	0.88 x 0.88 x 1.50	0.88 x 0.88 x 1.10
acquisition time	12.6	13.4	35.9

	pelvis	upper legs	lower legs
repetition time msec	4.8	4.9	5.8
echo time msec	1.42	1.44	1.68
flip angle (degrees)	25	25	25
field of view (mm)	451	451	451
rectangular field of view (%)	100	100	100
slab thickness (mm)	135	94.05	83.3
image matrix	400 x 300	416 x 312	464 x 348
partition	90	95	170
k space acquisition order	linear	linear	linear
acquired voxel (mm)	1.13 x. 1.48 x 1.50	1.08 x 1.42 x0.99	0.97 x 0.97 x 0.49
reconstructed voxel (mm)	0.88 x 0.88 x 1.50	0.88 x 0.88 x 0.88	0.52 x 0.52 x 0.49
acquisition time	100	110	174

Figure 2. MR-angiographic protocol. Sequence flow of the combined first-pass and steady-state MR angiographic protocol and technical parameters of T1-weighted gradient-echo sequences for first-pass and steady-state MR angiography.

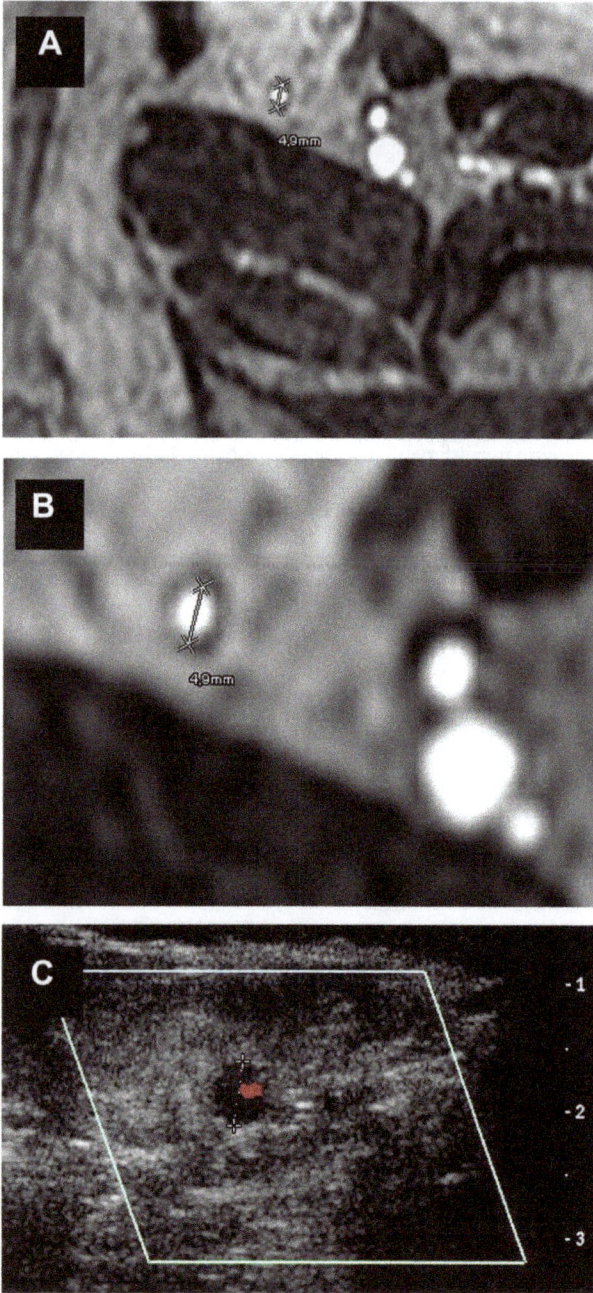

Figure 3. MR-angiographic and duplex sonographic images of the great saphenous vein. Magnetic resonance imaging (BPCA-MRA) and color-coded duplex sonography in the proximal level of the left GSV of a 63 year old female patient who suffered from PAOD stage III and was referred to the radiological department for assessment of the arterial status prior to a proposed bypass surgery. (a, b) Axial multiplanar reformat of contrast-enhanced T1-weighted gradient-echo images during the steady-state. (c) Axial color-coded duplex sonography.

Figure 4. MR-angiographic and duplex sonographic images of the great saphenous vein. Magnetic resonance imaging (BPCA-MRA) and color-coded duplex sonography in the distal level of the left GSV in a 69 year old male patient with PAOD stage IV. (a, b) Axial multiplanar reformat of contrast-enhanced T1-weighted gradient-echo images during the steady-state. (c) Axial color-coded duplex sonography.

integrated body coil served for image acquisition of the upper legs and pelvic region. Using a biphasic injection protocol, Gadofosveset trisodium was administered with an automatic power injector (Spectris; Medrad Europe, Beek, the Netherlands) at a flow rate of 1.2 ml/sec followed by a 25 ml saline flush at a flow rate of 0.6 ml/sec. As soon as the contrast medium was detected at the

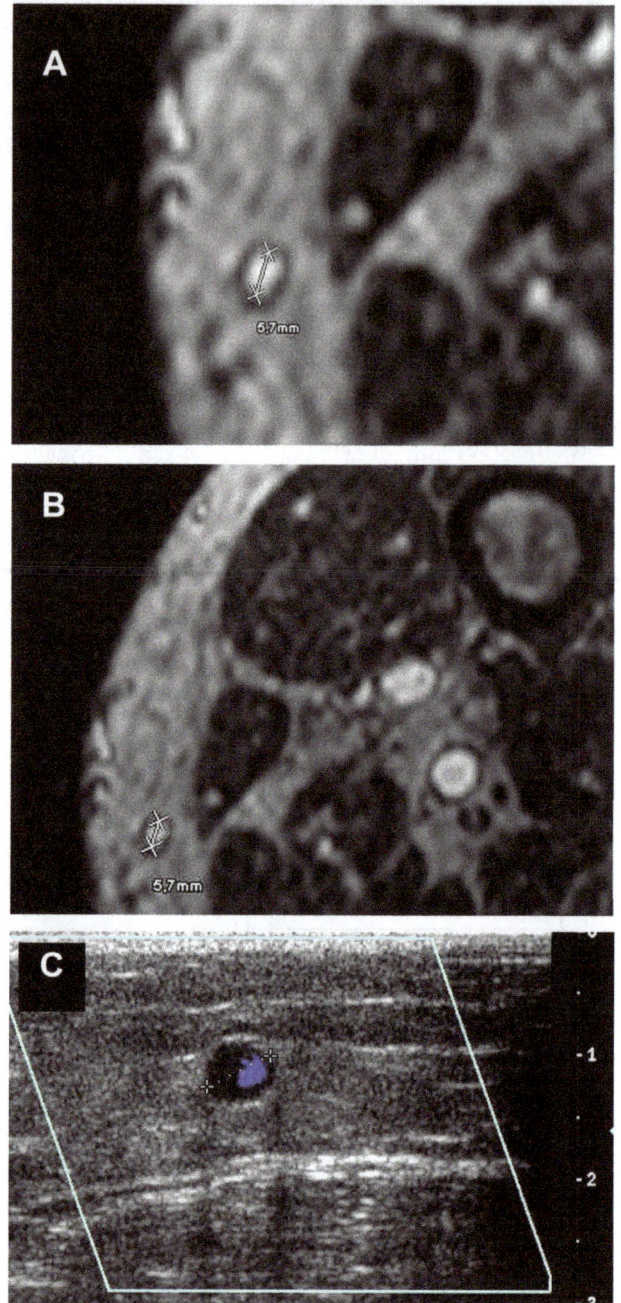

level of the common iliac arteries by means of fluoroscopic triggering, the acquisition of first pass images was started. The imaging protocol as well as technical parameters of the T1-weighted gradient-echo sequences that were used for first-pass and steady-state MR angiography are shown in figure 2 [31], [35]. Steady-state imaging followed first-pass imaging 4 minutes after contrast injection [36].

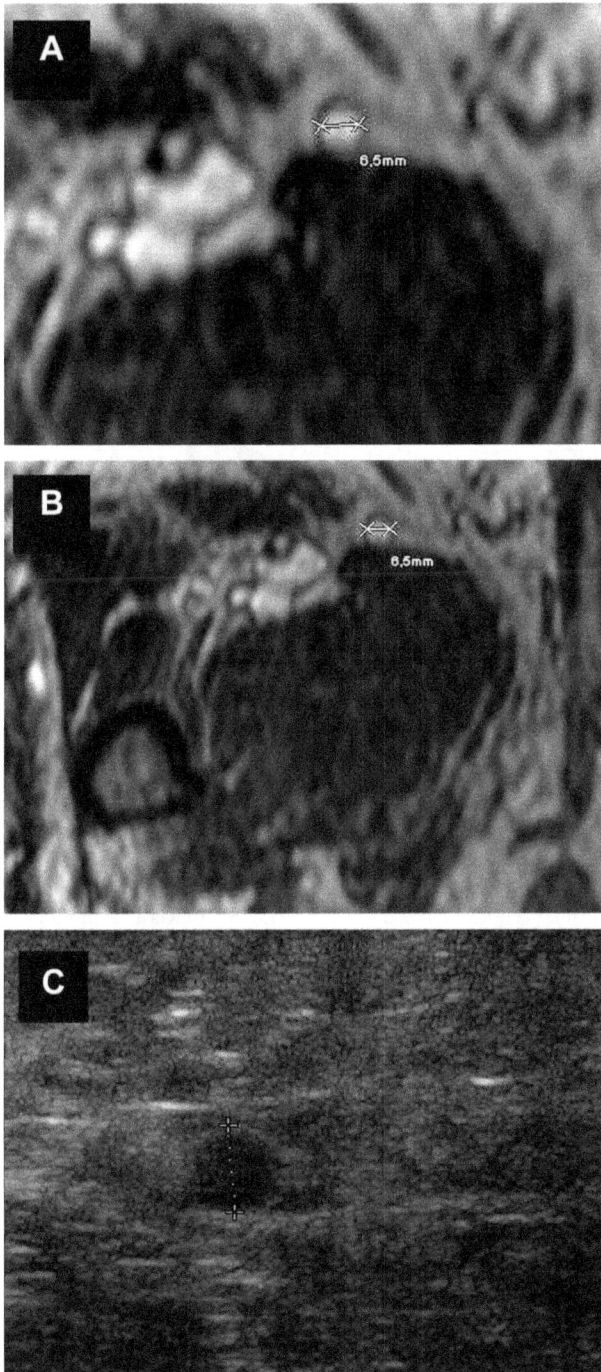

Figure 5. MR-angiographic and duplex sonographic images of the great saphenous vein. Magnetic resonance imaging (BPCA-MRA) and color-coded duplex sonography in the proximal level of the left GSV of a 69 year old male patient who suffered from ulcerations of the lower leg. (a, b) Axial multiplanar reformat of contrast-enhanced T1-weighted gradient-echo images during the steady-state. (c) Axial color-coded duplex sonography.

Contrast Agent

Gadofosveset trisodium (Vasovist, Bayer Healthcare, Leverkusen, Germany; discontinued, now available in the US and Canada as Ablavar, Lantheus Medical Imaging, N. Billerica, MA) was the first intravascular contrast agent approved for use with MRA in

the European Union, Switzerland, Turkey, Canada and Australia [37]. In 2008 it became the first contrast agent specifically approved for MR angiography in the US and Canada by the FDA in order to investigate aortoiliac occlusive disease. Due to an additional diphenylcyclohexyl group, this gadolinium-based contrast agent strongly but reversibly binds to human serum albumin resulting in a higher relaxivity ($r1 = 19$ L $*mmol^{-1} sec^{-1}$ at 1.5 T and 37°C in plasma) and an extended plasma half-life as compared to standard Gadolinium-containing contrast agents. A dose of 0.03 mmol/kg has been proven safe and effective for imaging of peripheral vascular disease [38] and was applied in all patients in our study.

Image analysis of MR Angiography

The maximum venous vessel diameter of the GSV (area of enhancing vessel lumen) was measured on cross-sectional images perpendicular to the flow axis by one radiologist (10 years of experience in vascular radiology) on multiplanar reformats of steady-state MR angiograms on a post-processing workstation (Viewforum; Philips Healthcare, Best, Netherlands) (figure 3–5). Each vein was measured at three levels: at the level just below the groin, at the level of the mid-thigh and 10 cm above the knee joint. To account for both the influence of the graft diameter on the patency rate and the influence of the graft length on the minimal diameter regarded as useable, [4] we decided to rate veins suitable which offered a diameter of at least 3.5 mm at one level and simultaneously a diameter of at least 3.0 mm at a neighboring level. In accordance to clinical practice we defined an upper limit of 10 mm. Nodular varicosities as well as other venous pathologies like thrombosis were exclusion criteria for use in bypass surgery. In order to minimize intraindividual measuring variability, three independent measurements were noted in each of the defined points and the mean was taken for comparison. Moreover a fixed magnification factor of 4 was applied. The reader was blinded regarding the patients names, clinical histories and the results of other diagnostic procedures, including color-coded duplex sonography.

Color-coded duplex sonography

Examinations were performed with the patient in supine position. A HD 11 ultrasound system (Philips Healthcare, Best, the Netherlands) with a 5–10 MHz ultrasonographic transducer was used to visualize the saphenous vein in transverse scans. Starting from the groin, the main trunk was tracked distally to the knee joint. Analogously to the MR angiographic image analysis, three independent measurements were taken from the cross-sectional scan at each level (figure 3–5) and the mean value was calculated. The reader of the DUS was blinded with regard to the results of the MRA.

Intraoperative Evaluation

The preparation of the GSV was carried out through an inguinal incision and a few auxiliary incisions along the saphenous vein. The vein was dissected and measured with a ruler as seen in figure 6. Branches were ligated, the vein was cut to size if necessary and anastomosed at its proximal and distal ends. Absolute values were not compared statistically because measurements were performed on dissected veins that are not in the same physiological condition as in vivo.

Statistical analysis

Students t-test for paired samples was used to test the differences between the diameters measured by DUS and MR angiography

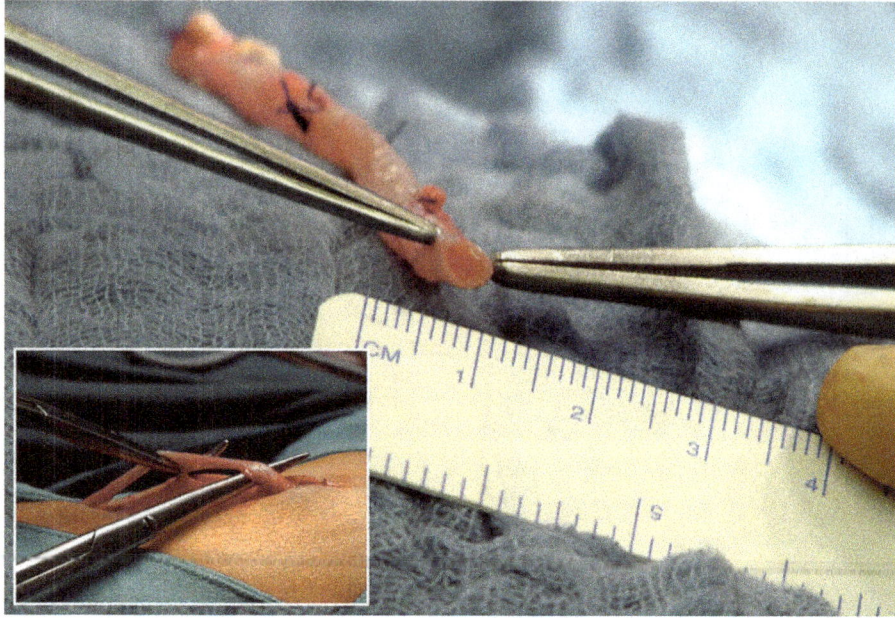

Figure 6. Intraoperative measurement of the dissected great saphenous vein.

based on a venous segment level. A *P* value of less than 0.050 was considered to indicate statistical significance. Correlation between the MR-tomographic and sonographic data was analyzed using Pearsons correlation coefficient. All statistical analyses were performed with the Statistical package for Social Sciences (SPSS) version 17.0 (SPSS, Chicago, Il, USA).

Results

3D steady-state MR angiography was successfully completed in 38 patients (76 assessable legs). Legs, which offered no measureable saphenous vein due to stripping of the saphenous vein (14/76), amputation at the level of mid-thigh (1/76) and absent definability in MRA as well as in sonography (no available level for comparison) (3/76) were excluded. Finally a total of 58 veins were available for intraindividual comparison at level 1, 54 veins for comparison at level 2, and 49 veins for comparison at level 3. The difference between the number of measurements available at the different levels is due to the fact that in some cases a segment (i.a. a

level) of the vein was not included in the scanned volume (5/13) or certain levels were not clearly definable in MRA and/or DUS (8/13). All segments containing the measuring points were satisfactorily displayed on steady-state MR angiography as well as with DUS. Altogether, 161 comparative measurements were performed (Table S1).

Mean venous diameters in MRA/DUS for level 1, 2 and 3 were 5.4±2.6 mm/5.5±2.8 mm, 4.7±2.7 mm/4.6±2.9 mm and 4.4±2.2 mm/4.5±2.3 mm respectively, without significant differences between the two modalities ($P = 0.207/0.806/0.518$, df = 57/53/48) (figure 7). The venous diameters measured were higher on steady-state MR angiography than on color-coded duplex sonography in 54 out of 161 measurements (33.54%) (overestimation) and lower on 82 out of 161 measurement (50.93%) (underestimation). In 25 out of 161 measurements (15.53%) the two methods yielded identical values. The mean values of the positive and negative differences (MRA-DUS) are 0,52±0,67 mm and −0,45±0,59 mm, respectively, with an overall mean of differences (MRA-DUS) of −0,06±0,72 mm.

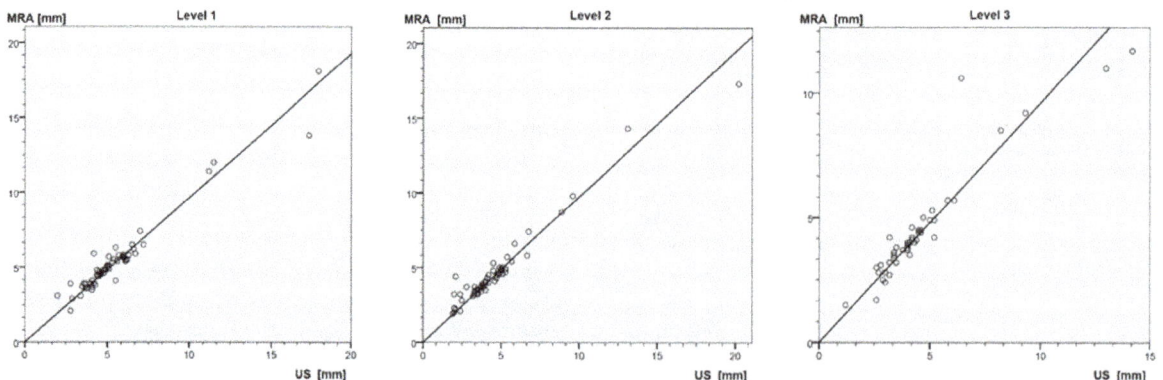

Figure 7. Correlation between MR-angiographic (MRA) and duplex sonographic (DUS) values in the three levels. Pearson correlation coefficients R^2: level 1: 0.989; level 2: 0.986, level 3: 0.973.

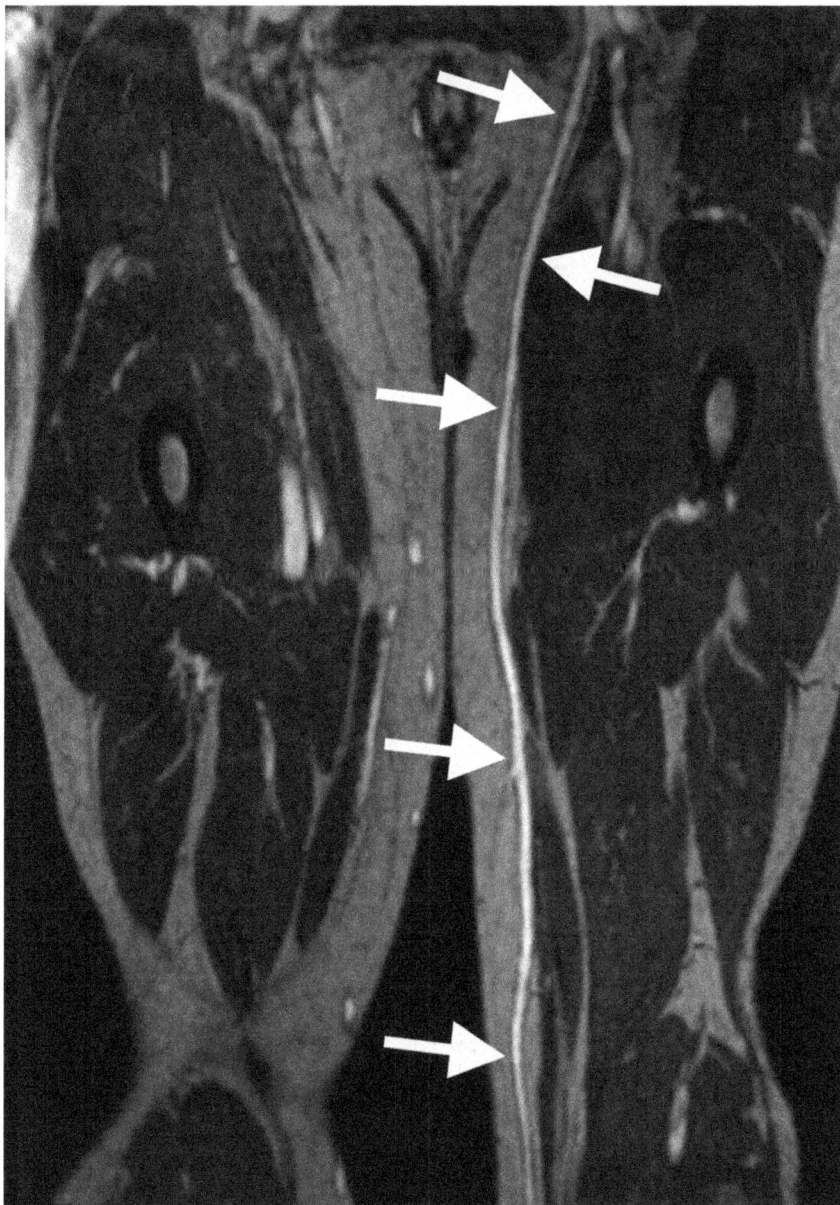

Figure 8. Multiplanar reformat of an MR-angiographic image of the great saphenous vein. The GSV displayed as a curved multiplanar reformat of high-spatial-resolution contrast-enhanced T1-weighted gradient-echo images during the steady-state of a 57 year old male patient suffering from PAOD stage III and thus being evaluated for bypass surgery.

27 of the 38 patients underwent subsequent bypass surgery. In all of these 27 patients, the MR-angiographic assessment and the independent sonographic evaluation showed the same results regarding the suitability of the vein which was considered as bypass conduit. A suitable saphenous vein was diagnosed in all of the 24/27 patients that received a venous bypass conduit. Intraoperative findings confirmed usability in these 24 patients (13 femoropopliteal, 6 popliteocrural and 5 femorocrural bypasses). Non-usability was found in 2/27 patients based on MRA/DUS: In one of these patients the diameter of the respective saphenous vein was too small, the second patient had nodular varicosities. A prosthetic graft was used for reconstruction in both patients. In 1/27 patients a prosthetic graft was utilized despite the usability of the great saphenous vein based on MRA and DUS findings. This decision was taken by the surgeons due to the

patients clinical condition and comorbidities (including coronary heart disease) in order to minimize the duration of the operation as well as to save the saphenous vein for a potential coronary bypass surgery. In 11 patients no bypass surgery was performed.

Discussion

Patients suffering from PAOD often present with concomitant venous disease [39].

In some patients that are evaluated for bypass surgery, veins or parts of them have already been removed due to varicosities or previous arterial surgery. Furthermore, the correct identification of a suitable vein helps to prevent unnecessary large dissections in already ischemic limbs [5], [40] and thereby reduces postoperative leg morbidity [13]. As such, the assessment of the usability of veins as a bypass graft is an indispensable part of the preoperative workup [41].

Our study demonstrates the diagnostic accuracy of MRA with a BPCA in comparison to DUS in the assessment of the luminal diameter of the GSV. Venous mapping was included in the MR-angiographic examination for arterial stenosis grading without the need of a change of examination parameters or any additional diagnostic step in the patient management. We compared sonographic and MR-angiographic measurements and tested the hypothesis that both modalities provide the same results concerning the usability of the GSV as a bypass conduit.

The visualization of the veins in the equilibrium phase of the MRA with Gadofosveset trisodium offered reliable results with regard to the luminal diameter of the GSV in our study population. Statistical analysis showed no significant differences between sonographic and MR-angiographic measurements. Usability (25/27) and non-usability (2/27) were diagnosed consistently by DUS as the standard of reference and MRA. Additionally, usability was verified by the intraoperative assessment of the vein in all patients that received a venous bypass conduit in subsequent bypass surgery.

MRA with the BPCA Gadofosveset trisodium has been proven to be safe, well-tolerated and highly efficient in patients with vascular disease [36], [42]. In 2000, a new disease which is now called nephrogenic systemic fibrosis (NSF) was first described [43]. In 2006, a link between NSF and the exposure to gadolinium-based contrast agents was observed [44], [45]. NSF is very rare and limited to patients with renal impairment [46], [47]. Following studies indicated that NSF almost exclusively occurs after administration of linear, non-ionic gadolinium-based contrast agents [44], [45]. Moreover a prolonged exposure to the contrast agent due to renal insufficiency is suggested as a factor in the pathogenesis of NSF [44], [45]. Although Gadofosveset trisodium is a gadolinium-based contrast agent with a linear structure and an extended plasma half life, so far no unconfounded cases of NSF after administration of a BPCA have been reported [44]. One reason for this might be the high efficiency of Gadofosveset trisodium which results in the use of a much lower Gadolinium concentration as compared to extracellular contrast agents [44]. Nevertheless, a responsible use of gadolinium-based contrast agents in patients with renal impairment is still obligatory.

The sequences needed for first pass and steady state MRA with a BPCA can be easily applied at any MR imaging system and allow for both arterial stenosis grading and the evaluation of venous diameters within the same scan with just a single-dose of contrast agent [35]. Traditionally, venous enhancement was considered a relative drawback of first-pass as well as of steady-state imaging because of impairment of arterial delineation [29], [30]. However, modern steady-state imaging with its increase in spatial resolution and the possibility to acquire isotropic voxels has proved to allow for a distinct analysis of arteries and veins without overlay [30], [31]. Our study lines with previous results that prove the potential of simultaneous visualization of arteries and veins, which was initially postulated in 1998 in view of examining the entire vasculature of the lower extremity in a single imaging procedure [29].

The accuracy of CE-MRA with a BPCA in arterial stenosis grading as compared with digital subtraction angiography (DSA) has already been demonstrated [31], [48]–[50]. Yet, few studies have investigated the inherent potential of the simultaneous visualization of arterial and venous structures in steady state imaging [33]–[35]. A recent study by Hadizadeh et al. showed that BPCA-MRA can reliably detect incidental venous thrombosis in patients undergoing peripheral MRA because of suspected PAOD

[35]. Having demonstrated the reliability of BPCA-MRA in the venous diameter measurement and thus the assessment of the GSV as a bypass conduit, our findings support the usability of BPCA-MRA for simultaneously grading arterial stenosis and visualizing the peripheral veins of the lower extremities in a diagnostically conclusive way.

Our study has several limitations. In the first place, the comparison of the mean venous diameters for the three levels as well as the comparison of the single measurements point out, that MRA in comparison to DUS tends to somewhat over- or underestimate the vessel diameter. However, the fact that the diagnosis of usability versus non-usability by MRA and DUS was consistent in all cases indicates that these slight differences of BPCA-MRA and DUS can practically be neglected. Still, it has to be taken into consideration that a larger study population will increase statistical power. Secondly, the fact that the MRA was carried out as a routine examination for the evaluation of the arterial system, in some cases resulted in the MR technologist accidently excluding the saphenous vein from the scan volume, leading to a reduced number of available segments for comparisons of level 2 (54/76) and 3 (49/76) diameters in comparison to level 1 (58/76). In relation to DUS [19], an inherent limitation of the MR-angiographic examination is the inability to preoperatively mark the course of the veins on the skin as a guide for bypass surgery [10]. However, similar to conventional venography (phlebography), MRA offers a 'roadmap' of the entire vascular system of the lower extremity for treatment planning [21], especially if curved multiplanar reformats are reconstructed (figure 8). In combination with the option to examine the vascular system in different planes, diagnostic analysis and treatment planning are facilitated [21] even in cases of difficult sonographic evaluation due to obesity, previous surgical interventions, multiple collaterals or varicosities. Moreover, in contrast to phlebography, the depth of the saphenous vein as well as the distinction between deep and superficial veins is clearly evident. Yet, the currently limited access to post-processing workstations might hamper the surgeons first-hand preoperative look at the saphenous vein.

In this context, the benefits of DUS are well known: it is a noninvasive, relatively cheap, mobile and adjustable procedure free of ionizing radiation and contraindications and risks related to strong magnetic fields [21]. Keeping this in mind, BPCA-enhanced MRA for assessment of the GSV may appear a rather expensive and inconvenient approach in relation to DUS. However, the MR-angiographic assessment of the GSV vein is not proposed as a separate examination but as an adjunct to MRA which is anyway implemented for evaluation of the run-off arteries. Since the 'add-on' only relates to image analysis and not to the MRA procedure itself, most of the advantages of DUS mentioned above are outweighed. The duration of performing the bilateral image analysis of the GSV by the radiologist, which in our cohort was between 3 to 8 minutes, is actually the only additional time and cost factor caused by the MR-angiographic evaluation of the GSV. The bilateral sonographic examination took between 5 to 15 minutes without calculating the patient or equipment transport required. Moreover, the MRA technique is less examiner-dependent than DUS, can be documented in a standardized way and can be reanalyzed at any time. Furthermore, the ability to assess arteries and veins at the same time within one single diagnostic test, reduces the number of examinations, simplifies preoperative diagnostics as well as patient management and may thus shorten the length of the hospital stay [35].

Another limitation of this study was due to the surgical practice that a vein identified as unusable by DUS did not undergo an additional intraoperative evaluation. An intraoperative evaluation of such veins would generally not yield an assessment differing from the ultrasonographic evaluation, which renders them unsuitable for bypass surgery. Its intraoperative exploration would therefore cause unnecessary trauma to the patient.

A final limitation of our study is the fact that in the bypass surgeries performed, the use of the GSV was often not limited to its supragenual segment. In several cases the length of the bypass required resulted in the additional intraoperative dissection and use of the infragenual segment of the GSV. Intraoperatively, in three patients the diameter of the infragenual segment of the vein turned out to be too small to be used as a bypass conduit. In these cases the GSV of the contralateral lower leg, the small saphenous vein of the contralateral lower leg and a prosthetic graft were used respectively to complement the supragenual GSV in order to acquire a bypass conduit which is long enough. This observation does not hamper the validity or significance of our results but retrospectively highlights that an extension of our preoperative mapping to the infragenual GSV could have presented useful additional information for the surgeons.

In conclusion, the MR-angiographic assessment of the suitability of the saphenous vein as a bypass conduit corresponded with the sonographic evaluation in all of the patients who underwent peripheral MRA and subsequent bypass surgery. With BPCA-MRA, a reliable assessment of the venous diameter of the GSV is possible and shows no significant differences in comparison to DUS as the standard of reference. Consequently, in patients with PAOD who in the preoperative workup undergo peripheral MRA to evaluate the arterial status, the inherent MR-angiographic imaging of autogenous saphenous veins can offer additional information regarding the suitability of the veins as a bypass conduit without the need of an additive ultrasound examination.

Author Contributions

Conceived and designed the experiments: ABJ AK WW. Performed the experiments: ABJ GK DH AK MSK WW. Analyzed the data: ABJ GK DH FT AK MSK FV WW HS. Wrote the paper: ABJ DH FT WW. Critical revision for important content: ABJ DH GK FT AK MSK FV HS WW.

References

1. Chaikhouni A (2010) The magnificient century of cardiothoracic surgery. Heart Views 11: 31–37.
2. Twine CP, McLain AD (2010) Graft type for femoro-popliteal bypass surgery. Cochrane Database Syst Rev CD001487. doi:10.1002/14651858.CD001487.pub2.
3. Klinkert P, Post PN, Breslau PJ, van Bockel JH (2004) Saphenous vein versus PTFE for above-knee femoropopliteal bypass. A review of the literature. Eur J Vasc Endovasc Surg 27: 357–362.
4. Schanzer A, Hevelone N, Owens CD, Belkin M, Bandyk DF, et al. (2007) Technical factors affecting autogenous vein graft failure: observations from a large multicenter trial. J Vasc Surg 46: 1180–1190.
5. Burnand KG, Senapati A, Thomas ML, Browse NL (1985) A comparison of preoperative long saphenous phlebography with operative dissection in assessing the suitability of long saphenous vein for use as a bypass graft. Ann R Coll Surg Engl 67: 183–186.
6. Mosley JG, Manhire AR, Raphael M, Marston JA (1983) An assessment of long saphenous venography to evaluate the saphenous vein for femoropopliteal bypass. Br J Surg 70: 673–674.
7. Shah DM, Chang BB, Leopold PW, Corson JD, Leather RP, et al. (1988) The anatomy of the greater saphenous venous system. J Vast Surg 3: 273–283. Tabrisky J, Christie SG, Nejdl RJ, Lindstrom RR (1976) The value of preoperative saphenous venography for graft evaluation in femoral arterial occlusive disease. J Can Assoc Radiol 27: 37–44.
8. Veith F, Moss C, Sprayregen S, Montefusco C (1979) Preoperative saphenous venography in arterial reconstructive surgery of the lower extremity. Surgery 85: 253–256.
9. Leopold PW, Shandall AA, Corson JD, Shah DM, Leather RP, et al. (1986) Initial experience comparing B-mode imaging and venography of the saphenous vein before in situ bypass. Am J Surg 152: 206–210.
10. McShane MD, Field J, Smallwood J, Chant AD (1988) Early experience with B mode ultrasound mapping of the long saphenous vein prior to femorodistal bypass. Ann R Coll Surg Engl 70: 147–149.
11. Buchbinder D, Semrow C, Friedell ML, Ryan T, Calligaro K, et al. (1987) B-mode ultrasonic imaging in the preoperative evaluation of saphenous vein. Am Surg 53: 368–372.
12. Luckraz H, Lowe J, Pugh N, Azzu AA (2008) Pre-operative long saphenous vein mapping predicts vein anatomy and quality leading to improved post-operative leg morbidity. Interact Cardiovasc Thorac Surg 7: 188–191.
13. Lemmer JH, Meng RL, Corson JD, Miller E (1988) Preoperative saphenous vein mapping for coronary artery bypass. J Card Surg 3: 237–240.
14. Head HD, Brown MF (1995) Preoperative vein mapping for coronary artery bypass operations. Ann Thor Surg 59: 144–148.
15. Seeger JM, Schmidt JH, Flynn TC (1987) Preoperative saphenous and cephalic vein mapping as an adjunct to reconstructive arterial surgery. Ann Surg 205: 733–739.
16. Leopold PW, Shandall A, Kupinski AM, Chang BB, Kaufman J, et al. (1989) Role of B-mode venous mapping in infrainguinal in situ veinarterial bypasses. Br J Surg 76: 305–307.
17. Towne JB, Schmitt DD, Seabrook GR, Bandyk DF (1991) The effect of vein diameter on patency of in situ grafts. J Cardiovasc Surg 32: 192–196.
18. Wengerter KR, Veith FJ, Gupta SK, Ascer E, Rivers SP (1990) Influence of vein size (diameter) on infrapopliteal reversed vein graft patency. J Vasc Surg 11: 525–531.
19. Puppinck P, Habi K, Ducasse E, Espagne P (1997) Evaluation of the venous network before arterial revascularization surgery. J Mal Vasc 22: 162–167.
20. Collins R, Cranny G, Burch J, Aguiar-Ibáñez R, Craig D, et al. (2007) A systematic review of duplex ultrasound, magnetic resonance angiography and computed tomography angiography for the diagnosis and assessment of symptomatic, lower limb peripheral arterial disease. Health Technol Assess 11: 1–184.
21. Lenhart M, Finkenzeller T, Paetzel C, Strotzer M, Mann S, et al. (2002) Contrast-enhanced MR angiography in the routine work-up of the lower extremity arteries. Rofo 174: 1289–1295.
22. Ruehm SG, Goyen M, Debatin JF (2002) MR angiography: first choice for diagnosis of the arterial vascular system. Rofo 174: 551–561.
23. Kroft LJ, de Roos A (1999) Blood pool contrast agents for cardiovascular MR imaging. J Magn Reson Imaging 10: 395–403.
24. Klessen C, Hein PA, Huppertz A, Voth M, Wagner M, et al. (2007) Firstpass whole-body magnetic resonance angiography (MRA) using the blood-pool contrast medium gadofosveset trisodium: comparison to gadopentetate dimeglumine. Invest Radiol 42: 659–664.
25. Maki JH, Wang M, Wilson GJ, Shutske MG, Leiner T (2009) Highly accelerated first- pass contrast-enhanced magnetic resonance angiography of the peripheral vasculature: comparison of gadofosveset trisodium with gadopentetate dimeglumine contrast agents. J Magn Reson Imaging 30: 1085–1092.
26. Frydrychowicz A, Russe MF, Bock J, Stalder AF, Bley TA, et al. (2010) Comparison of gadofosveset trisodium and gadobenate dimeglumine during time- resolved thoracic MR angiography at 3T. Acad Radiol 17: 1394–1400.
27. Lauffer RB, Parmelee DJ, Dunham SU, Ouellet HS, Dolan RP, et al. (1998) MS-325: albumin-targeted contrast agent for MR angiography. Radiology 207: 529–538.
28. Grist TM, Korosec FR, Peters DC, Witte S, Walovitch RC, et al. (1998) Steady-state and dynamic MR angiography with MS-325: initial experience in humans. Radiology 207: 539–544.
29. Goyen M (2008) Gadofosveset-enhanced magnetic resonance angiography. Vasc Health Risk Manag 4: 1–9.
30. Hadizadeh DR, Gieseke J, Lohmaier SH, Wilhelm K, Boschewitz J, et al. (2008) Peripheral MR angiography with blood pool contrast agent: prospective intraindividual comparative study of high-spatial-resolution steady-state MR angiography versus standard-resolution first-pass MR angiography and DSA. Radiology 249: 701–711.
31. Pfeil A, Betge S, Poehlmann G, Boettcher J, Drescher R, et al. (2012) Magnetic resonance VIBE venography using the blood pool contrast agent gadofosveset trisodium-An interrater reliability study. Eur J Radiol 81: 547–552.
32. Hoffmann U, Loewe C, Bernhard C, Weber M, Cejna M, et al. (2002) MRA of the lower extremities in patients with pulmonary embolism using a blood pool contrast agent: initial experience. J Magn Reson Imaging 15: 429–437.
33. Aschauer M, Deutschmann HA, Stollberger R, Hausegger KA, Obernosterer A, et al. (2003) Value of a blood pool contrast agent in MR venography of the lower extremities and pelvis: preliminary results in 12 patients. Magn Reson Med 50: 993–1002.

34. Hadizadeh DR, Kukuk GM, Fahlenkamp UL, Pressacco J, Schäfer C, et al. (2012) Simultaneous MR arteriography and venography with blood pool contrast agent detects deep venous thrombosis in suspected arterial disease. AJR Am J Roentgenol 198: 1188–1195.

35. Hartmann M, Wiethoff AJ, Hentrich HR, Rohrer M (2006) Initial imaging recommendations for Vasovist angiography. Eur Radiol 16 Suppl 2: B15–B23.

36. Goyen M (2007) Gadofosveset: the first intravascular contrast agent EU-approved for use with magnetic resonance angiography. Future Cardiol 3: 19–26.

37. Perreault P, Edelman MA, Baum RA, Yucel EK, Weisskoff RM, et al. (2003) MR angiography with gadofosveset trisodium for peripheral vascular disease: phase II trial. Radiology 229: 811–820.

38. Prandoni P (2007) Links between arterial and venous disease. J Intern Med 262: 341–350.

39. Cohn JD, Korver KF (2005) Optimizing saphenous vein site selection using Intraoperative venous duplex ultrasound scanning. Ann Thorac Surg 79: 2013–2017.

40. van Dijk LC, Wittens CH, Pieterman H, van Urk H (1996) The value of pre-operative ultrasound mapping of the greater saphenous vein prior to 'closed' in situ bypass operations. Eur J Radiol 23: 235–237.

41. Goyen M, Shamsi K, Schoenberg SO (2006) Vasovist-enhanced MR angiography. Eur Radiol 16 Suppl 2: B9–14.

42. Cowper SE, Robin HS, Steinberg SM, Su LD, Gupta S, et al. (2000) Scleromyxoedema-like cutaneous diseases in renal-dialysis patients. Lancet 356: 1000–1001.

43. Grobner T (2006) Gadolinium–a specific trigger for the development of nephrogenic fibrosing dermopathy and nephrogenic systemic fibrosis? Nephrol Dial Transplant 21: 1104–1108.

44. Marckmann P, Skov L, Rossen K, Dupont A, Damholt MB, et al. (2006) Nephrogenic systemic fibrosis: suspected causative role of gadodiamide used for contrast-enhanced magnetic resonance imaging. J Am Soc Nephrol 7: 2359–2362.

45. Breitschaft A, Stahlmann R (2009) Nephrogenic systemic fibrosis. Med Monatsschr Pharm 32: 377–382.

46. Braverman IM, Cowper S (2010) Nephrogenic systemic fibrosis. F1000 Med Rep 2: 84.

47. Anzidei M, Napoli A, Marincola BC, Nofroni I, Geiger D, et al. (2009) Gadofosveset-enhanced MR angiography of carotid arteries: does steady-state imaging improve accuracy of first-pass imaging? Comparison with selective digital subtraction angiography. Radiology 251: 457–466.

48. Bonel HM, Saar B, Hoppe H, Keo HH, Husmann M, et al. (2009) MR angiography of infrapopliteal arteries in patients with peripheral arterial occlusive disease by using Gadofosveset at 3.0 T: diagnostic accuracy compared with selective DSA. Radiology 253: 879–890.

49. Kos S, Reisinger C, Aschwanden M, Bongartz GM, Jacob AL, et al. (2009) Pedal angiography in peripheral arterial occlusive disease: first-pass i.v. contrast-enhanced MR angiography with blood pool contrast medium versus intraarterial digital subtraction angiography. AJR Am J Roentgenol 192: 775–784.

12

Magnetic Resonance Imaging (MRI) to Study Striatal Iron Accumulation in a Rat Model of Parkinson's Disease

Ana Virel[1]*, Erik Faergemann[1], Greger Orädd[2], Ingrid Strömberg[1]

1 Department of Integrative Medical Biology, Umeå University, Umeå, Sweden, **2** Department of Radiation Sciences, Umeå University, Umeå, Sweden

Abstract

Abnormal accumulation of iron is observed in neurodegenerative disorders. In Parkinson's disease, an excess of iron has been demonstrated in different structures of the basal ganglia and is suggested to be involved in the pathogenesis of the disease. Using the 6-hydroxydopamine (6-OHDA) rat model of Parkinson's disease, the edematous effect of 6-OHDA and its relation with striatal iron accumulation was examined utilizing *in vivo* magnetic resonance imaging (MRI). The results revealed that in comparison with control animals, injection of 6-OHDA into the rat striatum provoked an edematous process, visible in T2-weighted images that was accompanied by an accumulation of iron clearly detectable in T2*-weighted images. Furthermore, Prussian blue staining to detect iron in sectioned brains confirmed the existence of accumulated iron in the areas of T2* hypointensities. The presence of ED1-positive microglia in the lesioned striatum overlapped with this accumulation of iron, indicating areas of toxicity and loss of dopamine nerve fibers. Correlation analyses demonstrated a direct relation between the hyperintensities caused by the edema and the hypointensities caused by the accumulation of iron.

Editor: Yun Wang, National Health Research Institutes, Taiwan

Funding: This work was supported by grants from the Swedish brain foundation (Hjärnfonden), Swedish Research Council grant number 09917, Lars Hiertas Minne, Åhlén foundations, and Umeå University Medical Faculty Foundations. The funders had no role in study design, data collection and analysis, decision to publish, or preparation of the manuscript.

Competing Interests: The authors have declared that no competing interests exist.

* Email: ana.virel@umu.se

Introduction

Brain iron accumulation is a normal consequence of ageing. In neurodegenerative disorders this accumulation of iron seems to be augmented and has been proposed as a possible cause of neural death [1–3]. The mechanisms behind anomalous brain iron metabolism are not well understood. Previously, it was thought that abnormal accumulation of iron was a secondary event of neurodegeneration, but today several studies corroborate that abnormal brain iron deposition can originate from different sources such as misregulation of iron transport and storage or transcriptional modifications [1,3–5]. Ferrous iron can react with H_2O_2 via the Fenton reaction and lead to the formation of ferric iron (Fe^{+3}) and a hydroxyl radical. The hazard of the Fenton reaction is that the resulting reactive oxygen species (ROS) could participate in a cascade of events that lead to tissue oxidative stress [6–8]. Non-heme brain iron is mostly found in the ferric (+3) state bound to ferritin, and only a small amount of free intracellular ferrous iron is available [9,10]. Under non-pathological conditions cells have different mechanisms to protect themselves from the formation of these hazardous radicals. However, with age or in situations of abnormal iron accumulation, the availability of ferrous iron and formation of ROS is normally augmented [4,9].

In Parkinson's disease, an abnormal iron overload is present in the basal ganglia [11,12]. Indeed, new advances in the development of neuroprotective drugs to palliate this disorder are focused on the use of different iron chelators to remove toxic iron from brain tissue [13]. However, while much attention has been paid to the toxic effect of iron in the substantia nigra, little is known about the origin of iron deposition in other structures of the dopaminergic system. Iron can be taken up by neurons via the transferrin receptor [14] and then be axonally transported to iron-rich areas in the brain [15]. In dopaminergic neurons an excess of iron might constitute an extra threat since iron has the ability to react with dopamine and produce free radicals [4,16]. In parkinsonian patients, an inverse relationship between striatal iron levels and dopamine concentration has been found, suggesting a retrograde transport of iron from the nerve terminals in the striatum to the cell soma in the substantia nigra [17]. In fact, it has been postulated that degeneration in Parkinson's disease might first occur at the level of the striatal dopamine nerve fibers, and consequently trigger a slow retrograde degeneration of the dopamine neurons situated in the substantia nigra [18]. Therefore, it is important to investigate the possible causes of early dopamine nerve terminal loss in the striatum to clarify possible origins of this disorder.

In animal models of Parkinson's disease, iron levels are increased in the substantia nigra of N-methyl-4-phenyl-1,2,3,6-tetrahydropyridine (MPTP) and 6-hydroxydopamine (6-OHDA) injected animals [19–22]. Furthermore, high concentrations of iron can promote alpha-synuclein aggregation in dopaminergic cells, leading to the formation of Lewy bodies [23]. Novel studies have demonstrated that knockout tau mice accumulate iron in the substantia nigra and are more prone to develop parkinsonism, suggesting a role of tau protein as an iron export mediator [24]. However, due to the difficulties in diagnosing Parkinson's disease at early stages, most studies regarding iron accumulation and dopamine degeneration have been performed postmortem. In animal models, studies have been focused on the accumulation of iron in the substantia nigra after complete depletion of the dopamine neurons, thus, only mimicking late stages of the disorder [19,25]. It is therefore of great importance to investigate if iron overload can also be found at earlier phases of neurodegenerative diseases in other structures of the basal ganglia than in the substantia nigra to be able to hamper its toxic effects.

Magnetic resonance imaging (MRI) has emerged as one of the most promising techniques to study brain iron accumulation in neurodegenerative disorders [26–28]. Image contrast is characterized by proton density, together with the longitudinal and transverse proton relaxation. The effect of iron on the longitudinal relaxation is weak and will not be considered here. There exists three transverse relaxation rates, characterized by the transverse relaxation times T2, T2* and T2', and related by $1/T2* = 1/T2 + 1/T2'$. T2 and T2* governs the relaxation in spin-echo and gradient echo sequences, respectively and differ in that the effect of local magnetic field inhomogeneities are removed in the spin-echo sequence. Labile iron is hardly detectable in MRI. On the contrary, ferritin aggregates or hemosiderin greatly shortens the relaxation time of water protons resulting in hypointensities in T2- and T2*-weighted images (WI) [10,28–30]. Thus, each of these relaxation times can, and has indeed been used to characterize iron accumulation in biological tissue disorders [28], but no consensus on the best method has yet been reached, because of the disadvantages associated with each approach. The iron dependence on T2 has been used to some extent but, since also other factors, such as water content and biological structure, also affect T2, this relationship is not always easily exploited. The effect of iron on T2* is stronger due to the sensitivity to both the reversible and the irreversible effects of iron on the proton relaxation and is therefore considered a more sensitive and robust method to identify iron stores [29,31]. In fact, T2* analysis have been suggested as a biomarker to calculate iron deposition in Parkinsons disease [32]. On the downside, T2* is also affected by other sources of magnetic field variation, e.g. air-filled cavities that makes gradient echo imaging difficult in some parts of the brain, such as the substantia nigra. The susceptibility effect of the iron is also more spatially spread so that the affected area will be less defined in T2*-WI.

In parkinsonian patients, MRI analyses at advanced stages of the disease have shown evidence of iron accumulation based on shortening of relaxation times [32–34]. In animal models, there are only a few MRI reports on the neurotoxic effect of 6-OHDA or MPTP. These reports are basically focused on the use of T2-WI, to study the edematous effect of 6-OHDA [35,36]. Attempts have also been made to use T2 contrast to detect iron accumulation in the nigrostriatal structures, however, the results are not consistent, probably due to the small effect of iron on T2 [37,38]. While most studies to date have focused on iron accumulation in the substantia nigra, the present work is using MRI to monitor the effects of the neurotoxin 6-OHDA on striatal iron accumulation using T2*- and T2-WI. Unilateral injection of 6-OHDA into the striatum of young rats is commonly used as a model for early Parkinson's disease. When 6-OHDA is injected into the striatum, it is specifically taken up by catecholaminergic neurons and then autoxidized, producing reactive oxygen species (ROS) [39]. As a consequence, a slow retrograde degeneration of the dopamine system occurs which lasts over several weeks [40].

Here, the hemiparkinsonian rat model was used to monitor by MRI the effect of 6-OHDA on edema formation and its relation with brain iron accumulation in the striatum. Dopamine degeneration as well as microglia infiltration were also evaluated using immunohistochemistry, and the presence of iron was evaluated using Perls Prussian blue.

Materials and Methods

Animals and surgery

Female Sprague-Dawley rats were used in this study ($n = 19$). All animal experiments were performed in accordance with international accepted guidelines, and approved by the local ethics committee, Umeå Ethics Committee for Animal Studies (approval number A68/12). Animals were housed under a 12: 12 h light/dark cycle and provided with food and water *ad libitum*. All efforts were made to minimize animal suffering.

Dopamine lesions

Rats were anesthetized with isoflurane in O_2 (Baxter Medical AB, Kista, Sweden) and subjected for stereotaxic injections of 6-OHDA ($n = 10$) or vehicle ($n = 9$) into the right dorsal striatum. The following coordinates were used: 1.0 mm anterior, 2.8 mm lateral to bregma, and 5.0 mm below the dura. 6-OHDA injected animals received a dose of 20 µg of 6-OHDA, dissolved in 4 µL saline (0.9% NaCl) containing 0.02% ascorbic acid (pH 3.7). Control animals were injected with vehicle, consisting of 4 µL saline containing 0.02% ascorbic acid. Injections were performed at a rate of 1 µL/min using a Hamilton syringe with a 26 gauge stainless steel needle. The cannula was left in place for 4 min following injection.

In vivo MRI

MRI proton imaging experiments were performed at 9.4 T using a Bruker BioSpec 94/20 scanner equipped with a BG12S gradient set and running Paravision 5.1 software (Bruker, Ettlingen, Germany). Animals were anesthetized with isoflurane in O_2 and scanned utilizing a 40 mm quadrupolar volume coil (Bruker). Temperature and breathing rate were monitored during the course of the experiments using a SA physiological monitoring system (SA Instruments, Inc; Stony Brook, USA). Scans were performed 2 days, 1 week, 3 weeks, and 4 weeks after the intrastiatal injection. To calculate hypointensities and hyperintensities in the striatum T2 and T2* WI were executed: T2-WI were performed using a spin-echo sequence (RARE, TR/TE = 2500/33 ms, Matrix = 256, number of excitations = 4). For T2*-WI a gradient echo sequence was used (MGE, TR/TE = 1500/4, 10, 16, 22, 28, 34, 40, 46, 52, 58, 64, 70 ms, Matrix = 96, number of excitations = 2) from which T2*-maps were subsequently calculated. For both sequences a slice thickness of 0.30 mm with no interslice gap and a field of view of 2.88 cm, was used. The low resolution used for the creation of T2* parametric maps was motivated by the need of better signal to noise ratio for the fitting procedure. The rather low resolution will give rise to larger partial volume effects. However, we do not believe that this will affect the comparative analysis, especially when considering that the susceptibility contribution to T2* is less localized, therefore the effect will be more large-spread for T2* than for T2. For picture illustration an additional gradient echo sequence was utilized with higher in-plane resolution and thicker slices (TR/TE = 1500/22 ms, Matrix 256, Number of excitations = 2, slice thickness 0.53 mm, no interslice gap, Field of view = 3.00 cm). To analyze hypointensities in the substantia nigra a gradient echo sequence was used (TR/TE = 1500/10 ms, Matrix 256, Number of excitations = 2, slice thickness 0.53 mm, no interslice gap, Field of view = 3.00 cm).

Image analysis and quantifications in the striatum

Areas of affected relaxation times were quantified from T2-WI and T2*-WI using Paravision software 5.1 (Bruker) and expressed as pixel area (pu^2). The affected volumes were calculated similar to the method described in [35] by selecting voxels with intensities lying above (hyperintensities) or below (hypointensities) a threshold determined from the mean value for a control area (Fig. 1, ROI1). The cutoffs that gave the best signal to noise ratio were selected to process the pictures. Only voxels within a defined region of interest (Fig. 1, ROI2) were considered in the analysis. Total hypointense and hyperintense areas were calculated for each slice (0.3 mm thickness). When depicting the intensity values at each distance, each value represented the sum of two contiguous slices (0.6 mm).

T2-WI in the striatum (Fig. 1A–B). The control area (ROI1, 0.02 cm^2) was located in the contralateral striatum. Hyperintense voxels were defined as voxels within ROI2 having an intensity larger than 150% of the mean value in the control. For hypointense voxels the corresponding threshold was set to 65% of the control mean.

T2* maps in the striatum (Fig. 1C–D). T2* maps were calculated by fitting the voxel intensities to a single exponential decay for the different echo times, $I = I0*exp(-TE/T2*)$, using the fitting routines in Paravision 5.1 (Fig. 1E–H). The control area was located in the contralateral striatum (ROI1, 0.02 cm^2) and voxels with T2*-values lower than 75% of the mean of the control were defined as affected. This method is expected to give more accurate estimates compared to using voxel intensities for a single echo time. According to the equation above, voxels with low values of T2* will give rise to hypointensities in T2*-WI and, in this respect, we will use the term hypointensities both to denote voxels of lower intensity in T2*-WI and voxels of low T2* values in T2*-maps.

T2* WI in substantia nigra. The control ROI was drawn outside the substantia nigra. The region corresponding to the substantia nigra was located by correlating the MRI pictures with the atlas of *Paxinos et al*, and voxels in these regions were considered affected if the T2*-values were lower than 75% of the mean of the control.

Statistical analysis

To study hyperintensities caused by the presence of edema, non-parametric tests were used. Differences in hyperintensities between animal groups at each time point or position were analyzed using the Mann-Whitney test. To detect differences between distances from the injection site within each group, Kruskal-Wallis test was performed followed by a set of different Mann-Whitney tests using Bonferroni correction. To study differences in hyperintense area within each group at different time points Friedman Test was performed followed by Wilcoxon signed-rank tests.

To study differences in hypointensities between different distances from the injection, two-factor ANOVA was first performed to assess interactions between animal treatments (control/6-OHDA) and distances. Student's *t*-test was performed to determine differences in hypointensities at each distance between animal treatments. One-way ANOVA followed by Bonferroni *post hoc* were performed to detect differences in hypointensities at each distance within each group. To determine differences in hypointensities between 6-OHDA and control injected animals at each time point, mixed-design ANOVA was used. Student's *t*-test was performed to determine differences in hypointensities at each time point between animal groups. One-

way repeated measurements ANOVA followed by pairwise comparisons were performed to detect differences in hypointensities within each group. All results are expressed as mean values ± SEM. The significant level was set at p<0.05.

Pearson correlation and linear regression analysis were performed to correlate hyperintense and hypointense values. Scatter plots including the best linear fit were performed using Kaleidagraph 4.0 (Synergy software).

Histological analysis

Two days (n = 8) or 4 weeks (n = 11) after the striatal dopamine lesion, the rats were anesthetized with pentobarbital and transcardially perfused with Ca^{+2}-free Tyrode solution, followed by 4% paraformaldehyde in 0.1 M phosphate buffer (pH 7.4). The brains were then removed and postfixed in 4% paraformaldehyde in phosphate buffer (pH 7.4) overnight. Afterwards, the brains were stored at 4°C in 10% sucrose solution 0.01% NaN$_3$ in phosphate buffer (pH 7.4) until the brains were processed for sectioning (between 4 days and 3 months). Sucrose solution was changed regularly. The brains from all animals in the study (6-OHDA and controls) were frozen using CO$_2$ and axial sections (14 µm) from the striatum were collected. Sections were thawed onto gelatin-coated glass slides, and rinsed for 15 min in 0.1 M phosphate buffered saline (PBS; pH 7.4), prior to Perls staining or antibody incubations.

Perls Prussian blue staining and ED1 immunohistochemistry. To detect ferric iron in the sectioned brains, the Prussian blue method with DAB enhancement was used. Briefly, tissue sections from all animals were incubated in PBS (pH 7.4) for 3×5 min. Afterwards, endogenous peroxidase was blocked by incubating the samples in 1% H$_2$O$_2$ in PBS (pH 7.4) for 15 min and then washed 3×5 min in PBS (pH 7.4). The sections were then incubated in a fresh solution of equal parts of 2% HCl mixed with 2% potassium ferrocyanide in PBS (pH 7.4) for 45 min and then rinsed for 3×5 min in PBS (pH 7.4). DAB enhancement was performed by incubating in diaminobenzidine (DAB) solution (Sigma, Stockholm, Sweden) for 20 min. Samples were then washed 3×5 min in PBS (pH 7.4). After Prussian blue staining, the same sections were processed for immunohistochemical detection of active microglia. Microglial cells were visualized using antibodies raised against ED1 (mouse anti-rat, dilution 1:100 Millipore, Solna, Sweden) and secondary antibodies Alexa Fluor A488-conjugated antibodies (goat anti-mouse, diluted 1:200, Molecular Probes, Oregon, USA). Sections were cover-slipped in 90% glycerol in PBS (pH 7.4).

Immunoglobulin G (IgG) immunohistochemistry. To study the integrity of the blood-brain barrier (BBB) IgG immunohistochemistry was performed 2 days after the dopamine lesion [41]. Tissue sections were incubated for 1 hour at room temperature with antibodies specific for rat IgG (Alexa Fluor A594 rabbit anti-rat IgG, Invitrogen) dilution 1:200 in 0.3% Triton-X-100 in PBS (pH 7.4). Sections were rinsed 3×15 min in PBS (pH 7.4) and cover-slipped in 90% glycerol in PBS (pH 7.4).

Tyrosine hydroxylase (TH) immunohistochemistry. Dopamine denervation was evaluated using primary antibodies raised against tyrosine hydroxylase (TH; rabbit anti-rat, dilution 1:300, Millipore, Solna, Sweden), and secondary antibodies Alexa Fluor A594 (goat anti-rabbit, dilution 1:500 Molecular Probes, Oregon, USA). All antibodies were diluted in 0.3% Triton-X-100 in PBS (pH 7.4). Primary antibody incubations were performed for 48 hours at 4°C and secondary antibody incubations for 1 hour at room temperature. Preceding TH secondary antibody incubation, unspecific bindings were blocked with 5% goat serum for 15 min. Between antibody

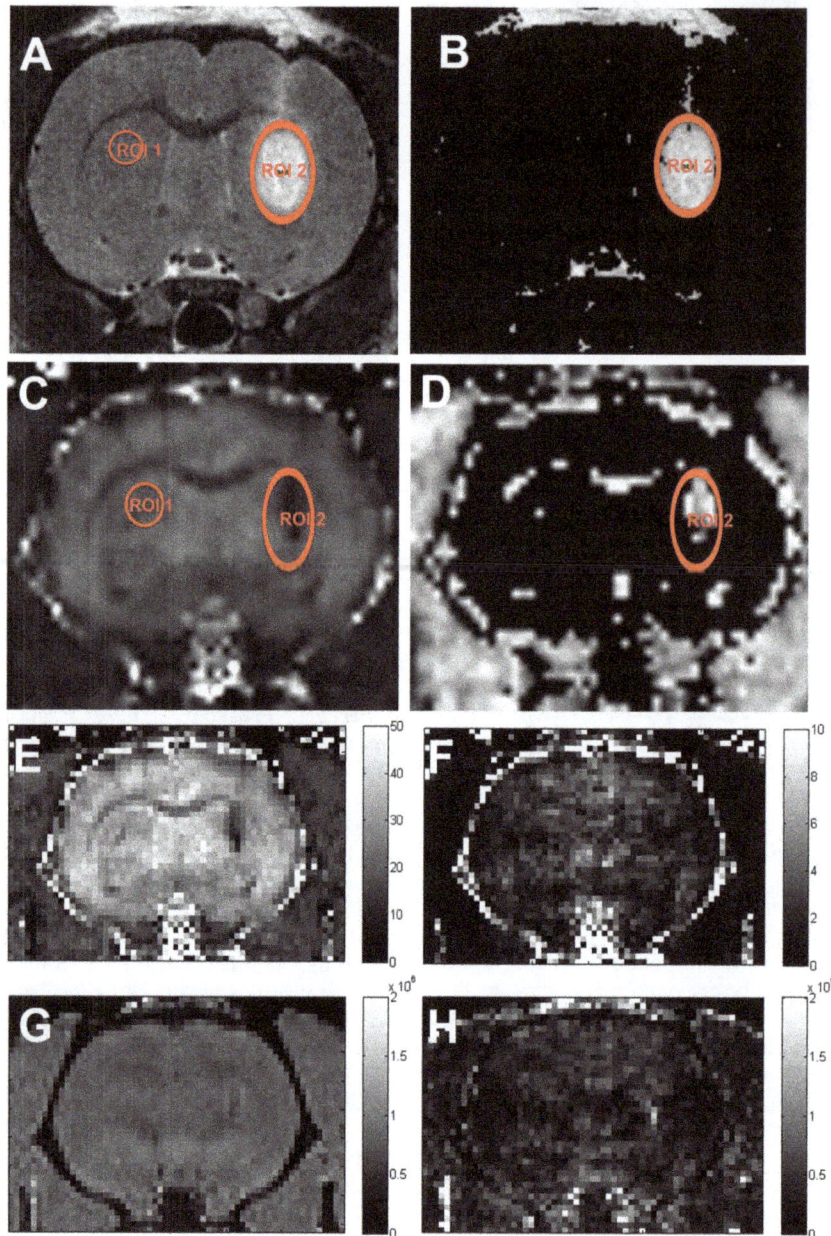

Figure 1. Image processing and ROI selection. T2-WI (A) and T2*-maps (C) were processed into thresholded intensity (B) and T2* maps (D) to calculate areas of affected relaxation times. A control (ROI1) was selected in the unprocessed image and the mean intensity value was used as a reference to select affected pixels (B, D). Only voxels within ROI2 were included in the analysis. Also included are the non-smoothed results of the fit, presented as T2* parametric maps (E) and its standard deviation (F) (scale bars in ms) and intensity (G) and its standard deviation (H) (scale bars in arbitrary units). Note that although figs. A–D are smoothed (Paravision default for image presentation), the ROI statistics are calculated on the non-smoothed data. High resolution T2*-WI of the same animal are represented in Fig. 7.

incubations, sections were rinsed 3×15 min in PBS (pH 7.4). Sections were cover-slipped in 90% glycerol in PBS (pH 7.4).

Giemsa staining. To evaluate the presence of hemorrhages at 2 days after the dopamine lesion, the sections were incubated in Giemsa solution for 5 min, and then washed in PBS. The sections were then mounted in 90% glycerol in PBS (pH 7.4).

Images were captured with Jenoptic, (Jena, Germany) or Retiga 4000RV CCD camera (Q-Imaging, Surrey, BC, Canada).

Results

Hyperintensities in the striatum

Two days after the striatal 6-OHDA injection T2-WI revealed a strong hyperintense signal around the site of injection, whereas this phenomenon was almost not noticeable in control animals (Figs. 2 and 3A). Mann-Whitney test revealed a significant difference in hyperintensities at 2 days between 6-OHDA and control animals ($U = 0.000$, $z = -2.739$ p<0.01). The hyperintensity appeared to be maximum at the injection site and spread at least 1 mm anterior-posteriorly (Fig. 3A). When comparing hyperintense

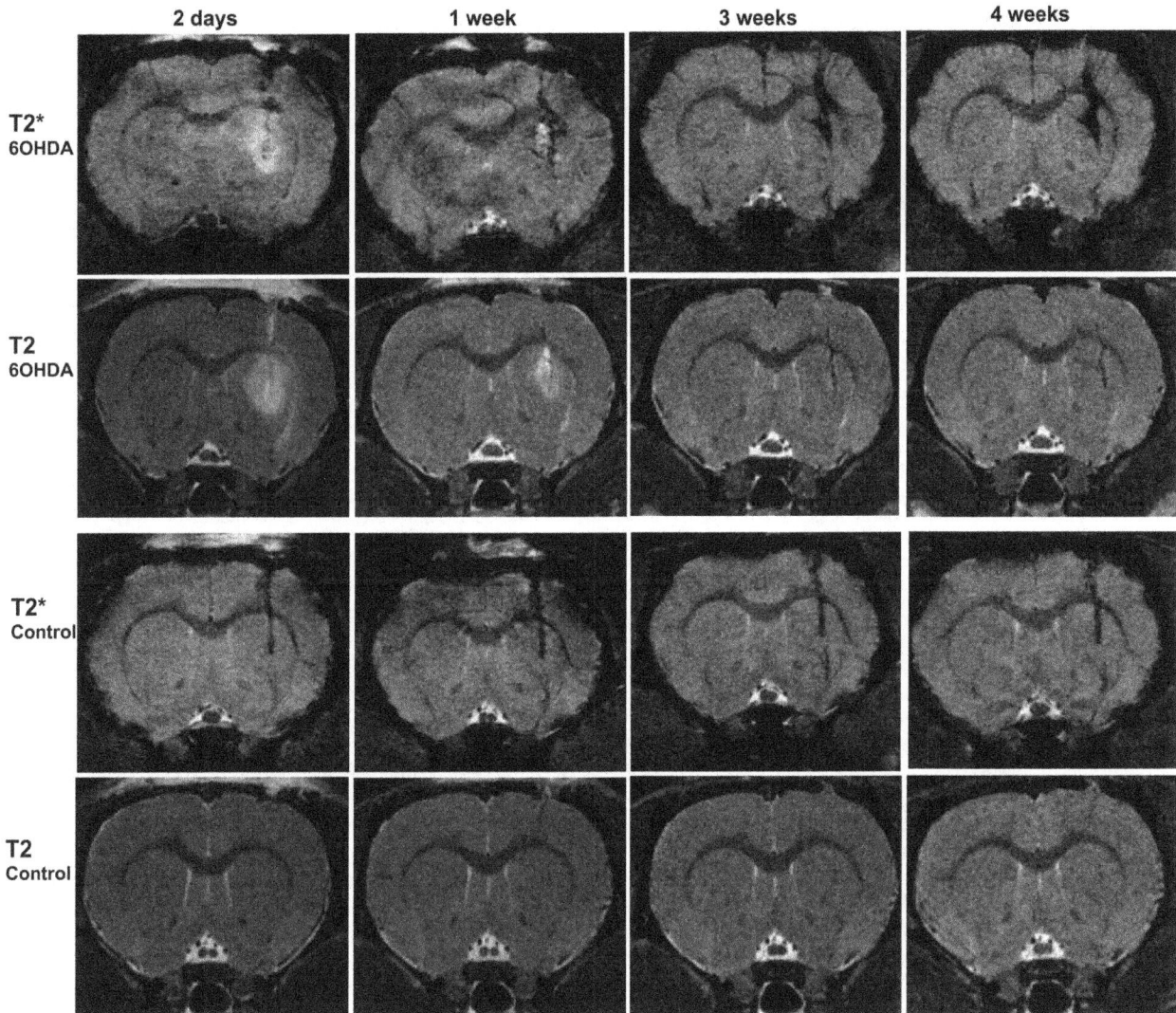

Figure 2. High resolution T2*- and T2 WI at different time points after striatal injections. Upper panels represent 6-OHDA injected animals and lower panels control animals. At two days a strong hyperintensity caused by the presence of edema is visible in T2 and T2*-WI in 6-OHDA- but not in control animals. T2*-WI from 1–4 weeks demonstrated a stronger and more widespread hypointense signal in 6-OHDA injected animals comparing with control animals.

values at different time points in the 6-OHDA injected animals, the peak value was observed at day two followed by a progressive decrease. At one week the hyperintense area had faded and it was vanished at three weeks (Fig. 3B).

Hypointensities in the striatum

To study hypointensities caused by the injection of 6-OHDA, T2*-WI and T2-WI were also performed in parallel to study the presence of hypointense areas (Fig. 4). T2*-WI were performed at different time points after 6-OHDA or vehicle injections. In 6-OHDA injected animals, T2*-WI revealed almost no hypointensities at 2 days after the lesion, instead a strong hyperintense signal was present, caused by the edema (Figs. 2 and 4A). One week postlesion, this T2*-hyperintensity was almost vanished and a hypointense signal was now visible at the place of the injection. This hypointense signal remained at least for 4 weeks (Figs. 2 and 4A). No significant differences in T2*-hypointensity values were found between the 1, 3, and 4 -week time points (F (2,10) = 1.146 p = 0.356, one-way repeated measurements ANOVA). In control

animals, albeit to a lesser extent than after 6-OHDA treatment, a hypointense signal was observed as early as at 2 days (Figs. 2 and 4A), which remained constant during the time points of the study (F(2,8) = 2.392 p = 0.153, one-way repeated measurements ANOVA). T2-hypointensities at different time points were also calculated (Fig. 4C). One-way repeated measurements ANOVA showed differences in T2-hypointensities between 1, 3, 4 weeks in 6-OHDA animals (F (2,10) = 10.759 p<0.01) but not in vehicle animals (F (2,8) = 1.459 p = 0.288).

T2* and T2 hypointense areas were calculated at different distances from the injection at 4 weeks (Fig 4 B and D respectively). The results revealed that in the 6-OHDA injected animals, the hypointense signal peaked at the injection site and spread approximately 1 mm anterior-posteriorly. On the other hand, in control animals, the hypointensity was located only to the level of the injection track (position 0.0 mm) without any further spreading. Two-way ANOVA demonstrated significant difference in the T2*-hypointense areas between 6-OHDA and control animals (F(1,45) = 41.360, p<0.001) with interactions between the

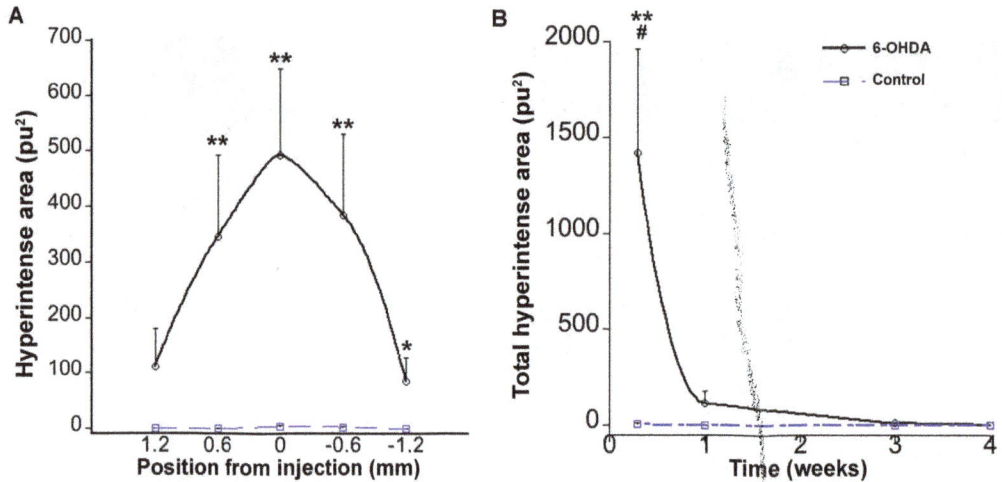

Figure 3. Hyperintense evaluations from T2-WI after striatal injections. A) Hyperintense distributions at 2 days postlesion in the striatum expressed as distances anterior (positive) and posterior (negative) to the injection site. Each point represents the summation of hyperintensities from two 0.3 mm-thick contiguous images. There are significant differences between control and 6-OHDA treated animals. B) Time course evolution of total hyperintense areas also differs from control animals. Continuous line represents 6-OHDA injected animals and broken line represents control animals. (*p<0.05, **p<0.01 compared between 6-OHDA and control animals, #p<0.05 compared between time points within 6-OHDA group).

factors (F(1,45) = 3.818, $p<0.05$). Further analyses confirmed that the hypointense areas close to the injection site had the greatest differences between the two groups (t(5.131) = 3.032 $p<0.05$, t(9) = 5.532 $p<0.001$, t(5.179) = 3.349 $p<0.05$, for coordinates 0.6, 0.0, −0.6 mm, respectively).

Correlation between hypointensities and hyperintensities

To demonstrate the correlation between edema and iron deposition, correlation and linear regression analyses were performed (Fig. 5). A first correlation analysis was performed to study the relation between edema and iron accumulation at different positions from the injection area. In 6-OHDA-lesioned animals, for each distance (1.2, 0.6, 0.0, −0.6, −1.2 mm from the injection site), mean hyperintense values at two days were plotted against the corresponding hypointense values at 4 weeks (Fig. 5A). Correlation for the data revealed that hypointensities and hyperintensities in the 6-OHDA were significantly related, (r = 0.92, p<0.05, two tailed). Additionally, total hyperintensities at two days were calculated for each animal in the study (control and 6-OHDA injected) and plotted against total hypointense values from the same animals at 4 weeks (Fig. 5B). The data revealed that total hypointensities and hyperintensities were correlated (r = 0.95, p<0.001 two tailed). Animals with high hyperintense values coincided with high hypointense values and vice versa.

Hypointensities in the substantia nigra

Hypointense evaluations in the ipsilateral substantia nigra were also quantified 4 weeks after the 6-OHDA striatal injections to study the possibility of iron accumulation. The results revealed that there were no significant differences in hypointensities between control- and 6-OHDA injected animals (t (8) = 1.248 p = 0.247).

Perls Prussian blue staining and ED1 immunohistochemistry

Histological Prussian blue staining of the perfused brains (control and 6-OHDA) followed by ED1 staining was performed at 2 days (Fig. 6 A, B, E, F) or 4 weeks (Fig. 6 C, D, G, H)

postinjection. The results revealed that at 2 days postlesion no iron was seen in 6-OHDA animals (Fig. 6 A) or in control animals (Fig. 6E) and only a small microglia reaction was detected (Fig. 6 B, F). On the other hand, at 4 weeks postlesion, a strong accumulation of iron was seen in the 6-OHDA injected animals (Fig. 6 C) compared with control animals (Fig. 6 G). At this time point ED1 imunohistochemistry showed a strong accumulation of reactive microglia in the center of the lesioned area, which was less pronounced in control animals (Figs. 6 D and H respectively). Most of ED1-positive cells overlapped with Prussian blue-positive deposits. However, other cells than ED1-positive microglia were positive for iron (Fig. 6, arrows). The presence of iron at four weeks was correlated with the T2* hypointensities observed at different distances from the injection of 6-OHDA (Fig. 7A, B, C). In control animals the presence of iron was almost absent (Fig. 7 D, E) which accordingly also coincided with the absence of hypointensities in these animals.

(IgG) immunohistochemistry

The integrity of the BBB was evaluated by studying infiltration of rat IgG in the striatum of control- and 6-OHDA-injected animals (Fig. 8 A and B, respectively). Two days after performing the dopamine lesions an enhanced IgG reactivity was found in the striatum of the lesioned- compared to vehicle-injected animals. In the controls, IgG infiltration was almost absent and only a weak reaction could be observed around the vehicle injection.

Tyrosine hydroxylase immunohistochemistry

In control animals, TH-positive nerve fibers were intact and no denervation was observed in the striatum. All animals injected with 6-OHDA showed a similar degree of nerve fiber denervation in the striatum (Figure S1).

Giemsa staining

Giemsa staining was performed to visualize hemorrhages that might have occurred from the injections. However, no red blood cells were found in the injection tracks at 2 days postlesion (Figure S2).

A

B

C

D

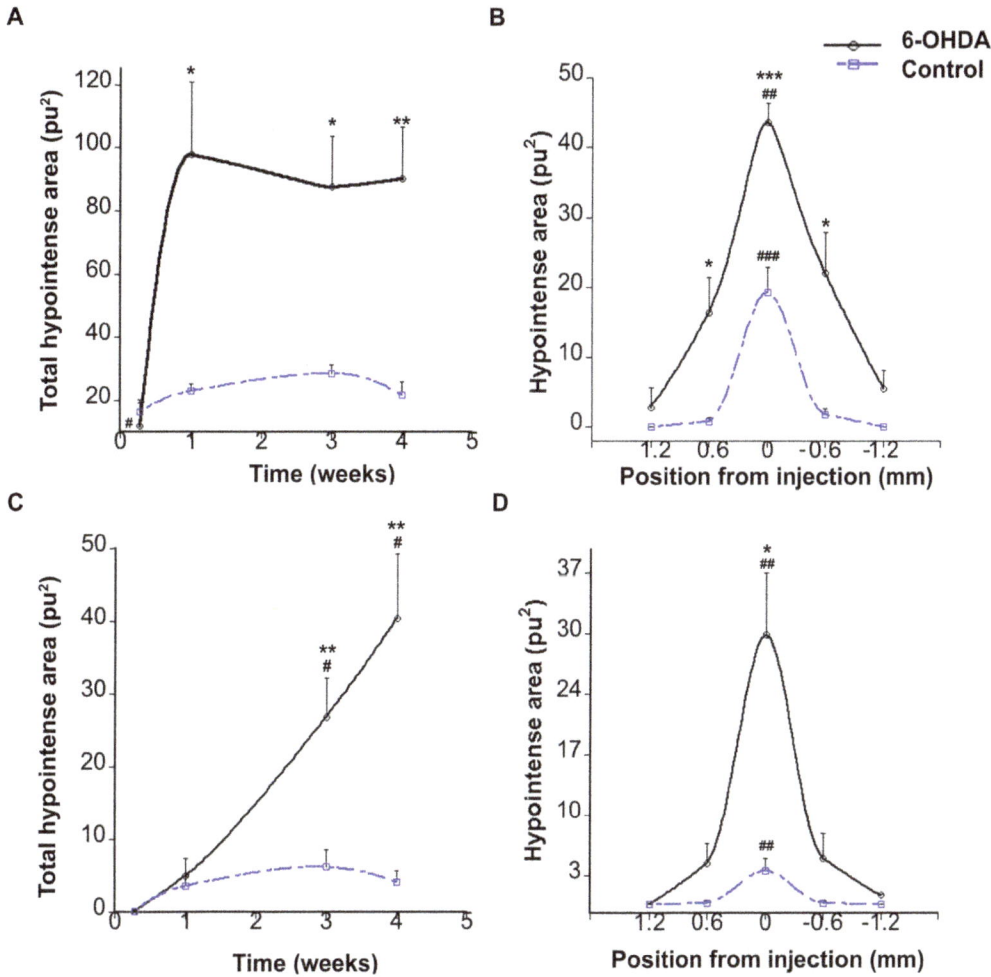

Figure 4. Hypointense evaluations from T2*- and T2 WI after striatal injections. A) Time course evolution of total T2*-hypointensities showed no significant differences between 1, 3 and 4 weeks, but showed differences between the two groups. B) T2*-hypointense distribution at 4 weeks expressed as distance anterior (positive) and posterior (negative) to the injection site. The results show a significant difference between 6-OHDA and control animals at different distances. C) Time course evolution of total T2-hypointensities D) T2-hypointense distribution at 4 weeks at different distances to the injection site. Continuous line represents 6-OHDA injected animals and broken line represents control animals. *p<0.05, **p<0.01, ***p<0.001 compared between control and 6-OHDA animals. #p<0.05, ##p<0.01, ###p<0.001 compared between different distances or time points within each group.

Discussion

MRI was used to follow possible iron accumulation in the intrastriatal 6-OHDA hemiparkinsonian rat. The results demonstrated that 2 days after the striatal 6-OHDA injection, a strong hyperintense signal was detected in T2-WI, which later was clearly associated with a hypointense region in T2*-WI. This hypointense area reached over several images in an anterior-posterior direction in 6-OHDA-lesioned animals while in control animals, the hypointensity was found mainly in one image, i.e. over the injection site, indicating that a larger volume was affected after the 6-OHDA lesion. The hypointensity was detected close to the injection track, in the center of the denervated area, and it was more pronounced and spread in 6-OHDA animals than in control animals. Prussian blue staining revealed accumulation of iron with similar volumetric spreading as found for the hypointensities at 4 weeks postlesion. In addition, ED-1-positive microglia was present in areas with accumulation of iron.

The presence of T2-hyperintensities after striatal injection of 6-OHDA has already been observed and described as an edematous

effect caused by 6-OHDA [35]. However, the origin and nature of this edema is still under debate [35,42,43]. To investigate the possibility that a vasogenic edema was caused by a disrupted BBB, an immunohistochemical method was used to detect extravasated IgG [41]. The results showed that the striatum surrounding the injection trace after 6-OHDA injection was positive to antibodies against rat IgG at 2 days suggesting the existence of a vasogenic edema and an altered (BBB). In fact, the existence of a disturbed BBB in Parkinson's disease has gained more acceptance during the last years [44] and has been proposed as one of the possible causes of neurodegeneration in Parkinson's disease [45]. Alterations in the BBB in the striatum after 6-OHDA injections have already been described, however these studies are focused at 10 and 34 days after the dopamine lesion [46]. Thus, our results demonstrate the presence of a disrupted BBB already during the first days after the neurotoxic lesion.

Another source of the edema might origin from the neurotoxin itself. A cytotoxic edema might originate not only from the substantial loss of dopamine fibers in the striatum but also from the void of astrocytes that is evident after the 6-OHDA injection

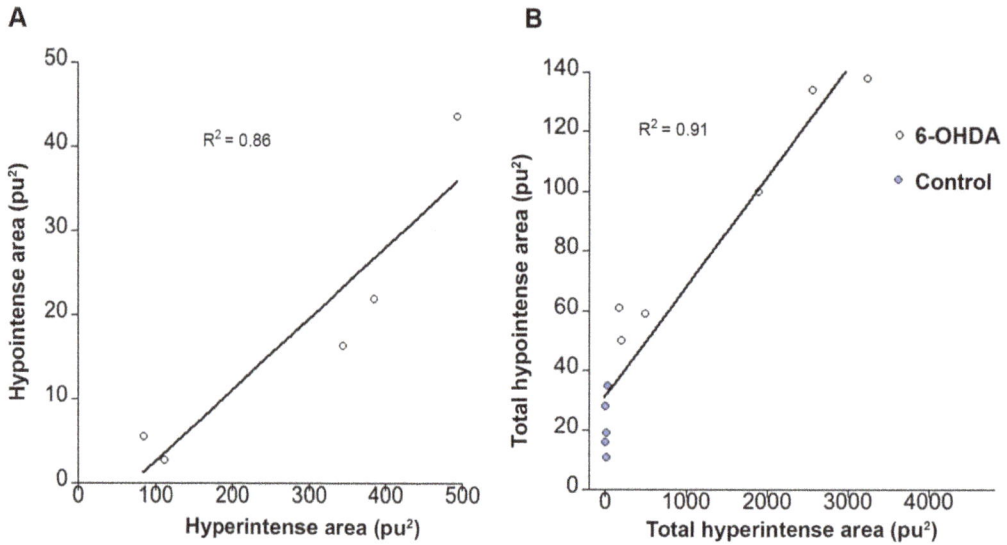

Figure 5. Correlations between edema and iron accumulation. A) Regression line showing the correlation between hyperintensities at day 2 and corresponding hypointensities at 4 weeks for different positions in the striatum (data points = 1.2 0.6, 0, −0.6, −1.2 mm from injection) of 6-OHDA injected animals. B) Regression line showing the correlation between total hyperintense areas at day 2 and corresponding hypointense areas at 4 weeks, calculated from control, and 6-OHDA groups (represented by blue and white dots respectively).

[42,47]. Interestingly, the time profile of the edematous process seen in the present study coincides with the time determined for astrocytic death after 6-OHDA injections. The loss of astrocytes after 6-OHDA reaches a maximum at day two, and a moderate increase in astrocytes start to be detected at day eight [47]. Degeneration of astrocytes might in fact affect the permeability of the BBB to iron since, astrocytes are reinforcing the tight junctions of the blood capillaries, acting as gatekeepers for the transport of

iron into the brain. Therefore, the edema might origin from a leakage in the BBB caused by the neurotoxin.

The small T2*-hypointense area found in both control and 6-OHDA-injected animals at 2 days using MRI was strictly located to the site of the injection. No iron accumulation could be found in sections stained with Prussian blue at this time point. This small hypointense area might represent hemoglobin-derived iron caused by the injection. However, neither iron accumulation nor

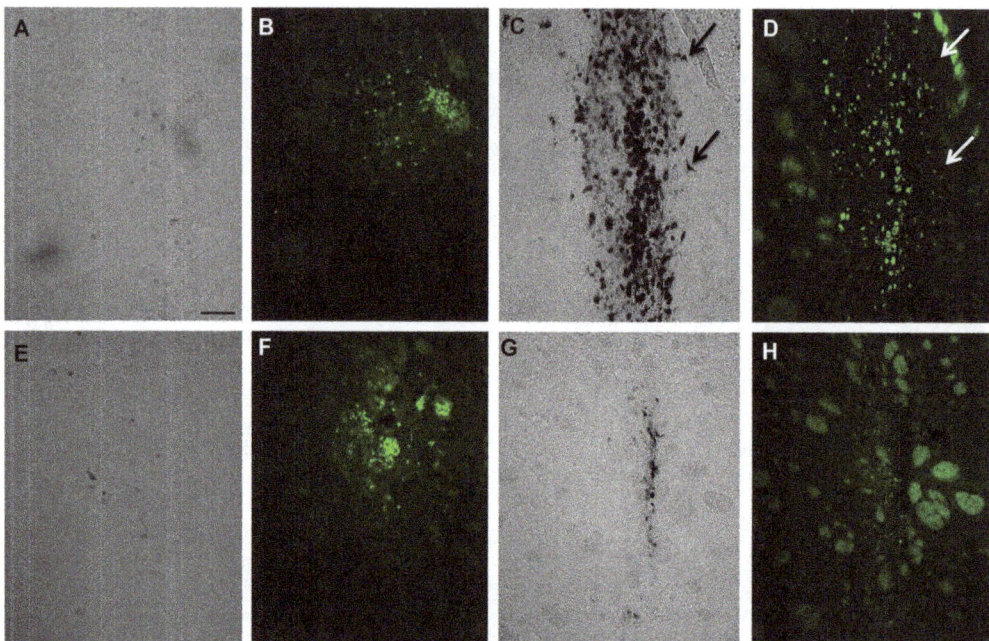

Figure 6. Histological analysis of hypointense areas. Prussian blue staining combined with ED1-inmunoreativity at 2 days postlesion (A, B, E, F) shows that in 6-OHDA injected animals (A, B) and control animals (E, F) iron (A and E) and microglia (B and F) are almost absent. At 4 weeks in 6-OHDA animals (C, D) the iron deposits are located to the same areas as active microglia (D). In control animals accumulation of iron (G) and activation of microglia (H) was less pronounced. Arrows show ED1-negative cells that were iron positive. Scale bar 50 μm.

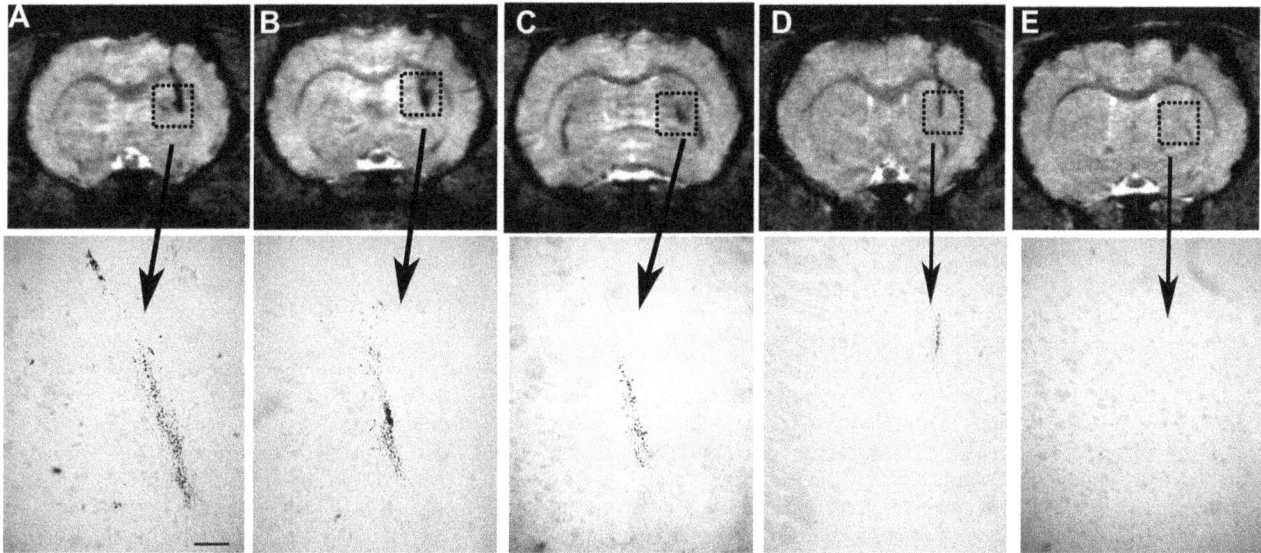

Figure 7. Correlations between T2*-hypointensities and iron accumulation. High resolution T2*-weighted images at four weeks after 6-OHDA injection showed a strong hypointense area at different positions in the striatum A) 0, B) −0.53 and C) −1.06 mm from the injection site which coincided with the presence of iron in Prussian blue histology. The hypointense area and the accumulation of iron was much smaller and more localized in control animals at 0 or −0.53 mm from the vehicle injection (D and E respectively). Scale bar 200 μm.

hemorrhages were found in the histological evaluations. The small hypointensities seen at this early time point might have other explanations than accumulation of iron. Other factors than iron that may affect T2* relaxation time may include increased tissue water, altered blood flow, or myelination [28]. On the other hand the influence of other metals on T2/T2* has probably no major influence since most of metallic ions found in the brain are nonmagnetic. It has been reported that a small increase of magnetic metals such as iron, manganese, copper, or zinc occurs after injecting 6-OHDA in the vicinity of the substantia nigra [48]. Nevertheless, these amounts were considerably lower than iron, and besides, some of them, such as for example manganese have rather an effect on T1 than T2 [10]. Thus, their effect on T2 is probably negligible. Therefore the amplified hypointensity found in the striatum of 6-OHDA-injected animals at later time points was more certainly derived from iron accumulation, since iron greatly affects T2* relaxivity, and moreover the hypointensities observed in T2*-WI coincided with the presence of iron as revealed by Prussian blue staining. Although some iron could have been chelated by the presence of phosphate in the perfusion buffer, no discrepancies were found between MRI hypointensities and patterns of distribution of histological iron. In the T2-WI of the dopamine-lesioned striatum, two effects influence the image contrast. The edema will increase T2 due to the change in water content, causing a hyperintense signal, while iron accumulation will act to decrease T2, resulting in a hypointense signal. The observed contrast will be due to both of these effects and therefore the time course from the T2-WI will be difficult to interpret. The same two effects will also influence on T2* but in this case the effect of iron accumulation will be larger and we therefore believe that the time course in Fig. 4A more closely resembles the actual change in iron concentration. The differences between T2 and T2* at one week observed in the 6-OHDA injected animals are probably due to the fact that in T2-WI the hyperintensities from the edema could be detected until 1 week in most animals therefore masking the small hypointensities from the presence of

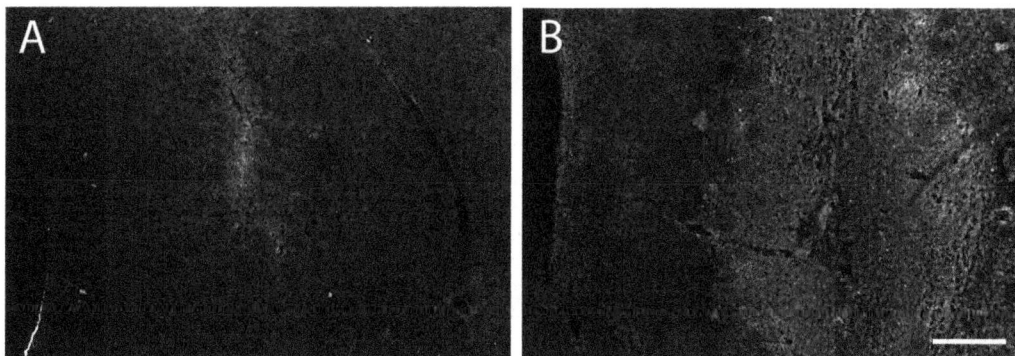

Figure 8. Immunoglobulin G (IgG) histochemistry. A) control- and B) 6-OHDA injected striatum at 2 days postlesion incubated with anti-rat IgG. Control animals showed almost not reactivity to IgG comparing with lesioned animals indicating that 6-OHDA provokes a disturbed BBB. Scale bar 100 μm.

iron. Thus, we believe that T2* are more reliable to measure hypointensities since there is a minor effect from the edema.

The mechanisms behind this accumulation of iron are yet not fully understood, but it might be correlated with misregulation of iron transporters [21] or the capacity of 6-OHDA to release iron from ferritin [19]. Recent studies have found the existence of iron in dopamine neuronal vesicles that are transported through the axons [49]. Thus, one source of abnormal iron accumulation in the 6-OHDA injected striatum might be the ferritin-bound iron or vesicular iron released from degenerated dopamine fibers. In addition, if the BBB is disturbed, which was the case in our study, the tight regulation of brain iron transport would be altered and as a consequence a leakage of serum iron might occur [17,50]. Our correlation analyses between hypointense and hyperintense areas in the striatum showed an evident relation between edema formation and iron deposition. The fact that an abnormal source of iron was accumulated precisely in the area of the edema further supports the hypothesis of a disturbed BBB and a leakage of iron.

It has previously been shown that 6-OHDA can promote iron deposition in the substantia nigra when injected in the medial forebrain bundle [19,22,25]. In fact, treatment with iron chelators can induce neuroprotection against 6-OHDA, demonstrating a participation of iron in the neurotoxic cascade induced by 6-OHDA [51]. Therefore, quantifications of hypointensities in the substantia nigra were performed. However, due to the interference of the bone cavities it was not possible to measure using the same T2*-maps as for the striatal measurements. Thus, higher resolution images with thicker slices were used for these measurements. No differences were found in hypointensities between 6-OHDA and control animals. These results were somehow expected since the 6-OHDA striatal lesion will only cause a partial depletion of the dopamine neurons in the substantia nigra. Thus, about 60% of the dopamine neurons in the substantia nigra are reported to remain after the striatal 6-OHDA injection [40]. Therefore a more substantial depletion might be required to detect iron accumulation in the substantia nigra [19,22,25]. Interestingly, it has been reported that this increase of iron in the substantia nigra does not occur until 7–10 days postlesion [48]. This might in part explain our results since a delayed increase in iron occurred when 6-OHDA was injected in the striatum.

Histological analyses using Prussian blue and ED1-immunohistochemistry, revealed an area of reactive microglia that was restricted to the region of iron accumulation. Other cells that were ED1-negative also seemed to accumulate iron. Thus, iron accumulation was not exclusively restricted to ED1- positive cells.

It is known that iron laden-microglia has been found in the brains of Parkinson's disease patients [52], 6-OHDA-induced animals [25], or other neurodegenerative diseases [53], suggesting a pathological role for iron-laden microglia. Therefore, the presence of activated microglia in the lesioned striatum probably represents an area where phagocytosis occurs induced by tissue damage and an excess of iron. The fact that iron accumulation and hypointensities were restricted to the same area as ED1 suggest that iron-laden microglia might account for a significant part of the MRI hypointensities.

Conclusions

The present study demonstrates by using *in vivo* MRI that iron accumulates in the striatum of a rat model of early Parkinson's disease where slow, retrograde neurodegeneration occurs. Injection of 6-OHDA in the rat striatum results in an edematous process accompanied with an abnormal accumulation of iron. In addition, this excess of iron is located in the same area as active microglia, suggesting a pathological role for this accumulation of iron. The association of iron overload with an edematous process suggests the presence of a vasogenic edema and a disrupted BBB as possible sources for this excess of iron.

Supporting Information

Figure S1   Tyrosine hydroxylase immunoreactivity. A) Control- and B) 6-OHDA injected striatum at 4 weeks after injections showing dopaminergic integrity or degeneration, respectively, around the injection track (black arrows). The size of the denervated zone appears similar in all lesioned animals. A and B represent composite images. Scale bar 200 µm.

Figure S2   Giemsa staining. A) control- and B) 6-OHDA injected striatum at 2 days postlesion incubated with Giemsa stain showed absence of red blood cells in both control- and 6-OHDA lesioned animals. Scale bar 200 µm.

Author Contributions

Conceived and designed the experiments: AV IS GO. Performed the experiments: AV EF. Analyzed the data: AV IS GO EF. Contributed to the writing of the manuscript: AV IS GO.

References

1. Sadrzadeh SM, Saffari Y (2004) Iron and brain disorders. Am J Clin Pathol 121 Suppl: S64–70.
2. Stankiewicz J, Panter SS, Neema M, Arora A, Batt CE, et al. (2007) Iron in chronic brain disorders: imaging and neurotherapeutic implications. Neurotherapeutics 4: 371–386.
3. Batista-Nascimento L, Pimentel C, Menezes RA, Rodrigues-Pousada C (2012) Iron and neurodegeneration: from cellular homeostasis to disease. Oxid Med Cell Longev 2012: 128647.
4. Nunez MT, Urrutia P, Mena N, Aguirre P, Tapia V, et al. (2012) Iron toxicity in neurodegeneration. Biometals 25: 761–776.
5. Hare D, Ayton S, Bush A, Lei P (2013) A delicate balance: Iron metabolism and diseases of the brain. Front Aging Neurosci 5: 34.
6. Rouault TA (2001) Systemic iron metabolism: a review and implications for brain iron metabolism. Pediatr Neurol 25: 130–137.
7. Ke Y, Ming Qian Z (2003) Iron misregulation in the brain: a primary cause of neurodegenerative disorders. Lancet Neurol 2: 246–253.
8. Cozzi A, Rovelli E, Frizzale G, Campanella A, Amendola M, et al. (2010) Oxidative stress and cell death in cells expressing L-ferritin variants causing neuroferritinopathy. Neurobiol Dis 37: 77–85.
9. Double KL, Maywald M, Schmittel M, Riederer P, Gerlach M (1998) In vitro studies of ferritin iron release and neurotoxicity. J Neurochem 70: 2492–2499.
10. Schenck JF (2003) Magnetic resonance imaging of brain iron. J Neurol Sci 207: 99–102.
11. Wallis LI, Paley MN, Graham JM, Grunewald RA, Wignall EL, et al. (2008) MRI assessment of basal ganglia iron deposition in Parkinson's disease. J Magn Reson Imaging 28: 1061–1067.
12. Berg D, Hochstrasser H (2006) Iron metabolism in Parkinsonian syndromes. Mov Disord 21: 1299–1310.
13. Mounsey RB, Teismann P (2012) Chelators in the Treatment of Iron Accumulation in Parkinson's Disease. Int J Cell Biol 2012: 12.
14. Moos T, Rosengren Nielsen T, Skjorringe T, Morgan EH (2007) Iron trafficking inside the brain. J Neurochem 103: 1730–1740.
15. Hill JM, Ruff MR, Weber RJ, Pert CB (1985) Transferrin receptors in rat brain: neuropeptide-like pattern and relationship to iron distribution. Proc Natl Acad Sci U S A 82: 4553–4557.
16. Hare DJ, Lei P, Ayton S, Roberts BR, Grimm R, et al. (2014) An iron-dopamine index predicts risk of parkinsonian neurodegeneration in the substantia nigra pars compacta. Chem Sci 5: 2160–2169.
17. Gerlach M, Ben-Shachar D, Riederer P, Youdim MB (1994) Altered brain metabolism of iron as a cause of neurodegenerative diseases? J Neurochem 63: 793–807.
18. Burke RE, O'Malley K (2013) Axon degeneration in Parkinson's disease. Exp Neurol 246: 72–83.

19. Wang J, Jiang H, Xie JX (2004) Time dependent effects of 6-OHDA lesions on iron level and neuronal loss in rat nigrostriatal system. Neurochem Res 29: 2239–2243.

20. Jiang H, Song N, Xu H, Zhang S, Wang J, et al. (2010) Up-regulation of divalent metal transporter 1 in 6-hydroxydopamine intoxication is IRE/IRP dependent. Cell Res 20: 345–356.

21. Lv Z, Jiang H, Xu H, Song N, Xie J (2011) Increased iron levels correlate with the selective nigral dopaminergic neuron degeneration in Parkinson's disease. J Neural Transm 118: 361–369.

22. Hare D, Reedy B, Grimm R, Wilkins S, Volitakis I, et al. (2009) Quantitative elemental bio-imaging of Mn, Fe, Cu and Zn in 6-hydroxydopamine induced Parkinsonism mouse models. Metallomics 1: 53–58.

23. Li W, Jiang H, Song N, Xie J (2011) Oxidative stress partially contributes to iron-induced alpha-synuclein aggregation in SK-N-SH cells. Neurotox Res 19: 435–442.

24. Lei P, Ayton S, Finkelstein DI, Spoerri L, Ciccotosto GD, et al. (2012) Tau deficiency induces parkinsonism with dementia by impairing APP-mediated iron export. Nat Med 18: 291–295.

25. He Y, Lee T, Leong SK (1999) Time course of dopaminergic cell death and changes in iron, ferritin and transferrin levels in the rat substantia nigra after 6-hydroxydopamine (6-OHDA) lesioning. Free Radic Res 31: 103–112.

26. Schipper HM (2012) Neurodegeneration with brain iron accumulation - clinical syndromes and neuroimaging. Biochim Biophys Acta 1822: 350–360.

27. Ohta E, Takiyama Y (2012) MRI findings in neuroferritinopathy. Neurol Res Int 2012: 197438.

28. Haacke EM, Cheng NY, House MJ, Liu Q, Neelavalli J, et al. (2005) Imaging iron stores in the brain using magnetic resonance imaging. Magn Reson Imaging 23: 1–25.

29. Wood JC (2011) Impact of iron assessment by MRI. Hematology Am Soc Hematol Educ Program 2011: 443–450.

30. Brass SD, Chen NK, Mulkern RV, Bakshi R (2006) Magnetic resonance imaging of iron deposition in neurological disorders. Top Magn Reson Imaging 17: 31–40.

31. Anderson LJ (2011) Assessment of Iron Overload with T2* Magnetic Resonance Imaging. Prog Cardiovasc Dis 54: 287–294.

32. Ulla M, Bonny JM, Ouchchane L, Rieu I, Claise B, et al. (2013) Is R2* a new MRI biomarker for the progression of Parkinson's disease? A longitudinal follow-up. PLoS One 8: e57904.

33. Rossi M, Ruottinen H, Soimakallio S, Elovaara I, Dastidar P (2013) Clinical MRI for iron detection in Parkinson's disease. Clin Imaging 37: 631–636.

34. Zhang J, Zhang Y, Wang J, Cai P, Luo C, et al. (2010) Characterizing iron deposition in Parkinson's disease using susceptibility-weighted imaging: an in vivo MR study. Brain Res 1330: 124–130.

35. Kondoh T, Bannai M, Nishino H, Torii K (2005) 6-Hydroxydopamine-induced lesions in a rat model of hemi-Parkinson's disease monitored by magnetic resonance imaging. Exp Neurol 192: 194–202.

36. Soria G, Aguilar E, Tudela R, Mullol J, Planas AM, et al. (2011) In vivo magnetic resonance imaging characterization of bilateral structural changes in experimental Parkinson's disease: a T2 relaxometry study combined with longitudinal diffusion tensor imaging and manganese-enhanced magnetic resonance imaging in the 6-hydroxydopamine rat model. Eur J Neurosci 33: 1551–1560.

37. Hall S, Rutledge JN, Schallert T (1992) MRI, brain iron and experimental Parkinson's disease. J Neurol Sci 113: 198–208.

38. Van Camp N, Vreys R, Van Laere K, Lauwers E, Beque D, et al. (2010) Morphologic and functional changes in the unilateral 6-hydroxydopamine lesion rat model for Parkinson's disease discerned with microSPECT and quantitative MRI. MAGMA 23: 65–75.

39. Sachs C, Jonsson G (1975) Mechanisms of action of 6-hydroxydopamine. Biochem Pharmacol 24: 1–8.

40. Sauer H, Oertel WH (1994) Progressive degeneration of nigrostriatal dopamine neurons following intrastriatal terminal lesions with 6-hydroxydopamine: a combined retrograde tracing and immunocytochemical study in the rat. Neuroscience 59: 401–415.

41. Schmidt-Kastner R, Meller D, Bellander BM, Stromberg I, Olson L, et al. (1993) A one-step immunohistochemical method for detection of blood-brain barrier disturbances for immunoglobulins in lesioned rat brain with special reference to false-positive labelling in immunohistochemistry. J Neurosci Methods 46: 121–132.

42. Wachter B, Schurger S, Schmid A, Groger A, Sadler R, et al. (2012) 6-Hydroxydopamine leads to T2 hyperintensity, decreased claudin-3 immunoreactivity and altered aquaporin 4 expression in the striatum. Behav Brain Res 232: 148–158.

43. Dhawan JK, Kumar VM, Govindaraju V, Raghunathan P (1998) Changes in Magnetic Resonance Imaging and Sex Behavior After 6-OHDA Injection in the Medial Preoptic Area. Brain Res Bull 45: 333–339.

44. Kortekaas R, Leenders KL, van Oostrom JC, Vaalburg W, Bart J, et al. (2005) Blood-brain barrier dysfunction in parkinsonian midbrain in vivo. Ann Neurol 57: 176–179.

45. Rite I, Machado A, Cano J, Venero JL (2007) Blood-brain barrier disruption induces in vivo degeneration of nigral dopaminergic neurons. J Neurochem 101: 1567–1582.

46. Carvey PM, Zhao CH, Hendey B, Lum H, Trachtenberg J, et al. (2005) 6-Hydroxydopamine-induced alterations in blood-brain barrier permeability. Eur J Neurosci 22: 1158–1168.

47. Stromberg I, Bjorklund H, Dahl D, Jonsson G, Sundstrom E, et al. (1986) Astrocyte responses to dopaminergic denervations by 6-hydroxydopamine and 1-methyl-4-phenyl-1,2,3,6-tetrahydropyridine as evidenced by glial fibrillary acidic protein immunohistochemistry. Brain Res Bull 17: 225–236.

48. Tarohda T, Ishida Y, Kawai K, Yamamoto M, Amano R (2005) Regional distributions of manganese, iron, copper, and zinc in the brains of 6-hydroxydopamine-induced parkinsonian rats. Anal Bioanal Chem 383: 224–234.

49. Ortega R, Cloetens P, Deves G, Carmona A, Bohic S (2007) Iron storage within dopamine neurovesicles revealed by chemical nano-imaging. PloS one 2: e925.

50. Zecca L, Youdim MBH, Riederer P, Connor JR, Crichton RR (2004) Iron, brain ageing and neurodegenerative disorders. Nat Rev Neurosci 5: 863–873.

51. Dexter DT, Statton SA, Whitmore C, Freinbichler W, Weinberger P, et al. (2011) Clinically available iron chelators induce neuroprotection in the 6-OHDA model of Parkinson's disease after peripheral administration. J Neural Transm 118: 223–231.

52. Jellinger K, Paulus W, Grundke-Iqbal I, Riederer P, Youdim MB (1990) Brain iron and ferritin in Parkinson's and Alzheimer's diseases. J Neural Transm Park Dis Dement Sect 2: 327–340.

53. Kwan JY, Jeong SY, Van Gelderen P, Deng HX, Quezado MM, et al. (2012) Iron accumulation in deep cortical layers accounts for MRI signal abnormalities in ALS: correlating 7 tesla MRI and pathology. PloS one 7: e35241.

13

Multi-Parametric Representation of Voxel-Based Quantitative Magnetic Resonance Imaging

Maria Engström[1,2]*, **Jan B. M. Warntjes**[2,3,4], **Anders Tisell**[2,5], **Anne-Marie Landtblom**[2,6], **Peter Lundberg**[2,5]

1 Division of Radiology, Department of Medical and Health Sciences, Linköping University, Linköping, Sweden, **2** Center for Medical Image Science and Visualization (CMIV), Linköping University, Linköping, Sweden, **3** Division of Cardiovascular Medicine, Department of Medical and Health Sciences, Linköping University, Linköping, Sweden, **4** SyntheticMR AB, Linköping, Sweden, **5** Division of Radiation Physics, Department of Medical and Health Sciences, Linköping University, Linköping, Sweden, **6** Division of Neurology, Department of Clinical and Experimental Medicine, Linköping University, Linköping, Sweden

Abstract

The aim of the study was to explore the possibilities of multi-parametric representations of voxel-wise quantitative MRI data to objectively discriminate pathological cerebral tissue in patients with brain disorders. For this purpose, we recruited 19 patients with Multiple Sclerosis (MS) as benchmark samples and 19 age and gender matched healthy subjects as a reference group. The subjects were examined using quantitative Magnetic Resonance Imaging (MRI) measuring the tissue structure parameters: relaxation rates, R_1 and R_2, and proton density. The resulting parameter images were normalized to a standard template. Tissue structure in MS patients was assessed by voxel-wise comparisons with the reference group and with correlation to a clinical measure, the Expanded Disability Status Scale (EDSS). The results were visualized by conventional geometric representations and also by multi-parametric representations. Data showed that MS patients had lower R_1 and R_2, and higher proton density in periventricular white matter and in wide-spread areas encompassing central and sub-cortical white matter structures. MS-related tissue abnormality was highlighted in posterior white matter whereas EDSS correlation appeared especially in the frontal cortex. The multi-parameter representation highlighted disease-specific features. In conclusion, the proposed method has the potential to visualize both high-probability focal anomalies and diffuse tissue changes. Results from voxel-based statistical analysis, as exemplified in the present work, may guide radiologists where in the image to inspect for signs of disease. Future clinical studies must validate the usability of the method in clinical practice.

Editor: Friedemann Paul, Charité University Medicine Berlin, Germany

Funding: The National Research Council (grant number VR/NT 2008-3368), Linköping University, and the County Council of Östergötland are acknowledged for financial support. The funders had no role in study design, data collection and analysis, decision to publish, or preparation of the manuscript. SyntheticMR AB provided support in the form of salary for author JBMW, but did not have any additional role in the study design, data collection and analysis, decision to publish, or preparation of the manuscript. The specific roles of these authors are articulated in the 'author contributions' section.

Competing Interests: The authors ME, AT, AML, and PL have declared that no competing interests exist. JBMW is part-time employed by SyntheticMR AB.

* Email: maria.engstrom@liu.se

Introduction

Magnetic resonance imaging (MRI) is frequently used for diagnosis of brain disorders, such as stroke, brain tumors, and multiple sclerosis (MS). Conventional clinical MRI is generally a qualitative method. This means that eventual tissue pathologies are detected as visible differences in image intensity between pathological and normal tissue. Diffuse pathologies can be particularly difficult to detect since there are no clear contrasting borders between pathological and normal tissue.

In recent years there has been an increasing interest in developing methods for quantitative MRI (qMRI), which provides information about structural differences in brain tissue [1]. Various methods for quantitative measurements of the tissue parameters, such as longitudinal relaxation time (T_1), transversal relaxation time (T_2) and/or proton density (PD); have been reported in the literature [2–10]. Previously, we reported a method for quick, simultaneous measurements of T_1, T_2, and PD, which also was optimized for clinical usage [11,12]. This method provides the possibility to compare objective measures of tissue

structure within subjects in longitudinal studies and between subjects in comparative studies. As T_1, T_2, and PD are quantified in each image voxel, the qMRI method allows for voxel-based statistical comparisons within and between subjects. In a recent study, we showed that qMRI together with brain normalization to a standard template could be used to generate reference tissue maps of typical brain characteristics in healthy subjects [13]. In the present study we aimed to explore the feasibility of voxel-based qMRI to *identify T_1, T_2, and PD tissue properties in these groups*. We aimed to investigate if voxel-based statistical analysis of qMRI data can reveal features in tissue structure that are typical for certain pathologies. In some disease conditions there are discrepancies between radiological and clinical measures. A well-known example is the clinico-radiological paradox in MS [14]. A second aim was therefore to investigate if correlation between normalized qMRI data and *clinical measures* can provide additional information about anatomical location of the pathologies that are related to specific symptoms in a patient group.

MR images are most often represented using a geometric representation in anatomical space where eventual lesions are related to certain anatomical structures. The qMRI method provides alternative opportunities to represent data, which are only little investigated. Here, we explore the possibilities of *multi-parametric visualization* for the ability to provide information about trends in the development of brain pathologies, reflected by objective measures in a patient group. As many neurological disorders are caused by focal rather than global pathologies, we also aimed to investigate if analyses in *regions of interest* (ROIs) using a generally accessible, standard brain atlas can provide additional information about local pathological changes.

We hypothesized that voxel-based qMRI and multi-parametric representation could be used to detect disease-specific pathologies, for example 'lesion probability' and 'diffuse tissue' changes that are difficult to detect by conventional neuroimaging methods. In order to demonstrate the feasibility of the voxel-based qMRI method, we selected a small group of healthy individuals and a group of MS patients as benchmark samples. The reason for choosing MS as benchmark is that this disease is characterized both by discrete lesions with high lesion frequency in certain anatomical structures and diffuse, globally spread white matter changes [3].

This work is a continuation of previously published works on methods for fast qMRI acquisition [11,12] and voxel-based analyses in a healthy reference group [13]. The overall aim with the present work was to further explore the opportunities of voxel-based analysis and multi-parametric representations of qMRI data from two different groups. Here we show that qMRI can be used for differentiation of tissue properties in a group of MS patients, and that multi-parametric representations provide additional information compared to conventional geometric representations in anatomical space.

Results

Group-level Tissue Characterization

In Figure 1 the averaged, normalized R_1, R_2, and PD maps are shown for a single slice in the reference brain (top row) and the MS benchmark brain (bottom row). It is clearly seen that cerebrospinal fluid (CSF), WM, and GM have different characteristics and the maps can discriminate between the different tissue types using any of the three parameters. By inspecting the images it is, however, not completely evident to discriminate differences in tissue characteristics between the two groups. By voxel-based statistical analysis, on the other hand, distinct tissue differences between MS patients and the reference group were detected very clearly. In general, MS patients had lower R_1 and R_2, and higher PD as compared to the reference group. Figure 2 shows differences in R_1, R_2, and PD between MS patients and the healthy reference group using a statistical threshold of T = 2. By inspecting Figure 2, marked differences between MS patients and healthy subjects are shown in periventricular WM and in wide-spread areas encompassing especially central and sub-cortical WM structures. In peripheral brain, only a few structures with differences between the groups appeared, but a number of sulci, mainly in the frontal and parietal lobes were highlighted. Correcting for multiple comparisons, we observed significant differences, p < 0.05, when testing for R_1 and R_2 lower in MS, and PD higher in MS in all regions, except occipital white matter when testing for PD (p = 0.07). No significant results were observed for the reverse comparisons. The analysis of the three different tissue structure parameters, R_1, R_2, and PD, yielded similar, but not identical results, which will be discussed further below.

The intracranial volume was similar in both groups: 1400 ± 131 mL and 1357 ± 95 mL in the reference group and in MS patients, respectively. The difference in intracranial volume

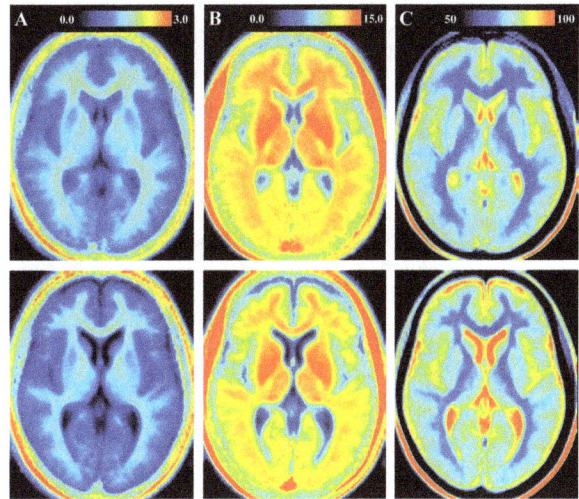

Figure 1. Geometrical representation of quantitative tissue parameters. The figure shows a selected slice of the quantitative tissue maps in the reference group of healthy subjects (top row) and the group of multiple sclerosis (MS) patients (bottom row). A) longitudinal relaxation rate (R_1) on a scale 0–3 s^{-1}; B) transversal relaxation rate (R_2) on a scale 0–15 s^{-1}; C) proton density (PD) on a scale 50–100%, where 100% corresponds to pure water at 37°C.

between the groups ($= 43$ mL) was not significant (p = 0.3). The brain parenchymal fraction, however, was $89.9 \pm 2.4\%$ for the reference group and $82.1 \pm 4.5\%$ for the MS group: a significant difference of 7.7% (p < 0.0001). The ventricular fraction was $1.0 \pm 0.5\%$ for the reference group and $2.5 \pm 1.2\%$ for the MS group: a significant difference of 1.5% (p < 0.0001).

Relation to Clinical Measures

In Figure 3, the geometrical representations of the correlation between tissue parameters and a clinical measure, the Expanded Disability Status Scale (EDSS), are shown. When comparing the EDSS correlation maps with the results in Figure 2, which shows voxel-based differences between MS patients and the reference group, some overlap was observed, especially in periventricular WM and the corona radiata. However, there were also features with distinct differences between the two representations. Notably, MS-related tissue pathology in frontal WM in, and adjacent to, the corpus callosum was highly correlated with EDSS, while WM changes in the posterior corpus callosum were highlighted in the group difference representations. These features are most clearly visualized in the sagittal images in Figures 2 and 3, which show uncorrected results. In this study, the differences between MS patients and the reference group were significant when correcting for multiple comparisons, whereas the EDSS correlations were not significant at the corrected level.

The partial overlap between the results of Figure 2 and Figure 3 suggests a weak correlation between group differences (Figure 2) and the MS-EDSS relation (Figure 3). To confirm this, we performed a linear regression of the T-maps presented in Figure 2 and the slope data presented in Figure 3. All data were included in the analysis, also non-significant data not plotted in Figures 2 and 3. The goodness of fit R^2 of the regression was 0.50 for R_1, 0.48 for R_2, and 0.46 for PD. The observed slopes were 0.53, 0.49, and 0.50 for R_1, R_2, and PD, respectively.

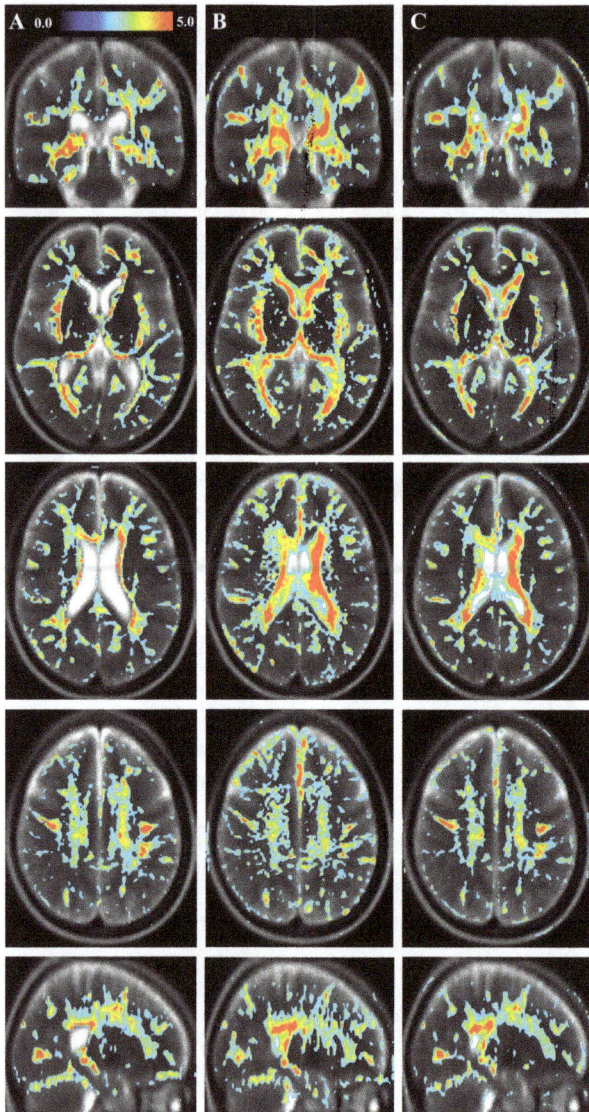

Figure 2. Geometrical representation of tissue parameter differences between groups. The figure shows differences in tissue parameters between the group of Multiple Sclerosis (MS) patients and the reference group. Shown as the color overlay is the T-statistics of the voxel-based differences between groups. A) longitudinal relaxation rate (R_1); B) transversal relaxation rate (R_2); C) proton density (PD) in one coronal, three axial and one sagittal slice. The color scale represents T = 0.0–5.0. The figure shows uncorrected statistics, thresholded at T = 2. In the background a synthetic T2-weighted image of the same slice is displayed for visual guidance.

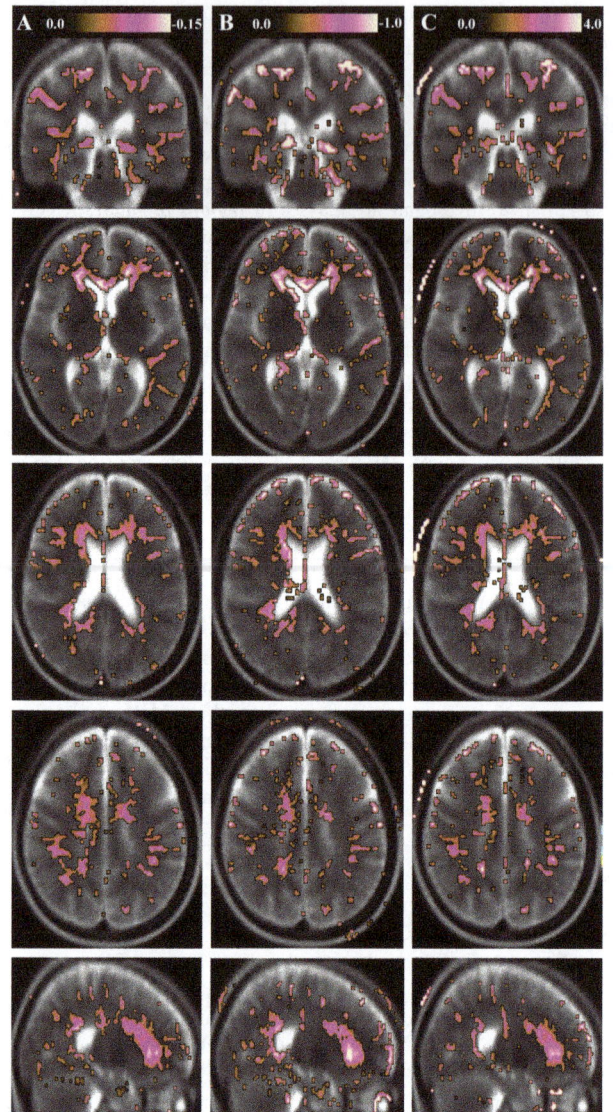

Figure 3. Geometrical representation of the correlation of tissue parameters and clinical measures. The figure shows the geometrical representation of the correlation of R_1–R_2–PD values with a clinical measure for the group of Multiple Sclerosis (MS) patients. Shown as the color overlay is the slope of the voxel-based correlation with Expanded Disability Status Scale (EDSS). A) longitudinal relaxation rate (R_1) on a scale r = 0.0 to -0.15; B) transversal relaxation rate (R_2) on a scale r = 0.0 to -1; C) proton density (PD) on a scale r = 0.0–4.0. The correlation images are shown in the same slices as in Figure 2. The figure shows uncorrected statistics, thresholded at T = 2. In the background synthetic T2-weighted images of the MS group in the same slices are displayed for visual guidance.

Multi-parametric visualization

In Figure 4 the multi-parametric representations of tissue parameters of the whole brain are projected as 2-dimensional graphs for each R_1-R_2, R_1-PD, and R_2-PD pair. The differences between the reference group and the MS group are visualized in two colors in the multi-parametric representations. The blue color scale indicates a larger number of voxels with a specific parametric location in the reference group compared to the MS group. Correspondingly, the red scale indicates a larger number of voxels in the MS group. Only voxels with signal intensity higher than 10% of the maximum signal intensity (*e.g.* 395451 out of 510340 voxels) were taken into account. In this way, differences between the groups are visualized in the multi-parametric space and indications of the direction of disease-specific tissue changes are provided. In Figure 4A, it can be seen that the direction of change due to MS is towards lower R_1 and R_2 values. In Figures 4B and 4C the MS-specific changes point towards higher PD values.

In Figure 5, the parametric representation in R_1-R_2 space is visualized for three selected ROIs: the caudate nucleus, the thalamus, and the total WM. Each ROI was reduced with 2 mm in comparison to the ROIs in the standard atlas to avoid large influence of partial volume at the ROI edges. Since the multi-

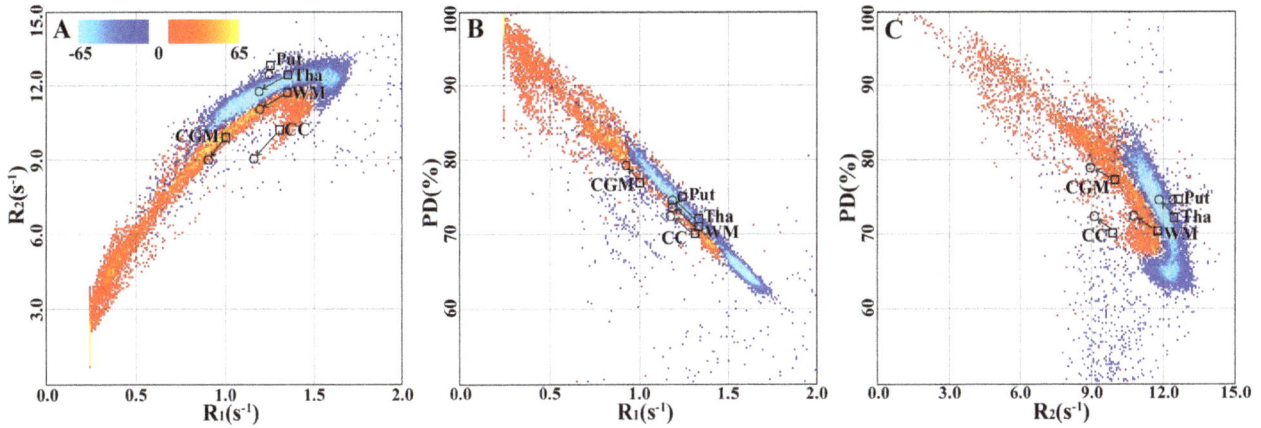

Figure 4. Multi-parametrical representation of tissue parameters in groups. The figure shows whole-brain differences in R_1-R_2-PD values between the group of Multiple Sclerosis (MS) patients and the reference group. A) R_1-R_2 values; B) R_1-PD values; C) R_2-PD values. The color scales indicate number of voxels. Blue color indicates a larger number of voxels in the reference group. Red color indicates a larger number of voxels in the MS group. The markers indicate the positions of the mean values in cortical grey matter (CGM), thalamus (Tha), putamen (Put), white matter (WM), and corpus callosum (CC). The mean values are taken from the decreased ROIs presented in Table 2. A square is used for the reference group and a circle for the MS group. The arrows point in the direction from the reference group to the MS group.

parametric representations in Figure 5 contained a far lower number of included voxels compared to the representations in Figure 4, the number of bins was chosen to 50 rather than 200 as in Figure 4.

Tissue properties in regions of interest

Figure 2 shows that the MS patients in general had lower R_1 and R_2, and higher PD compared to the reference group. In Table 1 and 2 it is seen that this general feature also apply to all investigated ROIs. The difference in tissue parameters between the reference group and MS patients were highly significant, $p < 0.001$. For the reduced ROIs (Table 2), we observed two tendencies: in some ROIs the magnitudes of the parametric values increased whereas in some ROIs the values decreased. For example, R_1 and R_2 increased and PD decreased with ROI reduction in the ventricles, whereas the opposite trend was observed for the corpus callosum and the pons.

In Figure 6 the trends regarding changes in R_1–R_2 values due to ROI reduction are visualized. The mean R_1–R_2 values in each ROI changed towards the R_1–R_2 values in the voxels most distant from the ROI surface upon ROI reduction. This feature is clearly seen for the thalamus (Figure 6B) and WM (Figure 6C).

Discussion

In this study we explored the ability of voxel-based image analysis of qMRI data to assess disease-specific features in groups. We showed that different multi-parametric representations could visualize different properties of brain structure in healthy individuals and MS patients.

Tissue characterization in groups

The advantage of voxel-based image analysis is the possibility of statistical descriptions of disease-specific features in groups of

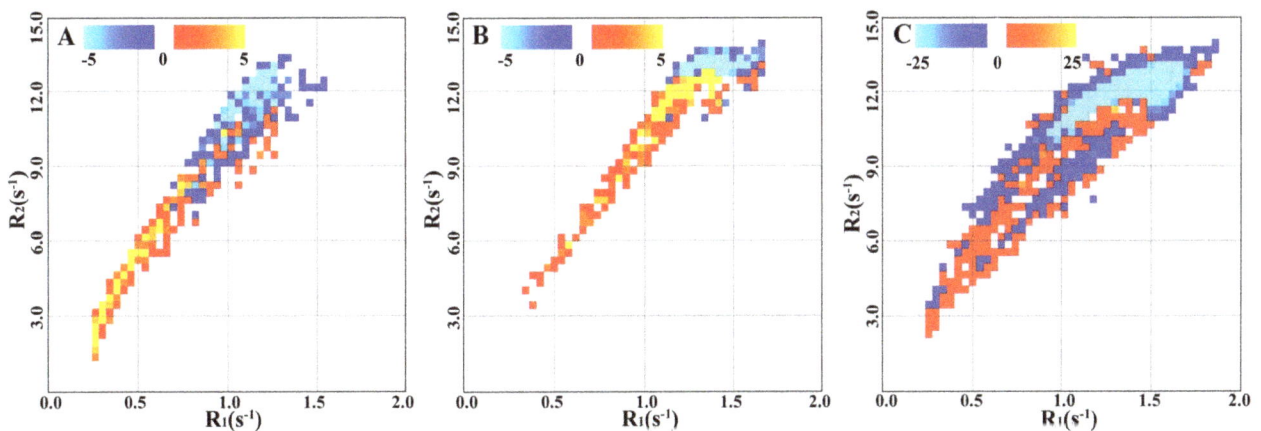

Figure 5. Multi-parametrical representation of tissue parameters in regions of interest (ROIs). The figure shows differences in R_1 and R_2 values between Multiple Sclerosis (MS) patients and the reference group for three separate cerebral ROIs. A) Caudate nucleus; B) Thalamus; C) Total white matter. The ROIs were all reduced with 2 mm to avoid partial volume effects at the edges. Only the R_1-R_2 projections of the R_1-R_2-PD space are shown. The color scales indicate number of voxels. Blue color indicates a larger number of voxels in the reference group. Red color indicates a larger number of voxels in the MS group.

Table 1. Descriptive data from the region of interest (ROI) analysis using standard templates.

Structure	ROI size (voxels)	Reference group R_1 (s^{-1})	R_2 (s^{-1})	PD (%)	Multiple Sclerosis group R_1 (s^{-1})	R_2 (s^{-1})	PD (%)
Lateral ventricles	2349	0.72 ± 0.56	6.6 ± 4.2	85 ± 14	0.40 ± 0.47	4.1 ± 3.7	92 ± 12
Insula	3628	0.94 ± 0.35	9.8 ± 2.7	80 ± 9	0.87 ± 0.39	9.0 ± 3.1	81 ± 10
Cingulate cortex	7655	1.09 ± 0.36	10.7 ± 2.2	77 ± 9	0.96 ± 0.39	9.7 ± 2.8	80 ± 10
Caudate nucleus	1956	1.08 ± 0.43	10.5 ± 3.4	78 ± 10	0.75 ± 0.51	7.4 ± 4.5	85 ± 11
Cortical gray matter	53401	1.02 ± 0.57	10.0 ± 3.2	75 ± 20	0.92 ± 0.61	9.1 ± 3.5	77 ± 20
Pons	2518	1.06 ± 0.43	9.8 ± 3.5	76 ± 11	0.94 ± 0.50	8.6 ± 4.2	78 ± 14
Putamen	2073	1.29 ± 0.18	12.9 ± 1.2	74 ± 5	1.25 ± 0.21	12.4 ± 1.5	74 ± 6
Mid brain	2289	1.18 ± 0.36	10.8 ± 3.0	74 ± 8	1.10 ± 0.39	10.1 ± 3.4	76 ± 9
Thalamus	2157	1.29 ± 0.25	12.1 ± 1.9	73 ± 7	1.12 ± 0.41	10.6 ± 3.5	76 ± 10
Occipital white matter	11077	1.22 ± 0.36	11.6 ± 1.9	74 ± 9	1.13 ± 0.34	11.1 ± 2.2	76 ± 9
Frontal white matter	40008	1.17 ± 0.46	10.8 ± 2.7	74 ± 14	1.05 ± 0.48	9.9 ± 3.1	77 ± 14
Parietal white matter	14362	1.18 ± 0.40	11.0 ± 2.5	74 ± 11	1.06 ± 0.42	10.2 ± 3.0	77 ± 12
Sublobar white matter	12855	1.25 ± 0.41	10.9 ± 2.8	73 ± 10	1.09 ± 0.48	9.6 ± 3.6	76 ± 12
White matter	106935	1.20 ± 0.41	11.1 ± 2.4	74 ± 12	1.07 ± 0.43	10.2 ± 2.9	77 ± 12
Corpus callosum	2685	1.20 ± 0.55	9.7 ± 3.7	73 ± 13	0.99 ± 0.59	8.1 ± 4.1	77 ± 14

The table shows ROI sizes, mean R_1, R_2, and proton density (PD) values, and standard deviations of 15 pre-defined structures in the Montreal Neurological Institute (MNI) standard brain template. All comparisons between the reference group and the multiple sclerosis group were highly significant, $p < 0.001$.

Table 2. Descriptive data from the region of interest (ROI) analysis using cropped templates.

Structure	ROI size (voxels)	Reference group R$_1$ (s^{-1})	R$_2$ (s^{-1})	PD (%)	Multiple Sclerosis group R$_1$ (s^{-1})	R$_2$ (s^{-1})	PD (%)
Lateral ventricles	96	0.29±0.33	3.4±2.9	96±9	0.20±0.17	1.7±1.4	99±5
Insula	1634	0.82±0.30	9.0±2.7	83±8	0.73±0.35	8.0±3.2	84±9
Cingulate cortex	7140	1.00±0.32	10.4±2.1	79±8	0.87±0.35	9.3±2.8	82±10
Caudate nucleus	1000	1.03±0.36	10.6±3.1	80±8	0.64±0.45	6.9±4.4	87±10
Cortical gray matter	306 1	.01±0.53	10.0±3.1	77±17	0.89±0.53	8.9±3.5	79±17
Pons	2654	1.06±0.43	9.8±3.5	76±11	0.94±0.50	8.6±4.2	78±14
Putamen	1252	1.29±0.18	12.9±1.2	74±5	1.25±0.21	12.4±1.5	74±6
Mid brain	2126	1.27±0.25	11.7±2.2	73±6	1.24±0.26	11.4±2.4	74±7
Thalamus	1998	1.34±0.15	12.7±1.1	72±5	1.22±0.28	11.7±2.4	75±7
Occipital white matter	4608	1.22±0.36	11.6±1.9	74±9	1.13±0.34	11.1±2.2	76±9
Frontal white matter	26450	1.30±0.37	11.6±1.9	72±10	1.13±0.39	10.8±2.4	74±10
Parietal white matter	6706	1.31±0.34	11.6±1.7	72±9	1.18±0.38	10.8±2.3	74±10
Sublobar white matter	3040	1.33±0.40	11.0±2.7	70±10	1.19±0.46	9.9±3.3	74±12
White matter	78549	1.35±0.34	11.7±1.7	71±9	1.22±0.37	10.8±2.3	74±12
Corpus callosum	770	1.31±0.53	10.3±3.4	70±12	1.13±0.53	9.3±3.6	72±13

The table shows ROI sizes, mean R$_1$, R$_2$, and proton density (PD) values, and standard deviations of 15 pre-defined structures in the Montreal Neurological Institute (MNI) standard brain template. The ROIs were cropped with 2 mm from the standard brain templates. All comparisons between the reference group and the multiple sclerosis group were highly significant, $p < 0.001$.

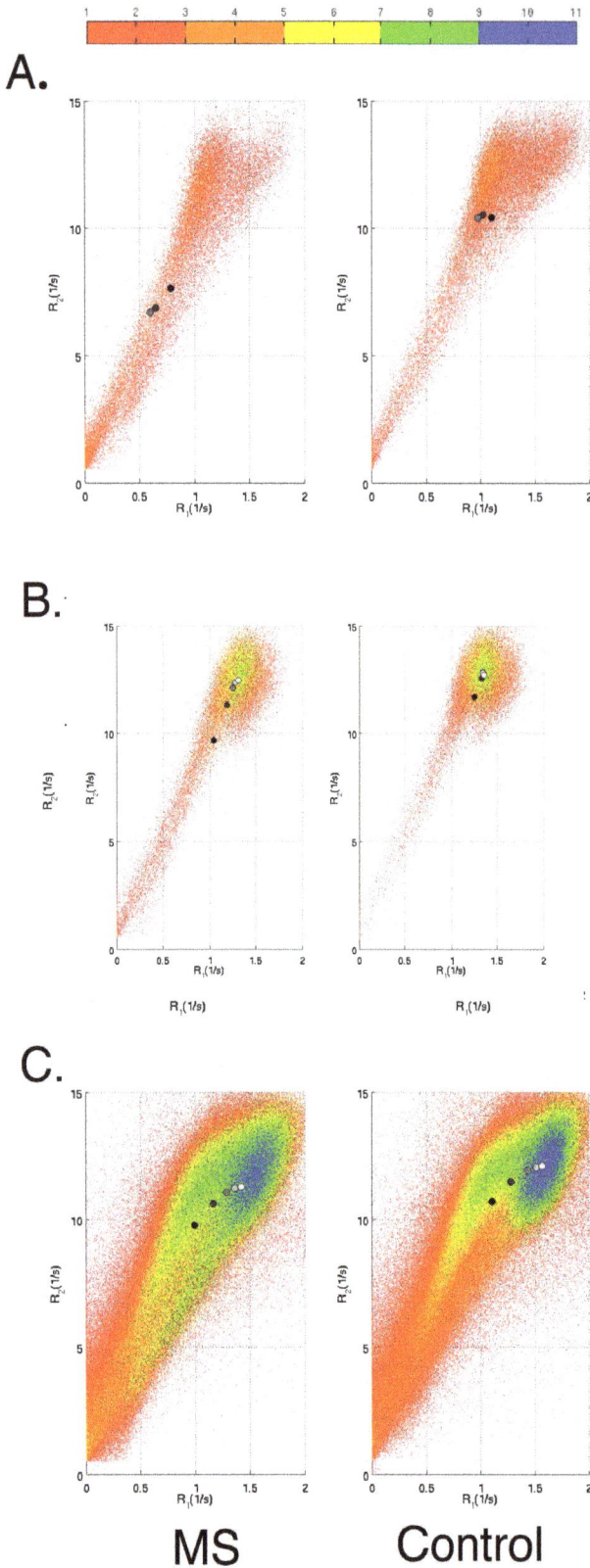

Figure 6. Effect of regions of interest (ROI) size on tissue parameters. The figure shows R_1–R_2 plots in ROIs for the Multiple Sclerosis (MS) and the reference group, respectively. A) Caudate nucleus; B) Thalamus; C) Total white matter. The color bar shows within-ROI distance from the ROI surface. The circles show mean R_1 and R_2 values in 0, 2, 4, 6, and 8 mm reduced ROIs. Black circles represent 0 mm reduction and white circles represent 8 mm reduction.

patients. This means that features that are common in several patients are highlighted whereas the impact of individual patients' focal changes is reduced. Using qMRI, such statistical descriptions typically result in 'lesion probability' maps where anatomical structures with the highest probability to find disease-specific lesions are visualized. The statistical treatment of qMRI data also provides a powerful tool to detect diffuse tissue changes that are difficult to distinguish by conventional MRI. Results from the group-level statistical analysis may guide radiologists where in the image to inspect for early signs of disease. However, future research have to validate the method by longitudinal clinical studies in larger study groups.

In this study, we observed distinct aberrations in periventricular white matter, corona radiata, and radiatio optica in MS patients compared to the reference group (Figure 2). Since the images are based on statistical analysis, they show the common pattern across the MS group. Individual lesions that are scattered in white matter and appear at different locations in each patient will be filtered away, and will therefore not show up in the images. If the prevalence of lesions at the same geometrical location is high, however, the average value can be significantly changed compared to the reference group. Therefore we interpret distinct aberrations in periventricular white matter, corona radiata, and radiatio optica to represent MS lesion probability. These locations coincide to a large extent with the lesion probability maps presented in the work by Hasan and co-workers [3].

By inspecting Figure 2, it is clear that MS patients had widespread white matter changes especially in central and sub-cortical WM structures. MS patients had reduced R_1 and R_2, and increased PD compared to the reference group. We interpret these findings to reflect diffuse changes in normal appearing WM. In previous studies, decreased R_2 in WM has been related to diffuse myelin or axonal pathology in MS [15,16]. The qMRI method, applied in the present work, opens up the possibilities to incorporate a myelin model to assess the degree of myelin damage [17]. This approach would enable more precise delineation of the neuropathological basis to the changes in qMRI parameters.

Abnormal relaxation rates and especially increased PD that was observed in the ventricles and cortical sulci of MS patients were probably related to brain atrophy causing enlarged ventricles and wider sulci. Although the brain normalization procedure tries to adjust for individual differences in brain volume, this procedure is not successful in all cases. Calculation of the ventricle fraction showed that the MS patients had significantly larger ventricles than the reference group prior to normalization. By inspecting individual images of MS patients, we observed that several patients had enlarged ventricles also after normalization (see section *Strengths and limitations* for further discussion on this topic).

Relation to clinical measures

Disorders of the brain are commonly diagnosed based on clinical, laboratory, and neuroimaging data. In MS, typical WM lesions, observed by MRI, are clear signs of disease and provide a solid ground for diagnosis [18]. Thus, conventional MRI provides important information for MS diagnosis and also about the lesion burden in MS. However, the correlation between the number of lesions and the degree of disability in MS is rather weak, and some patients have no visible lesions although they are diagnosed with MS based on clinical information and disease history. This discrepancy between radiological and clinical measures has been termed as the clinico-radiological paradox [14].

In the current study we investigated the possibility to correlate quantitative measures of brain tissue structure and clinical measures on a voxel-by-voxel basis. For this purpose we correlated the R_1, R_2, and PD values of each image voxel to the EDSS scores of each MS patient. By this method we showed that the tissue parameter values in frontal WM, especially in and adjacent to the corpus callosum, were correlated to the disease burden, as measured by the EDSS scores. This finding stands in contrast to the observation that WM in the posterior corpus callosum was commonly affected in the MS group independent of disability state. These results suggest that diffuse changes in frontal WM are severe for the individual patient and such information could therefore be indicative for prognosis and treatment strategies. In this context it is important to emphasize that the abnormal tissue parameter values detected by the qMRI method does not directly correspond to focal changes such as MS lesions. This issue is highlighted by the comparison between the present results and those of Kincses and co-workers who correlated MS lesion probability and EDSS [19]. They found that EDSS correlated with MS lesion probability most of all in the posterior periventricular WM.

In this study, we used MS as benchmark sample and EDSS as an example of a commonly used clinical scoring system. It must, however, be noted that EDSS is a rather coarse clinical measure, which especially relates to physical disability (motor dysfunction). The small sample size and the wide range of EDSS (disability scores) in this study, and the big variation of lesion localization in MS patients, must be kept in mind when interpreting the results of this study. Also, the mean MSSS being larger than mean EDSS indicates a proportion of severe cases in our benchmark sample.

Extending the voxel-based qMRI method for assessment of other disorders of the brain than MS, other clinical measures likely would be relevant, for example subjective symptom ratings, cognitive performance scores, or protein and genetic biomarkers, which may reflect significant deviations in other areas of the brain.

Multi-parametric visualization

In Figure 2, the qMRI parameters are visualized by the conventional geometric representation. Significant differences between two groups (in this case MS patients and healthy individuals) are shown in a data space represented by coronal, axial, and sagittal images. By the geometric representation it is, however, difficult to observe the relations between different qMRI parameters. Alternatively, multi-parametric representations of R_1, R_2, and PD pairs in 2-dimensional graphs provide visualization of different tissue types in segmented clusters. The parametric representation for a single patient has been presented previously by Alfano and co-workers [20]. They used this method to segment normal WM, GM, and CSF for volume calculations of individual subjects' brains. In our work, we extrapolated this method to comparisons of healthy and pathological brain tissue in groups, which to our knowledge have not been presented before. In this way we obtained additional information about disease-specific features.

In our benchmark case, we observed that MS patients had a larger number of voxels in the lower left quadrant in the R_1–R_2 space and in the higher left quadrant in the PD–R_1 and PD–R_2 spaces as compared to the reference group of healthy individuals. These representations show differences between MS patients and healthy individuals and highlight disease-specific features in the parameter space. Such multi-parametric representations could eventually be used for assessment of disease progression in individual patients using e.g. pattern recognition or deforming models.

Tissue properties in regions of interest

Brain normalization and voxel-based statistics of quantitative image data may form a way to automated pathology detection. Hasan and co-workers recently reported an atlas-based approach on multimodal MRI measuring volumetry, diffusimetry, relaxometry and lesion distribution in MS patients [3,21]. By this approach, they could demonstrate that cerebral pathology in MS is widespread and not limited to MRI visible lesions. Similar results were obtained in the current study, as will be discussed below.

Despite the convincing results, an indiscriminate use of atlas-based ROI analyses could be problematic, because brain normalization is always accompanied by registration errors and atlas-based ROIs are only approximate. Brain normalization is especially complex in patients with a high degree of lesion load and atrophy, which often occurs in MS. Results may also depend on the choice of reference group that is used for preparing the atlas. Yet another problem is the accurate definition of the ROIs: by applying a rather large ROI on a (by normalization) deformed brain will inevitably lead to partial volume effects and hence each ROI will to a certain extent contain information about different tissue types. In our study, we examined this by calculating the distributions of the quantitative measures in each ROI and also in reduced ROI sizes. We found, for example, that R_1 and R_2 decreased and PD increased in the ventricles upon ROI reduction. Simultaneously, the opposite behavior was observed for regions adjacent to CSF such as the corpus callosum and the pons. These findings indicate that partial volume effects in the ROI analyses were substantial, because reducing the ventricular ROI resulted in increased PD in the ventricles (and decreased R_1–R_2) significant of increased CSF fraction in the ventricular ROI. Correspondingly, reducing the corpus callosum and pons ROIs resulted in decreased PD (and increased R_1–R_2) indicating that the reduced ROIs contained a larger fraction of cerebral tissue.

Quantitative MRI in MS

Several quantitative MRI approaches have been used to assess pathological tissue in MS. The most widely used approaches are diffusion tensor imaging (DTI) [22] and magnetization transfer imaging (MTI) [23]. Both DTI [22,24,25] and MTI [26,27] allow for voxel-based statistical mapping and automated atlas-based analysis [28]. DTI measures and quantifies the diffusion of water molecules parallel or perpendicular to the axonal fibers, for example by calculating the fractional anisotropy (FA), which is a measure of the degree of diffusion directionality. In MS this can provide information about axonal damage and demyelination [22]. A low magnetization transfer ratio (MTR) is an indicator of reduced interaction between protons in free water and protons bound to macromolecules. In MS, demyelination is the most probable cause of an MTR reduction [23]. Quantitative MRI, which was utilized in the present study, provides information about the tissue parameters that give rise to the contrast in conventional MRI. PD gives information about the water content in tissue, and it is therefore sensitive to both edema and atrophy when brain tissue is replaced by CSF. R_1 and R_2 are the longitudinal and transversal relaxation rates, respectively, which magnitudes are affected by the tissue structure and the influence of magnetic exchange, especially with fast-relaxing myelin water. In this work only the main R_1 and R_2 components were measured. A potential extension of the technique might incorporate multi-exponential relaxation behavior as well.

Strengths and limitations

The strength of the qMRI method used in this study is the relatively short scanning time and the simultaneous acquisition of all three qMRI parameters in a single experiment. Depending on resolution the sequence requires 5 to 8 minutes, which enables readily introduction of qMRI sequences into conventional clinical routines. Additionally, by simultaneous measurements of all quantitative parameters the often problematic procedure of image registration in single subject imaging is avoided. Since qMRI is independent of scanner settings, such as echo time (TE) and repetition time (TR), and scanner imperfections, such as coil sensitivity of B_1 inhomogeneity, it is mapped on an absolute scale. This should improve the group statistics in comparison to conventional imaging, which is acquired on a relative scale. Moreover, qMRI forms a robust input for automatic brain segmentation procedures, which could provide complementary information about differences in brain volume [29,30].

Perhaps the main limitations of the present study are the rather large image voxel sizes and the non-isotropic image acquisition. These limitations have large impact on normalization quality. As discussed above, the normalization procedure failed to normalize ventricle sizes in MS patients. Non-optimized normalization was also observed in other cortical areas, especially in the occipital lobe, in some subjects. Various degrees of brain atrophy of the subjects generally constitute a problem for normalization procedures due to the complex geometry of the brain and the small, partial-volume areas filled with CSF. The relatively low resolution causes a relatively large partial volume effect, as demonstrated in Tables 1 and 2. Using smaller, isotropic voxels during image acquisition would substantially improve normalization and it would also allow refined normalization procedures for example using the method of nonlinear registration by local optimization as implemented in the DARTEL tool [31].

Conclusions

In the present study, we showed that multi-parametric representations of qMRI data could highlight deviations in cerebral structure in patients with brain disorders. The proposed method could visualize both high-probability focal anomalies and diffuse tissue changes. Thus, results from voxel-based statistical analysis, as exemplified in the present work, may guide radiologists where in the image to inspect for early signs of disease. Additionally, the fast imaging protocol facilitates the introduction of the qMRI method into clinical practice.

Materials and Methods

Ethics statement

The study was approved by the Regional Ethical Review Board in Linköping (Dnr. M88-07) and written informed consent was obtained from all participants.

Subjects

For generating the reference tissue maps, 19 healthy controls were recruited to the study (5 were males and 14 were females). In addition, 19 patients that were diagnosed with clinically definite MS were included. Five patients were male and 14 females. The mean age of the MS patients was 47.7 ± 11.9 years. The mean age difference between the healthy controls and the MS patients was 1.1 ± 2.6 years. All 19 MS patients fulfilled the Barkhof-Tintorée criteria of MS diagnosis [32] in prior MRI examinations. The mean duration of disease was 15.1 ± 10.2 years. The disability status of the MS patients was rated with EDSS [33] and the

Multiple Sclerosis Severity Score (MSSS) [34]: mean EDSS = 3.7 (range = 1–8.5), mean MSSS = 4.2 (range = 0.5–9.6).

Scanning protocol

For qMRI the QRAPMASTER sequence [12] was used. QRAPMASTER is a multi spin-echo saturation recovery sequence with 4 saturation delays and 5 echoes. The saturation delays were at 100, 400, 1380, and 2860 ms with a TR of 2950 ms. TE was set to 14, 28, 42, 56, and 70 ms. Hence each acquisition resulted in a matrix of $4 \times 5 = 20$ images per slice with different effects of T_1 and T_2 relaxation on the image signal intensity. The in-plane resolution was 1×1 mm^2 over a field of view (FOV) of 210 mm. Thirty axial slices of 4 mm thickness (no gap) were collected in a scan time of 8:21 minutes. The MR-scanner was an Achieva 1.5 T (Philips Healthcare, Best, The Netherlands).

Image post-processing

Image data were analyzed with the SyMRI 7.0 software (SyntheticMR AB, Linköping, Sweden) to retrieve the $R_1 = 1/T_1$, $R_2 = 1/T_2$, and PD maps as described in Warntjes et al. [12]. Furthermore a stack of T2-weighted images was recreated based on the same dataset using the approach of synthetic MRI [35,36]. The R_1, R_2, and PD maps were normalized to a standard stereotactic space in Montreal Neurological Institute (MNI) co-ordinates using SPM8 (Wellcome Department of Imaging Neuroscience, University College, London, UK), as described in previous works by us [13,37]. Before normalization, the synthetic T2-weighted images were smoothed with an 8 mm Gaussian kernel to reduce the individual anatomical details, and thereafter used as source images to calculate the transformation matrices between individual images and the template. The normalization to the MNI space was done by a 12-parameter (translation, rotation, shear, zoom) affine registration followed by nonlinear deformations, defined by a linear combination of three-dimensional discrete cosine basis functions. The resulting transformation matrices were then applied to the WM, GM, and CSF maps. The resulting maps were re-gridded to $2 \times 2 \times 2$ mm^3 voxel size to obtain an isotropic dataset. Voxel-wise differences in R_1, R_2, and PD between MS patients and healthy controls were estimated by two-sample t-tests controlling for age. For the MS group, all voxels of the parameter maps (R_1, R_2, and PD) were correlated to EDSS with age as a nuisance variable.

Brain segmentation was performed on the intracranial volume, brain volume, and cerebrospinal fluid volume, using the automatic segmentation algorithm of SyMRI 7.0. In summary, the tissue classes white matter, grey matter and CSF are determined as a combination of specified R_1, R_2 and PD value ranges. Partial volume is estimated for intermediate R_1, R_2 and PD values. The brain volume is calculated as a contiguous volume containing white and grey matter. The intracranial volume is calculated a contiguous volume containing brain tissue and CSF. The ventricular volume was obtained by manually selecting the lateral ventricles in the provided cerebrospinal fluid map. The brain parenchymal fraction was calculated as the brain volume divided by the intracranial volume. The ventricular fraction was calculated as the ventricular volume divided by the intracranial volume.

Region of interest analysis

The Wake Forrest University (WFU) PickAtlas [28] defined in the standard MNI space was used to define ROIs in the cingulate cortex, insula, putamen, thalamus, pons, and the midbrain. We also made ROIs representing whole brain grey matter (GM) and regions of frontal, parietal, occipital, and sub-lobar white matter (WM) as well as ROIs representing the corpus callosum and the lateral ventricle.

Statistical significance of differences in R_1, R_2, and PD between the reference group and MS patients, as well as the EDSS correlation in the MS group, was assessed by small volume corrections in brain parenchyma ROIs. Results were considered significant if $p < 0.05$, family wise error (FWE) rate corrected for multiple comparisons regarding the number of voxels in each ROI and the number of ROIs used in each test.

Differences in mean R_1, R_2 and PD were evaluated using a mixed linear model in R [38] using the lme4 [39] package. Group was used as a fixed factor and each subject and voxel were treated as random samples.

Since it was expected that these standardized ROIs would involve substantial partial volume effects, we also did the ROI analyses in reduced ROIs. We reduced the ROI volumes by eroding all voxels that had a distance of 2 mm or lower to the edge of the ROI. The ROI reduction was performed in steps of 2 mm and we calculated the mean R_1, R_2, and PD in each reduced ROI. The reduction was performed on the data after normalization to standard MNI isotropic 2 mm resolution.

Author Contributions

Conceived and designed the experiments: JBMW PL. Performed the experiments: AT. Analyzed the data: AT ME JBMW. Contributed reagents/materials/analysis tools: AML. Wrote the paper: ME. Revised the manuscript for important intellectual content: ME JBMW AT AML PL.

References

1. Tofts P, editor (2003) Quantitative MRI of the brain. Wiley.
2. Kumar R, Delshad S, Woo MA, Macey PM, Harper RM (2012) Age-related regional brain t2-relaxation changes in healthy adults. J Magn Res Imag 35: 300–308.
3. Hasan KM, Walimuni IS, Abid H, Wolinsky JS, Narayana PA (2012) Multimodal quantitative MRI investigation of brain tissue neurodegeneration in multiple sclerosis. J Magn Res Imag 35: 1300–1311.
4. Draganski B, Ashburner J, Hutton C, Kherif F, Frackowiak RSJ, et al. (2011) Regional specificity of MRI contrast parameter changes in normal ageing revealed by voxel-based quantification (VBQ). NeuroImage 55: 1423–1434.
5. Neema M, Stankiewicz J, Arora A, Dandamudi VS, Batt CE, et al. (2007) T1- and T2-based MRI measures of diffuse gray matter and white matter damage in patients with multiple sclerosis. J Neuroimag 17: 16S–21S.
6. Neeb H, Zilles K, Shah NJ (2006) A new method for fast quantitative mapping of absolute water content in vivo. NeuroImage 31: 1156–1168.
7. Oh J, Cha S, Aiken AH, Han ET, Crane JC, et al. (2005) Quantitative apparent diffusion coefficients and T2 relaxation times in characterizing contrast enhancing tumors and regions of peritumoral edema. J Magn Res Imag 21: 701–708.
8. Deoni SCL, M PT, K RB (2005) High-resolution T1 and T2 mapping of the brain in a clinically acceptable time with DESPOT1 and DESPOT2. Magn Res Med 53: 237–241.
9. Deichmann R (2005) Fast high-resolution T1 mapping of the human brain. Magn Res Med 54: 20–27.
10. Larsson HB, Frederiksen J, Petersen J, Nordenbo A, Zeeberg I, et al. (1989) Assessment of demyelination, edema, and gliosis by in-vivo determination of T1 and T2 in the brain of patients with acute attack of multiple sclerosis. J Magn Reson Med 11: 337–338.
11. Warntjes J, Dahlqvist O, Lundberg P (2007) A novel method for rapid, simultaneous t_1, t_2^* and proton density quantification. Magn Res Med 57: 528–537.
12. Warntjes J, Dahlqvist Leinhard O, West J, Lundberg P (2008) Rapid magnetic resonance quantification on the brain: Optimization for clinical usage. Magn Res Med 60: 320–329.
13. Warntjes J, Engström M, Tisell A, Lundberg P (2012) Brain characterization using normalized quantitative magnetic resonance imaging. Plos One 8: e70864.
14. Barkhof F (2002) The clinico-radiological paradox in multiple sclerosis revisited. Curr Opin Neurol 15: 239–245.
15. Neema M, Goldberg-Zimring D, Guss ZD, Healy BC, Guttmann CRG, et al. (2009) 3 T MRI relaxometry detects T2 prolongation in the cerebral normal-appearing white matter in multiple sclerosis. NeuroImage 46: 633–641.
16. Whittall KP, MacKay AL, Li DKB, Vavasour IM, Jones CK, et al. (2002) Normal-appearing white matter in multiple sclerosis has heterogeneous, diffusely prolonged T2. Magn Res Med 47: 403–408.
17. Levesque R, Pike GB (2009) Characterizing healthy and diseased white matter using quantitative magnetization transfer and multicomponent T_2 relaxometry: A unified view via a four-pool model. Mag Reson Med 62: 1487–1496.
18. Filippi M, Agosta F (2010) Imaging biomarkers in multiple sclerosis. J Magn Res Imag 31: 770–788.
19. Kincses ZT, Ropele S, Jenkinson M, Khalil M, Petrovic K, et al. (2010) Lesion probability mapping to explain clinical deficits and cognitive performance in multiple sclerosis. Mult Scler J 17: 681–689.
20. Alfano B, Brunetti A, Covelli EM, Quarantelli M, Panico MR, et al. (1997) Unsupervised, automated segmentation of the normal brain using a multispectral relaxometric magnetic resonance approach. Magn Res Med 37: 84–93.
21. Hasan KM, Walimuni IS, Abid H, Datta S, Wolinsky JS, et al. (2012) Human brain atlas-based multimodal MRI analysis of volumetry, diffusimetry, relaxometry and lesion distribution in multiple sclerosis patients and healthy adult controls: Implications for understanding the pathogenesis of multiple sclerosis and consolidation of quantitative MRI results in MS. J Neurol Sci 313: 99–109.
22. Roosendaal S, Geurts J, Vrenken H, Hulst H, Cover K, et al. (2009) Regional DTI differences in multiple sclerosis patients. NeuroImage 44: 1397–1403.
23. Filippi M, Rovaris M (2000) Magnetisation transfer imaging in multiple sclerosis. J Neuro Virol 6: 115–120.
24. Ceccarelli A, MA R, Pagani E, Ghezzi A, Capra R, et al. (2008) The topographical distribution of tissue injury in benign MS: A 3T multiparametric MRI study. NeuroImage 39: 1499–1509.
25. Bodini B, Khaleeli Z, Cercignani M, Miller D, Thompson A, et al. (2009) Exploring the relationship between white matter and gray matter damage in early primary progressive multiple sclerosis: An in vivo study with TBSS and VBM. Hum Brain Map 30: 2852–2861.
26. Audoin B, Ranjeva JP, Van Au Duong M, Ibarrola D, Malikova I, et al. (2004) Voxel-based analysis of MTR images: A method to locate gray matter abnormalities in patients at the earliest stage of multiple sclerosis. J Magn Res Imag 20: 765–771.
27. Jure L, Zaaraoui W, Rousseau C, Reuter F, Rico A, et al. (2010) Individual voxel-based analysis of brain magnetization transfer maps shows great variability of gray matter injury in the first stage of multiple sclerosis. J Magn Res Imag 32: 424–428.
28. Maldjian JA, Laurienti PJ, Kraft RA, Burdette JH (2003) An automated method for neuroanatomic and cytoarchitectonic atlas-based interrogation of fMRI data sets. NeuroImage 19: 1233–1239.
29. Vågberg M, Lindqvist T, Warntjes JBM, Sundström P, Birgander R, et al. (2013) Automated determination of brain parenchymal fraction in multiple sclerosis. Am J Neuroradiol 34: 498–504.
30. Ambarki K, Lindqvist T, Wåhlin A, Petterson E, Warntjes M, et al. (2012) Evaluation of automatic measurement of the intracranial volume based on quantitative MR imaging. Am J Neuroradiol 33: 1951–1956.
31. Ashburner J (2007) A fast diffeomorphic image acquisition algorithm. NeuroImage 38: 95–113.
32. McDonald WI, Compston A, Edan G, Goodkin D, Hartung HP, et al. (2001) Recommended diagnostic criteria for multiple sclerosis: guidelines from the international panel on the diagnosis of multiple sclerosis. Ann Neurol 50: 121–127.
33. Kurtzke J (1983) Rating neurologic impairment in multiple sclerosis: An expanded disability status scale (EDSS). Neurology 33: 1444–1452.
34. Roxburgh R, Seaman SR, Masterman T, Hensiek AE, Sawcer SJ, et al. (2005) Multiple sclerosis severity score. using disability and disease duration to rate disease severity. Neurology 64: 1144–1151.
35. Bobman S, Riederer S, Lee J, Suddarth S, Wang B, et al. (1985) Cerebral magnetic resonance image synthesis. Am J Neuro Rad 6: 265–269.
36. Riederer S, Lee J, Farzeneh F, Wang H, Wright R (1986) Magnetic resonance image synthesis: Clinical implementation. Acta Radiol 369: 466–468.
37. West J, Blystad I, Engström M, Warntjes JBM, Lundberg P (2013) Application of quantitative MRI for brain tissue segmentation at 1.5 T and 3.0 T field strengths. Plos One 8: e74795.
38. Team RC (2013) R: A language and environment for statistical computing. R Foundation for Statistical Computing, Vienna, Austria. Http://www.R-project.org.
39. Bates D, Maechler M, Bolker B, Walker S (2013) lme4: Linear mixed-effects models using Eigen and S4, R package version 1.0-4 edition. Http://CRAN.R-project.org/package=lme4.

14

Low Message Sensation Health Promotion Videos Are Better Remembered and Activate Areas of the Brain Associated with Memory Encoding

David Seelig[1,9], An-Li Wang[1,9], Kanchana Jaganathan[2], James W. Loughead[2], Shira J. Blady[2], Anna Rose Childress[2], Daniel Romer[1], Daniel D. Langleben[1,2]*

1 Annenberg Public Policy Center, Annenberg School for Communication, University of Pennsylvania, Philadelphia, Pennsylvania, 19104, United States of America,
2 Department of Psychiatry, School of Medicine, University of Pennsylvania, Philadelphia, Pennsylvania, 19104, United States of America

Abstract

Greater sensory stimulation in advertising has been postulated to facilitate attention and persuasion. For this reason, video ads promoting health behaviors are often designed to be high in "message sensation value" (MSV), a standardized measure of sensory intensity of the audiovisual and content features of an ad. However, our previous functional Magnetic Resonance Imaging (fMRI) study showed that low MSV ads were better remembered and produced more prefrontal and temporal and less occipital cortex activation, suggesting that high MSV may divert cognitive resources from processing ad content. The present study aimed to determine whether these findings from anti-smoking ads generalize to other public health topics, such as safe sex. Thirty-nine healthy adults viewed high- and low MSV ads promoting safer sex through condom use, during an fMRI session. Recognition memory of the ads was tested immediately and 3 weeks after the session. We found that low MSV condom ads were better remembered than the high MSV ads at both time points and replicated the fMRI patterns previously reported for the anti-smoking ads. Occipital and superior temporal activation was negatively related to the attitudes favoring condom use (see Condom Attitudes Scale, Methods and Materials section). Psychophysiological interaction (PPI) analysis of the relation between occipital and fronto-temporal (middle temporal and inferior frontal gyri) cortices revealed weaker negative interactions between occipital and fronto-temporal cortices during viewing of the low MSV that high MSV ads. These findings confirm that the low MSV video health messages are better remembered than the high MSV messages and that this effect generalizes across public health domains. The greater engagement of the prefrontal and fronto-temporal cortices by low MSV ads and the greater occipital activation by high MSV ads suggest that that the "attention-grabbing" high MSV format could impede the learning and retention of public health messages.

Editor: Martin Walter, Leibniz Institute for Neurobiology, Germany

Funding: This work was supported by the National Institute on Drug Abuse R03 DA035683 and National Institutes of Allergy and Infectious Diseases Penn Center for AIDS Research (CFAR) P30 AI 045008. The funders had no role in study design, data collection and analysis, decision to publish, or preparation of the manuscript" to the appropriate location in the manuscript.

Competing Interests: The authors have declared that no competing interests exist.

* Email: langlebe@upenn.edu

9 These authors contributed equally to this work.

Introduction

Health-related video public service announcements (PSAs) and commercial advertisements promoting health-related products and healthy behaviors, are an important component of public health campaigns to reduce the incidence of sexually transmitted infections (STI) and addictions [1,2,3]. To facilitate objective evaluation of health-related video advertisements (further "ads"), researchers have developed several standardized measures of video ad characteristics. "Message sensation value" (MSV), which quantifies video ad features that are arousing and engage attention, is one of the best validated of such measures [4,5,6,7]. Data support MSV's construct validity and value in predicting behavioral outcomes of video ads [8,9,10]. While there is no objective algorithm for development of effective video ads, a long held consensus has been that high MSV is likely to increase video ad effectiveness by capturing more attention [4]. This consensus was also in-line with the "distraction hypothesis" stating that diversion of attention from an ad core message to its other features (i.e., distraction), may actually *enhance* message effectiveness by impeding a viewer's ability to argue against an ad's arguments [11]. An alternative point of view was that attention-grabbing audio-visual features that confer higher salience may actually compete with ad's content for limited cognitive resources, thus reducing the processing of an ad's message [6,12,13,14,15,16]. In line with the latter overstimulation interpretation, a functional Magnetic Resonance Imaging (fMRI) study of anti-smoking video ads [17] found that compared to high MSV ads, low MSV ads were associated with better recognition of still frames extracted from these ads after a short delay and were more likely to activate the middle temporal gyrus during viewing, one of the brain regions associated with memory formation (i.e., encoding) [18,19]. In addition, low MSV ads were more likely to activate areas of the prefrontal cortex associated with top-down attention and cognitive processing [20,21,22]. In contrast, high MSV ads were associated with greater activation of the occipital cortex, a region associated with initial processing of visual information [23,24].

The above findings suggest that high MSV ads may interfere with memory encoding, perhaps due to the increased allocation of the limited cognitive resources to visual processing. Consistent with this hypothesis, medial temporal and prefrontal response to low MSV anti-tobacco video ads was positively correlated with subsequent frame recognition accuracy [17].

Despite the evidence that high MSV may disrupt the processing of ad arguments, campaign designers often include high MSV inputs to capture attention and without considering possible negative effects of these distractors [25]. The present research was designed to provide a further test of the "limited cognitive resources" explanation for the poorer recognition accuracy of high MSV ads. In particular, we investigated the relationship between regions associated with sensory stimulation during ad viewing (primarily occipital cortex) and the prefrontal and temporal regions associated with cognitive processing and memory encoding. If the "limited cognitive resources" explanation is valid, we would expect the connectivity between these regions to be weaker under high MSV than low MSV. The presence of such a system is supported by anatomical evidence of a direct occipito-temporal network [26], as well as functional demonstrations of an association between these regions during encoding of sensory information [27,28,29].

A second goal of the research was to determine whether the superiority of low MSV ads previously demonstrated for anti-tobacco video ads [17] would extend to another important public health domain, namely safe sex. We anticipated that prior findings of superior encoding of low MSV ads would generalize to safe sex video ads promoting condom use. Generalization of the findings from anti-tobacco video ads to an entirely different topic would replicate the prior finding and suggest that it is relevant to a wider range of health topics. We hypothesized that low MSV ads will be recognized on subsequent tests of recognition memory better than high MSV ads. Furthermore we hypothesized that low MSV will preferentially activate temporal and prefrontal cortices, while high MSV ads would preferentially activate the occipital cortex. To explore our hypothesis that low MSV ads are associated with a greater degree of occipito-temporal connectivity than high MSV ads, we examined the psychophysiological interaction (PPI) between the occipital and the prefronto-temporal regions. Such a relationship would suggest that video ads with excessive visual stimulation prevent the efficient transfer of information from regions involved in visual processing to downstream regions associated with storage of this information in memory.

Materials and Methods

Participants

Thirty-nine healthy subjects were recruited through advertising and screened for psychiatric, neurological or medical illnesses. Exclusion criteria included presence of DSM-4-TR Axis 1 psychiatric disorder [30], chronic medical or neurological illness or treatment that could alter cerebral structure or metabolism, and safety-related contraindications for MRI scanning. All participants reported sexual experience. Data from 34 subjects (17 F), aged from 19 to 31 years (Mean 23.4, SD 2.9), with an average of 15.2 (SD 1.7) years of education, all right handed, were included in the final analysis. Among these participants, 11 (33%) self-identified as African American, 16 (47%) as European American and 7 (21%) as Asian American. All participants reported having been sexually active in the past three months with an average of 1.4 (SD 0.7) sexual partners. Six (2 M) reported having sexual partners of both genders and 10 (4 M) reported never using condoms. Each participant gave written informed consent to participate in the study. The study protocol and consent form were approved by the University of Pennsylvania Institutional Review Board.

Stimulus selection

We identified 71 ads that encouraged condom use by populations at-risk for unplanned pregnancy or sexually transmitted Diseases (STDs). Most of the ads were commercials produced by condom manufacturers (e.g., Trojan, Durex), who share a common goal with government-sponsored programs to encourage their target audiences to engage in safe-sex practices. Any references to particular manufacturer brand names were cut or digitally blurred. All 71 videos were scored for MSV by two raters who were trained on using the validated rating procedure [31,32]. Briefly, MSV is an aggregate measure of audio and visual format features of video messages, derived from Zuckerman's theory of sensation-seeking [33]. The rated features include cuts, special effects, intense graphic imagery, saturated colors, loud sounds, animation and so on. The specific MSV rating procedure used in this study has been described in Morgan et al [31] and validated in multiple previous studies [15,34], including studies with neurophysiological correlates [17,32,35]. In the present study, the MSV of each ad was coded independently by two raters following the procedure described by Morgan et al. (2003). Rating are based on features described above, adjusted for ad length [31]. An ads' total score is a composite of both qualitative (Present/Absent) and categorical (number of occurrences) ratings. The inter-rater correlation for the total score ratings in the present set of ads was very high (Pearson r = 0.96). The rare divergent ratings were reconciled by consensus between the two raters and a 3rd similarly trained individual.

We selected 32 complete ads (ranging between 26 to 66 [$\bar{x}$ = 42.2] seconds in length) from the set of 71 drawn equally from above and below the collection's median MSV score of 6 (mean 6.2, SD = 2.9). The length of the ads was not different between high and low MSV categories (high MSV: 40.81±12.06; low MSV: 40.75±13.64; t = 0.01, df = 30, p = 0.99). We created two sets of 16 ads, each consisting of 8 "high MSV" and 8 "low MSV" ads, with no difference in MSV between these two sets (t = 0.30, df = 30, p = 0.68). The mean MSV of the low subgroup was 3.6 (SD = 1.2, range = 1–5), and the mean MSV of the high subgroup was 8.8 (SD = 1.3, range = 7–10). MSV values were significantly different between low and high MSV ads (t = −11.3, df = 30, p < 0.001). Four of the selected videos were produced by firms that sell condoms (e.g., Trojan, Durex), while the rest were developed by non-profit or government public health agencies (e.g., Centers for Disease Control) for network and cable broadcast (e.g. MTV).

Wang et al. [35] found an interaction between MSV and the persuasive strength of an ad's argument (AS). As the goal of the current study was to compare the effects specifically associated with variation in MSV, we assessed whether AS was balanced between the two MSV conditions, using a previously employed questionnaire [32,36] immediately prior to the end of their participation in the first session of the study. The mean AS scores of high MSV ads did not significantly differ from the mean AS of low MSV ads (t = −0.007, df = 30, p = 0.994).

Video task

Subjects were given the task (see Figure 1) of viewing one of the sets of 16 videos presented in a random sequence. Each ad was preceded and followed by an 18-second interstimulus interval (ISI) during which a homogenous black background with a grey fixation point ("+") was displayed. These ISI's were used as baseline periods for the purpose of imaging data analysis. Stimuli were not repeated and total task duration was 13 min 28 s.

Frame Recognition Test

Five minutes after the video task, subjects were given the Frame Recognition Test (FRT), a forced-choice recognition memory task designed to probe episodic memory of the videos they had seen in the scanner. This task was adapted from an electroencephalography study of the retention of TV commercials [37]. The FRT used in the current study consisted of 3 still-frame targets extracted from each of the 16 videos seen by the subject and 3 still-frame foils from each of 16 videos not seen by the subject (96 frames in total). To construct the frame recognition task (FRT) we used the approach of Wang (2013), Langleben (2009), and Silberstein (2001). Briefly, six frames, sampled at equal time intervals from each other to ensure that they were representative of the full length of the ad, were extracted from each ad. Then we randomly chose 3 frames from each video for the initial and follow up recognition tests. Frame stimuli were presented for 3 second each, in an optimized pseudo-random order [38] that included a variable ISI (0.25 to 16.25 s) during which a fixation point was present (see previous section above). For each trial, participants were instructed to respond "Yes" or "No" to the question "Have you seen this ad?", using a two-button keypad (FORP, Current Design Inc., Philadelphia, PA). The question intentionally implied the ad as a whole though only a single frame was displayed. Stimuli were not repeated, and the total task run time was 9 min 22 s.

Delayed Frame Recognition Test

Three weeks following the fMRI session, participants returned for a second Frame Recognition Test to examine decay and to assess whether initial differences between high MSV and low MSV ads remained. The FRT presented during this session ("delayed FRT") used the same design as the FRT that immediately followed the ad-viewing task. However, each participant was presented with a different set of 96 still-frames (also extracted from the same viewed and unviewed videos as the first FRT).

Condom Attitude Scale (CAS)

Subjects were questioned about their attitudes towards condoms immediately before and after viewing the video task using an abridged version of the Condom Attitude Scale (CAS) [39]. The abridged CAS contains 17 items that query three factors: condom efficacy in preventing sexually transmitted diseases (STDs) and perceived risks of STD, interpersonal impact of condom use, and the effect of condoms on sexual experience. Participants were instructed to indicate the extent to which they agree or disagree with each statement on a 1–6 scale (1 = Strongly Disagree, 6 = Strongly Agree). Two-way repeated-measures ANOVA assessed the main effect, on CAS, of the within-subjects variable (before vs. after task) and the between-subject variable (male vs. female), as well as their possible interaction.

Procedure

All visual tasks were programmed in the Presentation (Neuro-behavioral Systems Inc., Albany, CA) stimulus presentation package and rear-projected to the center of the visual field using a PowerLite 7300 Video projector system (Epson America, Inc., Long Beach, CA) that was viewed through a mirror mounted on the scanner head coil. The video soundtrack was delivered through Silent Scan 2100 MRI-compatible headphones (Avotec Inc., Stuart, FL). Before the imaging session, participants were instructed to watch all the videos carefully, that their memory of the videos would be tested after a delay and that their performance on this test was an integral part of the experiment. Participants performed the FRT approximately five minutes after the video task. The FRT was repeated 3 weeks later at a second session.

Behavioral data analysis

Statistical analyses were performed using the IBM Statistical Package for the Social Sciences (IBM SPSS version 21). Subjects' performance on the FRT was evaluated using the Discrimination Index, $Pr = Z_{Correct\ target\ recognition} - Z_{False\ alarms}$, which reflects how well subjects correctly distinguish targets from foils [40]. All subjects performed above chance level ($Pr \geq 0$), so none were excluded from analyses. Subject tendency to respond "Yes" or "No" under uncertainty was evaluated using the Response Bias measure, $Br = Z_{Correct\ target\ recognition} + Z_{False\ alarms}$. $Br = 0$ indicates no bias, $Br < 0$ indicates liberal bias (i.e. tendency of saying "Yes" when uncertain), $Br > 0$ indicates conservative bias (i.e. tendency of saying "No" when uncertain). Paired t-tests were performed comparing subject performance on Session 1 vs. Session 2 FRT (immediate vs. delayed sessions), and high MSV vs. low MSV. Independent t-tests were performed comparing gender performance.

fMRI data acquisition

MRI data were collected on the University of Pennsylvania's Siemens Trio (Erlangen, Germany) 3 Tesla whole body system using a 32-channel head coil. BOLD fMRI gradient-echo echo-planar sequence was acquired with the following parameters: TR = 3000 ms, TE = 32 ms, flip angle = 90, matrix = 64×64, FOV = 220 mm × 220 mm, slice thickness/gap = 3.4/0 mm, 46 slices. After BOLD fMRI, a 5-min magnetization prepared, rapid acquisition gradient echo T1-weighted image (MPRAGE,

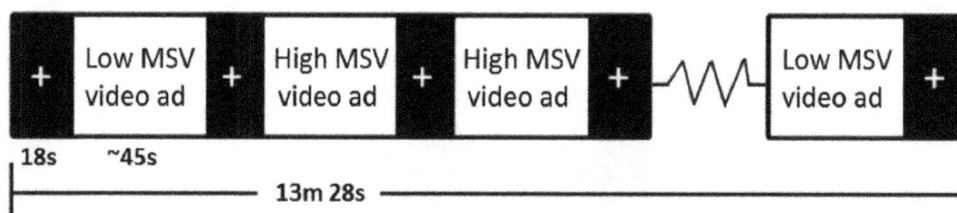

Figure 1. Design of the video message task. The actual task displays 16 video messages (8 high MSV and 8 low MSV) in pseudorandom order (the order presented above is one possible organization).

TR = 1620 ms, TE = 3.87 ms, FOV 250 mm, Matrix 192×256, effective voxel resolution of 1×1×1 mm) was acquired covering the whole brain for spatial normalization and anatomical overlay of functional data [41].

fMRI data preprocessing

fMRI data were preprocessed and analyzed using FEAT(fMRI Expert Analysis Tool), part of FSL (FMRIB's Software Library, www.fmrib.ox.ac.uk/fsl). Images were slice time-corrected, motion-corrected to the median image using tri-linear interpolation with six degrees of freedom [42], high-pass filtered (100 s), spatially smoothed (5 mm FWHM, isotropic) and scaled using mean-based intensity normalization. The median functional and anatomical volumes were co-registered and then transformed into standard space (T1 MNI template) using tri-linear interpolation [42,43]. BET (Brain Extraction Tool) [44] was used to remove non-brain areas. Data sets with motion or signal-to-noise ratio exceeding 2 standard deviations from the average were excluded (5 of 39 initial subjects). Coordinates were converted to Talairach space [45] for tables and figures.

Subject-level Analysis

Subject-level time series statistical analysis was carried out using FILM (FMRIB's Improved Linear Model) with local autocorrelation correction [46]. High MSV and low MSV video messages were modeled using a canonical hemodynamic response function for all subjects based on the order of stimulus presentation for each subject. Six rigid body movement parameters from the motion correction were modeled as nuisance variables. Second level analysis was performed on the contrast images generated from the subject level analysis including: high MSV>low MSV; low MSV>high MSV; All videos>baseline. Age, gender, educational level and condom use status were entered as covariates of no interest. Group statistical maps were thresholded at z = 2.3. To control for Type 1 error, group maps were cluster corrected for multiple comparisons at p<0.05, using the Family-wise Error Rate based on Gaussian Random Fields (GRF) theory. Brain response to high and low MSV ads was compared between African American and Caucasian participants. Lastly, we analyzed the correlation between brain activation during ad viewing and the change in CAS after the fMRI session, calculated as ΔCAS = CAS_post – CAS_pre, which was entered as a covariate of interest for the All videos>baseline contrast, resulting in positive and negative correlation maps (z>2.3 p<0.05).

Psychophysiological Interaction (PPI) Analysis

The PPI analysis was designed to test the hypothesis that greater visual processing would interfere with memory encoding of the ads. Thus, brain regions most associated with visual stimulation (specified by the **high** MSV>**low** MSV contrast) would have a weaker or negative functional relationship with the brain regions required for successful memory encoding of the videos, specified by the low MSV>high MSV contrast in the High MSV condition than the low MSV condition. In the first step of this analysis, based on methods detailed by Gitelman et al. [47], we computed individual average time-series to modeled interactions (for the two MSV conditions separately) between each voxel in the brain and a seed region specified by a functional bilateral mask. This mask was created by using the voxels surviving cluster correction (z>2.3 p< 0.05) in the high MSV>low MSV contrast. As seen by the blue-tinted voxels in the left half of Fig. 2, this seed mask was also nearly identical to the anatomically-defined occipital cortex. The seed time-courses for each subject were deconvolved based on the canonical hemodynamic response function (HRF) used by Gitel-

man et al [47] to construct a time series of neural activity in this region for each MSV condition. We then estimated a GLM with three regressors specifically during video-viewing segments: (1) A binary indicator function specifying low MSV vs. high MSV trials, (2) Average BOLD time-series for the seed (OCC mask) described above, and (3) An interaction between neural activity in the OCC seed and the indicator function described in #1. The second and third regressors were convolved with the HRF.

As our hypothesis was restricted to interactions between regional networks functionally defined by our task (i.e., brain areas associated with sensory stimulation vs. those associated with strong memory encoding), we utilized a second functional bilateral mask as a target region of interest (ROI). This seed mask was created by using the voxels surviving cluster correction (z>2.3 p< 0.05) in the low MSV>high MSV contrast. As seen by the red-tinted voxels in Fig. 2, this mask primarily covers the medial temporal gyrus (MTG) with a smaller proportion of voxels covering the inferior frontal gyrus (IFG). Our subsequent analysis examined the magnitude and valence (positive or negative) of each voxel in the ROI target based on its interaction with the seed during our task (i.e., we did not investigate any seed-voxel interactions outside of the target ROI mask).

To compare the strength and direction of averaged interactions involving the OCC (seed) and the MTG/IFG (ROI target) between low MSV vs. high MSV conditions, we performed a second-level t-test analysis using a procedure modified from Hartley et al [48]. As each subject (N = 34) possessed a pair of average OCC – MTG/IFG interaction values for the low MSV and high MSV conditions respectively, we calculated a two-tailed paired t-test to look for significant interaction differences between the two conditions.

To further characterize differences between the two PPI distributions, we divided both conditions' voxel distributions into two sets of 5 quintiles and used paired t-tests to compare the means within each pair of corresponding quintiles. This analysis involved the following procedure: Using the OCC mask as the seed region, a PPI z-score was determined for each voxel within the MTG/IFG (target region of interest, ROI) for each subject. Within the target ROI, the voxel/seed PPI distributions were broken into two sets of quintiles, one set for each condition.

The goal of this analysis was to determine whether differences in interaction between low MSV versus high MSV were driven by (1) a relative increase in positively interacting voxels during low MSV, (2) a relative increase in negatively interacting voxels during high MSV, or (3) a combination of these mechanisms. We also sought to determine if low MSV's more positive PPI mean could be associated with a weaker overall associative relationship between the seed and target ROI relative to high MSV, a result which would disprove our hypothesis that low MSV videos improve the cooperation between regions involved in input of sensory information and downstream encoding of this information.

Results

Behavioral data

A two-way repeated ANOVA revealed that memory performance was significantly better during the immediate post-task FRT session than the 3-week delayed session (F = 101.13, df = 1, p<0.001), and low MSV ads were bettered remembered than high MSV ads (F = 60.68, df = 1, p<0.001), but no interaction between Session and MSV (F = 2.20, df = 1, p = 0.15). Subjects responded significantly less conservatively during low MSV than high MSV ads (Br = −0.099 vs. 0.24, t = −7.045, df = 33, p<0.001). There were no significant bias differences between sessions (Br = 0.15 vs.

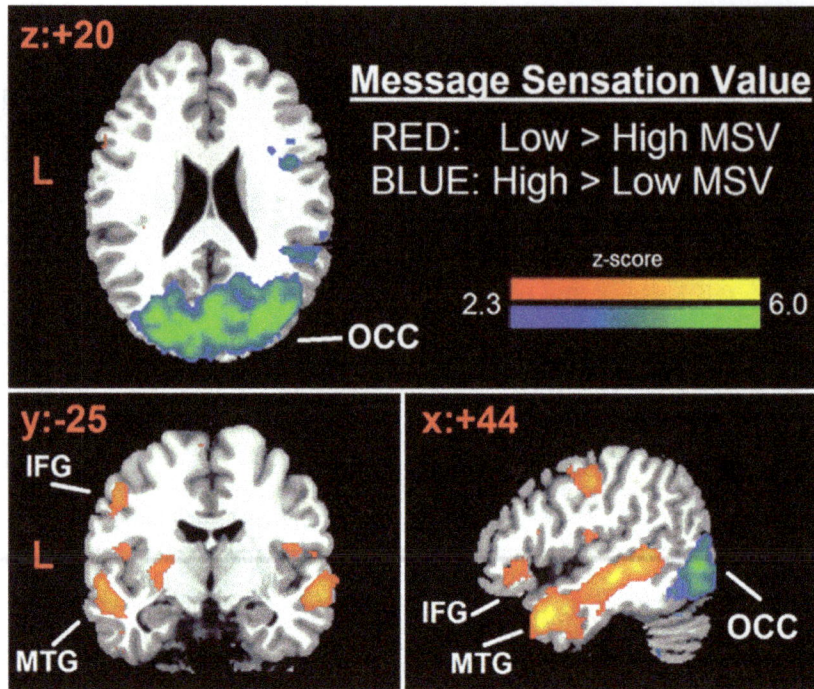

Figure 2. Brain response to safe-sex video messages. Middle temporal gyrus (MTG) and inferior frontal gyri (IFG) (red) have increased response for Low MSV>High MSV items. Occipital cortex (OCC) (blue) has increased response for High MSV>Low MSV ads. Statistical maps are displayed over the Montreal Neurological Institute (MNI) brain template and thresholded at Z=2.3, cluster-corrected for multiple comparisons at p<0.05. Coordinates converted to Talairach space [45].

0.69, t = 1.36, df = 33, p = 0.183). An independent t-test on gender revealed no significant differences between males vs. females in discrimination or response bias (Pr = 2.05 vs 2.20, t = −0.775, df = 32, p = 0.444; Br = 0.033 vs. 0.18, t = −1.67, df = 32, p = 0.104). Examining the pre- and post-task CAS measure, there was no main effect of PSA exposure (F = 0.546, df = 1, p = 0.465) or interaction of task and gender (F = 0.076, df = 1, p = 0.784). There was a strong main effect of gender, with females exhibiting more positive condom attitudes than men (F = 10.3, df = 1, p< 0.005).

fMRI data

Data were thresholded at Z = 2.3 and cluster-corrected for multiple comparisons at p<0.05. Compared to the high MSV videos, low MSV videos were associated with greater response in the prefrontal cortex, including the inferior and middle frontal gyri, and the temporal cortex, including the bilateral middle temporal gyrus (Table 1a, Figure 2 [red-yellow activation]). The high MSV videos were associated with greater activity in occipital cortex, including the cuneus and the fusiform and lingual gyri, when contrasted with low MSV videos (Table 1b, Figure 2 [blue-green activation]). In addition, changes in the Condom Attitude Scale (ΔCAS) in favor of condom use were negatively correlated with brain activation in the bilateral Fusiform and Superior Temporal Gyri (Table 2). There were no significant differences in between African American (N = 11) and Caucasian (N = 16) participants response to either high or low MSV ads.

Primary PPI analyses

Averaging the z-scores (interaction with OCC seed) across all MTG/IFG voxels revealed that both conditions shared a negative overall PPI, with low MSV less negative than high MSV (−0.46

vs. −0.95). This finding was marginally significant (p = 0.060, two-tailed, n = 34).

The analysis by quintiles revealed an asymmetrical voxel distribution, as reflected by the increasing asymmetry between low MSV and high MSV from Quintile 1 to Quintile 5. That is, while the MTG/IFG voxels with the most negative z-score interactions with OCC during the low MSV condition did not differ from that during high MSV (Quintile 1: −2.83 vs. −2.86, p = 0.94), the most positive quintile of voxels was significantly greater during low MSV than high MSV (Quintile 5:1.96 vs. 1.12, p = 0.0089). As seen in Table 3, proceeding from Quintile 1 to Quintile 5, a gradual divergence between low MSV and high MSV ads was observed, with low MSV interactions increasingly becoming more positive than their high MSV counterparts.

Discussion

This study extends findings from anti-smoking PSAs [17] to videos promoting safe sex through condom use. First, we confirmed our hypothesis that videos low in MSV would be better recognized both immediately and 3 weeks after the viewing session. This finding confirms the observation that high MSV video ads are not as well remembered as low MSV video ads [17] and suggests that the empirical strategy of capturing attention, i.e., "buying the eyeballs" [49,50] may come at the expense of learning the content and therefore the message of the ad. In line with our hypotheses regarding the brain systems-level mechanism of this phenomenon, we found that video ads low in MSV activated the middle temporal gyrus (MTG), a brain region engaged in episodic memory encoding [18,51] as well as the dorsal prefrontal cortex, a region associated with working memory and attention

Table 1.

Region[a]	Hem[f]	BA[b]	Size[c]	z-max[d]	X[e]	Y[e]	Z[e]
a) Low MSV>High MSV							
Middle Temporal Gyrus	L	21	3729	6.98	−54	−25	−4
Middle Temporal Gyrus	R	22	3149	6.56	44	−32	−2
Postcentral Gyrus	L	3	434	4.83	−50	−16	40
Lentiform Nucleus	L	N/A	433	3.84	−28	−4	−3
Medial Frontal Gyrus	L	6	431	4.49	−1	−3	59
Inferior Frontal Gyrus	L	47	414	4.08	−46	24	1
Insula	L	13	317	4.16	−45	−13	13
Precentral Gyrus	R	4	274	4.68	50	−13	39
b) High MSV>Low MSV							
Occipital Cortex	L	33	39498	6.88	−33	−70	−16
Middle Frontal Gyrus	R	6	933	4.25	29	−6	45
Caudate (head)	L	NA	932	4.1	−16	30	−2

[a]Location of the cluster's and the local maxima of the BOLD fMRI signal change. $Z > 2.3$ cluster corrected at $p < 0.05$.
[b]Brodmann area.
[c]Number of voxels.
[d]z-MAX values represent peak activation for the cluster.
[e]Talairach (1988) coordinates.
[f]Hemisphere.
For clarity, clusters with less than 150 voxels are not reported in this table.

Table 2.

Region[a]	Hem[f]	BA[b]	Size[c]	z-max[d]	X[e]	Y[e]	Z[e]
Lingual Gyrus	R	18	833	4.05	25	-77	-9
Superior Temporal Gyrus	R	13	567	3.72	48	-42	15
Fusiform Gyrus	L	37	437	3.35	-41	-41	-14
Superior Temporal Gyrus	L	13	403	3.69	-41	-24	9

[a] Location of the clusters and the local maxima of BOLD fMRI signal change correlated with changes in Condom Use Attitude. $Z > 2.3$ cluster corrected at $p < 0.05$.
[b] Brodmann area.
[c] Number of voxels.
[d] Z-MAX values represent peak activation for the cluster.
[e] Talairach (1988) coordinates.
[f] Hemisphere.

[19,20,21,22] and considered to be a predictor of long-term message efficacy in several studies [35,52,53,54]. By contrast, video ads high in MSV activated the occipital cortex (OCC), a region involved in primary processing of visual information [23,24].

The symmetrically bilateral occipitoparietal activation associated with high MSV ads, extends findings first reported in Langleben et al. [17] and confirmed by Wang et al. [35] in studies of anti-tobacco ads. The occipital activation evoked by high MSV videos could reallocate processing resources away from encoding of ad messages [55], reflected in the lower MTG activation and reduced recognition memory for the high MSV compared to the low MSV ads. In addition, the negative correlation between increased CAS in favor of condom use and activation in the bilateral Fusiform and Superior Temporal Gyri also suggests that visual input could interfere with the cognitive processing of video ads' message.

Finally, we used PPI to explore the hypothesis that relative to high MSV videos, low MSV videos allow for more efficient transfer of visual information inputs processed in the OCC and subsequently encoded in the MTG (also facilitated by co-activating attentional networks based in the IFG). By contrast, we hypothesized that high MSV videos should be associated with reduced interaction between these regions by reallocating brain processing resources away from the regions involved in processing and remembering ad messages [17,56]. In support of the overstimulation hypothesis, we found that despite an overall negative level of interaction between these regions, the distribution of interactions was progressively more positive while viewing low MSV ads.

For the most part, the distribution of PPI z-scores was negative between the regions of interest during viewing of either high MSV or low MSV videos. Studies disagree to what extent the negative interactions between the occipital and rostral cortices are part of normal brain activity. There is some evidence that negative interactions may imply a dysfunctional inhibitory process. For example, relative to healthy control subjects, hyperactivation of the ventrolateral prefrontal cortex in patients with schizophrenia has been found to diminish top-down cognitive control normally mediated by the anterior cingulate cortex [57]. However, other fMRI studies consider negative interactions to be evidence of a more functional or efficient system. For example, a recent study, which examined the connectivity between the lateral and ventromedial prefrontal cortex, was characterized by primarily negative interactions, which the authors interpreted to be evidence of a complex dynamic system involving reciprocal interactions [58]. These findings are consistent with a hypothesis [59] that reduced negative interaction between cortical and limbic systems is a marker of major depression.

Despite the controversy about whether to interpret negative interactions as evidence of increased or decreased functional connectivity, our PPI analysis shows the negative interaction between the OCC and MTG/IFG regions to be weaker during the low MSV than high MSV at a marginally significant ($p < 0.06$) level. This was especially prominent at the upper end of the PPI distribution (Table 3), suggesting that the former's smaller mean (closer-to-zero) is a result of a shift towards more positive interactions during low MSV ads (rather than more negative interactions during high MSV). These findings provide support for the hypothesis that high MSV inhibits memory encoding as a result of increased activation of the primary sensory cortices, while low MSV videos may facilitate more efficient transfer of sensory information processed by OCC to

Table 3.

Quintile	high MSV z-score PPI voxel average	low MSV z-score PPI voxel average	Difference	p-value two-tailed t-test (n = 34)	Standard Error (n = 34)
Quint 1 (Lowest 20%)	−2.86	−2.83	0.03	0.94	+/−0.20
Quint 2 (Lower 20%)	−1.74	−1.42	0.32	0.25	+/−0.19
Quint 3 (Middle 20%)	−1.01	−0.49	0.52	0.055	+/−0.20
Quint 4 (Higher 20%)	−0.24	0.47	0.71	0.012	+/−0.24
Quint 5 (Highest 20%)	1.12	1.96	0.84	0.0089	+/−0.33

Psychophysiological Interaction (PPI) between regional masks derived from the High>Low MSV (Occipital Cortex, OCC) and High>Low Recognition Memory (Middle temporal and Inferior frontal gyri, MTG/IFG) under conditions of High MSV and Low MSV, averaged within quintiles of MTG/IFG voxels.

downstream brain regions involved in encoding and attention (MTG, IFG). These results are consistent with theories modeling persuasion as a step-wise process that begins with attracting audience's attention, followed by comprehension [25], where an excess of attention-grabbing devices could interfere with comprehension. They are also in-line with theories of dual-processing of information, such as the Elaboration Likelihood Model [6] and Limited Capacity theories, which postulate that sensory input could compete for the limited cognitive resources available to process various types of information in the message and interfere with subsequent processing that leads to successful encoding [60]. This conclusion also weighs on an earlier debate between the proponents and critics of the "distraction hypothesis" suggesting that distracting elements in an ad improve persuasiveness by reducing the resistance to persuasive messages [11,61]. Our results complement the largely inconclusive behavioral studies of comparative effectiveness of the high and low MSV safe-sex video messages [3,7,62].

Although our results suggest that low MSV ads are more efficacious than the high MSV ads, they come with a number of caveats and limitations. Similarly to prior neuroimaging studies [37] [17], we used immediate and delayed recognition memory as a proxy outcome variable for the video ads' behavioral impact. As the ultimate goal of neuroimaging research in the context of communications is to elucidate the mechanisms by which video ads effect sustained behavioral change and apply this knowledge towards improving video ad effectiveness, future research is necessary to confirm the link between remembering an ad and actually changing behavior in accordance with an ad's message. The present study did not include in-depth standardized evaluation of sexual behaviors and participants' emotional reaction of the video ads, both of which should be taken into account in future neuroimaging studies of safe-sex ad processing. While both ad and audience characteristics are important for the overall ad effect, the present study focused on ad characteristics, i.e. the MSV and accounted for the socio-demographic variables [63,64,65,66,67,68] in the analysis. Future studies should

investigate the influence of audience variables on ad effectiveness. Third, to preserve ecological validity, we used authentic previously aired ads of varying lengths, in their entirety. Though the high and low MSV categories did not differ on ad length, there remains a possibility that ad length variability could have confounded the Frame Recognition Test performance. Future research could consider alternative approaches, such as producing ads specifically for the purpose of research study or editing existing ads to standard size. Finally, since CAS is only a proxy outcome variable, longitudinal assessment of actual condom use following ad exposure would be required to determine the translational significance of our findings.

In conclusion, we confirmed prior reports [17] that high MSV video ads are more likely to interfere with and be less effective at conveying their messages than low MSV ads. Our neuroimaging findings suggest that the potential mechanism for this advantage may be that low MSV ads enable more efficient cross-brain communication between the brain regions involved in early processing of visual information and regions involved in downstream processing and encoding of this information into long-term memory. The fact that these behavioral and neuroimaging findings generalize across message genres justifies further efforts to incorporate neuroimaging in the evaluation and design of public health communications.

Acknowledgements

Authors thank Dr. Rick Zimmerman for assistance in acquiring safe sex video ads and Dr. Lewis Donohew for comments on an earlier version of the paper.

Author Contributions

Conceived and designed the experiments: JWL DR DDL. Performed the experiments: SJB DR DDL. Analyzed the data: DS ALW KJ ARC DDL. Contributed reagents/materials/analysis tools: DS ALW KJ ARC DR DDL. Contributed to the writing of the manuscript: DS ALW KJ DR DDL.

References

1. Emery SL, Szczypka G, Powell LM, Chaloupka FJ (2007) Public health obesity-related TV advertising: lessons learned from tobacco. Am J Prev Med 33: S257–263.

2. Biener L, McCallum-Keeler G, Nyman AL (2000) Adults' response to Massachusetts anti-tobacco television advertisements: impact of viewer and advertisement characteristics. Tob Control 9: 401–407.

3. Zimmerman RS, Palmgreen PM, Noar SM, Lustria ML, Lu HY, et al. (2007) Effects of a televised two-city safer sex mass media campaign targeting high-

sensation-seeking and impulsive-decision-making young adults. Health Educ Behav 34: 810–826.

4. Harrington N, Lane DR, Donohew L, Zimmerman RS, Norling GR, et al. (2003) Persuasive strategies for effective anti-drug messages. Communication Monographs 70: 16–38.

5. Palmgreen P, Donohew L, Lorch E, Rogus M, Helm D, et al. (1991) Sensation seeking, message sensation value, and drug use as mediators of PSA effectiveness. Health Communication 3: 217–227.

6. Petty R, Cacioppo J (1986) Communication and persuasion: Central and peripheral routes to attitude change New York: Springer Verlag. 262 p.

7. Stephenson M, Southwell B (2006) Sensation Seeking, the activation model, and mass media health campaigns: Current findings and future directions for cancer communication. Journal of Communication 56: S38–S56.

8. D'Silva MU, Palmgreen P (2007) Individual differences and context: factors mediating recall of anti-drug public service announcements. Health Commun 21: 65–71.

9. Helme DW, Donohew RL, Baier M, Zittleman L (2007) A classroom-administered simulation of a television campaign on adolescent smoking: testing an activation model of information exposure. J Health Commun 12: 399–415.

10. Van Stee SK, Noar SM, Allard S, Zimmerman R, Palmgreen P, et al. (2012) Reactions to safer-sex public service announcement message features: attention, perceptions of realism, and cognitive responses. Qualitative health research 22: 1568–1579.

11. Festinger L, Maccoby N (1964) On Resistance to Persuasive Communications. Journal of abnormal psychology 68: 359–366.

12. Lang A (2006) Using the Limited Capacity Model of Motivated Mediated Message Processing to Design Effective Cancer Communication Messages. Journal of Communication 56: S57–S80.

13. Bolls PD, Muehling DD, Yoon K. (2003) The effects of television commercial pacing on viewers' attention and memory. Journal of Marketing Communications 9: 17–28.

14. Indovina I, Macaluso E (2007) Dissociation of stimulus relevance and saliency factors during shifts of visuospatial attention. Cereb Cortex 17: 1701–1711.

15. Kang Y, Cappella JN, Fishbein M (2006) The attentional mechanism of message sensation value: Interaction between message sensation value and argument quality on message effectiveness. Communication Monographs 73: 351–378.

16. Romer D (1979) Distraction, couterarguing and the internalization of attitude change. European Journal of Social Psychology 9: 1–17.

17. Langleben DD, Loughead JW, Ruparel K, Hakun JG, Busch-Winokur S, et al. (2009) Reduced prefrontal and temporal processing and recall of high "sensation value" ads. NeuroImage 46: 219–225.

18. Hannula DE, Ranganath C (2008) Medial temporal lobe activity predicts successful relational memory binding. J Neurosci 28: 116–124.

19. Buschman TJ, Miller EK (2007) Top-down versus bottom-up control of attention in the prefrontal and posterior parietal cortices. Science 315: 1860–1862.

20. D'Esposito M (2007) From cognitive to neural models of working memory. Philos Trans R Soc Lond B Biol Sci 362: 761–772.

21. Knudsen EI (2007) Fundamental components of attention. Annu Rev Neurosci 30: 57–78.

22. Murray LJ, Ranganath C (2007) The dorsolateral prefrontal cortex contributes to successful relational memory encoding. J Neurosci 27: 5515–5522.

23. Johnson JA, Zatorre RJ (2006) Neural substrates for dividing and focusing attention between simultaneous auditory and visual events. Neuroimage 31: 1673–1681.

24. Indovina I, Macaluso E (2004) Occipital-parietal interactions during shifts of exogenous visuospatial attention: trial-dependent changes of effective connectivity. Magn Reson Imaging 22: 1477–1486.

25. McGuire WJ (1989) Theoretical foundations of campaigns. In: Rice RE, CK A, editors. Public communication campaigns. 2 ed. Newbury Park, CA: Sage Publications. 43–65.

26. Guhn A, Dresler T, Hahn T, Muhlberger A, Strohle A, et al. (2012) Medial prefrontal cortex activity during the extinction of conditioned fear: an investigation using functional near-infrared spectroscopy. Neuropsychobiology 65: 173–182.

27. Plaud JJ (2003) Pavlov and the foundation of behavior therapy. Span J Psychol 6: 147–154.

28. Wolpe J (1963) Quantitative relationships in the systematic desensitization of phobias. The American journal of psychiatry 119: 1062–1068.

29. Milad MR, Rauch SL, Pitman RK, Quirk GJ (2006) Fear extinction in rats: implications for human brain imaging and anxiety disorders. Biol Psychol 73: 61–71.

30. First M, editor (2002) Diagnostic and statistical manual of mental disorders, 4th Edition, Text Revision. Washington, DC: American Psychiatric Association.

31. Morgan SE (2003) Associations between message features and subjective evaluations of the sensation value of antidrug public service announcements. Journal of Communication 53: 512–526.

32. Strasser AA, Cappella JN, Jepson C, Fishbein M, Tang KZ, et al. (2009) Experimental evaluation of antitobacco PSAs: effects of message content and format on physiological and behavioral outcomes. Nicotine Tob Res 11: 293–302.

33. Zuckerman M (1979) Sensation seeking: Beyond the optimal level of arousal. Hillsdale, NJ: Lawrence Erlbaum. 449 p.

34. Everett M, Palmgreen P (1995) Influences of sensation seeking, message sensation value, and program context on effectiveness of anticocaine public service announcements. Health Communication 7: 225–248.

35. Wang AL, Ruparel K, Loughead JW, Strasser AA, Blady SJ, et al. (2013) Content matters: neuroimaging investigation of brain and behavioral impact of televised anti-tobacco public service announcements. The Journal of neuroscience : the official journal of the Society for Neuroscience 33: 7420–7427.

36. Fishbein M, Hall-Jamieson K, Zimmer E, von Haeften I, Nabi R (2002) Avoiding the boomerang: Testing the relative effectiveness of antidrug public

37. Rossiter JR, Silberstein RB (2001) Brain-imaging detection of visual scene encoding in long-term memory for TV commercials. Journal of Advertising Research 41: Mar-Apr 2001.

38. Dale AM (1999) Optimal experimental design for event-related fMRI. Hum Brain Mapp 8: 109–114.

39. Sacco WP, Levine B, Reed DL, Thompson K (1991) Attitudes about condom use as an AIDS-relevant behavior: Their factor structure and relation to condom use. Psychological Assessment 3: 265–272.

40. Snodgrass JG, Corwin J (1988) Pragmatics of measuring recognition memory: applications to dementia and amnesia. Journal of experimental psychology General 117: 34–50.

41. Lancaster JL, Woldorff MG, Parsons LM, Liotti M, Freitas CS, et al. (2000) Automated Talairach atlas labels for functional brain mapping. Hum Brain Mapp 10: 120–131.

42. Jenkinson M, Bannister P, Brady M, Smith S (2002) Improved optimization for the robust and accurate linear registration and motion correction of brain images. Neuroimage 17: 825–841.

43. Jenkinson M, Smith S (2001) A global optimisation method for robust affine registration of brain images. Med Image Anal 5: 143–156.

44. Smith SM (2002) Fast robust automated brain extraction. Hum Brain Mapp 17: 143–155.

45. Talairach J, Tournoux P. (1988) Co-planar stereotaxic atlas of the human brain. 3-dimensional proportional system: an approach to cerebral imaging. New York: Thieme Medical Publishers.

46. Woolrich MW, Ripley BD, Brady M, Smith SM (2001) Temporal autocorrelation in univariate linear modeling of FMRI data. NeuroImage 14: 1370–1386.

47. Erlich JC, Bush DE, Ledoux JE (2012) The role of the lateral amygdala in the retrieval and maintenance of fear-memories formed by repeated probabilistic reinforcement. Front Behav Neurosci 6: 16.

48. Hartley CA, Fischl B, Phelps EA (2011) Brain structure correlates of individual differences in the acquisition and inhibition of conditioned fear. Cereb Cortex 21: 1954–1962.

49. Chattopadhyay A, Laborie J-L (2005) Managing Brand Experience: The Market Contact Audit (TM). Journal of Advertising Research 45: 9–16.

50. Russell CA, Belch M (2005) A Managerial Investigation into the Product Placement Industry. Journal of Advertising Research 45: 73–92.

51. Thrasher JF, Rousu MC, Anaya-Ocampo R, Reynales-Shigematsu LM, Arillo-Santillan E, et al. (2007) Estimating the impact of different cigarette package warning label policies: the auction method. Addictive behaviors 32: 2916–2925.

52. Chua HF, Ho SS, Jasinska AJ, Polk TA, Welsh RC, et al. (2011) Self-related neural response to tailored smoking-cessation messages predicts quitting. Nature neuroscience 14: 426–427.

53. Chua HF, Liberzon I, Welsh RC, Strecher VJ (2009) Neural correlates of message tailoring and self-relatedness in smoking cessation programming. Biol Psychiatry 65: 165–168.

54. Miettunen J, Lauronen E, Kantojarvi L, Veijola J, Joukamaa M (2008) Inter-correlations between Cloninger's temperament dimensions– a meta-analysis. Psychiatry Res 160: 106–114.

55. Akyurek EG, Vallines I, Lin EJ, Schubo A (2010) Distraction and target selection in the brain: an fMRI study. Neuropsychologia 48: 3335–3342.

56. Lang A, Bradley SD, Park B, Shin M, Chung Y (2006) Parsing the Resource Pie: Using STRTs to measure attention to mediated messages. Media Psychology 8: 369–394.

57. Schlosser RG, Koch K, Wagner G, Nenadic I, Roebel M, et al. (2008) Inefficient executive cognitive control in schizophrenia is preceded by altered functional activation during information encoding: an fMRI study. Neuropsychologia 46: 336–347.

58. Longe O, Senior C, Rippon G (2009) The lateral and ventromedial prefrontal cortex work as a dynamic integrated system: evidence from FMRI connectivity analysis. Journal of cognitive neuroscience 21: 141–154.

59. Mayberg HS (1997) Limbic-cortical dysregulation: a proposed model of depression. The Journal of neuropsychiatry and clinical neurosciences 9: 471–481.

60. Lang A (2000) The limited capacity model of mediated message processing. Journal of Communication 50: 46–70.

61. McGuire WJ (1966) Attitudes and opinions. Annual review of psychology 17: 475–514.

62. Noar SM, Palmgreen P, Chabot M, Dobransky N, Zimmerman RS (2009) A 10-Year Systematic Review of HIV/AIDS Mass Communication Campaigns: Have We Made Progress? J Health Commun 14: 15–42.

63. Reitman D, St Lawrence JS, Jefferson KW, Alleyne E, Brasfield TL, et al. (1996) Predictors of African American adolescents' condom use and HIV risk behavior. AIDS Educ Prev 8: 499–515.

64. St Lawrence JS, Eldridge GD, Reitman D, Little CE, Shelby MC, et al. (1998) Factors influencing condom use among African American women: implications for risk reduction interventions. American journal of community psychology 26: 7–28.

65. Johnson WD, Diaz RM, Flanders WD, Goodman M, Hill AN, et al. (2008) Behavioral interventions to reduce risk for sexual transmission of HIV among men who have sex with men. Cochrane database of systematic reviews: CD001230.

service announcements before a national campaign. American Journal of Public Health 92: 238–245.

66. Protogerou C, Johnson BT (2014) Factors Underlying the Success of Behavioral HIV-Prevention Interventions for Adolescents: A Meta-Review. AIDS Behav 18: 1847–1863.

67. Thurston IB, Dietrich J, Bogart LM, Otwombe KN, Sikkema KJ, et al. (2014) Correlates of sexual risk among sexual minority and heterosexual South African youths. American journal of public health 104: 1265–1269.

68. Widman L, Noar SM, Choukas-Bradley S, Francis DB (2014) Adolescent sexual health communication and condom use: A meta-analysis. Health psychology : official journal of the Division of Health Psychology, American Psychological Association 33: 1113–1124.

15

Mitochondrial DNA (mtDNA) Haplogroups Influence the Progression of Knee Osteoarthritis. Data from the Osteoarthritis Initiative (OAI)

Angel Soto-Hermida[1], Mercedes Fernández-Moreno[1], Natividad Oreiro[1], Carlos Fernández-López[1], Sonia Pértega[2], Estefania Cortés-Pereira[1], Ignacio Rego-Pérez[1]*, Francisco J. Blanco[1]*

1 Grupo de Genómica, Servicio de Reumatología, Instituto de Investigación Biomédica de A Coruña (INIBIC), Complexo Hospitalario Universitario de A Coruña (CHUAC), Sergas, Universidade da Coruña (UDC), A Coruña, España, **2** Unidad de Epidemiología. Instituto de Investigacion Biomedica de A Coruña (INIBIC), Complexo Hospitalario Universitario de A Coruña (CHUAC), Sergas, Universidade da Coruña (UDC), A Coruña, España

Abstract

Objective: To evaluate the influence of the mtDNA haplogroups on knee osteoarthritis progression in Osteoarthritis Initiative (OAI) participants through longitudinal data from radiographs and magnetic resonance imaging (MRI).

Methods: Four-year knee osteoarthritis progression was analyzed as increase in Kellgren and Lawrence (KL) grade, in addition to increase in OARSI atlas grade for joint space narrowing (JSN), osteophytes and subchondral sclerosis in the tibia medial compartment of 891 Caucasian individuals from the progression subcohort. The influence of the haplogroups on the rate of structural progression was also assessed as the four-year change in minimum joint space width (mJSW in millimetres) in both knees of (n = 216) patients with baseline unilateral medial-tibiofemoral JSN. Quantitative cartilage measures from longitudinal MRI data were those related to cartilage thickness and volume with a 24 month follow-up period (n = 381).

Results: During the four-year follow-up period, knee OA patients with the haplogroup T showed the lowest increase in KL grade (Hazard Risk [HR] = 0.499; 95% Confidence Interval [CI]: 0.261–0.819; p<0.05) as well as the lowest cumulative probability of progression for JSN (HR = 0.547; 95% CI: 0.280–0.900; p<0.05), osteophytes (HR = 0.573; 95% CI: 0.304–0.893; p<0.05) and subchondral sclerosis (HR = 0.549; 95% CI: 0.295–0.884; p<0.05). They also showed the lowest decline in mJSW (standardized response means (SRM) = −0.39; p = 0.037) in those knees without baseline medial JSN (no-JSN knees). Normalized cartilage volume loss was significantly lower in patients carrying the haplogroup T at medial tibia femoral (SRM = −0.33; p = 0.023) and central medial femoral (SRM = −0.27; p = 0.031) compartments. Cartilage thickness loss was significantly lower in carriers of haplogroup T at central medial tibia-femoral (SRM = −0.42; p = 0.011), medial tibia femoral (SRM = −0.32; p = 0.018), medial tibia anterior (SRM = +0.31; p = 0.013) and central medial femoral (SRM = −0.19; p = 0.013) compartments.

Conclusions: Mitochondrial genome seems to play a role in the progression of knee osteoarthritis. mtDNA variation could improve identification of patients predisposed to faster or severe progression of the disease.

Editor: Mario D. Cordero, University of Sevilla, Spain

Funding: This study was supported by grants from Fundacion Española de Reumatologia (programa GEN-SER) and from Fondo Investigacion Sanitaria (CIBERCB06/01/0040)-Spain, Fondo Investigacion Sanitaria-PI 08/2028, Ministerio Ciencia e Innovacion PLE2009-0144, with a contribution of funds from FEDER (European Community). IRP was supported by Contrato Miguel Servet-Fondo Investigacion Sanitaria (CP12/03192). The authors would like to thank the participants, principal investigators, coinvestigators and staff of the OAI. The Osteoarthritis Initiative (OAI) is a public-private partnership comprised of five contracts (N01-AR-2-2258; N01-AR-2-2259; N01-AR-2-2260; N01-AR-2-2261; N01-AR-2-2262) funded by the National Institutes of Health, a branch of the Department of Health and Human Services, and conducted by the OAI Study Investigators. Private funding partners include Pfizer, Inc.; Novartis Pharmaceuticals Corporation; Merck Research Laboratories; and GlaxoSmithKline. Private sector funding for the OAI is managed by the Foundation for the National Institutes of Health. This manuscript was prepared using an OAI public use data set and does not necessarily reflect the opinions or views of the OAI investigators, the NIH, or the private funding partners. This manuscript has received the approval of the OAI Publications Committee based on a review of its scientific content and data interpretation. The funders had no role in study design, data collection and analysis, decision to publish, or preparation of the manuscript.

Competing Interests: The authors have the following interests. The Osteoarthritis Initiative (OAI) is a public-private partnership comprised of five contracts. Private funding partners include Pfizer, Inc.; Novartis Pharmaceuticals Corporation; Merck Research Laboratories; and GlaxoSmithKline. There are no patents, products in development or marketed products to declare.

* Email: fblagar@sergas.es (FJB); Igancio.rego.perez@sergas.es (IRP)

Introduction

Osteoarthritis (OA), the most common joint disease related to ageing, is characterized by the degeneration of articular cartilage, affecting subchondral bone and soft tissue and leading to joint destruction and severe impairment of mobility [1]. OA is also the leading cause of permanent work incapacitation and one of the most common reasons for visiting primary care physicians. OA is a multifactorial disease in which a combination of both environmental and genetic factors interact [2–4].

At present, therapies available to treat OA are limited. Most current treatments are designed only to relieve pain and reduce or prevent the disability caused by bone and cartilage degeneration. Furthermore, clinical testing of new therapies is complicated by the highly variable way OA manifests in individual patients; it is established that some OA patients remain relatively stable over time, while others progress more rapidly to severe structural deterioration often leading to joint replacement. The usefulness of both genetic and protein biomarkers in OA is to predict, not only the risk of OA at an earlier stage of the disease [5], but also which OA patients are more likely to progress to severe disease. Some studies have evaluated the role of genetic factors in the severity or progression of OA [6–9] and, to date, relatively little is known about risk factors for radiographic knee OA progression, despite their great clinical importance.

The Osteoarthritis Initiative (OAI) is a public-private partnership that provides new resources and commitment to help find biochemical, genetic and imaging biomarkers for onset and progression of knee OA. One of the important goals of the OAI is to support development and validation of imaging and biochemical markers that indicate either the presence of OA, or an increased risk for OA, even when radiograph changes are minimal or absent, and which can accurately predict the subsequent course of disease. An essential step to achieve these goals is the assessment of biomarkers in longitudinal studies, over a period of time in which clinical change can be clearly defined, in large, well-characterized populations of persons with OA or who are developing OA.

The OAI cohort study has a public archive of data, biological samples and joint images collected over time from a clinically well characterized population of individuals comprising two subgroups, i) those with clinically significant knee OA who are at risk of disease progression; and ii) individuals who are at high risk for developing clinically significant knee OA. Participants are followed for four years for changes in the clinical status of the knee and other joints, including worsening and onset of symptoms and disabilities, worsening and onset of knee structural abnormalities, and changes in other imaging and biochemical markers of knee OA. Therefore, the use of this cohort of samples confers an extra degree of exceptionality to this work.

In recent years, a growing body of evidence suggests the implication of the mitochondria in the pathogenesis of OA [1,10–12]; mitochondrial function is altered in OA chondrocytes [13] and the mitochondrial dysfunction increases inflammatory responsiveness to cytokines in normal human chondrocytes [14,15]. Besides, the apoptotic mitochondrial pathway is one of the major cellular pathways for apoptosis of OA chondrocytes [16] and the inhibition of complexes III and V of the mitochondrial respiratory chain (MRC) causes an increased inflammatory response potentially related to the production of reactive oxygen species (ROS) [14]. Mitochondrial free radical production compromises chondrocyte function [17,18], causing mtDNA damage and reduced mtDNA capacity for repair [19].

In addition to mitochondrial dysfunction, mitochondrial genetics seems to play a role in the OA disease too. Mitochondrial DNA (mtDNA) haplogroups, defined as individual groups characterized by the presence of a particular set of single nucleotide polymorphisms (SNPs) in the mtDNA sequence [20], have been shown to be related to OA at different levels: i) prevalence of the disease in Spanish [6,21] and Asian [22] populations; ii) complementary genetic markers for the serum levels of collagen type II molecular biomarkers [23] and proteolytic enzymes [24]; and iii) lower nitric oxide (NO) production in human articular chondrocytes as well as higher telomere length [25].

In consideration of this background and the discovery of the role of mitochondria in OA, the aim of this study is to evaluate the occurrence of the mtDNA haplogroups in the progression of knee OA. For this purpose, we used the longitudinal data obtained from radiographs and magnetic resonance images (MRI) of knee OA patients belonging to the progression subcohort of the OAI.

Materials and Methods

Data used in the preparation of this article were obtained from the Osteoarthritis Initiative (OAI) database, which is available for public access at http://www.oai.ucsf.edu/. The Osteoarthritis Initiative (OAI) is a public-private partnership comprised of five contracts (N01-AR-2-2258; N01-AR-2-2259; N01-AR-2-2260; N01-AR-2-2261; N01-AR-2-2262) funded by the National Institutes of Health, a branch of the Department of Health and Human Services, and conducted by the OAI Study Investigators. Private funding partners include Pfizer, Inc.; Novartis Pharmaceuticals Corporation; Merck Research Laboratories; and GlaxoSmithKline. Private sector funding for the OAI is managed by the Foundation for the National Institutes of Health. The study was reviewed and approved by Comite Etico de Investigación Clínica de Galicia (Ref# 2008/144). Specific datasets used are the 0.2.2 clinical dataset and 0.6, 1.6, 3.5, 5.3, 5.5, 6.3, 0.5 and 1.5 imaging datasets.

Participants

DNA from all the participants, provided by the OAI, was previously isolated from buffy coat from plasma samples. All the participants analyzed in this study (N = 891) were of Caucasian ancestry and belonged to the progression subcohort of the OAI (**Table 1**). This subcohort includes patients with symptomatic tibiofemoral knee OA at baseline with frequent knee symptoms (pain, aching or stiffness) and radiographic tibiofemoral knee OA defined as tibiofemoral osteophytes (OARSI atlas grades 1–3 [26], equivalent to Kellgren and Lawrence (KL) grade ≥2) on the fixed flexion radiographs.

The follow-up period was 48 months for radiographic data and 24 months for magnetic resonance imaging (MRI) data.

All the clinical centers of the OAI have made provisions to ensure the safety, confidentiality and ethical treatment of study participants according to the Declaration of Helsinki. In this sense, all the OAI participants signed an informed consent.

mtDNA haplogroups genotyping

The mtDNA haplogroups of all OA patients were assessed following DNA isolation using a previously described assay [6]. Briefly, a multiplex polymerase chain reaction (PCR) was performed to amplify six mtDNA fragments that contain each of the informative SNPs that characterize the most common European mtDNA haplogroups (H, V, HV*, Uk, J and T). The resulting PCR fragments were further purified and analyzed by the Single Base Extension (SBE) assay and the informative SNPs were

Table 1. Demographic characteristics of the study population at baseline grouped by mitochondrial DNA (mtDNA) haplogroups in the progression subcohort of the OAI.

mtDNA haplogroups

Characteristic	H (N=341, 38.27%)	J (N=89, 9.99%)	T (N=85, 9.54%)	Uk (N=228, 25.6%)	Others (N=148, 16.61%)	p-value	Total (N=891)
Age at baseline (years)	62.2±9.1	60.3±9.9	61.6±9.5	62.4±9.5	61.4±9.6	0.378*	61.9±9.4
Gender:						0.792#	
Male	164 (48.1)	41 (46.1)	45 (52.9)	111 (48.7)	66 (44.6)		427 (47.9)
Female	177 (51.9)	48 (53.9)	40 (47.1)	117 (51.3)	82 (55.4)		464 (52.1)
BMI (Kg/m^2)	29.6±4.5	29.6±4.8	29.6±4.5	29.2±4.9	29.2±4.4	0.596*	29.4±4.6
BMI≤30	192 (56.3)	50 (56.2)	50 (58.8)	138 (60.5)	92 (62.2)	0.721#	522 (58.6)
BMI>30	149 (43.7)	39 (43.8)	35 (41.2)	90 (39.5)	56 (37.8)		369 (41.4)
KL grade at baseline (*worst knee*)**						0.851#	
0–I	45 (14.0)	9 (10.8)	9 (11.3)	31 (14.8)	21 (14.9)		115 (13.8)
II–IV	277 (86.0)	74 (89.2)	71 (88.8)	179 (85.2)	120 (85.1)		721 (86.2)
KL grade at baseline (*less severe knee*)						0.538#	
0–I	142 (44.1)	39 (47.0)	34 (42.5)	105 (50.0)	71 (50.4)		391 (46.8)
II–IV	180 (55.9)	44 (53.0)	46 (57.5)	105 (50.0)	46 (57.5)		445 (53.2)
mJSN at baseline (*worst knee*)						0.777#	
0–I	179 (55.6)	43 (51.8)	46 (57.5)	113 (53.8)	84 (59.6)		465 (55.6)
II–III	143 (44.4)	40 (48.2)	34 (42.5)	97 (46.2)	57 (40.4)		371 (44.4)
mJSN at baseline (*less severe knee*)						0.885#	
0–I	280 (87.0)	73 (88.0)	67 (83.8)	180 (85.7)	119 (84.4)		719 (86.0)
II–III	42 (13.0)	10 (12.0)	13 (16.3)	30 (14.3)	22 (15.6)		117 (14.0)
Osteophytes tibia medial (*worst knee*)						0.046#	
0–I	192 (67.4)	39 (52.7)	41 (56.9)	107 (57.5)	82 (66.7)		461 (62.3)
II–III	93 (32.6)	35 (47.3)	31 (43.1)	79 (42.5)	41 (33.3)		279 (37.7)
Osteophytes tibia medial (*less severe knee*)						0.577#	
0–I	267 (93.7)	68 (91.9)	66 (91.7)	174 (93.5)	119 (96.7)		694 (93.8)
II–III	18 (6.3)	6 (8.1)	6 (8.3)	12 (6.5)	4 (3.3)		46 (6.2)
Sclerosis tibia medial (*worst knee*)						0.131#	
0–I	181 (63.5)	37 (50.0)	46 (63.9)	110 (59.1)	83 (67.5)		457 (61.8)
II–III	104 (36.5)	37 (50.0)	26 (36.1)	76 (40.9)	40 (32.5)		283 (38.2)
Sclerosis tibia medial (*less severe knee*)						0.494#	
0–I	268 (94.0)	66 (89.2)	65 (90.3)	168 (90.3)	112 (91.1)		679 (91.8)
II–III	17 (6.0)	8 (10.8)	7 (9.7)	18 (9.7)	11 (8.9)		61 (8.2)

Values are mean±standard deviation or number of patients with percentage in parentheses; OAI: osteoarthritis initiative; (*) Kruskal-Wallis non-parametric test for comparison between mtDNA haplogroups; (#) Chi-square test; BMI: body mass index; KL: Kellgren and Lawrence; mJSN: Joint space narrowing in medial compartment; (**) The worst knee and the less severe knee at baseline were designated, respectively, as the knee with the highest and lowest KL (Kellgren andLawrence) grade, OARSI JSN (joint space narrowing) grade, OARSI osteophytes grade or OARSI sclerosis grade, as appropriate on each case; significant p-values are in bold.

visualized after loading the purified SBE product into an ABI 3130 XL genetic analyzer (Applied Biosystems, Foster City, CA, United States). The less common haplogroups (W, I, X and others) were assessed using PCR-restriction fragment length polymorphism (RFLP) according to the hierarchical scheme previously described [6]. The assigned mtDNA haplogroups were verified by sequencing the entire mtDNA control region in 30% of the samples and analysing some of the key SNPs described in phylotree (http://www.phylotree.org).

Progression criteria

We analyzed radiographic knee OA progression during the follow-up period (48 months) in terms of the KL grade, defining progression as an increase of at least one KL grade in either knee. Additionally, we also analyzed the development or progression of i) joint space narrowing in the medial compartment (mJSN), ii) osteophytes in the tibia medial compartment and iii) subchondral sclerosis in the tibia medial compartment. The progression criterion for each of these three features was an increase of at least one OARSI atlas grade in either knee.

We also analyzed the influence of the mtDNA haplogroups on the rate of structural progression in both knees of patients with baseline unilateral medial JSN (OARSI atlas grade 1–3) and no JSN in the lateral compartment (OARSI atlas grade <1). For this purpose, we analyzed the four-year change in radiographic medial joint space width (mJSW) at the minimum JSW in the medial compartment of both knees (baseline JSN knees and baseline no-JSN knees) of 216 OA patients that met the eligibility criteria.

Description of the MRI data

For this study, we analyzed the data obtained from measurements of cartilage volume and thickness from serial knee MRI scans performed by Felix Eckstein's group in Germany (Chondrometrics, Gmbh, Ainring) or Austria (Paracelsus University, Salzburg) (http://www.chondrometrics.com/) and contained in different datasets (Projects) of the OAI. These data consisted in a longitudinal study with a 24 month follow-up period of 381 knee OA patients (190 right knees and 191 left knees) in the progression subcohort (namely Project 9). We analyzed data from measurements of the femoral region defined as the 75% of the distance between trochlear notch and the posterior of the femoral condyle (**Figure S1**).

The image analysis relied on sagittal DESS (double echo steady-state) sequence of either the right or left knee [27,28]. Segmentation of the cartilages was performed at the image analysis center (Chondrometrics GmbH, Ainring, Germany).

Sample size of the study

The sample size of n = 891 patients allows the probability of OA progression to be estimated with ±3.3% precision using a 95% confidence interval. Additionally, "protective" hazard ratios (HR) < = 0,6 associated with an haplogroup present in at least 10% of the population will be detected as statistically significant with 80% power using a significant level of 0,05. This assumes a censoring probability of 60%.

To analyze the four-year change in medial JSW in patients with unilateral medial JSN, n = 216 OA patients were included in the analysis. Assuming a standard deviation of ±1, this sample size will allow us to detect as statistically significant mean differences of 0.6 or higher for the less frequent haplogroup (n = 24), with 80% power and a significant level of 0.05

For the analysis of cartilage integrity from MRI, data on n = 381 patients are available. This sample size will allow to detect as statistically significant a standardized mean difference of 0,35 or higher in the variables analyzed between the most and the less frequent haplogroup (assuming a ratio 1:4), with a 95% confidence level and 80% statistical power.

Statistical analysis

Briefly, for the multivariate analysis of radiographic progression and MRI data, comparisons between haplogroups were performed considering the most common mtDNA haplogroup, H, as the reference group. Therefore, in order to introduce mtDNA haplogroups in the models, a dummy coding was used, with the haplogroup H as the reference group. Since there was no interest in all possible pair-wise comparisons, no additional adjusting for multiple comparisons was done.

Statistical analyses were performed using IBM-SPSS software, release 19 (IBM, Armonk, NY, USA) and R software v3.0.2 (The R Foundation for Statistical Computing). All comparisons were two-sided, with p<0.05 defined as statistically significant.

Analysis of radiographic progression. Because the status of a patient was prospectively evaluated at predefined intervals (12, 24, 36 and 48 months), the precise date at which progression occurred could not be determined; it always occurred between visits. Only the interval during which the conversion occurred was observed, therefore such information is said to be interval-censored [29].

To avoid potential biases associated with the use of standard survival analysis in this context, interval-censored data analysis methods were used [29]. Turnbull's extension of the Kaplan-Meier curve to interval-censored data was used to estimate the cumulative probability of progression over time (survivor function) according to the mtDNA haplogroups [30]. An extended Cox proportional hazard model using the iterative convex minorant algorithm was used for multivariate analysis adjusting for the confounder effects of gender, age, BMI, radiographic status of the worst knee (highest KL grade, highest JSN OARSI grade, highest osteophytes OARSI grade or highest sclerosis OARSI grade, as appropriate on each case) and previous surgery, all of them at baseline [31]. Due to difficulties in deriving the asymptotic behavior of statistic tests based on interval-censored data, statistical significance was tested by confidence intervals (CIs) for the hazard ratios (HR) by means of resampling methods. Therefore, CIs were obtained using the bootstrap methodology (1000 replicates) with the percentile method.

To analyze the influence of the mtDNA haplogroups on four-year change in medial JSW (mJSW) from baseline, we focused on patients with unilateral medial JSN and no JSN in the lateral compartment. The JSN knees and no-JSN knees were modeled separately. The mean comparison of the difference between mJSW at baseline and mJSW at final visit (4 years) was further performed by means of an analysis of covariance (ANCOVA) comparing each of the mtDNA haplogroups with the rest pooled together and adjusting for the confounder effects of gender, age and BMI at baseline. Previously, we tested for possible significant associations of the mtDNA haplogroups with KL grade and mJSN at baseline for both JSN and no-JSN knees in this cohort of (n = 216) patients by means of chi-square analyses. Additionally, the standardized response means (SRM), defined as the mean change divided by the standard deviation (SD) of change, was used to measure the sensitivity to change.

Analysis of MRI data in the OAI cohort. The parameters analyzed were those related to both cartilage volume and thickness in representative subregions of the joint (**Figure S2**). The parameters for cartilage volume were: cartilage volume in the medial tibia femoral compartment (MFTC.VC) and central medial femoral (cMF.VC) and normalized cartilage volume in the medial tibia femoral compartment (MFTC.VCtAB) and the central medial femoral (cMF.VCtAB). We also analyzed the mean cartilage thickness in the central medial tibia femoral compartment (weight bearing) (cMFTC.ThCtAB), medial tibia femoral compartment (MFTC.ThCtAB), medial tibia (anterior) (aMT.ThCtAB) and central medial femoral (center) (ccMF.ThCtAB).

The mean change (MC) and standard deviation (SD) of change between baseline (T_0) and 24 months (T_2) were used as a measure of progression. The SRM was used as a measure of sensitivity to change. The influence of mtDNA haplogroups on changes over time in quantitative MRI scans data, between T_0 and T_2, was evaluated though a linear mixed-effects random-intercept and random-slope repeated measures analysis [32]. This model assumes that patient effects (intercepts) and time effects (slopes—MRI data changes over time) are random among patients, taking into account the correlation among repeated measurements in the same individual. Regression coefficients were also estimated for the interaction between time and mtDNA haplogroup, allowing the rate of change to vary from one haplogroup to another. Models

Table 2. Cumulative probability of osteoarthritis progression according to mitochondrial DNA (mtDNA) haplogroups and results of the extended Cox proportional hazard model.

Variables	KL grade			JSN			Osteophytes			Subchondral sclerosis		
	N(%Progressors)*	HR	95% CI#	N(%Progressors)*	HR	95% CI#	N(%Progressors)*	HR	95% CI#	N(%Progressors)*	HR	95% CI#
Gender (male)		0.672	0.528–0.859*		1.006	0.755–1.335		0.843	0.650–1.081		1.021	0.791–1.343
Age (years)		1.011	0.999–1.024		0.998	0.982–1.013		0.993	0.980–1.007		1.008	0.994–1.023
BMI (Kg/m²)		1.045	1.020–1.069*		1.052	1.021–1.084*		1.028	1.004–1.055*		1.027	0.996–1.056
Previous surgery		0.909	0.702–1.190		0.686	0.487–0.909		0.981	0.739–1.282		1.054	0.788–1.378
Worst knee at bl±		0.937	0.687–1.305		4.993	3.700–7.373*		1.799	1.405–2.314*		1.396	1.050–1.827*
mtDNA haplogroups												
H (n=341)	145 (42.5%)	1		111 (32.6%)	1		164 (48.0%)	1		136 (39.8%)	1	
J (n=89)	40 (44.3%)	1.147	0.731–1.655	28 (31.4%)	0.891	0.581–1.404	45 (51.1%)	1.090	0.715–1.611	29 (32.5%)	0.764	0.487–1.230
Uk (n=228)	100 (44.1%)	0.986	0.760–1.356	64 (28.4%)	0.741	0.530–1.049	106 (46.8%)	0.906	0.684–1.203	66 (29.1%)	0.632	0.436–0.879
T (n=85)	19 (22.0%)	0.499	0.261–0.819*	17 (19.7%)	0.547	0.280–0.900*	25 (29.0%)	0.573	0.304–0.893*	21 (25.0%)	0.549	0.295–0.884*
Others (n=148)	53 (36.0%)	0.786	0.542–1.099	35 (23.7%)	0.699	0.445–1.051	50 (34.1%)	0.687	0.500–1.013	52 (35.1%)	0.847	0.563–1.220

KL: Kellgren and Lawrence; JSN: joint space narrowing; BMI: body mass index; bl: baseline; (*): cumulative osteoarthritis progression rate after 48 months of follow-up; HR: hazard ratio; CI: confidence interval; (#): confidence intervals for the hazard ratios obtained using the bootstrap methodology by the percentile method; (±): the worst knee at baseline refers to the radiological status of the knee attending to (highest) KL grade, JSN grade, osteophytes grade or sclerosis grade, as appropriate on each case; (*): statistical significance declared at p≤0.05.

Table 3. Mean differences in mJSW change over 4 years at minimum mJSW among the mitochondrial DNA (mtDNA) haplogroups in 216 OA patients.

mtDNA haplogroups	JSN knees (N = 216)			No-JSN knees (N = 216)		
	Mean change±SD	SRM	p-value[#]	Mean change±SD	SRM	p-value[#]
H (N = 87)	−0.52±0.68	−0.77	0.688	−0.56±1.07	−0.52	0.754
J (N = 24)	−0.75±0.86	−0.87	0.217	−0.62±0.78	−0.79	0.578
T (N = 24)	−0.56±0.77	−0.73	0.919	−0.14±0.37	−0.39	0.034*
Uk (N = 44)	−0.53±0.68	−0.77	0.995	−0.61±1.12	−0.59	0.336
Others (N = 37)	−0.48±0.68	−0.71	0.662	−0.45±0.65	−0.69	0.886

Data are mean±standard deviation, in millimetres (mm); mJSW: medial joint space width; JSN: joint space narrowing; SD: standard deviation; SRM: standardized response means (mean divided by SD); (#) multivariate (ANCOVA) analysis, adjusting for gender, age and body mass index (BMI) at baseline; (*) indicates statistical significance at $p \leq 0.05$.

were also adjusted for potential confounding factors, including age, gender and BMI.

Results

Influence of the mtDNA haplogroups on radiographic knee OA progression

No significant differences in baseline characteristics, including age, gender and BMI of the study population, as well as the radiographic variables at baseline, were detected among the different mtDNA haplogroups, even when analyzed the *worst knee* and the *less severe knee*, except for the presence of osteophytes in the worst knee (p = 0.047) (**Table 1**). The *worst knee* and the *less severe knee* at baseline were designated, respectively, as the knee with the highest and lowest KL grade, OARSI JSN grade, OARSI osteophytes grade or OARSI sclerosis grade, as appropriate on each case. We then analyzed the increase of KL grade in knee OA patients as well as the radiographic progression or development of JSN, osteophytes and subchondral sclerosis.

After adjusting for age, gender, BMI, previous surgery and radiographic status of the worst knee at baseline, the results showed that the percentage of patients that experienced any increase in the KL grade during the follow-up period was significantly lower in carriers of the mtDNA haplogroup T (HR = 0.499; 95% CI: 0.261–0.819; p<0.05); in addition, these patients also showed less development of JSN (HR = 0.547; 95% CI: 0.280–0.900; p<0.05), osteophytes (HR = 0.573; 95% CI: 0.304–0.893; p<0.05) and subchondral sclerosis (HR = 0.549; 95% CI: 0.295–0.884; p<0.05) (**Table 2**).

BMI at baseline was found to be a risk factor for radiographic progression (p<0.05) in terms, not only of KL grade (HR = 1.045; 95% CI: 1.020 – 1.069), but also JSN (HR = 1.052; 95% CI: 1.021–1.084) and osteophytes (HR = 1.028; 95% CI: 1.004–1.055) besides, radiographic status of worst knee at baseline significantly associates (p<0.05) with increased development of JSN (HR = 4.993; 95% CI: 3.700–7.373), osteophytes (HR = 1.799; 95% CI: 1.405–2.314) and sclerosis (HR = 1.396; 95% CI: 1.050–1.827) during the follow-up period; male gender was also associated with lower risk for disease progression (p<0.05) in terms of KL grade (HR = 0.672; 95% CI: 0.528–0.859) (**Table 2**).

The analysis of the influence of the mtDNA haplogroups on the rate of structural progression in no-JSN knees, assessed by means of the minimum mJSW, showed carriers of the mtDNA haplogroup T with the lowest decline over time (SRM = −0.39; p = 0.037) (**Table 3**). Additionally, no significant differences were detected in KL grade and mJSN at baseline, in both JSN and no-

JSN knees, among the mtDNA haplogroups in this cohort of 216 patients (data not shown).

Influence of the mtDNA haplogroups on knee cartilage integrity. Data from MRI

Longitudinal analysis of cartilage volume. A significant decline in knee cartilage volume over time was detected (p<0.001). Patients that carry the mtDNA haplogroup T showed significantly lower declines in volume over time in medial tibia femoral (p = 0.015) (MC = $-0.02 \times 10^3 \pm 0.12$ mm^3) and central medial femoral (p = 0.015) (MC = $-0.01 \times 10^3 \pm 0.08$ mm^3) compartments compared with the most common mtDNA haplogroup H (MC = $-0.11 \times 10^3 \pm 0.25$ mm^3 and $-0.07 \times 10^3 \pm 0.15$ mm^3, respectively). When the normalized cartilage volume (cartilage volume divided by total area of subchondral bone) of these two subregions was analyzed, the results obtained were similar and carriers of the mtDNA haplogroup T also showed significantly lower declines in normalized volume in medial tibia femoral (p = 0.023) (MC = -0.04 ± 0.12 mm) and central medial femoral (p = 0.031) (MC = -0.03 ± 0.10 mm) compartments (MC = -0.12 ± 0.25 mm and -0.08 ± 0.18 mm, respectively) (**Figure 1a**, **Table 4** and **Table S1**). No differences were found in the rate of change between mtDNA haplogroup H and the other mtDNA haplogroups.

Longitudinal analysis of cartilage thickness. A significant decline in cartilage thickness over time was observed (p<0.001). When compared with carriers of mtDNA haplogroup H, patients with haplogroup T had significantly lower declines in thickness over time in central medial tibia femoral (weight bearing) (MC = -0.08 ± 0.18 mm *versus* -0.24 ± 0.41 mm, p = 0.011), medial tibia femoral (MC = -0.04 ± 0.12 mm *versus* -0.13 ± 0.26 mm, p = 0.018), medial tibia (anterior) (MC = $+0.02 \pm 0.08$ mm *versus* -0.02 ± 0.10 mm, p = 0.013) and central medial femoral (center) (MC = -0.03 ± 0.14 mm *versus* -0.13 ± 0.29 mm, p = 0.013) compartments (**Figure 1b**, **Table 4** and **Table S1**). Similar to cartilage volume, no differences in the loss rate of knee cartilage thickness over time were detected between mtDNA haplogroup H and the other haplogroups.

Discussion

To our knowledge, this is the first study to use the well characterized follow-up OAI cohort to analyze the influence of genetic factors on disease progression. Specifically, this study attempts to analyze the influence of mtDNA haplogroups on the progression of knee OA. The results obtained reveal that patients

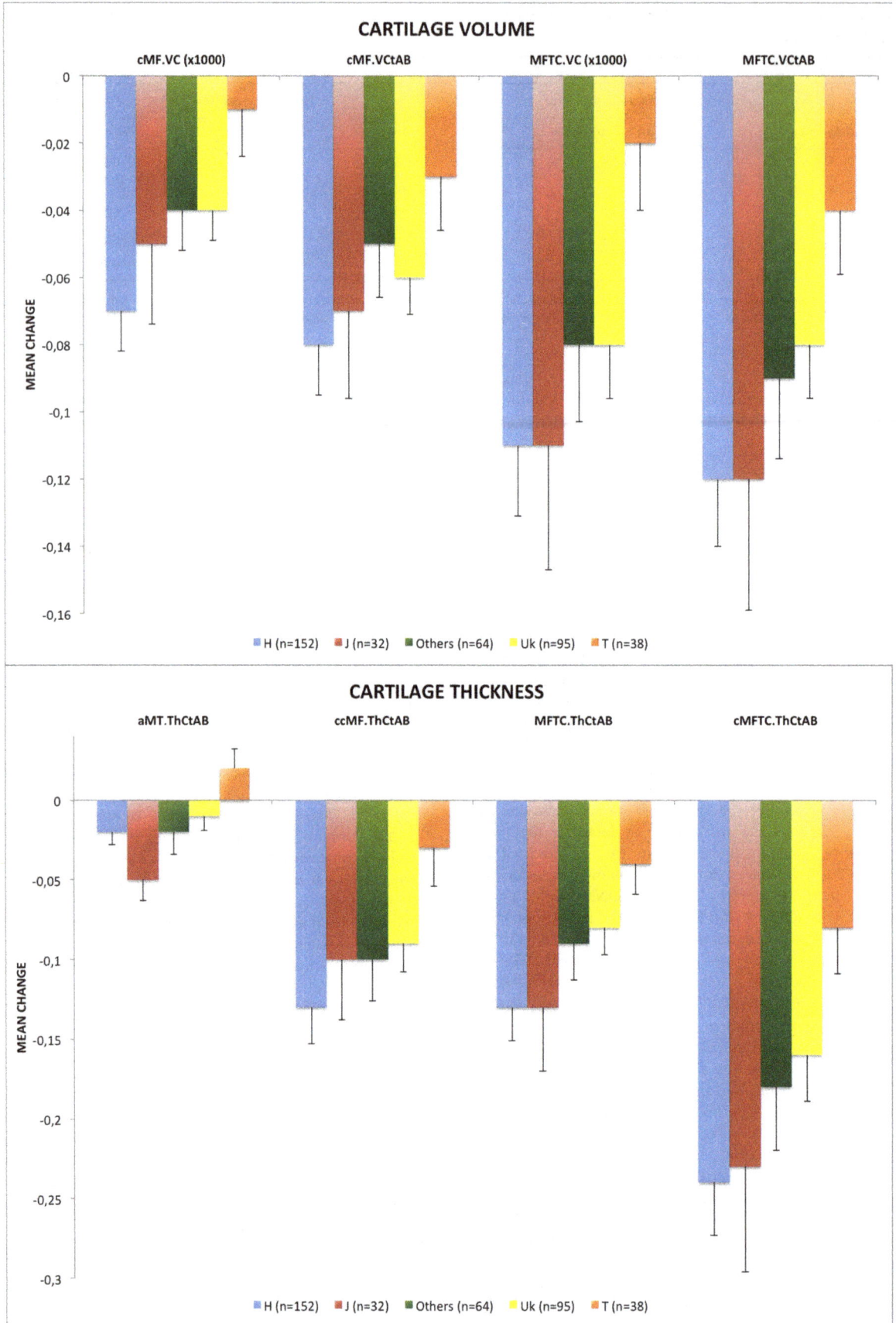

CARTILAGE VOLUME

CARTILAGE THICKNESS

Figure 1. Figure 1a. Longitudinal change between baseline and 24 months in cartilage volume grouped by mitochondrial DNA (mtDNA) haplogroups. MFTC.VCtAB: normalized cartilage volume in medial tibia femoral compartment; cMF.VCtAB: normalized cartilage volume in central medial femoral; MFTC.VC: cartilage volume in medial tibia femoral compartment; cMF.VC: volume of cartilage in central medial femoral. MFTC.VC and cMF.VC that are shown in cubic millimeters (mm3) and MFTC.VCtAB and cMF.VCtAB are shown in square centimeters (cm2); (*) indicates statistical significance (p<0.05). Values are mean change+SE (standard error). **Figure 1b.** Longitudinal change between baseline and 24 months in cartilage thickness grouped by mitochondrial DNA (mtDNA) haplogroups. cMFTC.ThCtAB: mean cartilage thickness in central medial tibia femoral compartment (weight-bearing); MFTC.ThCtAB: mean cartilage thickness in medial tibia femoral compartment; aMT.ThCtAB: mean cartilage thickness in medial tibia (anterior); ccMF.ThCtAB: mean cartilage thickness in central medial femoral (center). All of them represented in millimeters (mm); (*) indicates statistical significance (p<0.05). Values are mean change+SE (standard error).

in the progression subcohort carrying mtDNA haplogroup T show not only a significantly lower cumulative probability of progression in KL grade, but also less development of mJSN, osteophytes and subchondral sclerosis in the medial tibia. These observations were further strengthened by analyzing the evolution of cartilage integrity over two years showing a significantly reduced loss of knee cartilage thickness and volume in carriers of mtDNA haplogroup T too.

Previous findings reported in a Spanish cohort showed that patients with haplogroups belonging to cluster TJ had slower radiographic OA progression attending to KL grade [33]. Interestingly, an association study between haplogroups and OA prevalence in Spanish populations revealed a significant overrepresentation of the cluster TJ in radiological knee healthy subjects [6]. This association was further partially replicated in a larger cohort of hip OA patients from the same location, showing an association of the mtDNA haplogroup J with lower prevalence of hip OA [21]. Moreover, in another recent work, the mtDNA haplogroup T appeared overrepresented in knee healthy subjects from the United Kingdom after performing a regression model adjusting for gender and age [34].

To date, the study presented here is the first and most complete progression study involving the mtDNA haplogroups and OA using the cohort of the OAI; the results obtained should not be interpreted as discrepant in relation to previous findings, not only because this work does not analyze the association of mtDNA haplogroups with the prevalence of OA, but also because both above-mentioned mtDNA haplogroups T and J are considered "sister" haplogroups that share the same phylogenetic origin (the mtDNA cluster TJ) [35,36] that comprises a set of uncoupling mutations which, in combination with certain nuclear backgrounds, have been described to have common functional characteristics in their OXHPOS system such as decreased ATP production and reduced ROS generation [37–39].

A recent work by Hudson and co-workers found no evidence of an association between mtDNA variants and the prevalence of OA [40]. However, some points could explain this; first, as postulated by the authors, the relative contribution of specific mtDNA variants could vary in different ethnic groups by means of homoplasy and/or geographic differences in the finer details of sub-haplogroup structures of mtDNA [40]. In this sense, population-specific associations of the mtDNA haplogroups, probably due to their interaction with environmental factors [41] as a result of their adaptation to colder climates [35,36,42], have also been described [43,44]; second, as the authors describe in their manuscript, the GWAS study performed by the arcOGEN consortium also failed to replicate previous associations involving other genes described in OA at genome-wide significance levels, such as GDF5, chromosome 7q22 and MCF2L [45]; third, control samples from the arcOGEN study are only asymptomatic with no radiographic information, thus the selection of adequate healthy controls for association studies in the OA disease is a crucial for successfully conclusions.

The risk of structural progression in a knee without baseline JSN (no-JSN knee) is higher when the contralateral knee has already lost some space (JSN-knee); therefore, some authors suggest that the no-JSN knee would be the target knee in clinical trials because it would be expected to have less damage than a JSN knee but may have a significant progression over time due to the prevalence of contralateral JSN [46,47]. In order to evaluate the feasibility of detecting drug effects in clinical trials, we have quantified the mJSW following a similar approach to that described by Benichou and co-workers [48]. Results showed that OA patients with the mtDNA haplogroup T had lower rate of structural progression in no-JSN knees. These results point to take into consideration the mtDNA haplogroups when clinical trials in this population are performed.

The medial compartment is generally heavily loaded and knee OA affects this compartment more often than the lateral one [49,50]; therefore the analysis of MRI images carried out in this work was performed in regions/subregions that were previously characterized among the most sensitive to change in knee OA: the central medial tibia femoral compartment and medial tibia femoral compartment [28,51–54], as well as other regions of interest such as the central medial femoral condyle and medial tibia (anterior). The conclusion drawn is that OA patients carrying the mtDNA haplogroup T had a significantly lower decline of cartilage thickness and volume over time in these medial subregions.

A key part of the variation in different clinical forms of OA is attributable to genetics [55]. In relation to OA progression, previous studies by other investigators reported that genetic variants of genes, such as interleukin-1 receptor antagonist (IL1RN) [9,56,57] or cartilage intermediate-layer protein (CILP) [7], influence the severity and progression of OA. A functional polymorphism in the 5'-UTR of the growth differentiation factor-5 (GDF-5) gene has also been consistently associated with OA susceptibility and was part of a prediction model for knee OA based on genetic and clinical information [58,59]. The results of the present study strengthen the role of genetic variation, including mitochondrial genetics, in OA as previously described [1,3].

This study has some points that must be clarified; i) in relation to confounding factors, the analyses were finally adjusted for potential confounders such as age, gender, BMI and, in the radiographic progression, previous surgery and the radiographic status of the worst knee at baseline. Other predictors of OA occurrence or progression over time, such as bone marrow lesions or meniscal lesions, were also analyzed but finally not taken into account because of the small number of patients without missing data. On the other hand, ii) a key strength of this study is the analysis performed; the use of interval-censored data analysis to determine the probability of knee OA progression according to the mtDNA haplogroups avoids biases associated with the use of standard survival analysis in this context. Moreover, the use of linear mixed models in the analysis of MRI data allows us to take into account all available observations for each patient over time,

Table 4. Random-coefficients linear mixed model to analyze the influence of mtDNA haplogroups on change in cartilage volume (upper) and thickness (lower) over time in 381 knee OA patients in the progression subcohort of the OAI.

	Normalized cartilage volume in medial tibia femoral compartment			Normalized cartilage volume in central medial femoral			Cartilage volume in medial tibia femoral compartment			Cartilage volume in central medial femoral		
	B	SE	p-value[#]	B	SE	p-value[#]	B	SE	p-value[#]	B	SE	p-value[#]
Age	−0.011	0.003	0.001*	−0.008	0.002	<0.001*	−10.432	4.044	0.010*	−6.470	2.196	0.003*
Gender (Female)	−0.498	0.062	<0.001*	−0.294	0.042	<0.001*	−1211.529	71.933	<0.001*	−510.377	39.069	<0.001*
BMI	−0.008	0.006	0.193	−0.008	0.004	0.064	−0.34	7.543	0.964	−0.994	4.097	0.808
Haplogroup[†]												
H (n = 152)	0			0			0			0		
J (n = 32)	−0.239	0.120	0.047*	−0.173	0.080	0.032*	−353.483	135.435	0.009*	−191.118	74.039	0.010*
T (n = 38)	0.008	0.112	0.936	0.023	0.075	0.756	−66.358	126.596	0.600	−14.524	69.205	0.840
Uk (n = 95)	0.037	0.080	0.641	0.023	0.054	0.671	8.972	91.019	0.921	−6.14	49.759	0.902
Others (n = 64)	−0.112	0.092	0.222	−0.067	0.062	0.276	−239.768	103.953	0.022*	−120.847	56.828	0.034*
Time (years)	−0.061	0.008	<0.001*	−0.042	0.006	<0.001*	−57.915	8.369	<0.001*	−33.201	4.979	<0.001*
Time x Haplogroup*												
Time x H	0			0			0			0		
Time x J	0.002	0.020	0.927	0.008	0.014	0.552	1.708	20.069	0.932	5.474	11.940	0.647
Time x T	0.043	0.019	0.023*	0.029	0.013	0.030*	45.808	18.715	0.015*	27.020	11.134	0.015*
Time x Uk	0.021	0.013	0.121	0.013	0.010	0.155	17.160	13.495	0.204	11.489	8.029	0.153
Time x Others	0.016	0.015	0.292	0.015	0.011	0.183	18.899	15.375	0.219	13.807	9.148	0.132

	Mean cartilage thickness in central medial tibia femoral compartment			Mean cartilage thickness in medial tibia femoral compartment			Mean cartilage thickness in medial tibia (anterior)			Mean cartilage thickness in medial tibia			Mean cartilage thickness in central medial femoral (center)		
	B	SE	p-value[#]	B	SE	p-value[#]	B	SE	p-value[#]	B	SE	p-value[#]	B	SE	p-value[#]
Age	−0.012	0.005	0.022*	−0.011	0.003	0.002*	−0.011	0.003	0.002*	−0.007	0.003	0.042*			
Gender (Female)	−0.641	0.095	<0.001*	−0.481	0.063	<0.001*	−0.481	0.063	<0.001*	−0.377	0.059	<0.001*			
BMI	−0.018	0.010	0.077	−0.009	0.006	0.180	−0.010	0.006	0.180	−0.013	0.006	0.029			
Haplogroup[†]															
H (n = 152)	0			0			0			0			0		
J (n = 32)	−0.265	0.186	0.154	−0.226	0.121	0.062	−0.226	0.121	0.062	−0.188	0.114	0.998			
T (n = 38)	0.099	0.174	0.570	0.020	0.113	0.858	0.020	0.112	0.858	0.088	0.107	0.408			
Uk (n = 95)	0.102	0.125	0.412	0.044	0.081	0.585	0.044	0.081	0.585	0.041	0.077	0.592			
Others (n = 64)	−0.117	0.143	0.413	−0.105	0.093	0.260	−0.105	0.092	0.257	−0.043	0.088	0.623			
Time (years)	−0.119	0.014	<0.001*	−0.064	0.009	<0.001*	−0.064	0.009	<0.001*	−0.067	0.009	<0.001*			
Time x Haplogroup*															
Time x H	0			0			0			0			0		

Table 4. Cont.

	Mean cartilage thickness in central medial tibia femoral compartment			Mean cartilage thickness in central femoral compartment			Mean cartilage thickness in medial tibia (anterior)			Mean cartilage thickness in central medial femoral (center)		
	B	SE	p-value#	B	SE	p-value#	B	SE	p-value#	B	SE	p-value#
Time x J	0.006	0.034	0.852	0.001	0.021	0.970	0.001	0.021	0.969	0.018	0.023	0.424
Time x T	0.08⁻	0.032	0.011*	0.045	0.019	0.019*	0.045	0.019	0.018*	0.053	0.021	0.013*
Time x Uk	0.040	0.023	0.076	0.023	0.014	0.104	0.022	0.014	0.104	0.021	0.015	0.156
Time x Others	0.028	0.026	0.285	0.020	0.016	0.204	0.020	0.016	0.204	0.017	0.017	0.323

BMI: body mass index; B: regression coefficient; SE: standard error; (†) the coefficient of each haplogroup represents the mean difference between a particular haplogroup and the reference haplogroup and the reference haplogroup H at baseline; (¥) shows the interaction between the mtDNA haplogroups and the loss rate of cartilage volume and thickness over time; (#) linear mixed-effects random-intercept and random-slope repeated measures analysis adjusting for gender, age and BMI at baseline and considering the most common mtDNA haplogroup, H, as the reference group; (*): indicates statistical significance at $p \leq 0.05$.

therefore providing more accurate results and higher statistical power.

In summary, the results obtained in this work are of special interest because they show not only significant smaller longitudinal radiographic changes in patients carrying the mtDNA haplogroup T, but also significant lower decline in thickness and volume over time in weight bearing cartilage. A possible physiological explanation for these results, in line with what it was described above, is the mtDNA haplogroup T shows higher capacity to cope with oxidative stress than haplogroup H do [37] and oxidative stress is involved in the pathogenesis of OA [60]. This differential behavior is probably related with the origin of the mtDNA haplogroups, which are the result of a process of adaptive selection that permitted humans to adapt to colder climates when emigrated out from Africa [35,36]. Based on this theory, some of these mtDNA variants, specifically the mtDNA haplogroup H, are highly efficient in transforming the dietary calories into ATP, generating minimum heat and increased ROS; meanwhile, other mtDNA variants, such as mtDNA haplogroups T and J, are less efficient in converting dietary calories into ATP, therefore producing more heat and less ROS [61]. However, these mtDNA variants that have been critical for human adaptation to different global environments (not only temperature, but also changes in food or caloric supply, seasonal variation in climate or even infections) and would have favored survival and reproduction of populations residing in a particular climate zone might be maladaptive in a different environment with new lifestyles [62]. Hence, mtDNA haplogroups have been correlated with predisposition to a wide range of metabolic and degenerative diseases, obesity, cancers and longevity in a population-specific manner [42,63,64].

In conclusion, the results obtained in this work point to a possible role of mtDNA variation in the radiographic progression of OA and could improve identification of patients predisposed to faster or more severe progression of the disease. If further validated in additional prospective and well-characterized cohorts, the inclusion of mtDNA haplogroup assignment may also be useful for clinical trials.

Supporting Information

Figure S1 Sagittal RM images (DESSwe sequence) with the cartilage of MF being divided into cMF and pMF at 60% (left) and 75% (right) of the distance between the trochlear notch and the posterior end of the femoral condyle; MT: medial tibia; MF: medial femoral condyle; cMF: central (weight bearing) medial femoral condyle; pMF: posterior medial femoral condyle.

Figure S2 Representative subregions of the knee used to track changes in cartilage thickness and volume. cMF: central (weight-bearing) medial femoral condyle; MT: medial tibia; cLF: central (weight-bearing) lateral femoral condyle; LT: lateral tibia; ccMF: central subregion of central (weight-bearing) medial femur; cMFTC: central medial femoro-tibial compartment; cMT: central subregion of medial tibia; aMT: anterior subregion of medial tibia.

Table S1 Longitudinal change between baseline (T0) and 24 months (T2) in quantitative parameters of cartilage integrity (volume and thickness) grouped by mitochondrial DNA (mtDNA) haplogroups.

Table S2 Cross-sectional differences among the mitochondrial DNA (mtDNA) haplogroups in quantitative parameters of cartilage structure collected in an additional and different cohort of (n = 326) knee OA patients in the progression subcohort of the OAI with no follow-up (namely Project 18).

Acknowledgments

We would like to thank the participants, principal investigators, co-investigators and staff of the OAI.

References

1. Blanco FJ, Rego I, Ruiz-Romero C (2011) The role of mitochondria in osteoarthritis. Nature Reviews Rheumatology 7(3): 161–169.

2. Fernandez-Moreno M, Rego I, Carreira-Garcia V, Blanco FJ (2008) Genetics in Osteoarthritis. Current Genomics 9(8): 542–547.

3. Valdes AM, Spector TD (2011) Genetic epidemiology of hip and knee osteoarthritis. Nat Rev Rheumatol 7(1): 23–32.

4. Rego-Perez I, Fernandez-Moreno M, Soto-Hermida A, Fenandez-Lopez C, Oreiro N et al. (2013) Mitochondrial genetics and osteoarthritis. Front Biosci (Schol Ed) 5: 360–368.

5. Garnero P, Delmas PD (2003) Biomarkers in osteoarthritis. Curr Opin Rheumatol 15(5): 641–646.

6. Rego-Perez I, Fernandez-Moreno M, Fernandez-Lopez C, Arenas J, Blanco FJ (2008) Mitochondrial DNA haplogroups role in the prevalence and severity of knee osteoarthritis. Arthritis Rheum 58(8): 2387–2396.

7. Valdes AM, Hart DJ, Jones KA, Surdulescu G, Swarbrick P et al. (2004). Association study of candidate genes for the prevalence and progression of knee osteoarthritis. Arthritis Rheumatism 50(8): 2497–2507.

8. Kamarainen OP, Solovieva S, Vehmas T, Luoma K, Riihimaki H et al. (2008) Common interleukin-6 promoter variants associate with the more severe forms of distal interphalangeal osteoarthritis. Arthritis Res Ther 10(1): R21

9. Attur M, Wang HY, Kraus VB, Bukowski JF, Aziz N et al. (2010) Radiographic severity of knee osteoarthritis is conditional on interleukin 1 receptor antagonist gene variations. Arthritis Rheum 69(5): 856–861.

10. Cillero-Pastor B, Rego-Perez I, Oreiro N, Fernandez-Lopez C, Blanco FJ (2013) Mitochondrial respiratory chain dysfunction modulates metalloproteases -1, -3 and -13 in human normal chondrocytes in culture. BMC Musculoskelet Disord 14: 235.

11. Gavriilidis C, Miwa S, von Zglinicki T, Taylor RW, Young DA 2013 Mitochondrial dysfunction in osteoarthritis is associated with down-regulation of superoxide dismutase 2. Arthritis Rheumatism 65(2): 378–387.

12. Wu L, Liu H, Li L, Cheng Q, Li H et al. (2014) Mitochondrial Pathology in Osteoarthritic Chondrocytes. Curr Drug Targets 15(7): 710–719

13. Maneiro E, Martin MA, de Andres MC, Lopez-Armada MJ, Fernandez-Sueiro JL et al. (2003) Mitochondrial respiratory activity is altered in osteoarthritic human articular chondrocytes. Arthritis Rheumatism 48(3): 700–708.

14. Cillero-Pastor B, Carames B, Lires-Dean M, Vaamonde-Garcia C, Blanco FJ et al (2008). Mitochondrial dysfunction activates cyclooxygenase 2 expression in cultured normal human chondrocytes. Arthritis Rheumatism 58(8): 2409–2419.

15. Vaamonde-García C, Riveiro-Naveira RR, Valcárcel-Ares MN, Hermida-Carballo L, Blanco FJ et al. (2012) Mitochondrial dysfunction increases inflammatory responsiveness to cytokines in normal human chondrocytes. Arthritis Rheumatism 64(9): 2927–2936.

16. Kim HA, Blanco FJ (2007) Cell death and apoptosis in osteoarthritic cartilage. Curr Drug Targets 8(2): 333–345.

17. Blanco FJ, Lopez-Armada MJ, Maneiro E (2004) Mitochondrial dysfunction in osteoarthritis. Mitochondrion 4(5–6): 715–728.

18. Henrotin Y, Kurz B (2007) Antioxidant to treat osteoarthritis: dream or reality? Curr Drug Targets 8(2): 347–357.

19. Grishko VI, Ho R, Wilson GL, Pearsall AW (2009) Diminished mitochondrial DNA integrity and repair capacity in OA chondrocytes. Osteoarthritis Cartilage 17(1): 107–113.

20. Torroni A, Huoponen K, Francalacci P, Petrozzi M, Morelli L et al. (1996) Classification of European mtDNAs from an analysis of three European populations. Genetics 144(4): 1835–1850.

21. Rego I, Fernandez-Moreno M, Fernandez-Lopez C, Gomez-Reino JJ, Gonzalez A et al. (2010) Role of European mitochondrial DNA haplogroups in the prevalence of hip osteoarthritis in Galicia, Northern Spain. Ann Rheum Dis 69(1): 210–213

22. Fang H, Liu X, Shen L, Li F, Liu Y et al. (2014) Role of mtDNA haplogroups in the prevalence of knee osteoarthritis in a southern Chinese population. Int J Mol Sci 15(2): 2646–2659.

23. Rego-Perez I, Fernandez-Moreno M, Deberg M, Pertega S, Fenandez-Lopez C et al. (2010) Mitochondrial DNA haplogroups modulate the serum levels of biomarkers in patients with osteoarthritis. Ann Rheum Dis 69(5): 910–917.

24. Rego-Perez I, Fernandez-Moreno M, Deberg M, Pertega S, Fernandez-Lopez C et al. (2011) Mitochondrial DNA haplogroups and serum levels of proteolytic enzymes in patients with osteoarthritis. Ann Rheum Dis 70(4): 646–652.

25. Fernandez-Moreno M, Tamayo M, Soto-Hermida A, Mosquera A, Oreiro N et al. (2011) mtDNA Haplogroup J Modulates Telomere Length and Nitric Oxide Production. BMC Musculoskeletal Disord 12(1): 283–289

26. Altman RD, Hochberg M, Murphy WA, Wolfe F, Lequesne M (1995) Atlas of individual radiographic features in osteoarthritis. Osteoarthritis Cartilage 3 Suppl A: 3–70.

27. Eckstein F, Maschek S, Wirth W, Hudelmaier M, Hitzl W et al. (2009) One year change of knee cartilage morphology in the first release of participants from the Osteoarthritis Initiative progression subcohort: association with sex, body mass index, symptoms and radiographic osteoarthritis status. Ann Rheum Dis 68(5): 674–679.

28. Eckstein F, Kwoh CK, Boudreau RM, Wang Z, Hannon MJ et al. (2013) Quantitative MRI measures of cartilage predict knee replacement: a case-control study from the Osteoarthritis Initiative. Ann Rheum Dis 72(5): 707–714.

29. Sun J (2006) The statistical analysis of interval-censored failure time data. New York. Springer

30. Turnbull B (1976) The empirical distribution function with arbitrarily grouped, censored and truncated data. Journal of the Royal Statistical Society 38: 290–295.

31. Pan W (1999) Extending the iterative convex minorant algorithm to the Cox model for interval censored data. Journal of Computational and Graphical Statistics 8: 109–120.

32. Brown H, Prescott R (2006) Applied mixed models in medicine. Second Edition ed: Chichester.

33. Soto-Hermida A, Fernández-Moreno M, Pértega-Díaz S, Oreiro N, Fernández-López C et al. (2014) Mitochondrial DNA haplogroups modulate the radiographic progression of Spanish patients with osteoarthritis. Rheumatol Int Epub ahead of print

34. Soto-Hermida A, Fernandez-Moreno M, Oreiro N, Fernandez-Lopez C, Rego-Perez I, et al. (2014) mtDNA haplogroups and osteoarthritis in different geographic populations. Mitochondrion 15: 18–23.

35. Mishmar D, Ruiz-Pesini E, Golik P, Macaulay V, Clark AG et al. (2003) Natural selection shaped regional mtDNA variation in humans. Proc Natl Acad Sci U S A 1: 171–176.

36. Ruiz-Pesini E, Mishmar D, Brandon M, Procaccio V, Wallace DC (2004) Effects of purifying and adaptive selection on regional variation in human mtDNA. Science 303(5655): 223–226.

37. Mueller EE, Brunner SM, Mayr JA, Stanger O, Sperl W et al. (2012) Functional differences between mitochondrial haplogroup T and haplogroup H in HEK293 cybrid cells. PLoS One 7(12): e52367.

38. Kenney MC, Chwa M, Atilano SR, Falatoonzadeh P, Ramirez C et al. (2014) Molecular and bioenergetic differences between cells with African versus European inherited mitochondrial DNA haplogroups: Implications for population susceptibility to diseases. Biochim Biophys Acta 1842(2): 208–219.

39. Kenney MC, Chwa M, Atilano SR, Pavlis JM, Falatoonzadeh P et al. (2013) Mitochondrial DNA variants mediate energy production and expression levels for CFH, C3 and EFEMP1 genes: implications for age-related macular degeneration. PLoS One 8(1): e54339.

40. Hudson G, Panoutsopoulou K, Wilson I, Southam L, Rayner NW et al. (2013) No evidence of an association between mitochondrial DNA variants and osteoarthritis in 7393 cases and 5122 controls. Ann Rheum Dis 72(1): 136–139.

41. Domínguez-Garrido E, Martínez-Redondo D, Martín-Ruiz C, Gómez-Durán A, Ruiz-Pesini E et al. (2009) Association of mitochondrial haplogroup J and mtDNA oxidative damage in two different North Spain elderly populations. Biogerontology 10(4): 435–442.

42. Wallace DC, Ruiz-Pesini E, Mishmar D (2003) mtDNA variation, climatic adaptation, degenerative diseases, and longevity. Cold Spring Harb Symp Quant Biol 68: 479–486.

43. Herrnstadt C, Howell N (2004) An evolutionary perspective on pathogenic mtDNA mutations: haplogroup associations of clinical disorders. Mitochondrion 4(5–6): 791–798.

44. Dato S, Passarino G, Rose G, Altomare K, Bellizzi D et al. (2004) Association of the mitochondrial DNA haplogroup J with longevity is population specific. Eur J Hum Genet 12(12): 1080–1082.

45. Zeggini E, Panoutsopoulou K, Southam L, Rayner NW, Day-Williams AG et al. (2012) Identification of new susceptibility loci for osteoarthritis (arcOGEN): a genome-wide association study. Lancet 380(9844): 815–823.

46. Mazzuca SA, Brandt KD, Katz BP, Ding Y, Lane KA et al. (2006). Risk factors for progression of tibiofemoral osteoarthritis: an analysis based on fluoroscopically standardised knee radiography. Ann Rheum Dis 65(4): 515–519.

47. Le Graverand MP, Vignon EP, Brandt KD, Mazzuca SA, Piperno M et al. (2008). Head-to-head comparison of the Lyon Schuss and fixed flexion radiographic techniques. Long-term reproducibility in normal knees and sensitivity to change in osteoarthritic knees. Ann Rheum Dis 67(11): 1562–1566.

Author Contributions

Conceived and designed the experiments: IRP FJB. Performed the experiments: ASH MFM ECP NO CFL. Analyzed the data: IRP FJB SP. Contributed reagents/materials/analysis tools: ASH MFM NO CFL ECP. Wrote the paper: IRP FJB.

48. Benichou OD, Hunter DJ, Nelson DR, Guermazi A, Eckstein F et al. (2010) One-year change in radiographic joint space width in patients with unilateral joint space narrowing: data from the Osteoarthritis Initiative. Arthritis Care Res 62(7): 924–931.

49. Ledingham J, Regan M, Jones A, Doherty M (1993) Radiographic patterns and associations of osteoarthritis of the knee in patients referred to hospital. Ann Rheum Dis. 52(7): 520–526.

50. Zhao D, Banks SA, D'Lima DD, Colwell CW, Fregly BJ (2007) In vivo medial and lateral tibial loads during dynamic and high flexion activities. J Orthop Res 25(5): 593–602.

51. Wirth W, Hellio Le Graverand MP, Wyman BT, Maschek S, Hudelmaier M et al. (2009) Regional analysis of femorotibial cartilage loss in a subsample from the Osteoarthritis Initiative progression subcohort. Osteoarthritis Cartilage 17(3): 291–297.

52. Wirth W, Nevitt M, Hellio Le Graverand MP, Benichou O, Dreher D et al. (2010) Sensitivity to change of cartilage morphometry using coronal FLASH, sagittal DESS, and coronal MPR DESS protocols–comparative data from the Osteoarthritis Initiative (OAI). Osteoarthritis Cartilage 18(4): 547–554.

53. Eckstein F, Nevitt M, Gimona A, Picha K, Lee JH et al. (2011) Rates of change and sensitivity to change in cartilage morphology in healthy knees and in knees with mild, moderate, and end-stage radiographic osteoarthritis: results from 831 participants from the Osteoarthritis Initiative. Arthritis Care Res 63(3): 311–319.

54. Eckstein F, Wirth W, Nevitt MC (2012) Recent advances in osteoarthritis imaging–the osteoarthritis initiative. Nat Rev Rheumatol 8(10): 622–630.

55. Zhai G, Hart DJ, Kato BS, MacGregor A, Spector TD (2007) Genetic influence on the progression of radiographic knee osteoarthritis: a longitudinal twin study. Osteoarthritis Cartilage 15(2): 222–225.

56. Kerkhof HJ, Doherty M, Arden NK, Abramson SB, Attur M et al. (2011) Large-scale meta-analysis of interleukin-1 beta and interleukin-1 receptor antagonist polymorphisms on risk of radiographic hip and knee osteoarthritis and severity of knee osteoarthritis. Osteoarthritis Cartilage 19(3): 265–271.

57. Wu X, Kondragunta V, Kornman KS, Wang HY, Duff GW et al. (2013) IL-1 receptor antagonist gene as a predictive biomarker of progression of knee osteoarthritis in a population cohort. Osteoarthritis Cartilage 21(7): 930–938.

58. Miyamoto Y, Mabuchi A, Shi D, Kubo T, Takatori Y et al. (2007) A functional polymorphism in the 5′ UTR of GDF5 is associated with susceptibility to osteoarthritis. Nat Genet 39(4): 529–533.

59. Takahashi H, Nakajima M, Ozaki K, Tanaka T, Kamatani N et al. (2010) Prediction model for knee osteoarthritis based on genetic and clinical information. Arthritis Res Ther 12(5): R187

60. Suantawee T, Tantavisut S, Adisakwattana S, Tanavalee A, Yuktanandana P et al. (2013) Oxidative stress, vitamin e, and antioxidant capacity in knee osteoarthritis. J Clin Diagn Res 7(9): 1855–1859.

61. Wallace DC (2013) Bioenergetics in human evolution and disease: implications for the origins of biological complexity and the missing genetic variation of common diseases. Philos Trans R Soc Lond B Biol Sci 368(1622): 20120267.

62. Wallace DC (2005) A mitochondrial paradigm of metabolic and degenerative diseases, aging, and cancer: a dawn for evolutionary medicine. Annu Rev Genet 39: 359–407.

63. Gómez-Durán A, Pacheu-Grau D, López-Gallardo E, Díez-Sánchez C, Montoya J et al. (2010) Unmasking the causes of multifactorial disorders: OXPHOS differences between mitochondrial haplogroups. Hum Mol Genet 19(17): 3343–3353.

64. Nardelli C, Labruna G, Liguori R, Mazzaccara C, Ferrigno M et al. (2013) Haplogroup T is an obesity risk factor: mitochondrial DNA haplotyping in a morbid obese population from southern Italy. Biomed Res Int 631082.

16

Percutaneous Resolution of Lumbar Facet Joint Cysts as an Alternative Treatment to Surgery

Feng Shuang[1,2], Shu-Xun Hou[1]*, Jia-Liang Zhu[1], Dong-Feng Ren[1], Zheng Cao[1], Jia-Guang Tang[1]*

1 Department of Orthopaedics, The First Affiliated Hospital of General Hospital of Chinese PLA, Beijing, China, **2** Department of Orthopedics, The 94th Hospital of Chinese PLA, Nanchang, China

Abstract

Purpose: A comprehensive review of the literature in order to analyze data about the success rate of percutaneous resolution of the lumbar facet joint cysts as a conservative management strategy.

Methods: A systematic search for relevant articles published during 1980 to May 2014 was performed in several electronic databases by using the specific MeSH terms and keywords. Most relevant data was captured and pooled for the meta-analysis to achieve overall effect size of treatment along with 95% confidence intervals.

Results: 29 studies were included in the meta-analysis. Follow-up duration as mean $\pm$ sd (range) was 16$\pm$10.2 (5 days to 5.7 years). Overall the satisfactory results (after short- or long-term follow-up) were achieved in 55.8 [49.5, 62.08] % (pooled mean and 95% CI) of the 544 patients subjected to percutaneous lumbar facet joint cyst resolution procedures. 38.67 [33.3, 43.95] % of this population underwent surgery subsequently to achieve durable relief. There existed no linear relationship between the increasing average duration of follow-up period of individual studies and percent satisfaction from the percutaneous resolutions procedure.

Conclusion: Results shows that the percutaneous cyst resolution procedures have potential to be an alternative to surgical interventions but identification of suitable subjects requires further research.

Editor: Sam Eldabe, The James Cook University Hospital, United Kingdom

Funding: This work was supported by the National Natural Science Foundation of China (No. 81071514). The funders had no role in study design, data collection and analysis, decision to publish, or preparation of the manuscript.

Competing Interests: The authors have declared that no competing interests exist.

* Email: jiaguangtang@yahoo.com.cn (JGT); houshuxun_2000@163.com (SXH)

Introduction

Facet joint cysts of lumbar spine (LFJCs) are benign degenerative outgrowths which are most usually associated with low back pain and radiculopathy. Two types of cysts recognized under this category are the synovial cysts and ganglion cysts [1]. The synovial cysts have vascularized lining filled with xanthochromic fluid and have communication with facet joint while the ganglion cysts are covered by fibrocartilagenous capsule filled with proteinaceous and gelatinous material and do not communicate with joint [2].

These cysts can arise because of the chronic hypermobility of the spinal segments leading to increased and more frequent loading of the zygapophyseal joint (Z-joint; a synovial joint). This causes the accumulation of fibrocartilaginous substances which provide raw material for cyst formation [3,4]. The Z-joint is thought to be involved in the genesis of cysts owing to a degenerative process, not fully understood, though herniation of synovial tissue is frequently perceived [5–7]. The LFJCs are associated with spinal stenosis, nerve root compression, neurogenic claudication and many other neurological disturbances by encroaching the local foramen [8,9].

Although, small scale studies indicate that the prevalence of LFJCs in symptomatic patients is 0.7 to 2.5% (Ayberg et al., 2008) [10], but it may be higher and even increase with increasing longevity. This neuropathological agent is strongly associated with late decades of life and females harbor more than males [1].

Diagnosis of the LFJCs utilize magnetic resonance imaging (MRI) or computed tomography (CT) and to some extent CT myelography. Seldom these cysts resolve spontaneously; mostly require treatment. Various management strategies include bed rest, non-steroidal anti-inflammatory drugs, analgesics, physical therapies, transcutaneous electrical nerve stimulation (TENS), intra-articular steroid injections/epidural steroid instillation with or without cyst rupture and CT or flouroscopy guided aspiration of the cyst materials and surgical interventions such as laminectomy, facetectomy, flavectomy, cyst excision and microsurgery.

Long term relief from the symptoms associated with the LFJCs can be achieved with surgery or percutaneous resolution procedures, however. Surgery is the most effective treatment noted so far but studies indicate that percutaneous cyst resolution procedures can be an alternative to surgery in a well-sized subgroup of patients. Moreover, older and high risk patients who are abstained from surgical interventions due to many reasons can

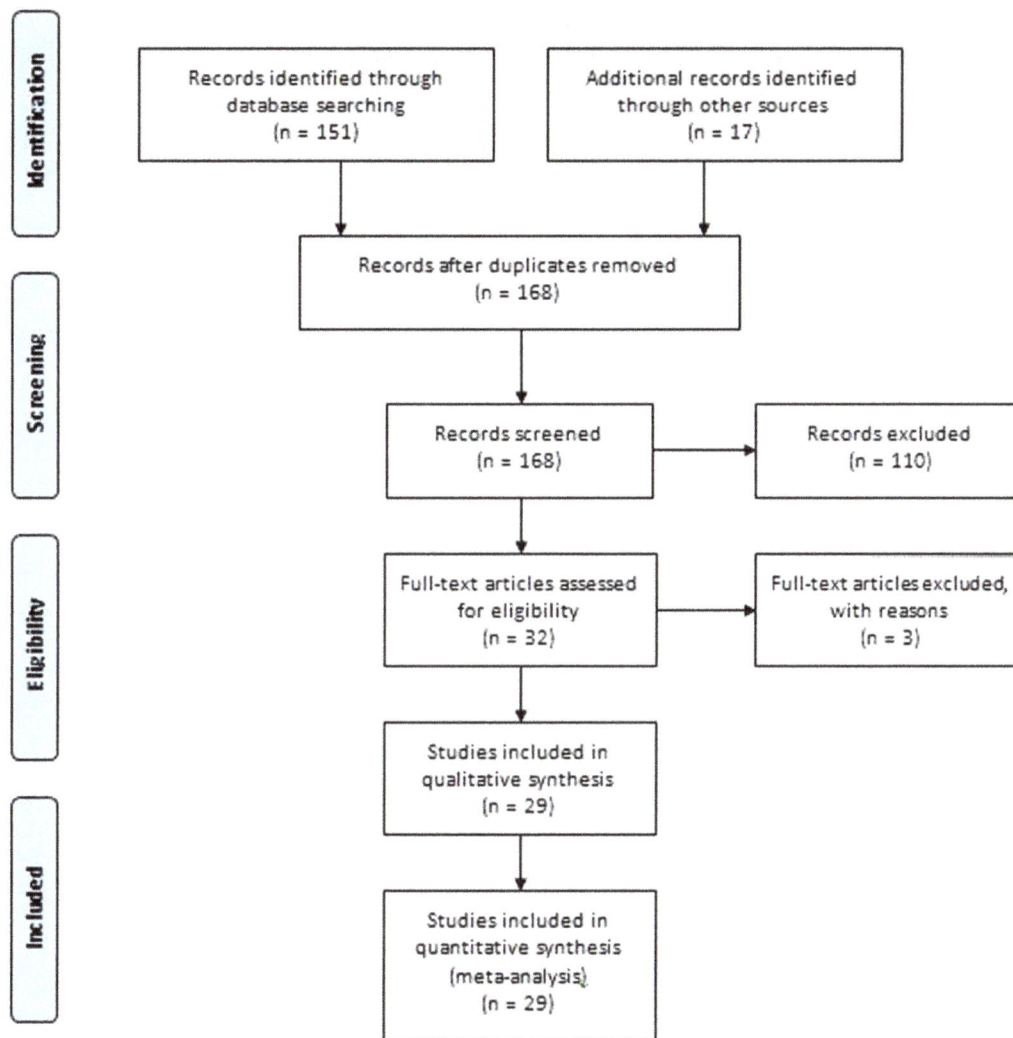

Figure 1. Flowchart of study screening and selection process.

also be benefited from later treatment regimen. In order to explore this avenue, this systematic review and meta-analysis is conducted to evaluate the success rate of percutaneous cyst resolution procedures in terms of durable relief and to attempt the identification of subgroup of patients in which chances success with this technique can be better than surgical intervention.

Materials and Methods

Study Identification

Detailed systematic search was made in several electronic databases including PubMed/Medline, Embase, EBSCO, CINAHL, Ovid SP, SCI Web of Science and Google Scholar under most relevant keywords. MeSH terms and keywords used in various logical combinations included: spinal, lumbar, cyst, synovial, ganglion, juxtafacet, facet, zygapophyseal, magnetic resonance imaging (MRI), computed tomography (CT), conservative management, percutaneous, puncture, rupture, steroid, injection, intra-articular, epidural, facet, joint, effusion. Literature search was restricted to a period from 1980 to May 2014. All retrospective analyses, prospective studies, and individual case reports were taken into consideration.

Selection criteria

The PRISMA guidelines were followed for this study. Because of the scarcity of well-designed clinical trials, selection of studies was made under a broader scope and all studies with prospective or retrospective designs and case reports were included. Inclusion criteria were: a) Studies mentioning percutaneous resolution procedures of LFJCs (synovial/ganglion) such as steroid injections, cyst rupture and cyst material aspiration by utilizing CT/ fluoroscopically guided instrumentation; b) studies mentioning a short-term or long-term follow-up of the outcomes and related details, including the provision of data of the subjects who underwent surgical procedures in case of failure of the interventions. Exclusion criteria were: a) studies/case reports intervening other types of similar spinal cyst pathologies such as discal cysts, vertebroplasty etc; b) studies involving percutaneous procedures for the purpose of diagnosis only; and c) studies/case reports utilizing percutaneous procedures for the alleviation of back pain without a diagnosis of LFJC/s; d) studies/case reports which did not contain sufficient details of the outcomes of interventions of interest.

Table 1. Quality Assessment Tool for Observational Cohort and Cross-Sectional Studies.

Criteria	12	13	14	15	16	17	18	19	20	21	22	23	24	25
1. Was the research question or objective in this paper clearly stated?	Y	Y	Y	Y	Y	Y	Y	Y	Y	Y	Y	Y	Y	Y
2. Was the study population clearly specified and defined?	Y	Y	Y	Y	Y	Y	Y	Y	Y	Y	Y	Y	Y	Y
3. Was the participation rate of eligible persons at least 50%?	Y	Y	Y	Y	Y	Y	Y	Y	Y	Y	Y	Y	Y	Y
4. Were all the subjects selected or recruited from the same or similar populations (including the same time period)? Were inclusion and exclusion criteria for being in the study prespecified and applied uniformly to all participants?	Y	Y	Y	Y	Y	Y	Y	Y	Y	Y	Y	Y	Y	Y
5. Was a sample size justification, power description, or variance and effect estimates provided?	N	N	N	N	N	N	Y	N	N	N	N	Y	N	N
6. For the analyses in this paper, were the exposure(s) of interest measured prior to the outcome(s) being measured?	NA	NA	NA	NA	NA	NA	NA	NA	NA	NA	NA	NA	NA	NA
7. Was the timeframe sufficient so that one could reasonably expect to see an association between exposure and outcome if it existed?	N	N	N	Y	Y	N	N	N	Y	N	N	N	N	N
8. For exposures that can vary in amount or level, did the study examine different levels of the exposure as related to the outcome (e.g., categories of exposure, or exposure measured as continuous variable)?	Y	Y	NA	Y	Y	NA	Y	Y	Y	Y	Y	Y	Y	Y
9. Were the exposure measures (independent variables) clearly defined, valid, reliable, and implemented consistently across all study participants?	Y	Y	Y	Y	Y	Y	Y	Y	Y	Y	Y	Y	Y	Y
10. Was the exposure(s) assessed more than once over time?	Y	Y	Y	Y	Y	NR	Y	Y	Y	Y	Y	NR	Y	NR
11. Were the outcome measures (dependent variables) clearly defined, valid, reliable, and implemented consistently across all study participants?	N	N	N	Y	Y	N	Y	N	Y	N	N	N	N	N
12. Were the outcome assessors blinded to the exposure status of participants?	N	N	N	N	N	N	N	N	N	N	N	N	N	N
13. Was loss to follow-up after baseline 20% or less?	CD	CD	CD	CD	CD	CD	CD	CD	CD	CD	CD	CD	CD	CD
14. Were key potential confounding variables measured and adjusted statistically for their impact on the relationship between exposure(s) and outcome(s)?	N	N	N	N	Y	N	Y	N	N	N	N	N	N	N

Legends: CD: Cannot be determined, NA: not applicable, NR: not reported, N: no, Y: yes.

Data extraction, synthesis and analysis

Data were extracted from each research article/case report regarding the demographics of patients, clinical and pathological characteristics, diagnostic tools, procedural features, follow-up period, and outcomes. Outcome measures were the percent satisfactory response of the patient after a reasonable follow-up and the percentage of patients who subsequently underwent surgery. Pooling of dichotomous data (satisfactory outcomes vs surgery requirement) was made by calculating standard errors and 95% confidence intervals (CI) of the data from individual studies and then overall effect size of the meta-analysis was calculated. Forest graphs were plotted manually on the spreadsheets from pooled data and the overall effect size. Descriptive data are presented as mean along with either standard deviation (sd) or range. Quality of the included studies was assessed by using Quality Assessment Tool for Observational Cohort and Cross-Sectional Studies [11].

Results

Search identified 29 articles [12–40] reporting 12 retrospective studies, 2 prospective studies and 15 case reports which are included in this analytical review. Study screening and selection process has been depicted in Figure 1. Quality assessment outcomes are presented in Table 1.

Major characteristics relevant to the manifesto of the present study are present in Table 2. Overall of the 544 subjects included in this meta-analysis, age of the participants as mean $\pm$ sd (range) was 62 ± 4.2 (28–87) years and proportion of females in this population was 64%. Spinal level of the cysts was L_{2-3} in 10, L_{3-4} in 69, L_{4-5} in 384 and L_5–S_1 in 96 cases (Figure 2). Size of the cyst ranged from 6×13 to 12×18 mm. Duration of symptoms before percutaneous resolution interventions ranged from 2 weeks to 60 months. Major conditions associated with the presence of LFJCs in these patients were lower back pain and radiculopathy, especially lower extremity radiculopathy. Symptomatic features at clinical presentation are presented in Table 3.

The procedures involved cyst puncture, rupture, aspiration, intra-articular steroid injection, epidural steroid injection, and local anesthetics injections. These procedures were performed under CT/fluoroscopic guidance, though, not all studies utilized each of these interventions. Arthrography was also performed in majority of cases. Majority of the subjects were diagnosed with MRI (about 85% vs CT about 15%) for harboring one or more

Table 2. Characteristics of the included studies which utilized percutaneous resolution of lumber facet joint cyst procedures.

Study/Design	Patients' characteristics	Pathology	Diagnosis	Intervention	Follow up	Outcome
Allen et al., 2009 [12]/ Retrospective cohort	n: 32; age: 66 (46–86) y; females: 18; Location (L$_{3-4}$/L$_{4-5}$/L$_5$–S$_1$): 2/22/8 (left 18, right 13, bilateral 1)	LBP/LER since 5 mo	MRI	FCR/ESI	12 (6–24) mo	Satisfactory: 19 (60%), Repeats: 11 (34%), Required Surgery: 6 (19%)
Amoretti et al., 2012 [13]/ prospective	n: 120; age: 68.2 (52–84) y; Location (L$_{3-4}$/L$_{4-5}$/L$_5$–S$_1$): 16/84/20; VAS change; mean ± sd: 7.2±1.2 to 2.9±1.2	Disabling LBP/radiculopathy	MRI	CTISI	12 mo	Satisfactory: 90 (75%), Repeats: 43 (36%), Required Surgery: 30 (25%)
Bjorkengren et al., 1987 [14]/ prospective	n: 3; age: 59 (44, 56 & 77) y; females: 2; Location: L$_{4-5}$ in all	LBP/LER	CT	CTISI	11 (6–14) mo	Satisfactory: 2 partially, Repeats: 1, Required surgery: 1/refused
Bureau et al., 2001 [17]/ retrospective	n: 12; age: 60 (45–79) y; females: 8; Location (L$_{3-4}$/L$_{4-5}$/L$_5$–S$_1$): 1/10/1; Cyst size: 11×13.6 (6–13×8–19)mm	LBP/radiculopathy	MRI	FCR/SI	23 (12–36) mo	Satisfactory: 9 (75%), Repeats: 7 (58%), Required Surgery: 3 (25%)
Cambron et al., 2013 [18]/ retrospective	n: 110; age: 63 (28–87) y; females: 71; Location (L$_{2-3}$/L$_{3-4}$/L$_{4-5}$/L$_5$–S$_1$): 6/17/89/22; Cyst size: 10.6 mm/intensity: H 48/L 65	LER	MRI	CT-guided FCR/SI	34 (7–93) mo	Satisfactory: 63 (57%), Repeats: 40 (36%), Required Surgery: 47 (43%)
Carrera, 1980 [19]/retrospective	n: 20; age (mean): 54 y; females: 12; Location (L$_{2-3}$/L$_{3-4}$/L$_{4-5}$/L$_5$–S$_1$): NA	LBP/symptomatic facet arthropathy	CT	IAFB	6–12 mo	Satisfactory: 6 (30%), Repeats: NA, Required Surgery: NA
Martha et al., 2009 [30]/ retrospective	n: 101; age: 59.8±1.3 y; females: 69; Location (L$_{2-3}$/L$_{3-4}$/L$_{4-5}$/L$_5$–S$_1$): 2/9/69/21	LBP/LER	MRI	FCR/SI	3.2±1.3 y (mean ± sd)	Satisfactory: 46 (46%), Repeats: 51 (51%), Required Surgery: 55 (55%)
Ortiz & Tekchandani, 2013 [32]/ retrospective	n: 20; age: 65.5 y average; females: 9; Location (L$_{2-3}$/L$_{3-4}$/L$_{4-5}$/L$_5$–S$_1$): 1/5/11/4; Cyst size: 7.3 (3–14) mm	LBP/LER	NA	CTISI/aspiration	18 (4–24)	Satisfactory: 18 (90%), Repeats: 4 (20%), Required Surgery: 2 (10%)
Parlier-Cuau et al., 1999 [33]/ retrospective	n: 30; age: 67 (44–82) y; females: 21; Location (L$_{2-3}$/L$_{3-4}$/L$_{4-5}$/L$_5$–S$_1$): 1/3/25/1; Symptom duration: at least 6 mo	Sciatic/femoral pain	CT: 27/MRI: 3/ arthrography	FISI	26 (8–50) mo	Satisfactory: 14 (47%), Repeats: 7 (23%), Required Surgery: 14 (47%)
Sabers et al., 2005 [35]/ retrospective	n: 23; age: 64 (28–81) y; females: 12; Location (L$_{3-4}$/L$_{4-5}$/L$_5$–S$_1$): 1/15/7; Symptom duration: 10.5 (2 wk–48 mo)	LBP/LER	MRI	FISI/aspiration	9.1 (1.5–21) mo	Satisfactory: 9 (50%), Repeats: 2 (1–4) per subject, Required Surgery: 9 (50%)
Sauvage et al., 2000 [36]/ retrospective	n: 13; age: 63 (42–87) y; females: 9; Location (L$_{3-4}$/L$_{4-5}$/L$_5$–S$_1$): 1/8/4; Cyst size: 9 (5–11) mm; largest 12×18 mm	radiculopathy	MRI	CTISI	9 (2–25) mo	Satisfactory: 6 (46%), Repeats: 6 (46%), Required Surgery: 3 (23%)
Schulz et al 2011 [37]/ prospective	n: 20; age: median 54.5 y; females: 17; Location (L$_{3-4}$/L$_{4-5}$/L$_5$–S$_1$): 1/19/0; Symptom duration: median 10.5 mo	radiculopathy	CT	CTISI	24 mo	Satisfactory: 8 (40%), Repeats: NA, Required Surgery: 12 (60%)
Shah and Lutz, 2003 [38]/ retrospective	n: 10; age: 60 (53–70) y; females: 8; Location (L$_{3-4}$/L$_{4-5}$/L$_5$–S$_1$): 0/8/2; Symptom duration: 7.9 (1–30) mo	LBP/LER	CT/MRI	FISI/aspiration/ESI	11.5 (3–30) mo	Satisfactory: 1 (10%), Repeats: 1 (10%), Required Surgery: 8 (80%)
Slipman et al., 2000 [40]/ retrospective	n: 14; age: 60.2 (39–87) y; females: 7; Location (L$_{3-4}$/L$_{4-5}$/L$_5$–S$_1$): 2/10/2; Symptom duration: 18.8 (3–60) mo	radiculopathy	CT/MRI	FISI/aspiration	1.4 (1–3) y	Satisfactory: 4 (40%), Repeats: NA, Required Surgery: 8(58%)
Case Reports						
Boissiere et al., 2013 [15]	57 y old male with cyst at L$_{4-5}$	Sciatica since 24 mo	CT	CTISI	6 mo	surgery (decompression + fusion)
Braza et al., 2005 [16]	48 y old man with cyst at L$_{4-5}$ (7 mm)	Thigh and calf pain (7 mo)	MRI	FISI/aspiration	2 mo	80% improvement in pain relief
Casselman et al 1985 [20]	65 y old woman with cyst at L$_{4-5}$	LBP/LER	CT	Intra-articular SI	3 mo	Underwent surgery

Table 2. Cont.

Study/Design	Patients' characteristics	Pathology	Diagnosis	Intervention	Follow up	Outcome
Chang et al 2009 [21]	63 y old woman with cyst at L5-S1 (7 mm)	Left-sided radiculopathy	MRI	CT-guided FISI	1 mo	Satisfactory relief
Foley, 2009 [22]	44 y old man with cyst at L4-5	LBP	MRI	FISI/rupture	1 mo	Satisfactory relief (0/10 VAS)
Gishen & Mill., 2001 [23]	65 y old woman with cyst at L5-S1	Hip osteoarthritis/left sciatica	MRI	CTISI/ESI	12 mo	Satisfactory (asymptomatic)
Hong et al., 1995 [24]	51 y old woman with cyst at L4-5	LBP/right knee pain (6 mo)	MRI	FCA, no SI	6 mo	Satisfactory (asymptomatic)
Imai et al., 1998 [25]	77/55 y old women with cysts at L4-5/L3-4	LBP/LER (15 mo/10 mo)	MRI	FISI/aspiration	5 d/2 mo	surgery for durable relief (both)
Kozar & Jer. 2014 [26]	77 y old man with cyst at L4-5 (3×5 mm)	LBP/LER (3 y)	MRI	CTISI/rupture	1 mo	Partial relief/surgery not feasible
Lim et al., 2001 [27]	67 y old woman with cyst at L4-5	LBP/right LER	MRI	CTISI	9 mo	Satisfactory (asymptomatic)
Lin et al, 2014 [28]	52 y old man with cyst at L4-5	LBP/right LER since 10 mo	MRI	UISI	18 mo	Satisfactory (asymptomatic)
Lutz and Shen, 2002 [29]	48 y old woman; cyst at L4-5 (7×15 mm)	LBP/right LER (4 mo)	MRI	FCA, no SI	1 mo	Satisfactory (asymptomatic)
Melfi & Aprill, 2005 [31]	72 y old woman with cyst at L4-5/L5-S1	Chronic LBP/LER (7 mo)	MRI	FISI	30 mo	Satisfactory (asymptomatic)
Rauchwerger 2011 [34]	70 y old woman with cyst at L5-S1	LBP/radiculopathy (1 y)	MRI	FISI	1 day	Partial relief
Shin et al., 2012 [39]	51 y old man with cyst at L4-5	LBP/LER (1mo)	MRI	FISI/aspiration	6 mo	Satisfactory (asymptomatic)

Values are presented as mean (range) unless otherwise stated. Abbreviations: CTISI (CT-guided Intra-cystic/Intra-articular SI), ESI (epidural SI), FCA (fluoroscopically-guided cyst aspiration), FCR (fluoroscopically guided cyst rupture), FISI (fluoroscopic intra-articular SI), IAFB (intra-articular facet block), LBP (lower back pain), LER (lower extremity radiculopathy), mo (month/s), NA (not available), SI (steroid injection), wk (week/s), y (year/s).

LFJCs. Cyst rupture outcomes were assessed by the loss of resistance method or by the extravasation of dye.

Follow-up duration as mean ± sd (range) was 16±10.2 (5 days to 5.7 years). Overall the satisfactory results (after short- or long-term follow-up) were achieved in 55.8 [49.5, 62.08] % (pooled mean and 95% CI) of the 544 patients subjected to percutaneous lumbar cyst resolution procedures (Figure 3). Repeat procedures were performed in 115 of 323 subjects at an average duration of 4.7 (range 0.06–26.3) months after first procedure (data from 7 studies only). On the other hand, 38.67 [33.3, 43.95] % of this population underwent surgery subsequently to achieve durable relief (Figure 4). Average time from percutaneous resolution procedure to surgery was 6.7 (range 0.13–34.4) months (data from six studies only).

There was no purposeful linear relationship between the increasing average duration of follow-up period of individual studies and percent satisfaction from the percutaneous resolutions procedure (correlation coefficient: 0.13; slope: 0.057; Figure 5). However, number of studies with around 1-year follow up was highest (10), with 2-year follow-up 4 and with 3-year follow-up 2 only. For this analysis individual case reports were lumped in to three groups according to follow-up period (1, 6 and 12 months). Only one case report had a follow-up of over 2-years duration (30 months).

Discussion

Usually, the LFJCs are found as rare incidental MRI findings of elderly patients (usually in their 6th or 7th decade) presenting with low back pain and lower extremity radiculopathy. However, discovery of LFJCs remains difficult because low back pain is one of the most common presentations in a visit to physician [41]. Frequently, small cohorts of patients often develop additional bony abnormalities, including instability and spondylolisthesis.

Previously, it was difficult to pinpoint a precise existence of a cyst. Rather, the physician relied on his/her clinical acumen. For example, bilateral examinations of L4, L5 and S1, supplying the knee, foot dorsiflexion and plantar flexion, respectively, could give quick insight into the functioning of these spinal nerve roots. Added to these were lumbosacral flexion-extension plain film radiographs that could provide basic information about vertebral anatomy. However, with the advent of modern imaging modalities like CT scans and MRI, primary care physicians as well as specialists started utilizing these techniques in order to obtain more reliable anatomical features leading to pathology. This has resulted in better insights of pathoanatomical diagnoses that can provide sustained and earlier relief.

The present study utilizes almost all relevant data to appraise the success rate of the percutaneous resolution of the LFJCs and finds perhaps the highest rate (56%) reviewed so far [2 e.g.]. This appears to be because of inclusion of 15 case reports which provide considerable power to analysis. Overall success rate noted in the case reports was 70%, whereas, in the pooled analysis of 14 studies the success rate was noted to about 50%. Although, follow-up period of the case reports was much less than the pooled analysis of 14 studies, yet, in the subset of 4 case reports with 9, 12, 18, and 30 months follow-up, the success rate was 100%. Overall association between the follow-up and satisfactory results was also not providing indication of declined success rate with increments in follow up period. Such a difference of success rate of percutaneous procedures in the retrospective analyses and case reports can be attributed to publication bias or scarcity of prospective studies will be clarified in future research. Nevertheless, this point is

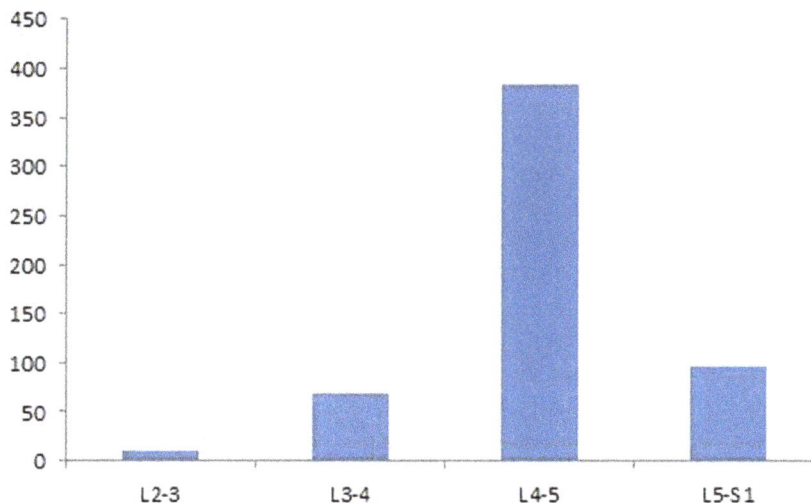

Figure 2. Spinal level of cysts diagnosed in the patients included in the meta-analysis.

encouraging enough to provide impetus for larger and longer trial/s to assess the potentials of this treatment strategy.

Natural history of the disease progression of LJFCs is not known. Frequently, patients with radicular pain may be advised for obtaining MRI scans and if there is incidental detection of LJC, detailed neurological examination is meritorious in order to seek insights into the associated pathophysiology. Patients presenting with any kind of radicular pain or associated claudication syndromes, cauda equina syndrome, or any lower extremity motor or sensory symptoms must be evaluated with advanced imaging like MRI. However, in order to avoid extra un-forecasted healthcare costs, there is sheer need of a good clinical examination at the presentation. Due to methodological issues, scarcity of categorical data and statistical power limitations, the present study could not arrive at an initiative of establishing criteria for the selection of suitable patients for percutaneous resolution procedures. Narrowing and ideally eliminating the gray areas of when to take the decision for percutaneous rupture versus the definitive strategy of cyst excision remains the hallmark of clinical research in this area. Surgical excision is precise, but is time consuming, expensive and still not risk-free. On the other hand complications may also develop following procedures such as paraplegia [42].

Because of a number of factors, the present study encounters significant limitations. Firstly, as the diagnosis of LJC remains incidental, there is only one considerable sized prospective study and all others are either retrospective analyses or case reports. Schulz et al. [37] utilized a prospective design to compare the efficacy of percutaneous resolution of LFJCs with microsurgery and noticed a clear-cut supremacy of microsurgery over percutaneous resolution attempts. Their study was not randomized but acts as a required initiative which noted satisfactory benefit of percutaneous treatment for 8 of 20 patients. Indeed, because of minimally invasiveness of this treatment, it remains a treatment of choice.

Secondly, follow-up period in the majority of studies was less than two years which makes it difficult to speculate long-term benefits of the intervention. Thirdly, data availability remained a major issue as it could be useful to apply meta-regression analyses for predicting factor by utilizing data such as age, gender cyst size, cyst type, cyst orientation/location, radiological intensity, pre-procedure duration of symptoms and previous history of treatment/s. Although, case reports were considerably detailed yet in many all relevant data was not available. Cambron et al. [18] studied the effect of low or high signal intensity of MRI on the success rate of percutaneous resolution of LFJCs and noted that patients with T2-hyperintene LFJCs can be more reliably benefited from percutaneous resolution procedures.

Table 3. Common presenting conditions of lumbar facet joint cysts.

Low back pain	Disc herniation
Unilateral or bilateral radiculopathy	Spinal stenosis
Myelopathy	Neural foraminal stenosis
Neurogenic claudication	Herniated nucleus pulposus
Caudaequina syndrome	Osteoarthritis
Intracystic or epidural hemorrhage	Arachnoiditis
Spondylolisthesis	Cauda equina compression from cyst
Trochanteric bursitis	High-intensity zone in disk
Peripheral neuropathy	

Study / Case reports	Benefitted subjects	Total	Percent benefitted subjects and 95% CI			Percent benefitted subjects and 95% CI
			Percentage	Upper limit	Lower limit	
Allen et al., 2009	19	32	59.37	32.68	86.07	
Amoretti et al., 2012	90	120	75.0	59.5	90.5	
Bjorkengren et 1987	1	3	33.33	-32.0	98.67	
Bureau et al., 2001	9	12	75.0	26.0	124.0	
Cambron et al 2013	63	110	57.27	43.13	71.42	
Carrera, 1980	6	20	30.0	5.995	54.0	
Martha et al., 2009	46	101	45.54	32.38	58.71	
Ortiz & Tekch., 2013	18	20	90.0	48.42	131.6	
Parlier-Cuau et 1999	14	30	46.66	22.22	71.11	
Sabers et al., 2005	9	23	39.13	13.57	64.7	
Sauvage et al., 2000	6	13	46.15	9.223	83.08	
Schulz et al., 2011	8	20	40.0	12.28	67.72	
Shah & Lutz, 2003	1	10	10.0	-9.6	29.6	
Slipman et al., 2000	4	14	28.57	0.571	56.57	
CR 1	4	8	50.0	1.0	99.0	
CR 2	2	3	66.66	-25.7	159.1	
CR 3	3	3	100	-13.2	213.2	
Summary	303	543	55.80	49.52	62.08	

-50   0   50   100 150 200

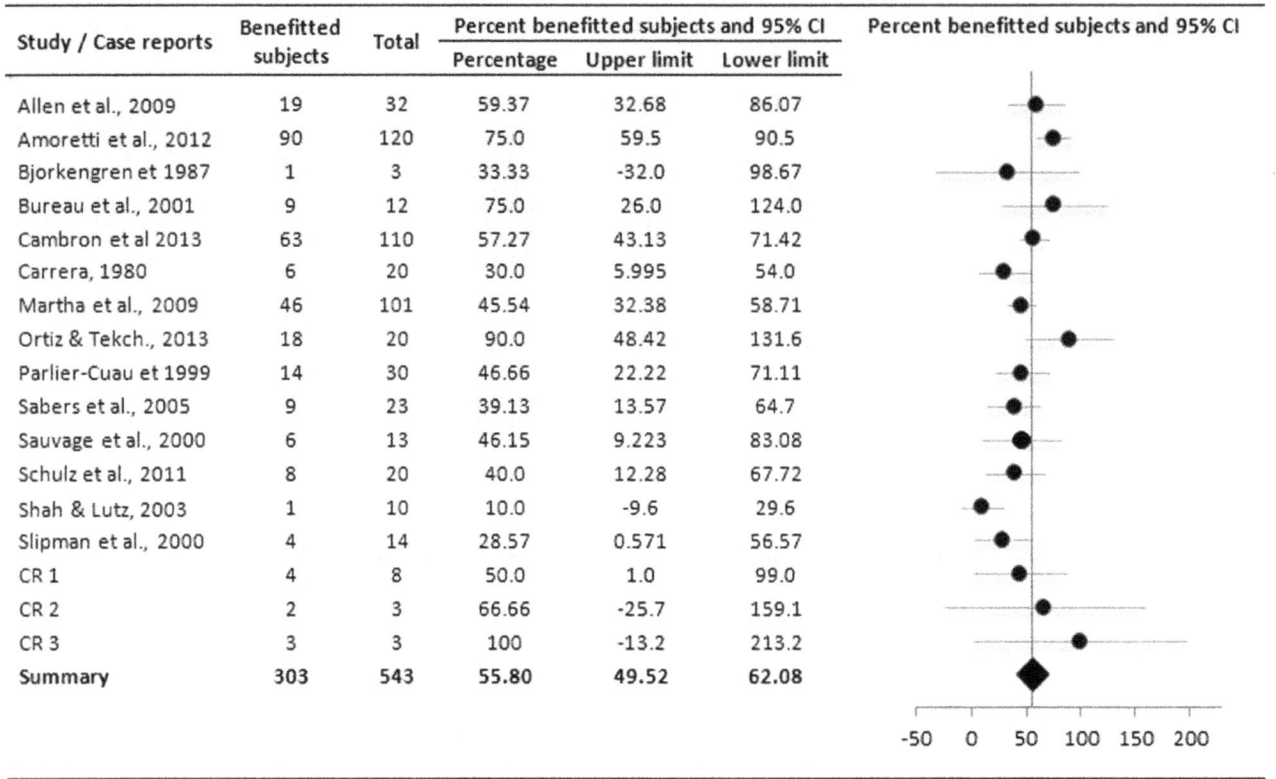

Figure 3. Forest plot showing effect sizes of satisfactory results of percutaneous treatments of the LFJCs after short- or long-term follow-up in individual studies (closed circles) and the overall effect size achieved in meta-analysis (diamond). CR 1 (follow-up 1 mo): Braza et al., 2005; Casselman et al., 1985; Chang, 2009; Foley, 2009; Imai et al., 1998; Kozar & Jeromal, 2014; Lutz and Shen, 2002; Rauchwerger et al., 2011/CR 2 (follow-up 6 month): Boissier et al., 2013; Hong et al., 1995; Shin et al., 2012/CR 3 (follow-up 1 year or more): Gishen et al., 2001; Lim et al., 2001; Lin et al., 2014; Melfi and Aprill, 2005.

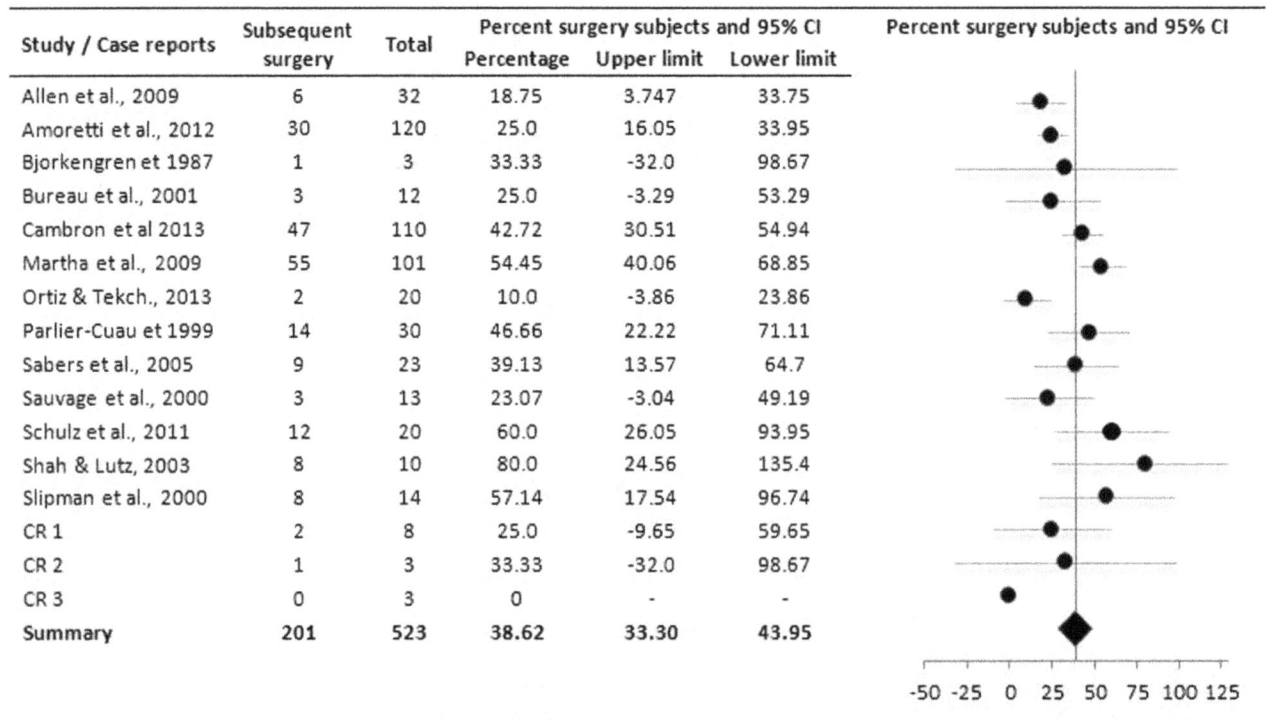

Study / Case reports	Subsequent surgery	Total	Percent surgery subjects and 95% CI			Percent surgery subjects and 95% CI
			Percentage	Upper limit	Lower limit	
Allen et al., 2009	6	32	18.75	3.747	33.75	
Amoretti et al., 2012	30	120	25.0	16.05	33.95	
Bjorkengren et 1987	1	3	33.33	-32.0	98.67	
Bureau et al., 2001	3	12	25.0	-3.29	53.29	
Cambron et al 2013	47	110	42.72	30.51	54.94	
Martha et al., 2009	55	101	54.45	40.06	68.85	
Ortiz & Tekch., 2013	2	20	10.0	-3.86	23.86	
Parlier-Cuau et 1999	14	30	46.66	22.22	71.11	
Sabers et al., 2005	9	23	39.13	13.57	64.7	
Sauvage et al., 2000	3	13	23.07	-3.04	49.19	
Schulz et al., 2011	12	20	60.0	26.05	93.95	
Shah & Lutz, 2003	8	10	80.0	24.56	135.4	
Slipman et al., 2000	8	14	57.14	17.54	96.74	
CR 1	2	8	25.0	-9.65	59.65	
CR 2	1	3	33.33	-32.0	98.67	
CR 3	0	3	0	-	-	
Summary	201	523	38.62	33.30	43.95	

-50 -25   0   25   50   75 100 125

Figure 4. Forest plot showing effect sizes of subjects underwent surgical treatments subsequent to failure of percutaneous treatments of the LFJCs in individual studies (closed circles) and the overall effect size achieved in meta-analysis (diamond). CR 1/CR 2/CR 3 as given in Figure 2.

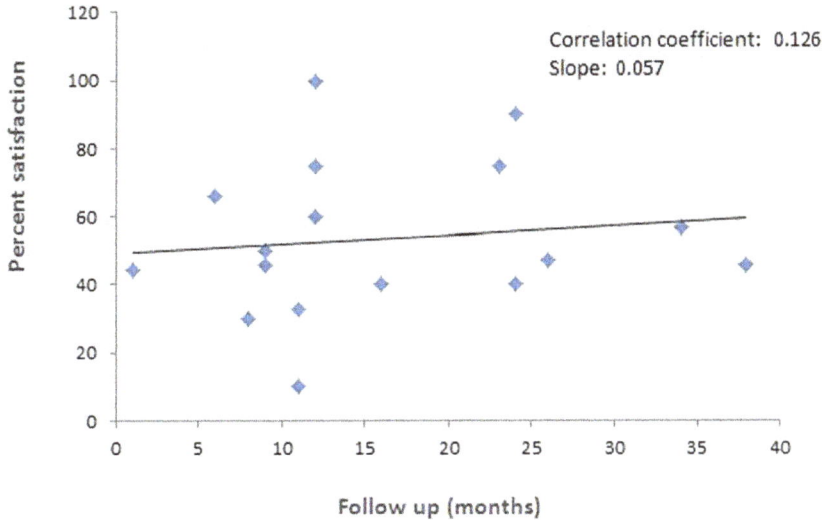

Figure 5. Scatter plot showing relationship between percent satisfaction of the subjects of percutaneous resolution procedures and follow-up duration in months.

It seems that the success rate of percutaneous resolution procedures will increase with the improvement in decision-making information and advancement in technology and skill training and exposure. However, of much importance is the availability of results of a few or a bigger, multi-center randomized controlled trial/s with adequate power to assess the success rate as well as the predicting factors for percutaneous resolution procedure selection. Without which as pointed out by Arnold et al. [43], patient is presented with the coin flip odds for percutaneous vs surgery choice.

Conclusion

By analyzing all available evidence pertaining to the efficacy of percutaneous cyst resolution procedures the present study finds

this therapeutic regimen as an alternative to surgical interventions but is unable to identify subgroup/s of patients that can be benefited more reliably with this technique and therefore urges to conduct comparative studies with longer follow-up periods.

Author Contributions

Conceived and designed the experiments: JGT SXH. Performed the experiments: SXH FS JLZ DFR ZC. Analyzed the data: FS SXH JLZ DFR ZC JGT. Wrote the paper: FS SXH.

References

1. Epstein NE, Baisden J (2012) The diagnosis and management of synovial cysts: Efficacy of surgery vs cyst aspiration. Surg Neurol Int 3: 157–66.
2. DePalma MJ (2009) Driving the lane: a clearer view of facet joint cyst intervention. Spine J 9: 921–3.
3. Shipley JA, Beukes CA (1998) The nature of spondylolytic defect. Demonstration of a communicating synovial pseudoarthrosis in the pars interarticularis. J Bone Joint Surg Br 80: 662–4.
4. Alicioglu B, Sut N (2009) Synovial cysts of the lumbar facet joints: a retrospective magnetic resonance imaging study investigating their relation with degenerative spondylolisthesis. Prague Medical Report 110: 301–9.
5. Budris DM (1991) Radiologic case study, intraspinal lumbar synovial cyst. Orthopedics 14: 618–20.
6. Gheyi GY, Uppot RN, Flores C, Koyfman YU (1999) Unusual case of lumbar synovial cyst. Clin Imaging 23: 394–6.
7. Boviatsis EJ, Staurinou LC, Kouyialis AT, Gavra MM, Stavrinou PC, et al. (2008) Spinal synovial cysts: pathogenesis, diagnosis and surgucal treatment in a series of seven cases and literature review. Eur Spine J 17: 831–7.
8. Abdullah AF, Chambers RW, Daut DP (1984) Lumbar nerve root compression by synovial cysts of the ligamentum flavum. Report of four cases. J Neurosurg 60: 617–20.
9. Kurz LT, Garfin SR, Unger AS, Thorne RP, Rothman RH (1985) Intraspinal synovial cyst causing sciatica. J Bone Joint Surg Am 67: 865–71.
10. Ayberg G, Ozveren F, Gok Yazgan A, Tosun H, Seçkin Z, et al. (2008) Lumbar synovial cysts: experience with nine cases. Neurol Med Chir 48: 298–303.
11. U.S. Department of Health & Human Services.Quality Assessment Tool for Observational Cohort and Cross-Sectional Studies. Available: http://www.nhlbi.nih.gov/health-pro/guidelines/in-develop/cardiovascular-risk-reduction/tools/cohort.htm. Accessed 2014 March.
12. Allen TL, Tatli Y, Lutz GE (2009) Fluoroscopic percutaneous lumbar zygapophyseal joint cyst rupture: a clinical outcome study. Spine J 9: 387–95.
13. Amoretti N, Huwart L, Foti P, Boileau P, Amoretti ME, et al. (2012) Symptomatic lumbar facet joint cysts treated by CT-guided intracystic and intra-articular steroid injections. Eur Radiol 22: 2836–40.
14. Bjorkengren AG, Kurz LT, Resnick D, Sartoris DJ, Garfin SR (1987) Symptomatic intraspinal synovial cysts: opacification and treatment by percutaneous injection. AJR Am J Roentgenol 149: 105–7.
15. Boissière L, Valour F, Rigal J, Soderlund C (2013) Lumbar synovial cyst calcification after facet joint steroid injection. BMJ Case Rep 2013. pii: bcr2012008029.
16. Braza DW, Dedianous D, Peterson B (2005) Lumbar synovial cyst. Am J Phys Med Rehabil 84: 911–2.
17. Bureau NJ, Kaplan PA, Dussault RG (2001) Lumbar facet joint synovial cyst: percutaneous treatment with steroid injections and distention—clinical and imaging follow-up in 12 patients. Radiol 221: 179–85.
18. Cambron SC, McIntyre JJ, Guerin SJ, Li Z, Pastel DA (2013) Lumbar facet joint synovial cysts: does T2 signal intensity predict outcomes after percutaneous rupture? AJNR Am J Neuroradiol 34: 1661–4.
19. Carrera GF (1980) Lumbar facet joint injection in low back pain and sciatica: preliminary results. Radiol 137: 665–7.
20. Casselman ES (1985) Radiologic recognition of symptomatic spinal synovial cysts. AJNR Am J Neuroradiol 6: 971–3.
21. Chang A (2009) Percutaneous CT-guided treatment of lumbar facet joint synovial cysts. HSS J 5: 165–8.
22. Foley BS (2009) Percutaneous rupture of a lumbar synovial facet cyst. Am J Phys Med Rehabil 88: 1046.
23. Gishen P, Miller FN (2001) Percutaneous excision of a facet joint cyst under CT guidance. Cardiovasc Intervent Radiol 24: 351–53.
24. Hong Y, O'Grady T, Carlsson C, Casey J, Clements D (1995) Percutaneous aspiration of lumbar facet synovial cyst. Anesthesiol 82: 1061–2.

25. Imai K, Nakamura K, Inokuchi K, Oda H (1998) Aspiration of intraspinal synovial cyst: recurrence after temporal improvement. Arch Orthop Trauma Surg 118: 103–5.

26. Kozar S, Jeromel M (2014) Minimally invasive CT guided treatment of intraspinal synovial cyst. Radiol Oncol 48: 35–9.

27. Lim AK, Higgins SJ, Saifuddin A, Lehovsky J (2001) Symptomatic lumbar synovial cyst: management with direct CT-guided puncture and steroid injection. Clin Radiol 56: 990–3.

28. Lin TL, Chung CT, Lan HH, Sheen HM (2014) Ultrasound-guided facet joint injection to treat a spinal cyst. J Chin Med Assoc 77: 213–6.

29. Lutz GE, Shen TC (2002) Fluoroscopically guided aspiration of a symptomatic lumbar zygapophyseal joint cyst: A case report. Arch Phys Med Rehabil 83: 1789–91.

30. Martha JF, Swaim B, Wang DA, Kim DH, Hill J, et al. (2009) Outcome of percutaneous rupture of lumbar synovial cysts: a case series of 101 patients. Spine J 9: 899–904.

31. Melfi RS, Aprill CN (2005) Percutaneous puncture of zygapophysial joint synovial cyst with fluoroscopic guidance. Pain Med 6: 122–8.

32. Ortiz AO, Tekchandani L (2013) Improved outcomes with direct percutaneous CT guided lumbar synovial cyst treatment: advanced approaches and techniques. J Neurointerv Surg doi: 10.1136/neurintsurg-2013-010891.

33. Parlier-Cuau C, Wybier M, Nizard R, Champsaur P, Le Hir P, et al. (1999) Symptomatic lumbar facet joint synovial cysts: clinical assessment of facet joint steroid injection after 1 and 6 months and long-term follow-up in 30 patients. Radiol 210: 509–13.

34. Rauchwerger JJ, Candido KD, Zoarski GH (2011) Technical and imaging report: fluoroscopic guidance for diagnosis and treatment of lumbar synovial cyst. Pain Pract 11: 180–4.

35. Sabers SR, Ross SR, Grogg BE, Lauder TD (2005) Procedure-based nonsurgical management of lumbar zygapophyseal joint cyst-induced radicular pain. Arch Phys Med Rehabil 86: 1767–71.

36. Sauvage P, Grimault L, Ben Salem D, Roussin I, Huguenin M, et al. (2000) Lumbar intraspinal synovial cysts: imaging and treatment by percutaneous injection. Report of thirteen cases. J Radiol 81: 33–8.

37. Schulz C, Danz B, Waldeck S, Kunz U, Mauer UM (2011) Percutaneous CT-guided destruction versus microsurgical resection of lumbar juxtafacet cysts. Orthopade 40: 600–6.

38. Shah RV, Lutz GE (2003) Lumbar intraspinal synovial cysts: conservative management and review of the world's literature. Spine J 3: 479–88.

39. Shin KM, Kim MS, Ko KM, Jang JS, Kang SS, et al. (2012) Percutaneous aspiration of lumbar zygapophyseal joint synovial cyst under fluoroscopic guidance - A case report. Korean J Anesthesiol 62: 375–8.

40. Slipman CW, Lipetz JS, Wakeshima Y, Jackson HB (2000) Nonsurgical treatment of zygapophyseal joint cyst-induced radicular pain. Arch Phys Med Rehabil 81: 973–7.

41. Deyo RA, Weinstein JN (2001) Low back pain. N Engl J Med 344: 363–70.

42. Kennedy DJ, Dreyfuss P, Aprill CN, Bogduk N (2009) Paraplegia following image-guided transforaminal lumbar spine epidural steroid injection: two case reports. Pain Med 10: 1389–94.

43. Arnold PM (2009) Efficacy of injection therapy for symptomatic lumbar synovial cysts. Spine J 9: 919–20.

17

Neuronal Correlates of a Virtual-Reality-Based Passive Sensory P300 Network

Chun-Chuan Chen[1], Kai-Syun Syue[1], Kai-Chiun Li[1], Shih-Ching Yeh[2]*

1 Graduate Institute of Biomedical Engineering, National Central University, Jhongli city, Taoyuan County, Taiwan, **2** Department of Computer Science and Information Engineering, National Central University, Jhongli city, Taoyuan County, Taiwan

Abstract

P300, a positive event-related potential (ERP) evoked at around 300 ms after stimulus, can be elicited using an active or passive oddball paradigm. Active P300 requires a person's intentional response, whereas passive P300 does not require an intentional response. Passive P300 has been used in incommunicative patients for consciousness detection and brain computer interface. Active and passive P300 differ in amplitude, but not in latency or scalp distribution. However, no study has addressed the mechanism underlying the production of passive P300. In particular, it remains unclear whether the passive P300 shares an identical active P300 generating network architecture when no response is required. This study aims to explore the hierarchical network of passive sensory P300 production using dynamic causal modelling (DCM) for ERP and a novel virtual reality (VR)-based passive oddball paradigm. Moreover, we investigated the causal relationship of this passive P300 network and the changes in connection strength to address the possible functional roles. A classical ERP analysis was performed to verify that the proposed VR-based game can reliably elicit passive P300. The DCM results suggested that the passive and active P300 share the same parietal-frontal neural network for attentional control and, underlying the passive network, the feed-forward modulation is stronger than the feed-back one. The functional role of this forward modulation may indicate the delivery of sensory information, automatic detection of differences, and stimulus-driven attentional processes involved in performing this passive task. To our best knowledge, this is the first study to address the passive P300 network. The results of this study may provide a reference for future clinical studies on addressing the network alternations under pathological states of incommunicative patients. However, caution is required when comparing patients' analytic results with this study. For example, the task presented here is not applicable to incommunicative patients.

Editor: Emmanuel Andreas Stamatakis, University Of Cambridge, United Kingdom

Funding: Chun-Chuan Chen and Shih-Ching Yeh are funded by National Science Council of Taiwan (NSC 101-2221-E-008 -003; NSC 103-2420-H-008 -001; NSC 102-2221-E-008 -077). The funder had no role in study design, data collection and analysis, decision to publish, or preparation of the manuscript.

Competing Interests: The authors have declared that no competing interests exist.

* Email: shihching.yeh@gmail.com

Introduction

Neuronal activities as measured with electroencephalogram (EEG)/MEG are the direct window for studying the living brain at work. Specifically, P300, a positive event-related potential (ERP) evoked at around 300 ms after stimulus [1] has been investigated intensively and thought to reflect the higher level cognitive processes like selective attention and memory updating [2,3]. P300 can be elicited reliably in an oddball paradigm using a variety of stimuli, such as visual, auditory or sensory stimuli. There are two types of P300: active and passive P300. Active P300 requires the subjects' attention to response, while passive P300 requires no intentional response [2]. Active P300 has been successfully applied to discriminate the abnormality from the healthy based on its amplitude and latency [3]. For example, P300 with prolonged latencies and markedly lower amplitudes are characteristic of patients with Alzheimer's disease [4,5]. Because of the medical significance of P300 activity, numerous studies have investigated the neuronal origin and the underlying mechanisms involved in generating active P300, although conclusions have been inconsistent. For instance, Downar et al. have identified the neuroana-

tomical correlates underlying the detection of changes in the sensory environment using event-related functional magnetic-resonance imaging (fMRI) and a modified oddball paradigm [6]. They concluded that a distributed, right-lateralized network-comprising temporoparietal junction (TPJ), inferior frontal gyrus (IFG), insula and left cingulate and supplementary motor areas (CMA/SMA) as well as the primary sensory cortex (SI)–responds to changes in multiple sensory modalities and the subsequent involuntary attention shift. The aforementioned areas correspond closely to lesions in hemineglect patients and are considered as the underlying mechanism of the P300 production. Crottaz-Herbette and Menon examined the attentional control network by using simultaneous fMRI and EEG data recorded while performing auditory and visual oddball attention tasks [7]. They showed that the anterior cingulate cortex (ACC), left premotor area (PMA), inferior parietal lobule (IPL), and the primary sensory areas formed a network underlying the generation of P300 and that the ACC plays a crucial role in the top-down modulation of sensory processing. In 2005, Huang et al., employed MEG to study the engagement of the distributed parietal-frontal network in a median-nerve oddball paradigm [8]. They found that the same parietal-frontal neuronal network activated by both visual and auditory changes can also be activated by somatosensory stimulation. Recently, Brazdil et al. further studied the effective connectivity between right IPL, ACC and lateral prefrontal cortex (PFC) using fMRI and Dynamic Causal Modelling (DCM) during a visual oddball task [9]. They concluded that bidirectional coupling occurs between the frontal and parietal regions and that the ACC exerts influence over PFC mediating the top-down attentional control. In summary, the frontal, parietal and temporal cortices, and primary sensory cortex are associated with the generation of active P300, though the engagement of brain areas is subjective to various stimuli and measurement modalities (for a more detail review, see Appendix S1). As for passive P300, numerous studies have shown that the passive oddball paradigm is adequately sensitive for probing the conscious state of incommunicative brain trauma or stroke patients [10,11,12]. Furthermore, passive P300 waves have been used in brain-computer interfaces (BCIs) because of its advantages of no training required and the results were significant [13,14]. Although active and passive P300 differ only in the amplitude but not in the latency and scalp distribution [15,16,17], it was suggested that different neuronal pathways and networks may be involved in the active and passive conditions. However, to our best knowledge, the mechanism underlying the passive P300 production has not been addressed. In particular, it remains unclear whether the passive conditions share the active P300-generating network architecture when no response is required.

Virtual reality (VR) is a computer-based environment that provides the users an immersive experience of a synthetic world. Since the development of VR, researchers have been applying VR technologies continually in various medical contexts, such as diagnosis, presurgical rehearsal and planning, as well as stroke rehabilitation [18]. VR provides a simulated environment and features controllable parameters, thereby facilitating the systemic testing of human functions in both healthy and diseased states [19,20]. Thus, we designed a VR-based passive sensory oddball task to elicit the passive P300 and investigated the underlying neuronal network by applying for ERP [21,22]. A passive sensory oddball task was selected for this study because sensory P300 can be evoked reliably and is suitable for BCI applications and consciousness probing. Traditional passive sensory oddball paradigms either apply only sensation to skin (ex. vibration or painless electrical stimulation), or use median nerve electrical stimulation that induces both sensory and motor responses at the same time. The common difficulty for a passive task is that there is no way to assure the attentive of the subjects. Lack of attention may decrease largely the amplitude of P300 and lead to a non-significant result [23]. Moreover, the hand movement produced by median nerve stimulation may cause a confound when investigating the underlying neuronal network since there exists a movement-related top-down modulation during a simple movement task [24]. Specifically, it has not been tested whether the backward modulation, if there has any, is engaged under a passive condition, or just is a reflection of movement-related top-down control. Therefore, in this study, we take the advantage of VR to design a task that can keep the subjects' attention and is still able to separate the movements from sensory change detection. We expect that, this task will evoke the somatosensory evoked potentials (SEPs) of P50, N80, and P200 [25] during the standard events, as well as passive P300 during the rare events. Based on this expectation, we aim to investigate this passive sensory P300 network by DCM for ERP. Importantly, the causal relationship of this passive P300 network and the changes in connection strength will be examined to address the possible functional roles. This paper is organized as follows; The subsequent section outlines the experimental protocol design and details the plausible dynamic causal models. The final section presents the results and the implications of the findings.

Materials and Methods

Written consent was obtained from all subjects for the experiment with a protocol approved by the institutional review board of Taipei Veterans General Hospital.

Subjects and Task

Ten healthy, right-handed male college students (22–29 years of age) were recruited for this study. Written consent was obtained from all subjects for the experiment with a protocol approved by the institutional review board of Taipei Veterans General Hospital, in accordance with the Declaration of Helsinki. The subjects sat comfortably wearing goggles, through which they viewed a virtual robot pitching a baseball toward them at 4 ± 0.5 second intervals (mean interval between trials = 4 seconds). The angle and speed of the ball varied between trials to prevent the subjects from anticipating the characteristics of the next pitch. They were instructed to catch the virtual ball by using a game controller held in their right hand, and no further instruction was given regarding the actions to be taken after catching it. This VR-based ball-catching task was performed under 2 conditions (standard and rare) characterized by different occurrence frequencies. The standard condition (480 trials; 80% occurrence) was designed to mimic the real-world conditions of a person catching a ball. When the subjects successfully caught the virtual ball, haptic stimuli (i.e. the sensory force feedback) were delivered through the game controller. The rare condition (120 trials; 20% occurrence) was designed to elicit passive P300 by removing the haptic stimuli, even when the subjects successfully caught the ball. In other words, a passive P300 will be produced by the occasional lack of haptic feedback, i.e. the rare conditions, while the SEPs will be evoked during the standard events. As the haptic feedback came after the movement finished (i.e. the ball has been caught), this task allows us to bypass the possible movement-related top-down modulation that may cause a confound [24].

EEG Acquisition and Processing

Thirty-channel EEG data (10–20 system montage; QuickAmp amplifier by Brain Products), referred to linked earlobes with a forehead ground, were recorded at a sampling rate of 250 Hz during the ball catch task. Waveforms were further re-referenced on-line by common average across all channels. The position of the EEG electrodes was measured using an optical 3D electrode digitizer system (Xensor) before starting the EEG-recordings. The locations of the subject-specific channels will be used in DCM for co-registration of the EEG coordinates with the canonical template MRI images in SPM. The data were epoched offline by using SPM8 (Wellcome Trust Centre for Neuroimaging, available at: http://www.fil.ion.ucl.ac.uk/spm/), with a peristimulus window from –500 to 1000 ms, where Time 0 denoted the moment the ball was caught. Poorly performed trials (i.e. when the subjects failed to catch the virtual ball) were excluded from further analysis, resulting in 467 ± 26 and 118 ± 6 trials for standard and rare events, respectively. EOG contamination (i.e. EEG amplitude >100 mV) was removed from the epochs by using a fully automated correction method [26] and these EOG-free trials were divided into standard and rare groups according to their occurrences. The epochs of both groups were lowpass filtered (cutoff frequency = 30 Hz), baseline corrected (–2000 ms) and

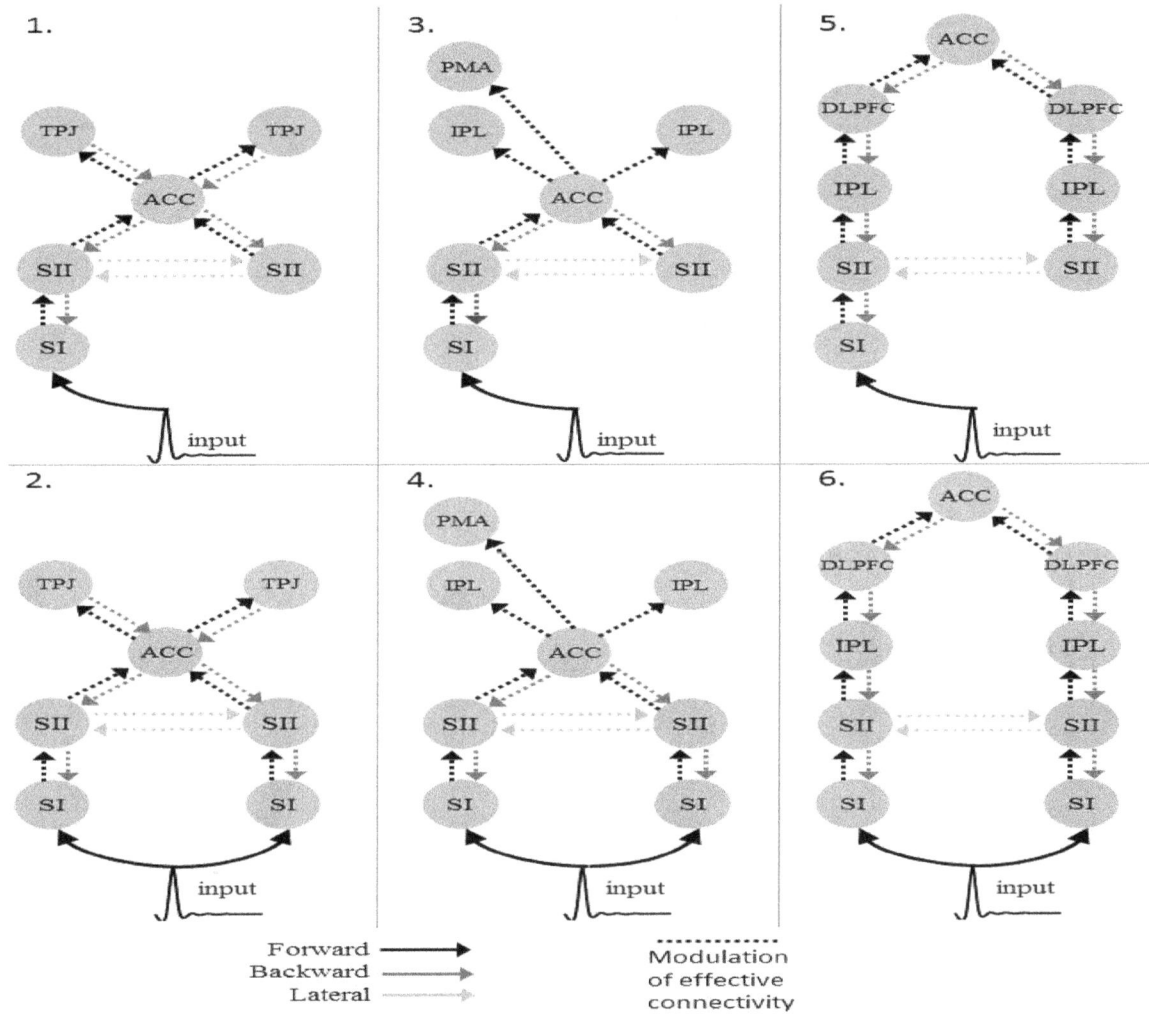

Figure 1. The architectures of the plausible model pairs. (SI : primary sensory area; SII : secondary sensor area; ACC : Anterior cingulate cortex; TPJ: Temporoparietal junction; IPL : Inferior parietal lobule; PMA : Premotor area;DLPFC: Dorsolateral prefrontal cortex).

averaged across trials. The mean ERPs in both groups were first examined phenomenonally to identify the SEPs and P300. Subsequently, the ERPs entered DCM of ERPs as the observations that the DCM models are trying to explain.

Model specification for DCM of ERP

In DCM for ERP analysis, we use only neuronal responses recorded between 0 and 900 ms, because these signals capture the entire stimulus duration and cortical responses for P300 as well as exclude the movement-related responses. To reduce the number of potential model combinations, we applied the following 2-step strategy. **Firstly**, we specified 3 plausible model pairs (Figure 1) to identify the most likely model hierarchy based on 3 previous studies discussed in the Introduction section [6,7,8]. Specifically, we addressed the following 2 factors: (1) whether the ACC is at the top of the passive network hierarchy; and (2) whether bilateral inputs are essential to generate activities in this sensory cognitive network as this task involves a unilateral stimulus only. These models share common structures, including SI ([-34 -31 56; 37-30 54]), secondary somatosensory areas (SII, [-59 -28 24; 50-28 25]) and ACC ([1 4 29]) [6], yet they differed in some higher areas and connections. Model 1 includes the bilateral TPJ ([-54 -48 10; 54-42

13]), which may be involved in detecting changes in the sensory environment [6]. Model 3 has bilateral IPL [-40 -38 56; 46-26 32] and left PMA [-32 -16 -64] for mediating the attentional control [7]. It should be noted that, in Crottaz-Herbette and Menon's study, SMA has been suggested as a node in this distributed network. Because the spatial resolution of our EEG system is not good enough to distinguish the activity of SMA from that of ACC, for simplicity, we used ACC here to represent the activities of ACC/SMA as the report of Downar et al. [6] shows. Model 5 specifies a distributed parietal-frontal network that is activated during the sensory oddball task using MEG data. This network comprises bilateral DLPFC ([-34 25 29; 37 23 30]) and IPL ([-37 50 46; 46 46 41]) [8]. Model 2, 4 and 6 differ from Model 1, 3 and 5 in the present of the sensory input to the right SI (Figure 1). These source locations in the models (in Talairach coordinate) were taken from the cited studies that motivated the models during an active oddball task. The task-related modulation in these networks was pre-assumed to be reciprocal in all connections. **Secondly**, once we have established the most likely network, we then further examine where the task specific modulation takes place. We altered the task-related modulation as forward (F), backward (B) or lateral (L), thereby constructing 5 additional

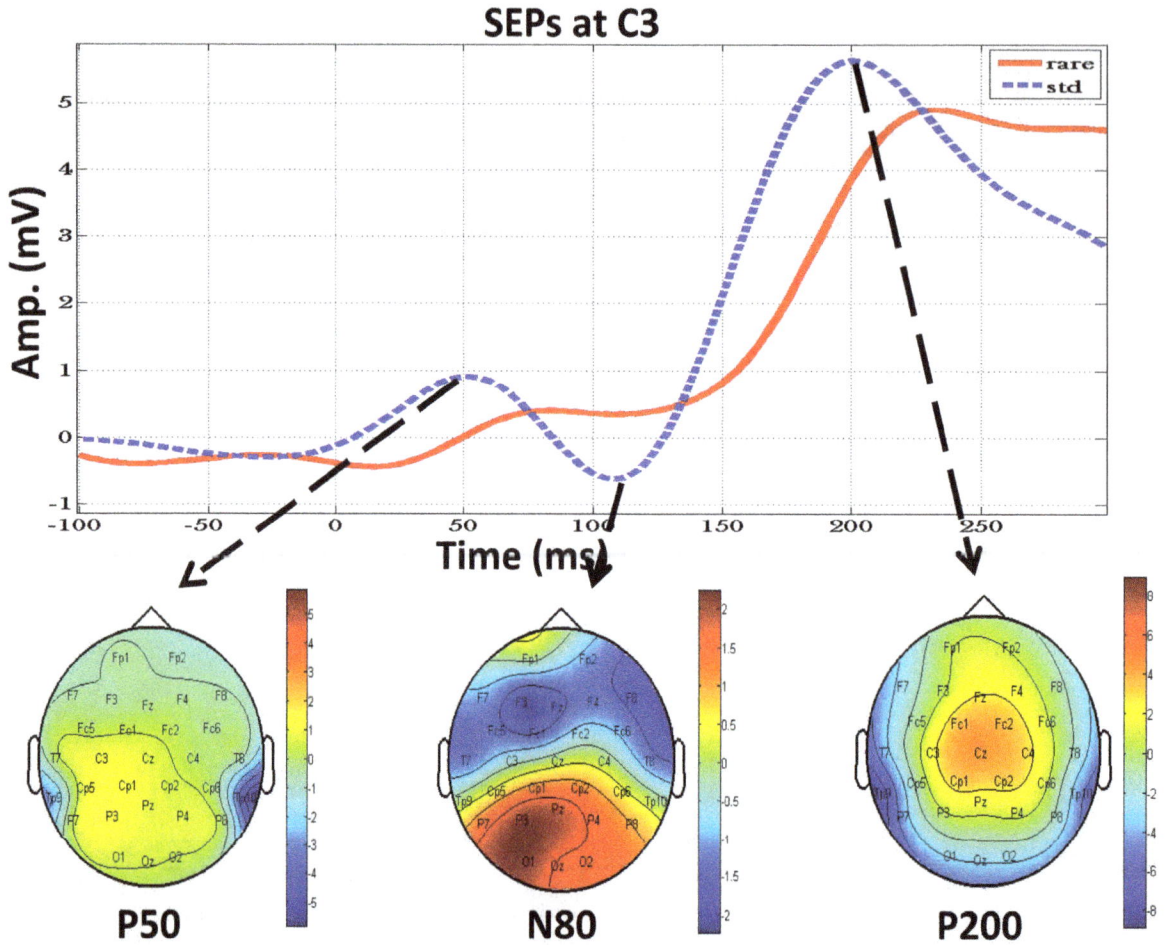

Figure 2. The time courses of the mean SEPs under standard (dash line) and rare (solid line) conditions at C3 and the mean topographic maps at the individual peak of P50, N80 and P200.

models (denoted as F, B, FB, FL and BL). In addition, we grouped the 6 models into 3 families: F (F+FL), B (B+BL) and FB (FB+FBL) to compare the model families to draw inferences on the importance of the directionality of the modulatory connection, independent of any uncertainty associated with the model structure [27]. Note that we also used a recently validated third-party software package [28] to accelerate the computation of DCM for ERPs.

Statistical Tests and Bayesian Model Selection

A repeated measures analysis of variance (rmANOVA) was applied to test the experimental factors (conditions x electrode locations; 230) given the peak amplitude of P300 over all 10

Table 1. The mean P300 peak amplitude and latency under the rare condition.

Electrode	Amplitude (μV) (mean ± standard deviation)	Latency (ms) (mean ± standard deviation)
FC1	6.09±3.50	403.67±215.88
FC2	5.46±3.78	408.67±171.38
Cz	7.34±3.19	442.33±143.58
CP1	7.65±2.72	544.67±119.01
CP2	7.28±2.51	521.67±127.54
Pz	8.15±3.49	549.33±108.47
P3	7.28±3.84	617.00±125.89
P4	6.59±3.25	563.33±129.75

subjects. The window of P300 was set to be between +250 to + 800 ms after the ball was caught. Post hoc tests (Bonferroni-Dunn correction) were performed to assess differences in peak amplitude among factors. Because the elicitation of SEPs is most reflective at primary somatosensory cortex, we used the paired t-test to examine the peak amplitudes of SEPs (P50, N80 and P200) at C3 within a window from 0 to 250 ms, of the standard and rare conditions to ensure that the haptic stimulus were delivered successfully in the standard condition. Results were considered statistically significant when P<.05 after correction for multiple comparisons (Bonferroni-Dunn correction).

For DCM analysis, we used Bayesian model selection (BMS) to identify the best models among the models being tested at the individual level under the fixed effects assumption (FFX) [29]. At the group level, we applied the random effects (RFX) assumption to accommodate inter-individual variability in the structure of models or functional architectures that gave rise to individual-specific brain activity while performing the task [27,30,31]. After identifying the wining model by BMS, we tested the modulatory effect of the experimental manipulation by performing a t test to identify significant modulatory network parameters.

Results

Behavioral Data and SEPs

The behavioral data revealed that the task performance of all subjects was consistent (mean miss rate = 3.5%, mean reaction time = 939.9±21.7 ms), indicating that all of the subjects were attentive. The SEPs (i.e. P50, N80, and P200) were examined to ensure that (1) the haptic stimulus was successfully delivered in the standard condition and (2) the absence of this stimulus elicited P300 activity. Figure 2 shows the time courses of the mean SEPs of all subjects under both standard and rare conditions at electrode C3 and the corresponding topographic maps at the individual peak of P50, N80 and P200 under the standard condition. The peak amplitudes of SEPs elicited under the standard condition were higher than those elicited under the rare condition, although the differences were non-significant for P50 ($P = .2$), N100 ($P = .06$), and P200 ($P = .07$). The scalp topographies of the P50 and N80 components were more prominent over the regions contralateral to the stimulation, whereas the P200 peak amplitude exhibited a centroparietal-dominant scalp distribution with maximal amplitudes at electrode Cz. The t test results of the SEPs amplitudes at electrode C3 and C4 under the standard condition confirmed that there is a significant lateralization effect

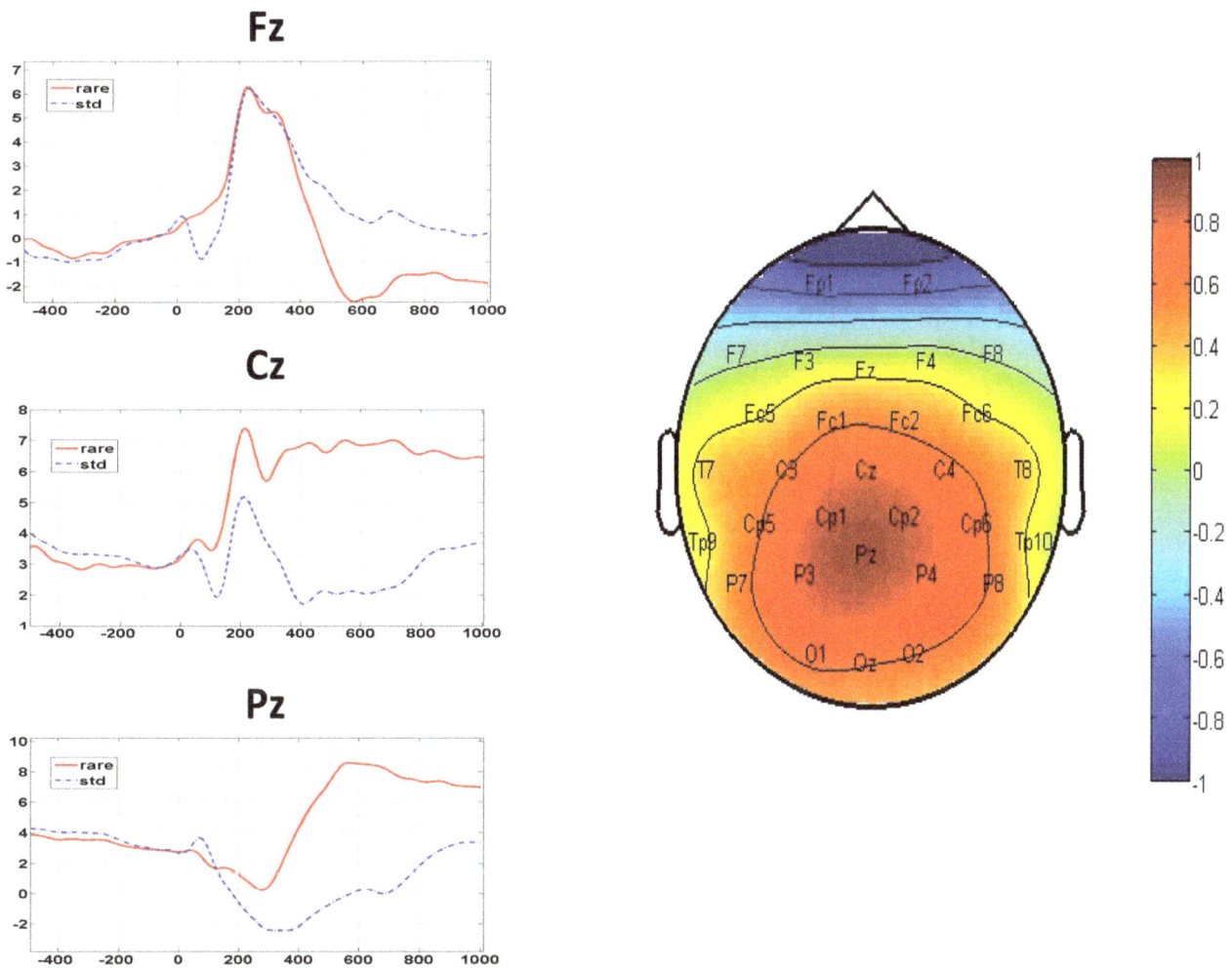

Figure 3. The time courses of the ERP at Fz, Cz and Pz averaged across subjects (left) and the mean topographic map at the individual peak of P300, normalized to the individual-specific maximum and minimum (right).

(P<0.004 for P50, P<0.031 for N100 and P<0.044 for P200). These results are in line with the previous study [25].

P300

Figure 3 shows the time courses of the mean ERPs at Fz, Cz and Pz (averaged across subjects; left side of the figure) and the mean topographic map at the P300 peak amplitudes for each subject (normalized to the individual-specific maximum and minimum; right side of the figure). The central-parietal areas (Cz and Pz) exhibited the greatest difference in mean amplitude between the 2 conditions but the difference was non-significant at Fz. The rmANOVA results of the P300 peak amplitudes of all 30 channels confirmed a significant effect on the condition (F[1.00, 9.00] = 6.638, $P = .0299$) and location (F[1.27, 11.44] = 4.781, $P = .0435$) as well as their interaction (condition × location; F[2.61, 23.46] = 11.411, $P = .0001$). Post-hoc paired t-test after correction for multiple comparisons further identified 8 channels, including FC1 (p = 0.0011), FC2 (p = 0.0003), Cz (p = 0.0001), CP1 (p = 0.0013), CP2 (p = 0.0001), Pz (p = 0.0001), P3 (p = 0.0005) and P4 (p = 0.0002) (Figure 4), supporting that the P300 component was elicited in this task. Table 1 summarizes the mean peak amplitudes and latencies across all subjects at the above 8 electrodes.

Inferences on Model Space

Six DCMs were inverted for each subject (Figure 1). Figure 5 shows the BMS results at the individual level under the FFX assumption. Seven out of ten subjects have the Model 6 as the best model. At the group level, the BMS results under FFX (Figure 6a) indicated that Model 6 was the winning model without outliers, and the BMS results under the RFX assumption (Figure 6b) confirmed this finding, with a remarkable exceedance probability of 0.7495. Having identified the best model in which the ACC is at the top of this network hierarchy, we then further investigated the task-related modulation mechanism by comparing Model 6 (i.e. FBL model) with 5 derivative models (Figure 7; see **Model Specification for DCM of ERP** section for details). Forward modulation was crucial in this task as the FL and FBL models were optimal for 5 and 4 subjects, respectively (Figure 8a). At the group level, the BMS result under the RFX assumption (Figure 8b) suggested that the FL model is the best (exceedance probabili-

ty = 0.6934), followed by the FB model (exceedance probability = 0.21). A comparison of the model families (Figure 9) revealed the importance of forward modulation. We observed that the F family was far superior to the B family, and the F and FB families exhibited almost equal exceedance probabilities (0.5005 and 0.4955, respectively). Collectively, forward modulation appeared to be more vital in this passive P300 network, despite the possibility that 2 optimal models could be applied to this task.

Inference on the Modulatory Effect

The modulation parameter matrix of the winning model from each subject entered the t test to verify the inter-individual consistency (i.e. the modulation gain is not equal to 1). We examined the modulation effect among all connections in both FL and FBL model since there was no significant difference between the two models at the individual level. Table 2 listed the statistical results of the modulatory coupling parameters. It can be seen that only forward modulations - from LIPL to LDLPFC and LDLPFC to ACC in the FL model and from LIPL to LDLPFC and RIPL-RDLPFC in the FBL model were were statistically significant.

Discussion

In this study, we have developed a VR-based sensory oddball task to elicit passive P300. The SEPs and P300 were examined to verify the elicitation of passive P300, and the neural network linked to this passive P300 production was identified using DCM and BMS.

Statistical Analysis of SEPs and P300

To elicit passive P300, we designed a passive sensory paradigm that enables a separation of pure change detection from the response control. The strongest P300 activity was observed at Pz (mean amplitude = 5.14 μV, mean latency = 544 ms), which is in agreement with the findings reported by Duncan et al (2009), Linden (2005), and Polich (2007), thereby supporting the hypothesis that the proposed novel task can reliably elicit P300 activity [2,3,32]. It is worth to point out that, despite the time course of the mean SEPs at C3 differed between the 2 conditions (Figure 2), the difference was non-significant. This may be attributed to the constant primary bottom-up sensory input as

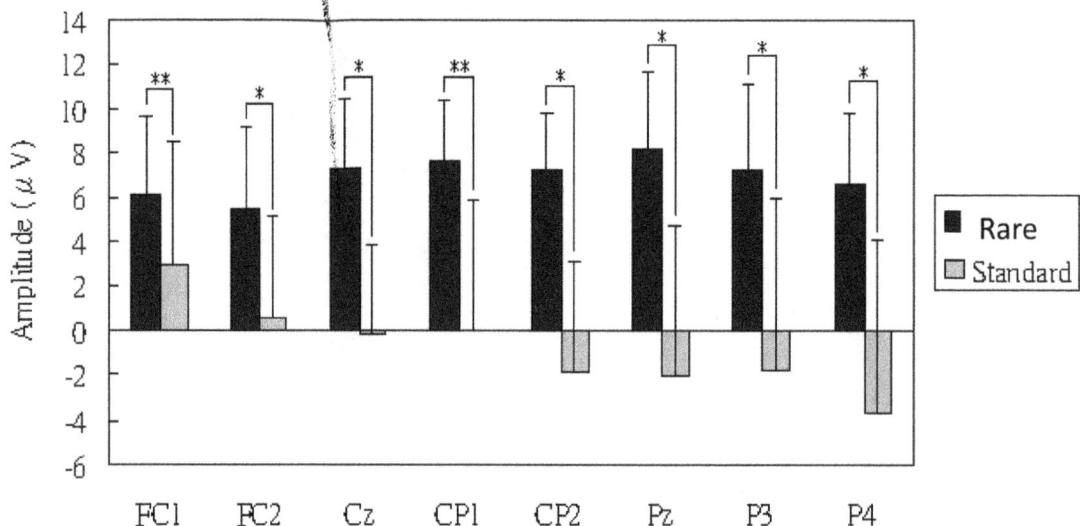

Figure 4. The statistic result revealed by the Post-hoc paired t-test on the P300 amplitude. (*: P<0.001, **: P<0.05).

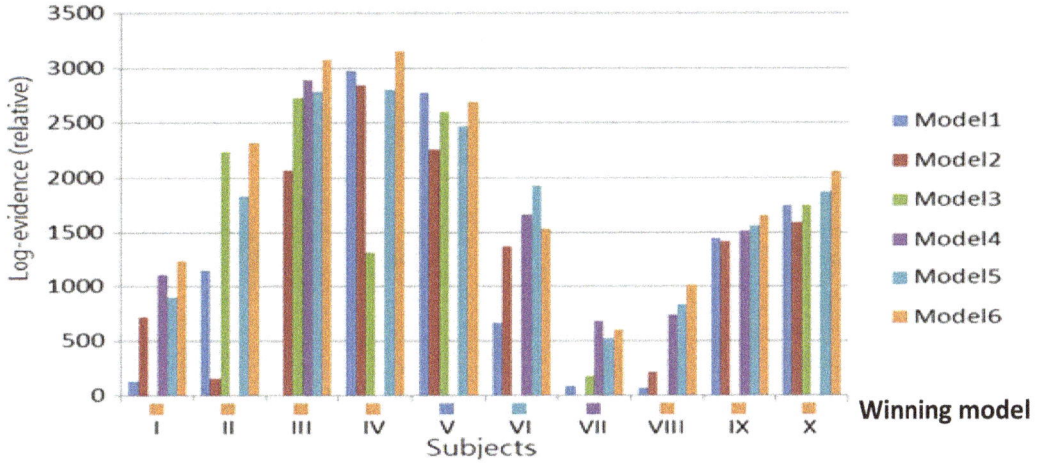

Figure 5. The result of BMS at the single subject level under FFX.

the subjects held the game controller throughout the experiment. Although the P values of the SEPs increased over time (i.e. $P = .2$ on P50, $P = .06$ on N100, and $P = .07$ on P200), the experimental effect of removing the haptic stimuli was indicated by the elicitation of P300 only, as evidenced by the statistical analysis results ($P<.05$). Similar results have been reported by several previous studies. Akatsuka et al (2007) employed a passive sensory oddball task to examine the effects of stimulus probability, and they observed a non-significant difference of the P50, N80, and P200 peak amplitudes between standard and deviant conditions when the occurrences of the deviant events were 30% and 50% [33]. Bekinschtein et al (2009) used a modified auditory oddball

task to probe the consciousness, and found that the only significant difference between the standard and deviant stimuli occurred in the P3b amplitudes [34].

The latency of P300 is thought to reflect, up to some degree, the time needed for processing information while performing the task. The variation in P300 latency is task- and condition-dependent [32]. For instance, P300 latency becomes longer when it is (1) elicited by a visual oddball paradigm than by an auditory one (Bennington and Polich, 1999), (2) elicited by a difficult task than by an easy task [35], (3) elicited under a passive condition than under an active condition [36], or (4) elicited under pathological states such as cognitive impairment [37,38,39] or normal aging

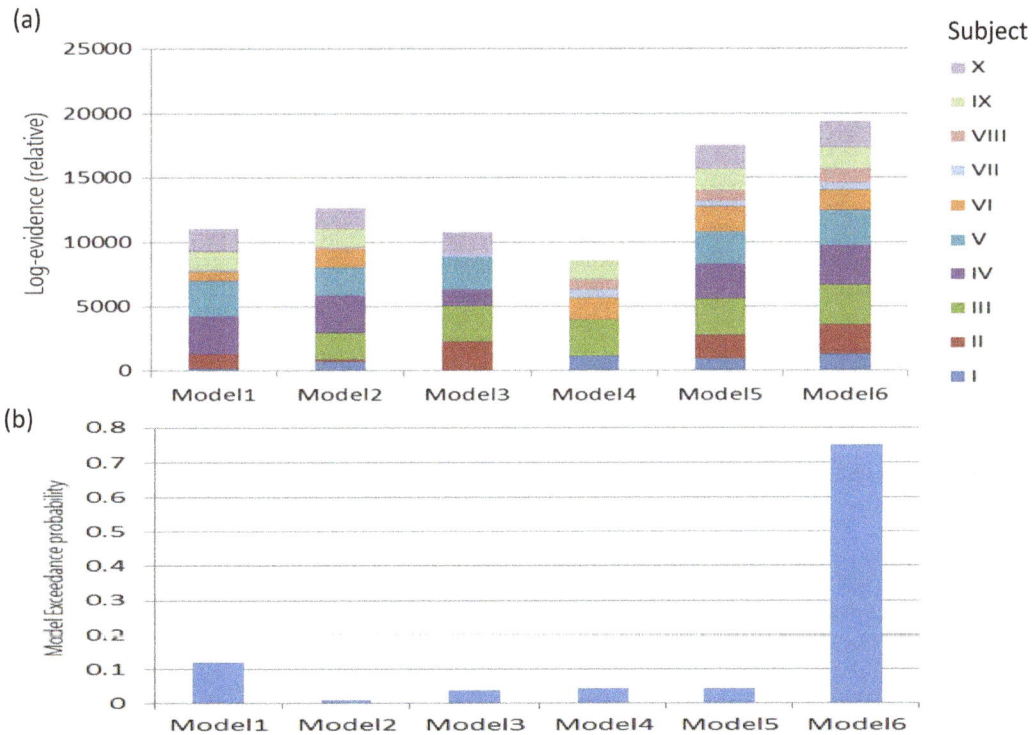

Figure 6. BMS results at the group level under FFX (a) and RFX (b) both confirmed that Model 6 is the most likely model hierarchy among tested models.

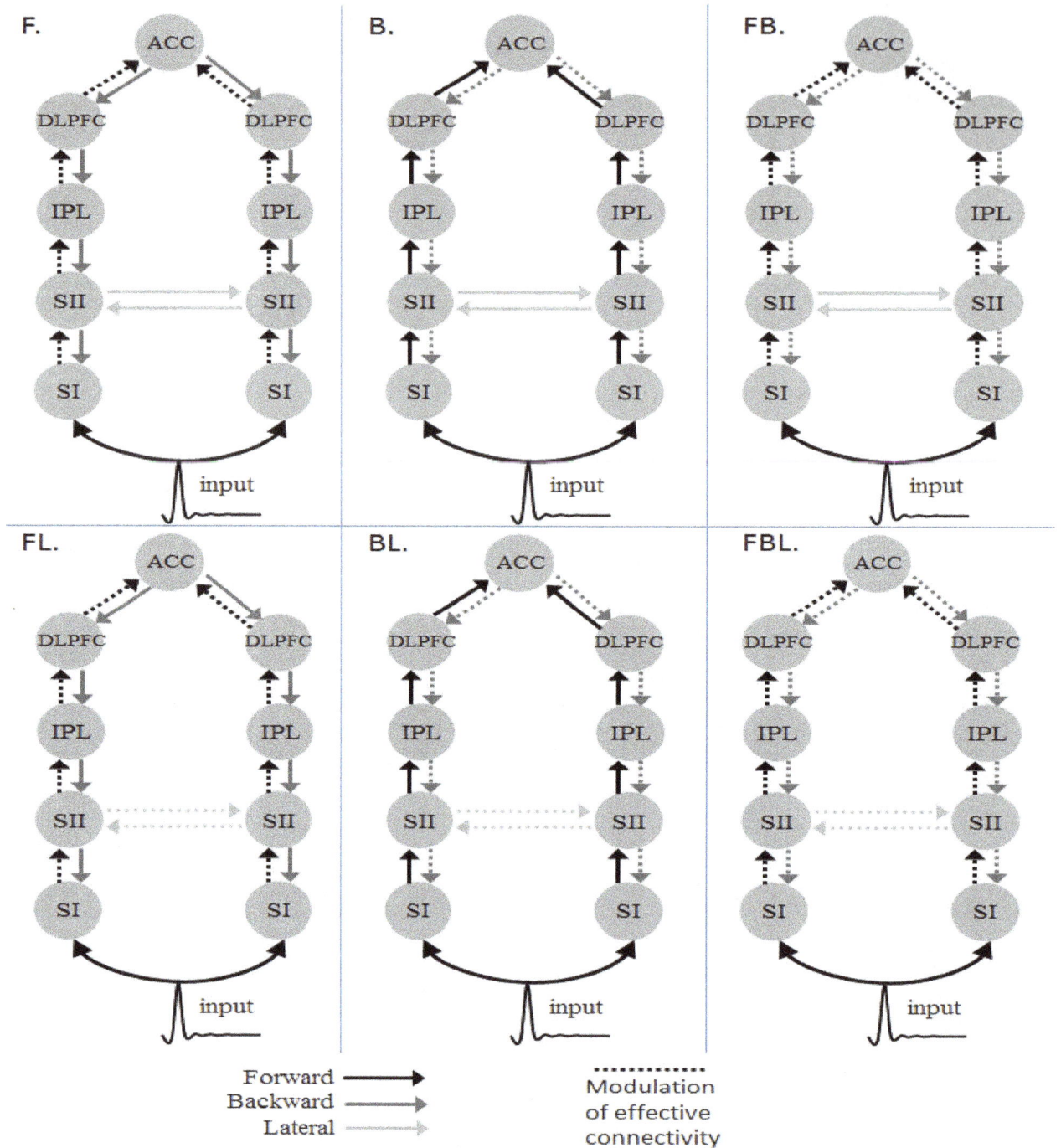

Figure 7. The models for testing the mechanism of the task-related modulation.

[40,41]. Nevertheless, a window of 300–800 ms for each electrode was proved to successfully identify the P300 component under a passive task [36] while a mean tactile P300 latency from 491 to 544 ms at Pz has been reported [41]. Taken together, it is reasonable that we obtained a mean latency of 544 ms of sensory P300 elicited in this passive task.

Novelty P3, Target P3 and Passive P300

Empirically, there are two subcomponents of P300, target P3/ P3b and novelty P3/P3a. Target P3/P3b can be evoked with

posterior foci over parietal area when subjects were responding to the target stimulus using a typical oddball paradigm; novelty P3/ P3a was identified maximally over frontal electrode when novel rare events were presented using a variant of the oddball paradigm, such as a passive or three-stimulus oddball task [32,42]. However, a passive paradigm can reliably elicit a comparable central-parietal maximal P3b that was usually obtained under an active condition by a proper task design (e.g. a long enough inter-trial interval in the range of 4–8 s) [36,43,44]. This implies that the elicitation of P3a and P3b was influenced

(a)

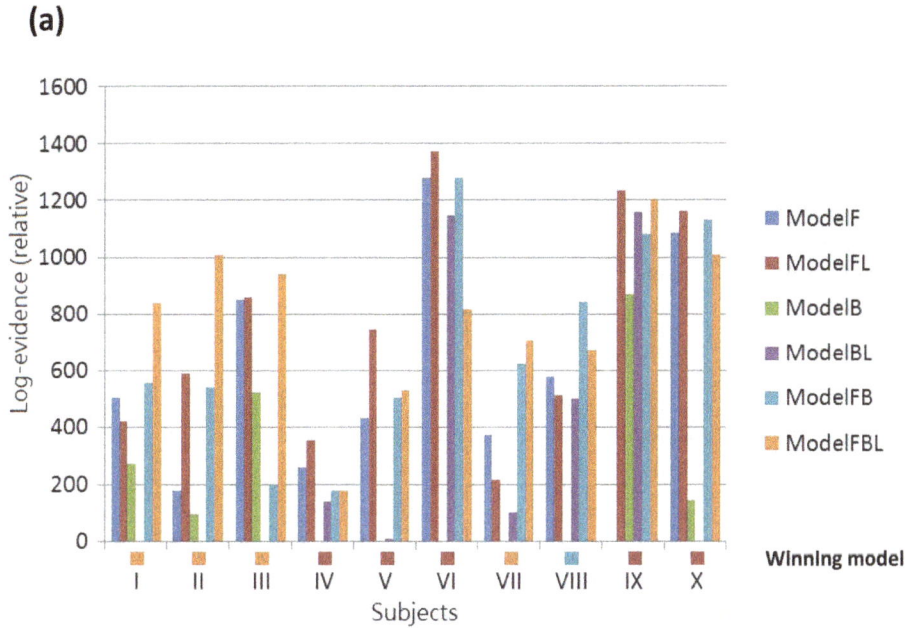

Figure 8. The BMS results of task-dependent modulations under FFX at the single subject level (a) and under RFX at the group level (b).

largely by the stimulus context [45,46]. Nevertheless, P3a and P3b can co-occur within the same ERP waveform [42], and they may reflect the output of a widely distributed neural network engaged in attention and memory updating [32,47,48]. Hence it seems to be more reasonable to study P3a and P3b as a whole when concerning the generating mechanism.

In this study, the passive P300 was elicited by occasional lack of haptic sensory feedbacks without giving any instruction prior to the experiment. This means that these deviant events were unexpected to the subjects and should be able to elicit the novelty P3a. On the other hand, the long inter-trial interval and the highly task-related infrequent events in this task were intended to produce the typical P3b under a passive condition. Therefore, the passive

P300 elicited in this study may comprise of both P3a and P3b, which were mainly manifest over parietal area, and we used a time window from –500 to 900 ms to cover them when modelling the network mechanism in DCM.

Neuronal Network for Passive P300

In this study, we identified a network comprising the ACC, DLPFC, and IPL, as well as the primary and associative sensory areas for generating passive sensory P300 activity using EEG data. This network has been identified in the previous study [8] for mediating the attentional control using an active somatosensory oddball task and MEG data. fMRI data as well showed the similar results [9,49]. Brazdil et al (2007) observed a bidirectional network

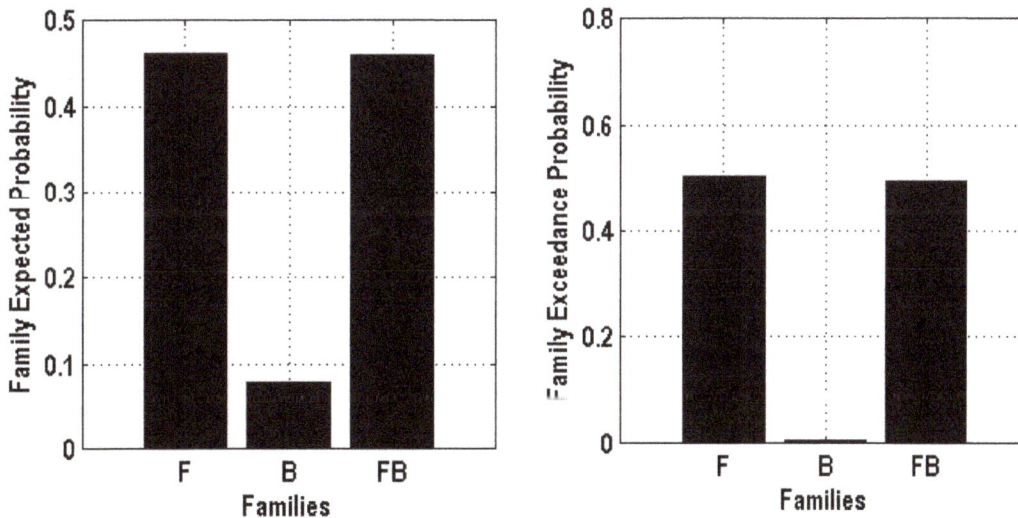

Figure 9. The BMS result of model families.

Table 2. The statistical results on the modulatory coupling parameters.

Model FL

Forward	P-Value	Lateral	P-Value
LS1-LS2	0.517	LS2-RS2	0.452
RS1-RS2	0.137	RS2-LS2	0.721
LS2-LIPL	0.538		
RS2-RIPL	0.876		
LIPL-LDLPFC	**0.029***		
RIPL-RDLPFC	0.071		
LDLPFC-ACC	**0.045***		
RDLPFC-ACC	0.990		

Model FBL

Forward	P-Value	Backward	P-Value	Lateral	P-Value
LS1-LS2	0.978	LS2-LS1	0.050	LS2-RS2	0.921
RS1-RS2	0.488	RS2-RS1	0.841	RS2-LS2	0.298
LS2-LIPL	0.453	LIPL-LS2	0.308		
RS2-RIPL	0.065	RIPL-RS2	0.941		
LIPL-LDLPFC	**0.011***	LDLPFC-LIPL	0.907		
RIPL-RDLPFC	**0.010***	RDLPFC-RIPL	0.689		
LDLPFC-ACC	0.497	ACC-LDLPFC	0.965		
RDLPFC-ACC	0.070	ACC-RDLPFC	0.175		

*$P < 0.05$.

of the ACC, PFC, and IPL for target stimulus processing and they associated this network with two parallel neuronal circuits- frontal (P3a system for top-down attentional control) and parietal circuits (P3b attentional/event encoding system) in target detection [9]. In addition, Asplund et al. (2010) showed that the lateral PFC plays a key role in converging goal-directed and stimulus-driven attention [49]. In other words, the ACC and DLPFC are probably the higher areas providing top-down modulation in the attentional control network. Our findings are in line with these studies specifically because we identified the ACC and DLPFC at top of this network. It is noted that, although the task employed in this study involved a unilateral sensory force input into the right hand, the BMS selects a model with bilateral exogenous inputs to SIs as the wining model. Zhu et al. reported that ipsilateral SI was also activated when using unilateral tactile stimulus [50]. The activity of ipsilateral SI was thought to provide information to SII and the parietal ventral area (PV) for spatiotemporal sensory integration. On the contrast, several studies using unilateral sensory stimuli have reported no significant ipsilateral SI activity though the bilateral SII activations are very evident [6,51,52]. The inconsistent results in the previous studies lead to a question whether the ipsilateral SII receives information from ipsilateral SI or contralateral SII or both. In our study, after comparing the models with and without exogenous input to ipsilateral SI (model 6 and 5, respectively) and without inter-hemispheric SII connection (data not shown), we found that information from both ipsilateral SI and contralateral SII are essential inputs to activate the ipsilateral SII.

In summary, our findings are in agreement with those reported by previous studies, implying that a common neural network architecture exists for P300 production, irrespective of the type of stimulus (i.e. sensory, auditory, or visual) or condition (i.e. active or passive).

Feed-forward Dominating Modulation for a Passive Task

In this study, by omitting haptic stimulus from some of the trials, the P300 was evoked passively through pure change detection, independent of the subjects' response or attentional control. The BMS results suggested a feed-forward modulatory effect underlying this passive network as evidenced by the exceedance probability values of the FL model under the RFX assumption. This may be explained heuristically; when no response is necessary, no regulation (i.e. the top-down modulation) is required. A study using fMRI data and DCM had shown that the bottom-up stimulus-driven responses, such as surprise processing, engage only the feed-forward connections from the IPL to the ACC and DLPFC, whereas conflict processing modulates only the backward information flow from the ACC and DLPFC to the IPL [8]. In other words, the functional role of forward modulation may indicate the delivery of the sensory information, automatic detection of difference, and the stimulus-driven attentional processes involved in performing the task. This could partly explain our finding of the wining FL model. However, a comparison of the model families under the RFX assumption provides similar evidence for both the F and FB model families, indicating that backward modulation may also play a role in this passive task. From previous studies, it has been shown that backward modulation is involved in attentional control/shifting and motor control [53,54]. But both the attentional control/shifting and motor control were absent from our experiment as a passive task and can provide only a minor contribution to our model. When taking into account the model parameters, it can be seen that only parameters governing forward modulations are significant. Taken together, this inconsistence may speak to the fact that there is individual variability in response to the experimental manipulation as reflected in two possible models but the most consistent inter-individual modulation effect was observed only in the feed-forward connections.

Conclusion

In this study, we developed a VR-based sensory oddball task to elicit the passive P300 and investigated the neural network linked to its production by DCM for ERP. The ERP results confirmed that the experimental protocol can reliably elicit passive P300. The DCM results suggested that the passive P300 uses the same parietal-frontal neural network for attentional control, which was identified under an active P300 task. The DCM results also showed that the model with feed-forward modulatory effect wins over the model with backward modulations. To our best knowledge, this is the first study to address the passive P300

network, and these results may provide a reference point for future clinical studies, for example, addressing the network alternations under pathological states of incommunicative patients. However, caution is required when comparing patients' analytic results with this study. For example, the task presented here is not applicable to incommunicative patients.

Author Contributions

Conceived and designed the experiments: CC SY. Performed the experiments: KL CC. Analyzed the data: CC KS KL. Contributed reagents/materials/analysis tools: CC KS KL SY. Wrote the paper: CC. Designed the VR scene: SY.

References

1. Sutton S, Braren M, Zubin J, John ER (1965) Evoked-potential correlates of stimulus uncertainty. Science 150: 1187–1188.
2. Duncan CC, Barry RJ, Connolly JF, Fischer C, Michie PT, et al. (2009) Event-related potentials in clinical research: guidelines for eliciting, recording, and quantifying mismatch negativity, P300, and N400. Clin Neurophysiol 120: 1883–1908.
3. Linden DE (2005) The p300: where in the brain is it produced and what does it tell us? Neuroscientist 11: 563–576.
4. Polich J, Corey-Bloom J (2005) Alzheimer's disease and P300: review and evaluation of task and modality. Curr Alzheimer Res 2: 515–525.
5. Yeung N (2010) Bottom-up influences on voluntary task switching: the elusive homunculus escapes. J Exp Psychol Learn Mem Cogn 36: 348–362.
6. Downar J, Crawley AP, Mikulis DJ, Davis KD (2000) A multimodal cortical network for the detection of changes in the sensory environment. Nat Neurosci 3: 277–283.
7. Crottaz-Herbette S, Menon V (2006) Where and when the anterior cingulate cortex modulates attentional response: combined fMRI and ERP evidence. J Cogn Neurosci 18: 766–780.
8. Huang MX, Lee RR, Miller GA, Thoma RJ, Hanlon FM, et al. (2005) A parietal-frontal network studied by somatosensory oddball MEG responses, and its cross-modal consistency. Neuroimage 28: 99–114.
9. Brazdil M, Mikl M, Marecek R, Krupa P, Rektor I (2007) Effective connectivity in target stimulus processing: a dynamic causal modeling study of visual oddball task. Neuroimage 35: 827–835.
10. Faugeras F, Rohaut B, Weiss N, Bekinschtein TA, Galanaud D, et al. (2011) Probing consciousness with event-related potentials in the vegetative state. Neurology 77: 264–268.
11. Perrin F, Schnakers C, Schabus M, Degueldre C, Goldman S, et al. (2006) Brain response to one's own name in vegetative state, minimally conscious state, and locked-in syndrome. Arch Neurol 63: 562–569.
12. Rappaport M, McCandless KL, Pond W, Krafft MC (1991) Passive P300 response in traumatic brain injury patients. J Neuropsychiatry Clin Neurosci 3: 180–185.
13. Mak JN, Arbel Y, Minett JW, McCane LM, Yuksel B, et al. (2011) Optimizing the P300-based brain-computer interface: current status, limitations and future directions. J Neural Eng 8: 025003.
14. Wolpaw JR, Birbaumer N, McFarland DJ, Pfurtscheller G, Vaughan TM (2002) Brain-computer interfaces for communication and control. Clin Neurophysiol 113: 767–791.
15. Herbert AM, Gordon GE, McCulloch DL (1998) A 'passive' event-related potential? Int J Psychophysiol 28: 11–21.
16. Mertens R, Polich J (1997) P300 from a single-stimulus paradigm: passive versus active tasks and stimulus modality. Electroencephalogr Clin Neurophysiol 104: 488–497.
17. Obuchi C, Harashima T, Shiroma M (2012) Auditory Evoked Potentials under Active and Passive Hearing Conditions in Adult Cochlear Implant Users. Clin Exp Otorhinolaryngol 5 Suppl 1: S6–9.
18. John N (2002) Basis and Principles of Virtual Reality in Medical Imaging. In: Caramella D, Bartolozzi, C., editor. 3D Image Processing: Springer Berlin Heidelberg. pp. 279–285.
19. Laver KE, George S, Thomas S, Deutsch JE, Crotty M (2011) Virtual reality for stroke rehabilitation. Cochrane Database Syst Rev: CD008349.
20. Rizzo A, Schultheis M, Kerns K, Mateer C (2004) Analysis of assets for virtual reality applications in neuropsychology. Neuropsych Rehab 14: 207–223.
21. Kiebel SJ, Garrido MI, Moran R, Chen CC, Friston KJ (2009) Dynamic causal modeling for EEG and MEG. Hum Brain Mapp 30: 1866–1876.

22. David O, Friston KJ (2003) A neural mass model for MEG/EEG: coupling and neuronal dynamics. Neuroimage 20: 1743–1755.
23. Duncan CC, Mirsky AF, Lovelace CT, Theodore WH (2009) Assessment of the attention impairment in absence epilepsy: comparison of visual and auditory P300. Int J Psychophysiol 73: 118–122.
24. Chen CC, Kiebel SJ, Kilner JM, Ward NS, Stephan KE, et al. (2012) A dynamic causal model for evoked and induced responses. Neuroimage 59: 340–348.
25. Montoya P, Sitges C (2006) Affective modulation of somatosensory-evoked potentials elicited by tactile stimulation. Brain Res 1068: 205–212.
26. Pullamsetti SS, Berghausen EM, Dabral S, Tretyn A, Butrous E, et al. (2012) Role of Src tyrosine kinases in experimental pulmonary hypertension. Arterioscler Thromb Vasc Biol 32: 1354–1365.
27. Stephan KE, Penny WD, Daunizeau J, Moran RJ, Friston KJ (2009) Bayesian model selection for group studies. Neuroimage 46: 1004–1017.
28. Wang WJ, Hsieh IF, Chen CC (2013) Accelerating Computation of DCM for ERP in MATLAB by External Function Calls to the GPU. PLoS One 8: e66599.
29. Penny WD, Stephan KE, Mechelli A, Friston KJ (2004) Comparing dynamic causal models. Neuroimage 22: 1157–1172.
30. Stephan KE, Harrison LM, Kiebel SJ, David O, Penny WD, et al. (2007) Dynamic causal models of neural system dynamics:current state and future extensions. J Biosci 32: 129–144.
31. Stephan KE, Penny WD, Moran RJ, den Ouden HE, Daunizeau J, et al. (2010) Ten simple rules for dynamic causal modeling. Neuroimage 49: 3099–3109.
32. Polich J (2007) Updating P300: an integrative theory of P3a and P3b. Clin Neurophysiol 118: 2128–2148.
33. Akatsuka K, Wasaka T, Nakata H, Kida T, Kakigi R (2007) The effect of stimulus probability on the somatosensory mismatch field. Exp Brain Res 181: 607–614.
34. Bekinschtein TA, Dehaene S, Rohaut B, Tadel F, Cohen L, et al. (2009) Neural signature of the conscious processing of auditory regularities. Proc Natl Acad Sci U S A 106: 1672–1677.
35. Kok A (2001) On the utility of P3 amplitude as a measure of processing capacity. Psychophysiology 38: 557–577.
36. Jeon YW, Polich J (2001) P3a from a passive visual stimulus task. Clin Neurophysiol 112: 2202–2208.
37. Goodin DS, Aminoff MJ (1992) Evaluation of dementia by event-related potentials. J Clin Neurophysiol 9: 521–525.
38. Lai CL, Lin RT, Liou LM, Liu CK (2010) The role of event-related potentials in cognitive decline in Alzheimer's disease. Clin Neurophysiol 121: 194–199.
39. Picton TW (1992) The P300 wave of the human event-related potential. J Clin Neurophysiol 9: 456–479.
40. Polich J (1996) Meta-analysis of P300 normative aging studies. Psychophysiology 33: 334–353.
41. Reuter EM, Voelcker-Rehage C, Vieluf S, Winneke AH, Godde B (2013) A parietal-to-frontal shift in the P300 is associated with compensation of tactile discrimination deficits in late middle-aged adults. Psychophysiology.
42. Friedman D, Cycowicz YM, Gaeta H (2001) The novelty P3: an event-related brain potential (ERP) sign of the brain's evaluation of novelty. Neurosci Biobehav Rev 25: 355–373.
43. Polich J, McIsaac HK (1994) Comparison of auditory P300 habituation from active and passive conditions. Int J Psychophysiol 17: 25–34.
44. Polich J (1989) P300 from a passive auditory paradigm. Electroencephalogr Clin Neurophysiol 74: 312–320.
45. Katayama J, Polich J (1996) P300, probability, and the three-tone paradigm. Electroencephalogr Clin Neurophysiol 100: 555–562.

46. Katayama J, Polich J (1998) Stimulus context determines P3a and P3b. Psychophysiology 35: 23–33.

47. Polich J (1988) Bifurcated P300 peaks: P3a and P3b revisited? J Clin Neurophysiol 5: 287–294.

48. Wang L, Liu X, Guise KG, Knight RT, Ghajar J, et al. (2010) Effective connectivity of the fronto-parietal network during attentional control. J Cogn Neurosci 22: 543–553.

49. Asplund CL, Todd JJ, Snyder AP, Marois R (2010) A central role for the lateral prefrontal cortex in goal-directed and stimulus-driven attention. Nat Neurosci 13: 507–512.

50. Zhu Z, Disbrow EA, Zumer JM, McGonigle DJ, Nagarajan SS (2007) Spatiotemporal integration of tactile information in human somatosensory cortex. BMC Neurosci 8: 21.

51. Maldjian JA, Gottschalk A, Patel RS, Pincus D, Detre JA, et al. (1999) Mapping of secondary somatosensory cortex activation induced by vibrational stimulation: an fMRI study. Brain Res 824: 291–295.

52. Robinson CJ, Burton H (1980) Somatotopographic organization in the second somatosensory area of M. fascicularis. J Comp Neurol 192: 43–67.

53. Hopfinger JB, Buonocore MH, Mangun GR (2000) The neural mechanisms of top-down attentional control. Nat Neurosci 3: 284–291.

54. Narayanan NS, Laubach M (2006) Top-down control of motor cortex ensembles by dorsomedial prefrontal cortex. Neuron 52: 921–931.

18

Diffusion Tensor Imaging of Parkinson's Disease, Multiple System Atrophy and Progressive Supranuclear Palsy

Amanda Worker[1,2,3], Camilla Blain[1,4], Jozef Jarosz[4], K. Ray Chaudhuri[1,2,3,4], Gareth J. Barker[1], Steve C. R. Williams[1,2], Richard G. Brown[1,2,3], P. Nigel Leigh[5], Flavio Dell'Acqua[1,2,3], Andrew Simmons[1,2,3]*

1 Institute of Psychiatry, King's College London, London, United Kingdom, 2 National Institute for Health Research Biomedical Research Centre for Mental Health at South London and Maudsley NHS Foundation Trust and Institute of Psychiatry, King's College London, London, United Kingdom, 3 National Institute for Health Research Biomedical Research Unit for Dementia at South London and Maudsley NHS Foundation Trust and Institute of Psychiatry, King's College London, London, United Kingdom, 4 King's College Hospital, London, United Kingdom, 5 Trafford Centre for Biomedical Research, Brighton and Sussex Medical School, University of Sussex, Falmer, Brighton, United Kingdom

Abstract

Although often clinically indistinguishable in the early stages, Parkinson's disease (PD), Multiple System Atrophy (MSA) and Progressive Supranuclear Palsy (PSP) have distinct neuropathological changes. The aim of the current study was to identify white matter tract neurodegeneration characteristic of each of the three syndromes. Tract-based spatial statistics (TBSS) was used to perform a whole-brain automated analysis of diffusion tensor imaging (DTI) data to compare differences in fractional anisotropy (FA) and mean diffusivity (MD) between the three clinical groups and healthy control subjects. Further analyses were conducted to assess the relationship between these putative indices of white matter microstructure and clinical measures of disease severity and symptoms. In PSP, relative to controls, changes in DTI indices consistent with white matter tract degeneration were identified in the corpus callosum, corona radiata, corticospinal tract, superior longitudinal fasciculus, anterior thalamic radiation, superior cerebellar peduncle, medial lemniscus, retrolenticular and anterior limb of the internal capsule, cerebral peduncle and external capsule bilaterally, as well as the left posterior limb of the internal capsule and the right posterior thalamic radiation. MSA patients also displayed differences in the body of the corpus callosum corticospinal tract, cerebellar peduncle, medial lemniscus, anterior and superior corona radiata, posterior limb of the internal capsule external capsule and cerebral peduncle bilaterally, as well as the left anterior limb of the internal capsule and the left anterior thalamic radiation. No significant white matter abnormalities were observed in the PD group. Across groups, MD correlated positively with disease severity in all major white matter tracts. These results show widespread changes in white matter tracts in both PSP and MSA patients, even at a mid-point in the disease process, which are not found in patients with PD.

Editor: Jan Kassubek, University of Ulm, Germany

Funding: Support for this study was provided by the NIHR Biomedical Research Centre for Mental Health and NIHR Biomedical Research Unit for Dementia at South London and Maudsley NHS Foundation Trust and Institute of Psychiatry, King's College London. The funders had no role in study design, data collection and analysis, decision to publish, or preparation of the manuscript.

Competing Interests: GJB has received honoraria for teaching for General Electric Healthcare, and acts as a consultant for IXICO.

* Email: andy.simmons@kcl.ac.uk

Introduction

Parkinson's disease (PD), Multiple System Atrophy (MSA) and Progressive Supranuclear Palsy (PSP) are neurodegenerative diseases that are characterized by very similar motor symptoms, making them difficult to distinguish in the early stages [1,2], despite having distinct molecular pathology [3–5].

A range of Magnetic Resonance Imaging (MRI) techniques have been used to identify regions of brain pathology in parkinsonian syndromes. Previous imaging studies have highlighted pathological changes in white matter, with some involvement of the cortex [6–10]. Diffusion tensor imaging (DTI) provides an indirect insight into white matter microstructure in disease [11]. Frequently used DTI measures include fractional anisotropy (FA) (directionality of water molecule movement within white matter fibers and axons) and mean diffusivity (MD) (degree to which water molecules move within tissues). Studies utilising FA, MD and other diffusion measures in PSP have described abnormalities in the superior longitudinal fasciculus, corpus callosum [12,13] and superior cerebellar peduncles [13–17], whilst in MSA white matter abnormalities have been identified in the putamen [8] and middle cerebellar peduncles [18,19]. In non-demented PD, white matter is thought to remain largely normal [20], however there have been reports of corpus callosum, superior cerebellar peduncles, cingulum and uncinate involvement [17].

Previous neuroimaging studies have often taken a Region of Interest (ROI) approach and few DTI studies have been carried out to characterize the whole brain white matter pathology of patients with Parkinson's Plus syndromes. Tract-Based Spatial Statistics (TBSS) is a whole-brain skeleton-based technique [21] that enables differences in measures such as FA and MD, that may reflect the microstructural properties of white matter tracts, to be identified, whilst avoiding the need for a priori regions of interest to be selected. TBSS also offers advantages over standard voxel-based analytic techniques by removing the need for spatial smoothing and minimizing the methodological pitfalls caused by misalignment and misregistration, consequently increasing the sensitivity and interpretability of findings.

The present study aimed to use TBSS to compare FA and MD values across PSP, MSA, PD and healthy controls, enabling the characterization of regions of abnormal white matter diffusion properties. We performed a series of analyses to test the hypothesis that white matter changes are present in the superior cerebellar peduncle, superior longitudinal fasciculus and corpus callosum in PSP, middle cerebellar peduncles and motor tracts in MSA, with fewer changes demonstrated in the PD group. To our knowledge this is the first study to assess PD, MSA, PSP and healthy controls in a single study using a whole brain approach.

Methods

Participants

Sixteen patients diagnosed with the Richardson's syndrome variant of PSP, seventeen with MSA and fourteen with PD, according to established criteria, [22–24] were recruited successively from the Movement Disorders Clinic at King's College Hospital and via referrals from clinicians in south east England. Both clinical variants of MSA were included; eleven probable MSA-P (predominant parkinsonian features) and five MSA-C (predominant cerebellar features). All PSP patients were classified as probable, [1] while all patients with PD fulfilled criteria for definite PD [23]. Eighteen healthy age-matched controls were also recruited (spouses and friends of patients) (see Table 1).

Ethics Statement

The project was approved by research ethics committees of King's Healthcare NHS Trust and the Institute of Psychiatry and South London and Maudsley NHS Trust. Written informed consent was given by all subjects before participation in the study.

Clinical and cognitive measures

Within 1 week of the MRI scan each participant was examined by the same clinician (CB). Disease severity was measured using Hoehn and Yahr (H&Y) [25], Schwab and England Activities of Daily Living (ADL) [26] and Unified Parkinson's Disease Rating Scale Part III (UPDRS-III) [27]. Cerebellar ataxia and occulo-motor dysfunction were assessed using the Parkinson's Plus Scale (PPS) [28]. A higher score on the UPDRS-III (0–108 points) and H&Y (stages 1–5) represents greater impairment, whilst a higher score on the Schwab and England ADL (0–100%) represents less impairment. Global cognitive function was assessed using the Mini-Mental State Examination (MMSE) [29] and Mattis Dementia Rating Scale (DRS) [30].

Image acquisition

All images were acquired with slices parallel to the anterior commissure–posterior commissure line, on a 1.5-T Signa LX NV/

i system (General Electric, Milwaukee, WI), with actively shielded magnetic field gradients (maximum amplitude 40 mTm^{-1}). A standard quadrature birdcage head coil was used for both RF transmission and reception.

Using a multislice, peripherally gated echoplanar imaging pulse sequence, each DTI volume was acquired from 60 contiguous 2.5 mm thick slices with field of view (FOV) 240×240 mm and matrix size 96×96, zero-filled to 128×128, giving an in-plane voxel size of 1.875×1.875 mm^2. Echo time was 107 ms, and effective repetition time was 15 R-R intervals. At each location, 7 images were acquired without diffusion weighting, together with 64 images with a weighting of 1,300 s mm^{-2} applied along directions uniformly distributed in space (Jones et al, 2002). Since acquisition of DTI data were cardiac-gated, scanning time varied according to each subjects pulse rate. For most subjects, scanning time was approximately 25 minutes. A semi-automated EPI quality control procedure was used [31].

Image processing

An additional visual inspection of diffusion data was further used to exclude data that did not meet quality requirements; one MSA patient and one healthy control subject were excluded due to corrupted scans. Data were then processed using ExploreDTI [32] to correct for the effects of eddy current distortions and head motion. For each subject the b-matrix was then re-oriented to provide a more accurate estimate of tensor orientations. The diffusion-tensor was estimated using a non-linear least square approach, with FA and MD calculated from the diffusion-tensor. Voxel-wise statistical analysis of FA and MD was carried out using TBSS v1.2 (tract-based spatial statistics) (http://www.fmrib.ox.ac.uk/fsl/tbss/) [21,33,34] to compare groups. First, each fractional anisotropy image was registered to standard MNI space using the non-linear registration tool in FSL (FNIRT), resulting in a standardised version of each FA image. These steps were repeated for the mean diffusivity data. A voxel-wise average of all subjects was used to create a study-specific mean fractional anisotropy image, which was then 'skeletonized' to create a mean fractional anisotropy skeleton, representing the centres of all white matter tracts. To exclude low anisotropic regions in the skeleton, a fractional anisotropy threshold of 0.2 was applied.

Statistical Analysis

Clinical Variables. Clinical variables were analysed using SPSS (version 20); one-way ANOVA with built-in post-hoc Bonferroni tests were used to assess between-group differences in age, duration of disease, UPDRS-III and cognitive measures (MMSE and DRS scores). Post-hoc t-tests were also performed to assess the difference in age between the PSP group and each other group.

A Kruskall-Wallis test was run to determine if there were differences between H&Y, Schwab and England ADL, PPS Occulomotor and Cerebellar scores between clinical groups. Pairwise comparisons were performed using Dunn's (1964) procedure with a Bonferroni correction for multiple comparisons.

Image Analysis. Whole-brain statistical analyses were performed using Randomise v2.1 (FSL). Differences in FA and MD between groups were assessed using a two-sample t test to compare FA and MD values. Clinical groups were first compared with a healthy control population, and then further compared to each other. Additional analyses were run on all subjects as a single group to assess associations between FA and MD values and measures of disease severity (H Schwab and England ADL; UDRS-III), PPS cerebellar and occulomotor scores and cognition (MMSE; DRS).

Table 1. Demographic and clinical data of control subjects and patients with PD, MSA and PSP.

	Control (n = 17)	PD (n = 14)	MSA (n = 16)	PSP (n = 16)	P-value
Age, mean (SD)	63.9 (8.4)	64.7 (6.9)	62.3 (7.3)	69.2 (6.2)	0.056
Sex, M:F	9:8	7:7	8:8	6:10	NA
Disease duration, mean (SD)	NA	6.6 (2.0)	5.1 (2.7)	5.2 (2.5)	0.181
H&Y* median score (range)	NA	2.5 (2.0–3.0)	3.0 (2.5–5.0)	4.0 (3.0–4.0)	<0.001
Schwab and England ADL* median score (range)	NA	90% (80–100%)	60% (40–80%)	45% (20–80%)	<0.01
UPDRS III, *mean +/− SD (range)	NA	21.8+/−9.6 (5–38)	37.6+/−13.5 (12–62)	35.9+/−6.6 (24–47)	<0.001
Occulomotor Score, †median (range)	NA	0 (0–3)	1.5 (0–5)	16 (7–20)	<0.001
Cerebellar Score, †median (range)	NA	0 (0–2)	7.5 (0–13)	2 (0–6)	<0.05
MMSE, mean (SD)	29 (1)	29.5 (1.1)	28 (2.7)	26 (2.7)	<0.001
DRS, mean (SD)	140 (3.4)	140 (2.9)	135.4 (8.9)	126 (10.2)	<0.001

*For patients taking levodopa drug treatment, scores given in the 'on' state.
†From Parkinson's Plus Scale (Cerebellar Score, maximum 24; Occulomotor Score, maximum 21).
MSA = multiple systems atrophy; PSP = progressive supranuclear palsy; PD = Parkinson's disease; MSA-P = multiple system atrophy parkinsonian variant; MSA-C = multiple system atrophy cerebellar variant; H&Y = Hoehn and Yahr; ADL = activities of daily living; UPDRS III = Unified Parkinson Disease Rating Scale–part III; MMSE = Mini Mental State Examination; DRS = Mattis Dementia Rating Scale.

Age and gender were de-meaned before analysis and used as covariates of no-interest within the voxel-based analysis. Threshold-free cluster enhancement (TFCE) was used in all statistical comparisons to correct for multiple comparisons across space; a non-parametric permutation test was used, in which group membership was permuted 5000 times to generate a null distribution for each contrast. Due to the number of statistical tests carried out an additional Bonferroni correction for multiple comparisons was applied dividing the alpha value by the number of tests each data set was included in. To localize significant voxel effects, contrast maps were subdivided according to the 48 regions of the JHU-ICBM-DTI-81 white matter atlas [35], allowing identification of regions of significance and peak voxels within clusters.

Results

Demographic and clinical variables

Diagnostic groups did not differ significantly in age, gender or disease duration in one-way ANOVA analyses. However, post hoc t-tests showed that the PSP group is significantly older than the MSA (p = 0.007) and HC (p = 0.048) groups. The PD group scored lower than the MSA and PSP groups on measures of disease severity; H&Y (p≤0.001), Schwab and England ADL (p≤0.01) and UPDRS III (p≤0.001). The MSA group had more severe cerebellar dysfunction (p≤0.05) than the other two clinical groups, while the PSP group had more severe occulomotor dysfunction (p≤0.001) and greater cognitive impairment; MMSE (p≤0.001) and DRS (p≤0.001) (Table 1).

PD, MSA and PSP versus healthy controls

First, the white matter maps of each clinical group (PD, MSA, PSP) were compared individually with the maps of age-matched healthy control subjects.

PSP. These comparisons revealed regions of reduced FA in PSP in the corpus callosum, anterior and superior corona radiata, superior longitudinal fasciculus/arcuate, and corticospinal tract bilaterally as well as the left posterior corona radiata (Figure 1; Table 2). Regions of increased MD were found in the PSP group in the corpus callosum, superior corona radiata, anterior thalamic radiation, superior cerebellar peduncle, medial lemniscus, cerebral peduncle and posterior limb of the internal capsule bilaterally (Figure 1; Table 3).

MSA. MSA patients showed increased MD in the corticospinal tract, middle and inferior cerebellar peduncles, and medial lemniscus (Figure 2; Table 3).

PD. There were no significant differences between the PD patients and healthy controls.

All results are Bonferroni corrected (corrected alpha = 0.0167).

Clinical group comparisons

PSP vs PD. Reduced FA was identified in the PSP group when compared to PD in the corpus callosum, corona radiata, corticospinal tract, anterior thalamic radiation, superior cerebellar peduncle, external capsule, retrolenticular and anterior limb of the internal capsule bilaterally, as well as the right superior longitudinal fasciculus, left posterior limb of the internal capsule and the right posterior thalamic radiation (Figure 1; Table 2). Increased MD was also seen in PSP compared to PD, affecting the corpus callosum, corona radiata, superior cerebellar peduncles, anterior thalamic radiation, superior longitudinal fasciculus, medial lemniscus, cerebral peduncle, posterior and anterior limbs of the internal capsule and the external capsule bilaterally (Figure 1; Table 3).

MSA vs PD. When compared to PD the MSA group displayed reduced FA in the body of the corpus callosum, anterior corona radiata, corticospinal tract, middle and inferior cerebellar peduncles, medial lemniscus, and posterior limb of the internal

Table 2. White matter regions of fractional anisotropy changes between PSP, MSA, PD and HC.

Region	Coordinates			PSP<HC	PSP<PD	MSA<PD
	X	Y	Z	P-value	P-value	P-value
Corpus callosum						
Genu	4	27	0	0.0008	0.0002	
Body	1	−21	23	0.0006	0.0002	0.0106
Splenium	−18	−47	27	0.0008	0.0002	
Corona Radiata						
Left anterior	−17	22	29	0.0011	0.0004	0.0166
Right anterior	18	16	29	0.0006	0.0002	0.0124
Left superior	−18	11	33	0.0008	0.0004	
Right superior	19	12	33	0.0006	0.0002	
Left posterior	−19	−33	33	0.0008	0.0023	
Right posterior	29	−57	20		0.0072	
Corticospinal						
Right	20	−31	50	0.0008	0.0006	0.0032
Left	−6	−55	−20	0.0008	0.0092	0.0032
Longitudinal fasciculus						
Left superior	−36	−31	34	0.0155		
Right superior	39	−6	30	0.0004	0.0006	
Thalamic radiation						
Right anterior	6	−13	14		0.0036	
Left anterior	−4	−14	14		0.0036	0.0096
Cerebellar peduncle						
Left superior	−7	−45	−29		0.0038	
Right superior	7	47	−32		0.0038	
Middle	14	−35	−30			0.0021
Left inferior	−11	−46	−30			0.0021
Right inferior	13	−46	−30			0.0021
Pontine crossing tract	2	−31	−30			0.0017
Lemniscus						
Left medial	−6	−38	−30			0.0025
Right medial	6	−37	−30			0.0025
External Capsule						
Left	−28	14	0		0.0062	
Right	31	12	0		0.0072	
Internal Capsule						
Left retrolenticular	−29	−21	0		0.0104	
Right retrolenticular	38	−28	0		0.0068	
Left posterior limb	−20	−14	0		0.0072	0.0077
Right posterior limb	19	−10	0			0.0196
Left anterior limb	−10	5	0		0.0072	0.0098
Right anterior limb	10	5	0		0.0134	
Thalamic Radiation						
Right posterior	30	−60	0		0.0068	

All results reported at p<0.05, TFCE and Bonferroni corrected (corrected alpha = 0.0167).

capsule bilaterally, as well as the left anterior limb of the internal capsule and left anterior thalamic radiation (Figure 2; Table 2). Increased MD was found in the superior corona radiata, corticospinal tract, superior, middle and inferior cerebellar peduncles, posterior limb of the internal capsule, cerebral peduncle and the external capsule bilaterally (Figure 2; Table 3).

PSP vs MSA. The PSP group showed increased MD when compared to MSA in the anterior thalamic radiation and superior cerebellar peduncles (Figure 1; Table 2).

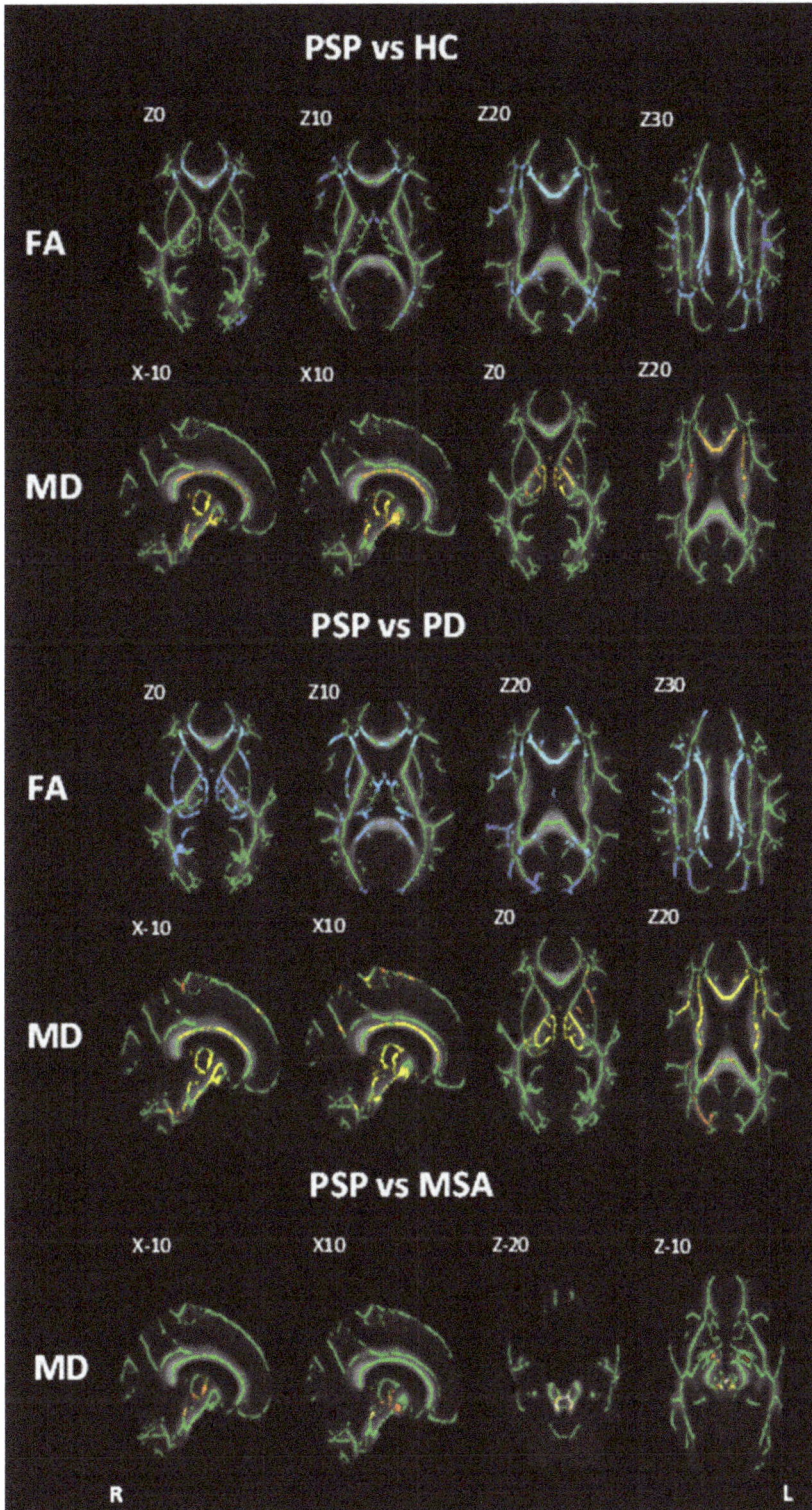

Figure 1. White matter maps showing regions of significant decreased fractional anisotropy and increased mean diffusivity in PSP patients when compared to healthy controls, PD and MSA (Bonferroni corrected alpha – 0.0167). Background image corresponds to the mean fractional anisotropy image of all subjects in standard MNI152 space (radiological view). Fractional anisotropy white matter skeleton is represented by green voxels. Blue voxels represent regions of decreased FA and yellow voxels represent regions of increased MD in the PSP group.

Table 3. White matter regions of mean diffusivity changes between PSP, MSA, PD and HC.

Region	Coordinates			HC<PSP	HC<MSA	PD<PSP	PD<MSA	MSA<PSP
	X	Y	Z	P-value	P-value	P-value	P-value	P-value
Corpus Callosum								
Body	0	14	20	0.005				
Genu	2	26	10	0.006		0.0002		
Splenium	14	−36	26	0.005		0.0002		
Corona Radiata								
Left anterior	−26	30	12			0.0017		
Right anterior	27	26	12			0.0002		
Left superior	−27	7	26	0.0145		0.0008	0.0040	
Right superior	27	9	26	0.0145		0.0002	0.0040	
Left posterior	−26	−32	27			0.0002		
Right posterior	26	−31	27			0.0013		
Corticospinal								
Left	−10	−23	−24		0.0028	0.0002	0.0004	
Right	10	−27	−27		0.0017		0.0004	
Longitudinal fasciculus								
Left superior	−32	−29	39			0.0006		
Right superior	35	4	27			0.0002		
Thalamic radiation								
Left anterior	4	−19	−7	0.0008		0.0002		
Right anterior	−6	−19	−1	0.0013		0.0002		0.0028
Cerebellar peduncle								
Left superior	−3	−29	−19	0.0006		0.0002	0.0025	0.0023
Right superior	4	−29	−19	0.0011		0.0002	0.0008	
Left inferior	−8	−53	−21		0.0015		0.0002	0.0021
Right inferior	8	−53	−21		0.0013		0.0002	0.0021
Middle	14	−35	−31		0.0008		0.0002	
Pontine crossing tract	4	−30	−28		0.0015		0.0002	
Lemniscus								
Left medial	−5	−35	−26	0.0008	0.0017	0.0002		
Right medial	6	−35	−25	0.0008	0.0008	0.0002		
Cerebral peduncle								
Left	−10	−26	−12	0.0013		0.0002	0.0008	
Right	12	−25	−12	0.0013		0.0002	0.0008	
Internal Capsule								

Table 3. Cont.

Region	Coordinates			HC<PSP	HC<MSA	PD<PSP	PD<MSA	MSA<PSP
	X	Y	Z	P-value	P-value	P-value	P-value	P-value
Left posterior limb	−10	−8	0	0.0013		0.0002	0.0041	
Right posterior limb	11	−8	0	0.0021		0.0002	0.0041	
Left anterior limb	−10	0	0			0.0002		
Right anterior limb	10	0	0			0.0002		
External capsule								
Right	33	−20	0			0.0028	0.0028	
Left	−30	−13	14			0.0028	0.0041	

All results reported at p<0.05, TFCE and Bonferroni corrected (corrected alpha 0.0167).

There were no regions in which PD showed significantly reduced FA or decreased MD compared to either MSA or PSP. All results passed bonferroni correction (corrected alpha = 0.0167).

Relationship between FA and MD values and clinical variables

Measures of disease severity showed significant correlation with MD values after Bonferroni correction. Disease severity as measured by the Schwab and England ADL correlated negatively with MD values in all main white matter tracts that showed changes in this study (see Table 2 and 3) with a right lateralisation of the corona radiata, corpus callosum and superior longitudinal fasciculus (Figure 3). MD values in the middle cerebellar peduncles also correlated positively with scores on the H&Y scale of disease severity (Figure 3).

Radial and Axial Diffusivity

As requested by one of the reviewers additional analyses were undertaken to assess group differences in radial and axial diffusivity. As these measures were not part of the hypothesis for this study we have included these results (see Table S1 and S2).

Discussion

To our knowledge this is the first study to investigate DTI indices consistent with white matter microstructural properties using a whole-brain automated technique to directly compare PD, MSA, PSP and healthy control subjects. We demonstrate changes in FA and MD measures that are consistent with white matter tract degeneration in PSP encompassing all of the main white matter tracts including the corpus callosum, superior longitudinal fasciculus, superior cerebellar peduncles and cingulum, in line with recent reports [12–17,36]. These results support the work of Agosta and colleagues, whilst also identifying additional regions that may be implicated in the disease process by using an exploratory whole-brain approach that does not rely on a priori regions of interest. Other regions showing changes in PSP included the corona radiata, thalamic radiation, medial lemniscus, cerebral peduncle, internal capsule and the external capsule. In MSA changes reflecting white matter tract degeneration were observed in the middle and inferior cerebellar peduncle, corticospinal tract, lemniscus, cerebral peduncle, left posterior limb of the internal capsule and left external capsule. Consistent with previous studies, white matter was found to be intact in PD [20,37–39].

Of particular interest is the superior cerebellar peduncles in PSP which showed significant changes that may be reflective of neurodegeneration. In contrast, patients with MSA displayed significant changes in the middle and inferior cerebellar peduncles compared to healthy controls and in the superior, middle and inferior cerebellar peduncles when compared with PD. These results are in line with a previous study that has reported the ability to differentiate between patients with PD, MSA and PSP based on diffusion measures in the middle cerebellar peduncles [9] – a region that appears to be particularly affected in MSA. In this study, MD values across the cerebellar peduncle also correlated with patients H&Y and Schwab and England ADL scores; measures of disease severity, which may mean that degeneration in this region could be used to assess disease progression and that cerebellar peduncle diffusion measures along with a network of other regions of high significance such as the corpus callosum and corona radiata may have the potential to be used to discriminate between MSA and PSP. Furthermore, these results confirm that degeneration of these tracts does not occur in PD.

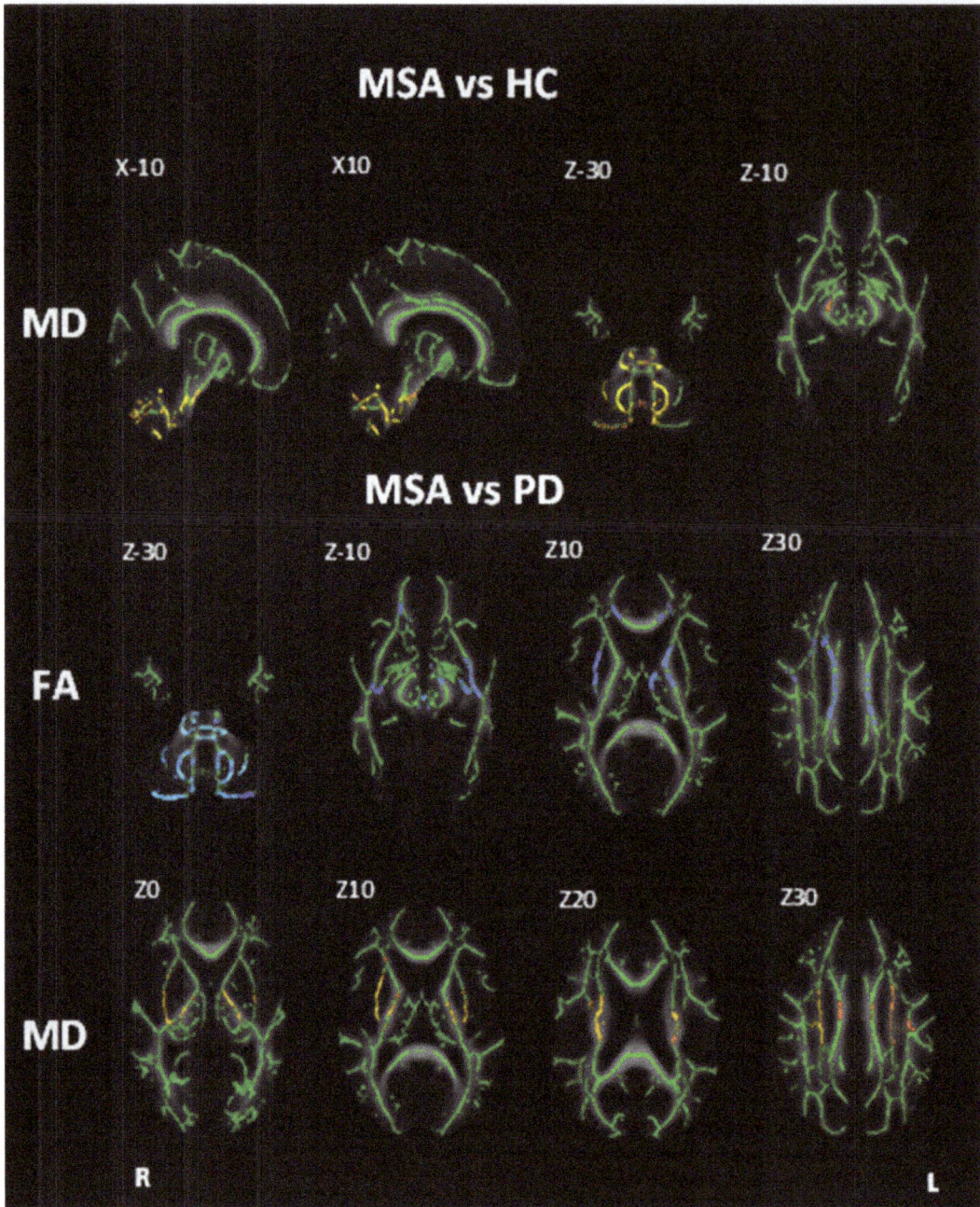

Figure 2. White matter maps showing regions of significant decreased fractional anisotropy and increased mean diffusivity in MSA patients when compared to healthy controls and PD (Bonferroni corrected alpha = 0.0167). Background image corresponds to the mean fractional anisotropy image of all subjects in standard MNI152 space (radiological view). Fractional anisotropy white matter skeleton is represented by green voxels. Blue voxels represent regions of decreased FA and yellow voxels represent regions of increased MD in the PSP group.

Interestingly, superior cerebellar peduncles abnormalities in PSP relative to PD, MSA and control subjects were found only for MD value, while reduced FA identified greater changes in the left peduncle relative to PD. This discrepancy between fractional anisotropy and mean diffusivity results could be due to differences in fiber architecture between subjects leading to increased variability of fractional anisotropy across groups – fiber architecture is a major determinant of anisotropy in healthy brains [40]. Mean diffusivity may provide a more direct measure of neuronal

integrity because it is believed to be less affected by the fiber architecture or its structural organisation.

Significantly reduced FA and MD were observed in PSP in the genu, body and splenium of the corpus callosum. These results are more widespread than in previous studies that have reported only partial involvement of the corpus callosum [12,14,36,41]. The fibres of the genu of the corpus callosum provide connections to the premotor and supplementary motor areas of the superior frontal gyrus – regions of grey matter that have been previously implicated in the disease [12,42,43] whilst the splenium of the

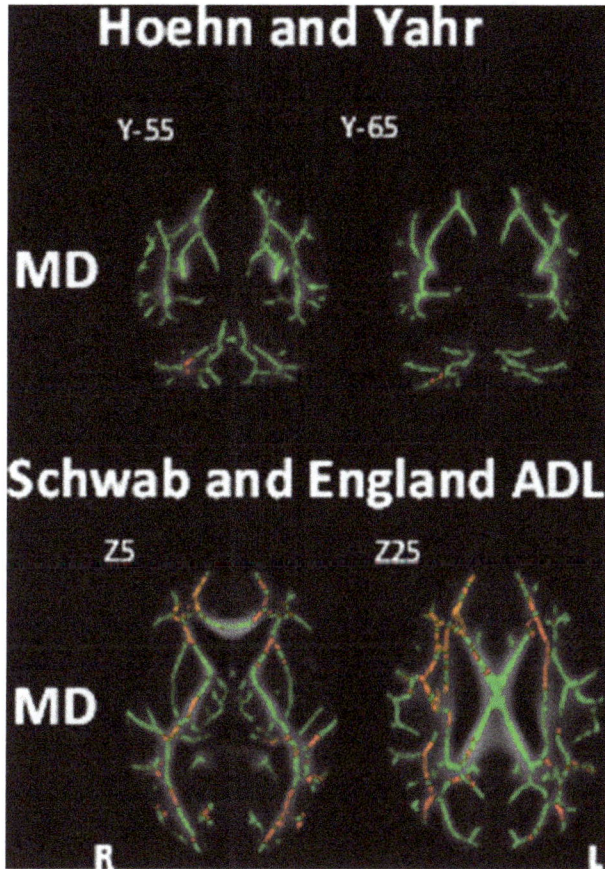

Figure 3. White matter maps showing regions of significant correlation between mean diffusivity and measures of disease severity (Bonferroni corrected alpha = 0.0167). Top row coronal view, bottom row axial view. Background image corresponds to the mean fractional anisotropy image of all subjects in standard MNI152 space (radiological view). Fractional anisotropy white matter skeleton is represented by green voxels. Blue voxels represent regions of decreased FA and yellow voxels represent regions of increased MD in the PSP group.

corpus callosum communicates somatosensory information between the parietal lobe and visual centre of the occipital lobe. FA and MD values in the corpus callosum did not correlate with any clinical variables. It could be that loss of integrity in these white matter tracts is a result of Wallerian degeneration, a secondary degeneration of axons following cortical grey matter atrophy in regions that have been found to be related to clinical symptoms and severity.

An alternative explanation to Wallerian degeneration could be activated microglia or tau deposition causing changes to the microstructural properties of these white matter tracts. The pattern of degeneration of white matter tracts in PSP seen in this study is consistent with the pattern of activated microglia found in a previous study [44]. The activation of microglia is a reactive response to pathology [45] and so is likely to indicate where pathology exists but not the cause of it. The presence of microglia in white matter tracts has been shown to correlate with tau burden in the cerebral peduncle and internal capsule, but not the superior cerebellar peduncle where microglial presence was higher. Thus in some regions microglia may become active in response to tau related pathology, whilst in others microgliosis may be related to degeneration that is not associated with tau

pathology, but another cause of initial degeneration, with microgliosis leading to further tissue pathology [46]. Similarly, in MSA, both activated microglia and glial cytoplasmic inclusion (GCI) are present in affected white matter tracts [44,47,48]. Further pathological studies are required to understand the impact of protein dysfunction, microgliosis and Wallerian degeneration on white matter integrity in these populations.

This study additionally identified lateralisation of FA changes in regions including the left posterior corona radiata, right superior longitudinal fasciculus and right posterior thalamic radiation in PSP and in the left anterior thalamic radiation, left anterior limb of the internal capsule in MSA patients. Hemispheric lateralisation has not been well studied in these patient samples and has not been reported in previous studies of this nature, thus these results will need to be verified in a larger sample size to ensure that this lateralisation is not an artefact.

Our study has a number of strengths. This is the first study to explore differences and similarities of DTI indices that are indicative of white matter tract degeneration in PD, MSA and PSP populations in a single study. Secondly, this is the first study to apply a whole-brain automated technique in these populations, avoiding the use of a priori defined ROIs. TBSS offers several other advantages over other methods, for example it removes the need for spatial smoothing and minimises the methodological pitfalls caused by misalignment and misregistration, consequently improving the sensitivity and interpretability of findings. The main limitation of this study is the sample size for each clinical group, the statistical power of the study would be increased with larger group sizes. In addition, results may have been affected by the slightly older age of the PSP patients, thus age was included as a nuisance factor in all analyses to account for this difference. It would also have been beneficial to run a battery of neuropsychological tests on all subjects to rule out confounding effects due to other disorders or conditions. Due to the inclusion of a series of statistical tests with the four groups, a Bonferroni correction was applied which is likely to have reduced the power of the results. Finally, in this study both subtypes MSA-C and MSA-P patients were included as a single MSA group, it is possible that there are subtle pathological differences between these groups, thus in future it would be interesting to look at both of these subtypes as separate groups.

It is clear from this study that in the established disease state PSP patients have profound and widespread white matter alterations. Similarly, MSA patients also display white matter changes in the later stages of the disease. Despite PD patients having longer mean disease duration than MSA and PSP, they scored significantly lower on measures of disease severity and displayed unaffected white matter. This evidence, along with positive correlations between disease severity and white matter changes, provides evidence for slower neurodegeneration along with slower symptom progression [1] in PD compared to other Parkinsonian syndromes. This study provides a comprehensive characterisation of white matter alterations in MSA and PSP that may be used to identify regions of particular interest in future studies assessing early stage disease and may in future aid in the identification of an in vivo biomarker. In conclusion, this work provides evidence for widespread changes in FA and MD that are consistent with white matter neurodegeneration in both MSA and PSP patients, whilst white matter remains preserved in PD. These disruptions are particularly evident in the cerebellar peduncles, supratentorial regions and association fibers.

Acknowledgments

The authors thank the people affected by MSA, PSP, and PD and healthy volunteers for their participation. They also thank consultant colleagues from the King's College Hospital Movement Disorders Group and south England for referring patients, and the Neuroprotection and Natural History in PSP and MSA (NNIPPS) consortium for allowing them to use the Parkinson's Plus Scale.

Author Contributions

Conceived and designed the experiments: CB KRC PNL AS. Performed the experiments: CB JJ KRC GJB SCRW RGB PNL AS. Analyzed the data: AW FD AS. Contributed reagents/materials/analysis tools: AW FD AS. Contributed to the writing of the manuscript: AW FD AS. Critically revised the manuscript and approved final version: CB JJ KRC GJB SCRW RGB PNL.

References

1. Litvan I, Bhatia KP, Burn DJ, Goetz CG, Lang AE, et al. (2003) SIC Task Force appraisal of clinical diagnostic criteria for parkinsonian disorders. Movement Disorders 18: 467–486.
2. Bensimon G, Ludolph A, Agid Y, Vidailhet M, Payan C, et al. (2009) Riluzole treatment, survival and diagnostic criteria in Parkinson plus disorders: the NNIPPS study. Brain 132: 156–171.
3. Braak H, Braak E (2000) Pathoanatomy of Parkinson's disease. Journal of Neurology 247: II3–II10.
4. Braak H, Tredici KD, Rüb U, de Vos RA, Jansen Steur EN, et al. (2003) Staging of brain pathology related to sporadic Parkinson's disease. Neurobiology of aging 24: 197–211.
5. Hauw J-J, Daniel S, Dickson D, Horoupian D, Jellinger K, et al. (1994) Preliminary NINDS neuropathologic criteria for Steele-Richardson-Olszewski syndrome (progressive supranuclear palsy). Neurology 44: 2015–2015.
6. Boxer AL, Geschwind MD, Belfor N, Gorno-Tempini ML, Schauer GF, et al. (2006) Patterns of brain atrophy that differentiate corticobasal degeneration syndrome from progressive supranuclear palsy. Archives of neurology 63: 81–86.
7. Price S, Paviour D, Scahill R, Stevens J, Rossor M, et al. (2004) Voxel-based morphometry detects patterns of atrophy that help differentiate progressive supranuclear palsy and Parkinson's disease. Neuroimage 23: 663–669.
8. Schocke M, Seppi K, Esterhammer R, Kremser C, Jaschke W, et al. (2002) Diffusion-weighted MRI differentiates the Parkinson variant of multiple system atrophy from PD. Neurology 58: 575–580.
9. Prodoehl J, Li H, Planetta PJ, Goetz CG, Shannon KM, et al. (2013) Diffusion tensor imaging of Parkinson's disease, atypical parkinsonism, and essential tremor. Movement Disorders 28: 1816–1822.
10. Pereira JB, Ibarretxe-Bilbao N, Marti MJ, Compta Y, Junqué C, et al. (2012) Assessment of cortical degeneration in patients with Parkinson's disease by voxel-based morphometry, cortical folding, and cortical thickness. Human brain mapping 33: 2521–2534.
11. Basser PJ, Mattiello J, LeBihan D (1994) MR diffusion tensor spectroscopy and imaging. Biophysical journal 66: 259–267.
12. Padovani A, Borroni B, Brambati SM, Agosti C, Broli M, et al. (2006) Diffusion tensor imaging and voxel based morphometry study in early progressive supranuclear palsy. Journal of Neurology, Neurosurgery & Psychiatry 77: 457–463.
13. Caso F, Agosta F, Volontè MA, Martinelli D, Sarro L, et al. (2014) Mapping Regional Grey and White Matter Damage in Patients with Progressive Supranuclear Palsy Syndrome (S57. 007). Neurology 82: S57. 007-S057. 007.
14. Whitwell JL, Master AV, Avula R, Kantarci K, Eggers SD, et al. (2011) Clinical correlates of white matter tract degeneration in progressive supranuclear palsy. Archives of neurology 68: 753–760.
15. Tsuboi Y, Slowinski J, Josephs KA, Honer WG, Wszolek ZK, et al. (2003) Atrophy of superior cerebellar peduncle in progressive supranuclear palsy. Neurology 60: 1766–1769.
16. Agosta F, Pievani M, Svetel M, Ječmenica Lukić M, Copetti M, et al. (2012) Diffusion tensor MRI contributes to differentiate Richardson's syndrome from PSP-parkinsonism. Neurobiology of aging 33: 2817–2826.
17. Agosta F, Galantucci S, Svetel M, Lukić MJ, Copetti M, et al. (2014) Clinical, cognitive, and behavioural correlates of white matter damage in progressive supranuclear palsy. Journal of neurology 261: 913–924.
18. Paviour DC, Thornton JS, Lees AJ, Jäger HR (2007) Diffusion-weighted magnetic resonance imaging differentiates Parkinsonian variant of multiple-system atrophy from progressive supranuclear palsy. Movement disorders 22: 68–74.
19. Blain C, Barker G, Jarosz J, Coyle N, Landau S, et al. (2006) Measuring brain stem and cerebellar damage in parkinsonian syndromes using diffusion tensor MRI. Neurology 67: 2199–2205.
20. Hattori T, Orimo S, Aoki S, Ito K, Abe O, et al. (2012) Cognitive status correlates with white matter alteration in Parkinson's disease. Human brain mapping 33: 727–739.
21. Smith SM, Jenkinson M, Johansen-Berg H, Rueckert D, Nichols TE, et al. (2006) Tract-based spatial statistics: voxelwise analysis of multi-subject diffusion data. Neuroimage 31: 1487–1505.
22. Gilman S, Low P, Quinn N, Albanese A, Ben-Shlomo Y, et al. (1999) Consensus statement on the diagnosis of multiple system atrophy. Journal of the neurological sciences 163: 94–98.
23. Hughes AJ, Ben-Shlomo Y, Daniel SE, Lees AJ (1992) What features improve the accuracy of clinical diagnosis in Parkinson's disease A clinicopathologic study. Neurology 42: 1142–1142.
24. Litvan I, Agid Y, Calne D, Campbell G, Dubois B, et al. (1996) Clinical research criteria for the diagnosis of progressive supranuclear palsy (Steele-Richardson-Olszewski syndrome) Report of the NINDS-SPSP International Workshop*. Neurology 47: 1–9.
25. Hoehn MM, Yahr MD (1998) Parkinsonism: onset, progression, and mortality. Neurology 50: 318–318.
26. Schwab RS, England AC (1969) Projection technique for evaluating surgery in Parkinson's disease; pp. 152–157.
27. Fahn S, Elton RL, Committee UD (1987) Unified Parkinson's disease rating scale. Recent developments in Parkinson's disease 2: 153–163.
28. Payan C, Vidailhet M, Lacomblez L, Viallet F, Borg M, et al. Neuroprotection and natural history in Parkinson plus syndromes (NNIPPS): construction and validation of a functional scale for disease progression assessment in Parkinson plus syndromes, progressive supranuclear palsy (PSP) and multiple system atrophy (MSA); 2002. WILEY-LISS DIV JOHN WILEY & SONS INC, 605 THIRD AVE, NEW YORK, NY 10158-0012 USA. pp. S256–S256.
29. Folstein MF, Folstein SE, McHugh PR (1975) "Mini-mental state": a practical method for grading the cognitive state of patients for the clinician. Journal of psychiatric research 12: 189–198.
30. Mattis S (1988) Dementia rating scale. Odessa, FL: Psychological Assessment Resources.
31. Simmons A, Moore E, Williams SC (1999) Quality control for functional magnetic resonance imaging using automated data analysis and Shewhart charting. Magnetic Resonance in Medicine 41: 1274–1278.
32. Leemans A, Jeurissen B, Sijbers J, Jones D (2009) Explore DTI: a graphical toolbox for processing, analyzing, and visualizing diffusion MR data; pp. 3537.
33. Smith SM, Jenkinson M, Woolrich MW, Beckmann CF, Behrens TE, et al. (2004) Advances in functional and structural MR image analysis and implementation as FSL. Neuroimage 23: S208–S219.
34. Smith SM (2002) Fast robust automated brain extraction. Human brain mapping 17: 143–155.
35. Hua K, Zhang J, Wakana S, Jiang H, Li X, et al. (2008) Tract probability maps in stereotaxic spaces: analyses of white matter anatomy and tract-specific quantification. Neuroimage 39: 336–347.
36. Knake S, Belke M, Menzler K, Pilatus U, Eggert KM, et al. (2010) In vivo demonstration of microstructural brain pathology in progressive supranuclear palsy: a DTI study using TBSS. Movement Disorders 25: 1232–1238.
37. Seppi K, Schocke MF, Prennschuetz-Schuetzenau K, Mair KJ, Esterhammer R, et al. (2006) Topography of putaminal degeneration in multiple system atrophy: a diffusion magnetic resonance study. Movement disorders 21: 847–852.
38. Rizzo G, Martinelli P, Manners D, Scaglione C, Tonon C, et al. (2008) Diffusion-weighted brain imaging study of patients with clinical diagnosis of corticobasal degeneration, progressive supranuclear palsy and Parkinson's disease. Brain 131: 2690–2700.
39. Tsukamoto K, Matsusue E, Kanasaki Y, Kakite S, Fujii S, et al. (2012) Significance of apparent diffusion coefficient measurement for the differential diagnosis of multiple system atrophy, progressive supranuclear palsy, and Parkinson's disease: evaluation by 3.0-T MR imaging. Neuroradiology 54: 947–955.
40. Pierpaoli C, Barnett A, Pajevic S, Chen R, Penix L, et al. (2001) Water diffusion changes in Wallerian degeneration and their dependence on white matter architecture. Neuroimage 13: 1174–1185.

41. Ito S, Makino T, Shirai W, Hattori T (2008) Diffusion tensor analysis of corpus callosum in progressive supranuclear palsy. Neuroradiology 50: 981–985.

42. Josephs KA, Xia R, Mandrekar J, Gunter JL, Senjem ML, et al. (2013) Modeling trajectories of regional volume loss in progressive supranuclear palsy. Movement Disorders 28: 1117–1124.

43. Brenneis C, Seppi K, Schocke M, Benke T, Wenning G, et al. (2004) Voxel based morphometry reveals a distinct pattern of frontal atrophy in progressive supranuclear palsy. Journal of Neurology, Neurosurgery & Psychiatry 75: 246–249.

44. Ishizawa K, Dickson DW (2001) Microglial activation parallels system degeneration in progressive supranuclear palsy and corticobasal degeneration. Journal of Neuropathology & Experimental Neurology 60: 647–657.

45. Kreutzberg GW (1996) Microglia: a sensor for pathological events in the CNS. Trends in neurosciences 19: 312–318.

46. Klegeris A MP (1997) Beta-amyloid protein enhances macrophage production of oxygen free radicals and glutamate. J Neurosci Res 49: 229–235.

47. Ishizawa K, Komori T, Sasaki S, Arai N, Mizutani T, et al. (2004) Microglial activation parallels system degeneration in multiple system atrophy. Journal of Neuropathology & Experimental Neurology 63: 43–52.

48. Stefanova N, Reindl M, Neumann M, Kahle PJ, Poewe W, et al. (2007) Microglial activation mediates neurodegeneration related to oligodendroglial α-synucleinopathy: Implications for multiple system atrophy. Movement Disorders 22: 2196–2203.

19

Azathioprine versus Beta Interferons for Relapsing-Remitting Multiple Sclerosis: A Multicentre Randomized Non-Inferiority Trial

Luca Massacesi[1,2]*, **Irene Tramacere**[3], **Salvatore Amoroso**[4], **Mario A. Battaglia**[5], **Maria Donata Benedetti**[6], **Graziella Filippini**[3], **Loredana La Mantia**[7], **Anna Repice**[2], **Alessandra Solari**[3], **Gioacchino Tedeschi**[8], **Clara Milanese**[3]

1 Dipartimento di Neuroscienze, Psicologia, Farmaco e Salute del Bambino Università di Firenze, Firenze, Italy, **2** Neurologia 2, Azienda Ospedaliero-Universitaria Careggi, Firenze, Italy, **3** Fondazione IRCCS Istituto Neurologico Carlo Besta, Milano, Italy, **4** Dipartimento di Neuroscienze, Sezione di Farmacologia, Università Politecnica delle Marche, Ancona, Italy, **5** Associazione Italiana Sclerosi Multipla (AISM), Fondazione Italiana Sclerosi Multipla (FISM), Genova, Italy, **6** Dipartimento Universitario di Neurologia, Azienda Ospedaliera Universitaria Integrata di Verona, Verona, Italy, **7** Unità di Neurologia - Multiple Sclerosis Center, I.R.C.C.S. Santa Maria Nascente Fondazione Don Gnocchi, Milano, Italy, **8** Clinica Neurologica, Università di Napoli, Napoli, Italy

Abstract

For almost three decades in many countries azathioprine has been used to treat relapsing-remitting multiple sclerosis. However its efficacy was usually considered marginal and following approval of β interferons for this indication it was no longer recommended as first line treatment, even if presently no conclusive direct β interferon-azathioprine comparison exists. To compare azathioprine efficacy versus the currently available β interferons in relapsing-remitting multiple sclerosis, a multicenter, randomized, controlled, single-blinded, non-inferiority trial was conducted in 30 Italian multiple sclerosis centers. Eligible patients (relapsing-remitting course; ≥2 relapses in the last 2 years) were randomly assigned to azathioprine or β interferons. The primary outcome was annualized relapse rate ratio (RR) over 2 years. Key secondary outcome was number of new brain MRI lesions. Patients (n = 150) were randomized in 2 groups (77 azathioprine, 73 β interferons). At 2 years, clinical evaluation was completed in 127 patients (62 azathioprine, 65 β interferons). Annualized relapse rate was 0.26 (95% Confidence Interval, CI, 0.19–0.37) in the azathioprine and 0.39 (95% CI 0.30–0.51) in the interferon group. Non-inferiority analysis showed that azathioprine was at least as effective as β interferons (relapse RR$_{AZA/IFN}$ 0.67, one-sided 95% CI 0.96; p<0.01). MRI outcomes were analyzed in 97 patients (50 azathioprine and 47 β interferons). Annualized new T2 lesion rate was 0.76 (95% CI 0.61–0.95) in the azathioprine and 0.69 (95% CI 0.54–0.88) in the interferon group. Treatment discontinuations due to adverse events were higher (20.3% vs. 7.8%, p = 0.03) in the azathioprine than in the interferon group, and concentrated within the first months of treatment, whereas in the interferon group discontinuations occurred mainly during the second year. The results of this study indicate that efficacy of azathioprine is not inferior to that of β interferons for patients with relapsing-remitting multiple sclerosis. Considering also the convenience of the oral administration, and the low cost for health service providers, azathioprine may represent an alternative to interferon treatment, while the different side effect profiles of both medications have to be taken into account.

Trial Registration: EudraCT 2006-004937-13

Editor: Klemens Ruprecht, Charite - Universitätsmedizin Berlin, Germany

Funding: The present study was funded by AIFA (Agenzia Italiana del Farmaco, www.agenziafarmaco.gov.it). The funder had no role in study design, data collection and analysis, decision to publish, or preparation of the manuscript.

Competing Interests: Dr. Solari, Dr. Massacesi and Dr. Tedeschi have read the journal's policy and have the following conflicts: Dr. Solari was a board member for Novartis, Biogenidec and Merck Serono, and has received speaker honoraria from Sanofi-Aventis. Dr. Massacesi has received reimbursements for meeting participation or educational grants from Biogen-Idec, Merk-Serono, Sanofi-Aventis and Novartis. In addition, he is a member of the Scientific Advisory Group Neurology of the European Medicine Agency (EMA) and of the Italian Medicine Agency (Agenzia Italiana del Farmaco, AIFA) Advisory Committee on Neurology, but the opinions included in this paper do not involve this activity. Dr. Tedeschi has received reimbursements for meeting participation or educational grants from Biogen-Idec, Merk-Serono, Sanofi-Aventis and Novartis. In addition, he was a member of the Italian Medicine Agency (Agenzia Italiana del Farmaco, AIFA) Advisory Committee on Neurology, but the opinions included in this paper do not involve this activity. All the other authors have declared that no competing interests exist.

* Email: massacesi@unifi.it

Introduction

For almost three decades azathioprine (AZA) has been used in many countries to treat relapsing-remitting multiple sclerosis (MS) based on placebo controlled randomized clinical trials (RCTs) [1–

4]. Efficacy however was usually considered marginal [5,6], and following approval of β interferons (IFNs) AZA was no longer recommended as first-line therapy [7]. Lack of MRI evaluation, methodological weaknesses and the low power of the trials may have fostered perception of the poor efficacy of AZA, whereas consistently efficacious and safe IFN trials in MS [8–11] have made IFN a drug of choice for this indication [7]. However, meta-analyses [12–14], new comparative RCTs [15,16], and MRI results [17,18] suggest a similar effect size of AZA in relapsing-remitting MS. Presently no conclusive direct IFN-AZA comparison exists. This paper documents an independent multicenter RCT evaluating the non-inferiority of the efficacy of AZA vs. IFNs on clinical and MRI measures of disease activity in relapsing-remitting MS.

Materials and Methods

The protocol for this trial and supporting CONSORT checklist are available as supporting information; see Protocol S1, Amendment S1, and Checklist S1.

Ethics statement

This study was approved by ethics committees in the coordinating center (Careggi University Hospital, Ethic Committee, Florence) and in each of the participating centers (**Fondazione IRCCS Istituto Neurologico Carlo Besta**, Milano; **Clinica Neurologica**, Novara; **Università "La Sapienza"**, Roma; **Policlinico "G. Rodolico" Azienda Ospedaliero-Universitaria**, Catania; **Clinica Neurologica 2**, Genova; **Azienda Ospedaliera Universitaria Integrata**, Verona; **Ospedale Clinicizzato "Colle Dall'Ara"**, Chieti; **Università di Sassari**, Sassari; **Università di Napoli**, Napoli; **Ospedale S. Antonio**, Padova; **Ospedale Civile S. Agostino-Estense**, Modena; **Ospedale Santa Maria**, Reggio Emilia; **Policlinico Universitario Mater Domini**, Catanzaro; **Ospedale S. Gerardo**, Monza; **Azienda Ospedaliero-Universitaria S. Anna**, Ferrara; **Ospedali Riuniti**, Ancona; **Istituto S. Raffaele "G. Giglio"**, Cefalù; **Azienda Ospedaliero San Giovanni Battista, Università di Torino**, Torino; **Ospedale Sacro Cuore**, Negrar; **Ospedale Santa Chiara**, Trento; **Ospedale Regionale**, Bolzano; **Azienda Ospedaliero-Universitaria Senese, Policlinico "Le Scotte"**, Siena; **Ospedale "Misericordia e Dolce"**, Prato; **Università degli Studi di Pisa**, Pisa; **Policlinico "G. Martino"**, Messina; **Università degli Studi di Palermo**, Palermo; **Università Cattolica, Policlinico Gemelli**, Roma; **Dipartimento Neuroriabilitativo ASL CN1**, Cuneo; **Luigi Gonzaga Hospital**, Orbassano Ethics Committees), adhered to Good Clinical Practice (GCP) guidelines and Declaration of Helsinki. The original trial was registered in 2006 in the EudraCT register (EUDRACT n.: 2006-004937-13) at a time that was prior to being accepted as a registry that fulfills the requirements by the International Committee of Medical Journal Editors (ICMJE) (http://www.icmje.org/faq_clinical.html). Since this registry was only considered to fulfill the requirements by the ICMJE since June 2011 and was not publicly available for several years after it was established, this precluded fulfilment of the requirements outlined by the ICMJE. We confirm that all ongoing and future trials are now registered.

Study design and patients

Designed as a multicenter, randomized, single-blinded, phase III clinical trial, the study assesses non-inferiority of AZA efficacy vs. IFNs over two years. Patients were recruited between February 2007 and March 2009 in 30 MS centers throughout Italy. Inclusion criteria were: age, 18–55 years; relapsing-remitting MS [19]; at least two clinical relapses in the preceding two years; a baseline Expanded Disability Status Scale (EDSS) [20] score from 1.0 to 5.5; effective female contraception and a signed informed consent. Exclusion criteria were: clinical relapses or steroid therapy 30 days prior to study entry; immunomodulatory or immunosuppressive treatments in the preceding year; concomitant diseases precluding IFN or AZA treatment; pregnancy or breastfeeding; cognitive decline preventing informed consent; pathological conditions interfering with MS evolution; non-steroidal anti-inflammatory drugs (NSAID) allergy or intolerance to AZA or IFNs.

The study was an independent academic initiative supported by the Italian Medicine Agency (Agenzia Italiana del Farmaco, AIFA) through a competitive Grant following a public call aimed to support independent Clinical Trials.

Randomization and blinding

Patients were selected for AZA or IFNs using a computer generated central randomization list (1:1 ratio), in blocks of four and stratified by disability score (EDSS≤3.5 or >3.5). Patients were assessed by an unblinded treating and a blinded examining neurologist at their centers. Brain MRI images were centrally analyzed by two blinded independent experts at the Image Analysis Centre of the University of Florence (Italy).

Interventions

Treatment was prescribed free of charge by treating neurologists and self-administered within one month after screening and one week after randomization.

Standard treatment. The IFN-treated patients were either administered 250 μg of IFNβ-1b subcutaneously on alternate days (Betaferon), 30 μg of IFNβ-1a IM, weekly (Avonex); 22/44 μg of subcutaneous IFNβ-1a thrice weekly (Rebif). The type of IFNβ (Betaferon, Avonex or Rebif) was selected by the treating neurologist. The standard dose was titrated over the first four weeks.

Experimental treatment. The AZA-treated patients were given an oral target dose of 3 mg/kg/day, individually adjusted to their differential white cell counts. The initial 50 mg/day dose was subsequently titrated for the first six to eight weeks, increasing 50 mg every fortnight to the target dose.

Treatment adjustment and discontinuation criteria. For all medications, treatment adjustment criteria included: reaching grade two for adverse events (AEs) of Common Toxicity Criteria (CTC) [21], including n<800/μl lymphocyte count and n<3000/μl white blood cells. For AZA in case of grade two AEs, a 25/50 mg dose reduction was required. When the AE occurred during dose titration the higher dose was not prescribed. Returning to the target dose after reduction or increasing dose during titration was allowed for AEs occurring only once, otherwise the low dose was maintained. The treatment monitoring, including hemato-chemical tests (erythrocytes, hemoglobin, leukocytes with differential count, platelets, ALT, AST, GGT, ALP, and bilirubin), were performed quarterly. These tests were performed every fortnight during the first two months of treatment (one month for the IFNs) and when a grade two AE occurred. Treatment was discontinued for grade two AEs persistent at two subsequent controls after dose reduction. Other withdrawal criteria were: a grade three AE or AEs considered intolerable by patients or treating neurologists; treatment failure (i.e., more relapses during the study than in the previous two years, or an equal number of relapses and increase of at least one EDSS point confirmed after six months, or shift to a secondary progressive course); pregnancy; and consent withdrawal.

Co-interventions. Symptomatic treatments were allowed and 1 g of I.V. methylprednisolone was given for three-five days for relapses, as prescribed by the treating neurologist.

Procedures

The treating neurologist oversaw the overall medical management of patients, including drug prescription and self-administration instruction, scheduled (quarterly) and unscheduled (i.e., at the onset of new symptoms or complications) follow-up visits where he/she recorded symptoms, blood test results, clinical AEs and their management, and any treatment decision, including discontinuation. The examining neurologist was responsible for the neurological examination and EDSS scoring at scheduled (every six months) and unscheduled visits, that were requested by the treating neurologist to confirm relapses. These included the onset of new neurological symptom(s), or worsening of pre-existing ones from MS, determining worsening of at least one point in one or more functional system or at least 0.5 EDSS points. A new symptom was considered part of a new relapse if it lasted at least 48 hours with no fever, and if reported at least 30 days from the end of a previous relapse. To discontinue treatment a final visit was planned within 30 days from the last dose.

A Contract Research Organization (CRO) visited all centers before enrolment and every four months thereafter.

Outcomes

Clinical efficacy. The primary outcome was annualized relapse rate ratio (RR) over two years. Secondary clinical outcomes were: a) annualized relapse rate during the first and second year; b) proportion of patients with 0, 1, and ≥ 2 relapses during the first and second year; c) proportion of patients with corticosteroid-treated relapses; d) time to first relapse after randomization; e) proportion of patients with no confirmed disability progression, i.e., without an increase of at least one EDSS point confirmed after at least six months over two years; f) mean EDSS change from baseline to the end of follow-up; g) number of treatment failures; h) mean change of the MSQOL-54 scale [22] over two years.

Brain MRI. Brain lesions were evaluated through MRI scans performed over 30 days prior to treatment (baseline) and at two years (study completion). In the MRI study participated 23 Centers, all identified prior to the beginning of the study. The primary MRI outcome was the number of new T2 brain lesions, defined as new or enlarging lesions on T2-weighted scans. Secondary outcomes were: a) proportion of patients with 0, 1–2, ≥ 3 new T2 brain lesions; b) combined new and enhancing lesions (CE); c) mean and median Gadolinium contrast enhancing (Gd+) lesions on T1-weighted scans; d) proportion of patients with 0, 1–2, ≥ 3 Gd+ lesions. New lesion numbers were evaluated through dedicated software packages (Analyze 10.0), comparing each scan obtained at study completion with the corresponding baseline scan [see Methods S1 in File S1 for details].

Safety. Data was collected on: 1) AEs and serious AEs (SAEs); 2) patients with any AE; 3) patient withdrawal after any AE; 4) severity of any AE and their correlation with treatments as judged by the treating neurologist. Frequency and severity of AEs were actively assessed every three months or upon patient request. Severity was graded using the National Cancer Institute Common Terminology Criteria for AE [21]. SAE notification was sent to a specifically appointed Pharmacological Surveillance Unit (PSU).

Non-inferiority margin, power and sample size

Non-inferiority margin. To compare treatment relapse rates, a non-inferiority margin (M) was calculated following published guidelines [23–25], as a fraction of the mean effect of IFNs vs. placebo ($E_{IFNvsPlacebo}$) on the same outcome measure in previous trials with the same inclusion criteria and follow-up period [8,9,11]. By next expressing the $E_{IFNvsPlacebo}$ as a relapse rate ratio, M was expressed as 50% of the excess to 1.0 of this rate ratio. Given the historical $E_{IFNvsPlacebo}$ of 1.46 ($= 2.55/1.75$, corresponding to the relapse rate reduction through IFN treatment), M = 1.23 was therefore selected [8,9]. The annualized new T2 lesion rate over two years was chosen as the primary MRI outcome, as this was the main MRI outcome available in the pivotal trial aimed at establishing the efficacy of IFNβ-1b vs. placebo and whose inclusion criteria and follow-up length were identical [8,11], thereby enabling precise evaluation of the $E_{IFNvsPlacebo}$ on new T2 lesion rates, as their ratio was 2.67 ($= 6.4/2.4$). Based on these data, a non-inferiority margin of M = 1.84 was established *a priori*, as 50% of the excess to 1.0 of the 2.67 historical ratio.

Power and sample size. Sample size was calculated to verify the non-inferiority of AZA against IFNs. With a power of 80%, α of 5% and under the hypothesis of no difference between the means of relapse rates (new T2 lesion rates for MRI), with an expected loss of 20% at follow-up, 360 patients (175/treatment arm) for relapse, and 192 patients (96/treatment arm) for MRI were needed. However, the sample size of the study was undermined by the revision of the Italian National Health System reimbursement criteria, that occurred during the recruitment period and allowed IFN therapy from the first MS attack, thus overcoming the required presence of at least two relapses during the previous two years, which was one of the inclusion criteria of this study. This change remarkably reduced the number of eligible patients and the recruitment slowed to such a low rate that the Steering Committee of the study judged the planned sample size not feasible any more. For this reason a protocol amendment, approved by the Independent Data and Safety Management Committee (IDSMC) and by the Ethic Committee of the Coordinating Center, recommended a 150 patient recruitment ceiling, accepting a power of 60–65% for relapses, and 80% for MRI outcome, under the hypothesis of no differences between the means of relapse/new T2 lesion rates [see Protocol S1 and Amendment S1 for details]. It is worth to note that the request of amendment was submitted by the Steering Committee exclusively on the basis of the observed accrual rate, when no data or codes were available.

Statistical analyses

Baseline characteristics. Baseline clinical and demographic characteristics were analyzed using χ^2 test for categorical, and t-test (or Mann-Whitney test in the absence of Normal distribution) for continuous variables.

Clinical outcome measures. AZA efficacy was judged non-inferior to IFNs if the upper limit (U_L) of the one-sided 95% confidence interval (95% CI) of the annualized relapse $RR_{AZA/IFN}$ over two years, calculated by Poisson regression, was $< M = 1.23$. Secondary outcomes were analyzed using χ^2 test with one degree of freedom for rate comparison (based on Poisson regression); χ^2 test with two degrees of freedom for number of relapsed patients; Kaplan-Meier curves, log-rank test and Cox proportional-hazards model for time to first relapse; Fisher's exact test for patients with no confirmed disability progression; and t-test for EDSS and MSQOL-54 score changes. For the annualized relapse rate, sensitivity analyses were performed adjusting for baseline covariates (number of relapses during the previous two years, baseline EDSS score, and disease duration from onset of symptoms), and excluding Avonex treated patients. An additional sensitivity analysis was performed to include in the analysis patients lost to follow-up, using two multiple imputation methods (monotone logistic regression and fully conditional specification [FCS] logistic regression method) [26–28], taking the randomized treatment as the covariate (i.e., incorporating possible different uncertainty due to different dropout rates between the two randomized treatment groups). All analyses were performed in the intention to treat (ITT) and per-protocol (PP, i.e. after excluding noncompliant patients and drop-outs) populations. In the analyses based on relapse rates and on proportion of patients with relapses or disability progression, patients lost to follow-up were excluded.

Brain lesions. AZAs were judged non-inferior to IFNs if the U_L of the one-sided 95% CI of the annualized new T2 lesion rate ratio over two years, calculated by Poisson regression, was <M = 1.84. Secondary outcomes were analyzed through χ^2 test with one degree of freedom for rate comparison (based on Poisson regression); χ^2 test with two degrees of freedom for number of patients with lesions; and Mann-Whitney test for Gd+ lesion number. All analyses were performed in the ITT and PP populations.

Adverse Events. AEs were analyzed as rates, in terms of patients with AEs and overall number of AEs, using χ^2 test based on Poisson regression for rate comparison, and χ^2 test for categorical variable comparison for discontinued interventions after AEs, AE severity and correlation of AE with treatment. SAEs were described reporting their postulated correlation with treatment and any consequent discontinuation.

Data were reported following the CONSORT guidelines [29].

Results

Characteristics of participants

Figure 1 presents patient allocation and follow-up. Of the 150 randomized patients 77 and 73 were AZA- and IFN-assigned respectively. In the IFN group, 26 (36%) were assigned to Avonex, 5 (7%) to Betaferon, 35 (48%) to Rebif 22, and 7 (10%) to Rebif 44. Of the 150 patients screened at baseline, 127 completed the ITT follow-up: 62 (81%) in the AZA group, and 65 (89%) in the IFN group (overall 85%). Eight patients, initially randomized to AZA, refused consent and received IFN (out of these, four were lost to follow up). Including losses to follow up, treatment discontinuations were respectively 30 in the AZA group (39%; with the patients who refused to begin the treatment, n = 8) and 19 in the IFN group (26%). The majority of the discontinuations under AZA occurred in the first year (n = 26; 87%) whereas those under IFN occurred in the second year (n = 12; 63%). The discontinuations were 22 (32%) and 18 (25%) respectively, if only patients who began the treatments are included in the analysis of pharmacological compliance.

Fourteen (47%) of 30 treatment discontinuations in the AZA group and 6 (32%) of 19 discontinuations in the IFN group were due to AEs; 2 (7%) of 30 patients in the AZA group and 3 (16%) of 19 patients in the IFN group discontinued for lack of efficacy. Demographic, clinical characteristics and MRI findings at baseline were highly comparable in both groups (Table 1), even considering the ITT (n = 127), the PP (n = 101), and the MRI (n = 97) populations who completed follow-up [data not shown]. Baseline characteristics were comparable even separately considering patients enrolled during the first and second year of recruitment [data not shown].

Efficacy - clinical outcomes

From the primary efficacy analysis, AZA emerges as significantly non-inferior to IFN (Fig. 2), as the upper limit (U_L) of the one-sided 95% CI for the annualized relapse $RR_{AZA/IFN}$ was 0.96, i.e., below the non-inferiority margin M (= 1.23; p<0.01). This U_L is also significantly (p = 0.03) below a more stringent non-inferiority margin M1 = 1.0, corresponding to 100% of the effect

of IFNs vs. placebo. The U_L of the one-sided 99% CI for the $RR_{AZA/IFN}$ (i.e., 1.12), corresponding to the 75% of the IFN effect vs. placebo, was also significantly below the non-inferiority margin of M = 1.23 (p<0.01). The annualized relapse rates observed over two years among the AZA and the IFN treated subjects were 0.26 and 0.39, respectively (p = 0.07, adjusted p = 0.06; Table 2). The corresponding $RR_{AZA/IFN}$ was 0.67 (95% CI, 0.43–1.03) based on the 127 patients who completed follow-up, 0.67 (95% CI, 0.40–1.12) based on 150 randomized patients and using the monotone logistic regression multiple imputation method, and 0.69 (95% CI, 0.43–1.10) using the FCS logistic regression multiple imputation method [data not shown]. Adjusted analysis gave similar results (Table 2), confirming the robustness of the findings. In addition, comparable results were obtained in a sensitivity analysis excluding the Avonex treated patients (the annualized relapse rate over two years among Betaferon or Rebif treated patients was 0.37, with a corresponding $RR_{AZA/IFN}$ of 0.70, 95% CI, 0.43–1.15) [data not shown]. No significant difference was noted between AZA and IFN in the proportion of patients with 0, 1, 2, ≥3 relapses over two years and separately in the first or the second year, the proportion of patients with corticosteroid-treated relapses, and the proportion of patients with no confirmed disability progression over two years. (Table 2). There were six treatment failures in the AZA group and five in the IFN group. For QOL, no difference was observed between the treatments, for both physical and mental-QOL (p = 0.94 and 0.93, respectively) [data not shown]. Figure 3 shows Kaplan-Meier curves of the time to first relapse: no significant difference was observed in terms of log-rank (p = 0.11) or Cox proportional-hazards model results, with a hazard ratio of 0.66 (95% CI, 0.40–1.10). Similar results were obtained in sensitivity analyses excluding Avonex treated patients (log-rank p = 0.15) [data not shown]. The analyses performed in the PP population yielded similar findings [data not shown].

Efficacy - MRI outcomes

Of the 122 patients given baseline MRI (61 per group), 97 completed the ITT follow-up: 50 (82%) in the AZA group, and 47 (77%) in the IFN group. The ratio of annualized new T2 lesion rates of AZA vs. IFNs was 1.10 (Fig. 4). The corresponding U_L of the 95% one-sided CI was 1.45, below the non-inferiority margin M = 1.84, indicating an AZA vs. IFN effect equivalent to at least 73% of the IFNs vs. placebo effect. Moreover, the U_L of the one-sided 99% CI for the new T2 lesion $RR_{AZA/IFN}$ (i.e., 1.63) was also significantly below the non-inferiority margin of M = 1.84 (p< 0.01). Table 3 summarizes the MRI outcomes: no significant difference was noted between AZA and IFNs for new T2, new CE, and Gd+ lesions. The annualized new T2 lesion rate was 0.69 (95% CI, 0.54–0.88) in the IFN and 0.76 (95% CI, 0.61–0.95) in the AZA patients (p = 0.75). Adjustments for inflammatory activity at baseline, expressed by the Gd+ lesion number confirmed these findings. Analyses performed in the PP population (81 patients: 40 in the AZA and 41 in the IFN group) confirmed these results [data not shown].

Safety comparison

The rate of patients with at least one AE was not different between the two groups (p = 0.28), however the rate of AEs was higher in the AZA group (p<0.01) (Table 4). The most frequently reported AEs were flu-like symptoms, more frequent in IFNs (p< 0.01), nausea/vomiting and abnormal blood count more frequent in AZA-treated patients (p<0.01). AE-related discontinued interventions were more frequent among AZA (20.3%) than IFN (7.8%) patients (p = 0.03). SAEs and other AEs are described in Tables S1 and S2 in File S1.

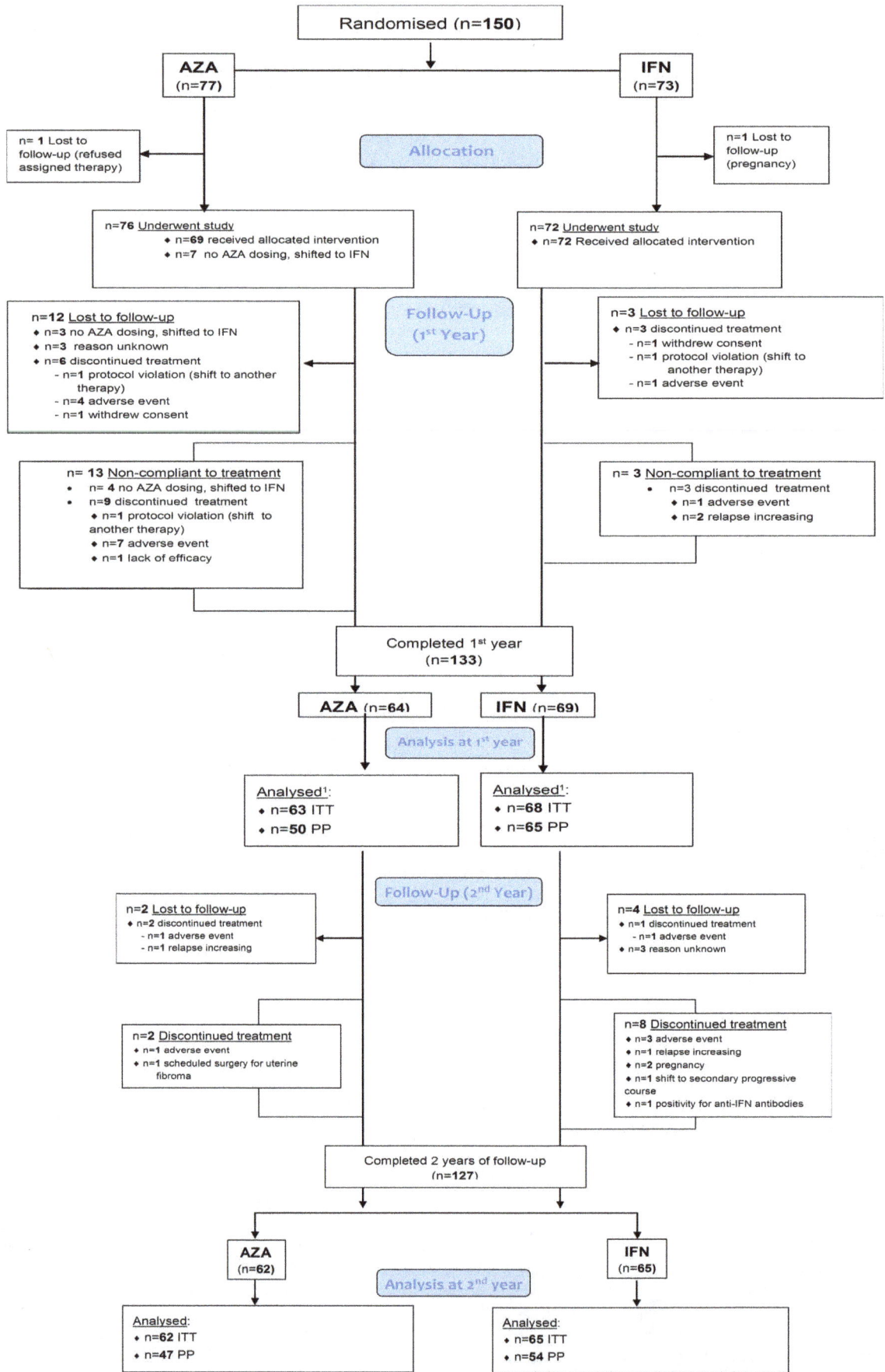

Randomised (n=**150**)

AZA (n=**77**)   IFN (n=**73**)

Allocation

n= **1** Lost to follow-up (refused assigned therapy)

n=**1** Lost to follow-up (pregnancy)

n=76 Underwent study
• n=69 received allocated intervention
• n=7 no AZA dosing, shifted to IFN

n=72 Underwent study
• n=72 Received allocated intervention

Follow-Up (1st Year)

n=**12** Lost to follow-up
• n=3 no AZA dosing, shifted to IFN
• n=3 reason unknown
• n=6 discontinued treatment
  - n=1 protocol violation (shift to another therapy)
  - n=4 adverse event
  - n=1 withdrew consent

n=**3** Lost to follow-up
• n=3 discontinued treatment
  - n=1 withdrew consent
  - n=1 protocol violation (shift to another therapy)
  - n=1 adverse event

n= **13** Non-compliant to treatment
• n= 4 no AZA dosing, shifted to IFN
• n=9 discontinued treatment
  • n=1 protocol violation (shift to another therapy)
  • n=7 adverse event
  • n=1 lack of efficacy

n= **3** Non-compliant to treatment
• n=3 discontinued treatment
  • n=1 adverse event
  • n=2 relapse increasing

Completed 1st year (n=**133**)

AZA (n=**64**)   IFN (n=**69**)

Analysis at 1st year

Analysed[1]:
• n=**63** ITT
• n=**50** PP

Analysed[1]:
• n=**68** ITT
• n=**65** PP

Follow-Up (2nd Year)

n=2 Lost to follow-up
• n=2 discontinued treatment
  - n=1 adverse event
  - n=1 relapse increasing

n=4 Lost to follow-up
• n=1 discontinued treatment
  - n=1 adverse event
• n=3 reason unknown

n=2 Discontinued treatment
• n=1 adverse event
• n=1 scheduled surgery for uterine fibroma

n=8 Discontinued treatment
• n=3 adverse event
• n=1 relapse increasing
• n=2 pregnancy
• n=1 shift to secondary progressive course
• n=1 positivity for anti-IFN antibodies

Completed 2 years of follow-up (n=**127**)

AZA (n=**62**)   IFN (n=**65**)

Analysis at 2nd year

Analysed:
• n=**62** ITT
• n=**47** PP

Analysed:
• n=**65** ITT
• n=**54** PP

Figure 1. Flow-chart: patient allocation and follow-up. Abbreviations: AZA, azathioprine; IFN, interferon; ITT, intention to treat; PP, per-protocol. [1]One missing CRF at month 12.

Discussion

Principal findings

This study directly compared AZA and IFN efficacy on clinical and MRI outcomes in relapsing-remitting MS patients. The results indicated that AZA was non-inferior to IFNs in reducing relapses and new brain lesions over two years. The effect size on the primary end point (annualized relapse rate ratio) was 0.67, with the upper CIs indicating that in the worst case scenario efficacy of AZA vs. placebo can be estimated as at least 100% (95% CI) or as

Table 1. Baseline characteristics of the patients.

Characteristic	AZA (N = 77)	IFN (N = 73)	p-value[1]
Demographic characteristics			
Female – No. (%)	49 (63.6%)	50 (68.5%)	p = 0.53
Age - Years			
Mean ± SD	38.1±8.9	36.6±8.8	p = 0.31
Median (range)	37.9 (21.3–56.5)	37.6 (19.1–58.8)	
Clinical characteristics			
Duration of disease from onset of symptoms - Years			
Mean ± SD	6.8±7.1	5.7±5.7	
Median (range)	3.4 (0.5–25.3)	3.4 (0.3–24.8)	p = 0.53
Relapses in previous 2 years			
Mean ± SD	2.38±0.78	2.41±0.89	
Median (range)	2 (0–5)	2 (0–6)	p = 0.91
No. patients with relapses in previous 2 years - No. (%)			
0–1[2]	3 (3.9%)	2 (2.7%)	
2	48 (62.3%)	47 (64.4%)	p = 0.91
≥3	26 (33.8%)	24 (32.9%)	
No. patients with previous histories of ... - No. (%)			
AZA treatment	1 (1.3%)	1 (1.4%)	p = 0.95
IFN treatment	4 (5.2%)	3 (4.1%)	
EDSS score[3]			
Mean ± SD	1.9±0.9	1.9±0.9	
Median (range)	1.5 (1.0–5.5)	1.5 (0.0–5.0)	p = 0.86
Patients with concomitant diseases – No. (%)[4]	5 (6.9%)	4 (5.8%)	p = 0.80
	AZA (N = 61)	**IFN (N = 61)**	**p-value[1]**
MRI findings			
Gd+ lesion number			
Mean ± SD	1.64±3.85	2.32±4.53	
Median (range)	0 (0–24)	1 (0–20)	p = 0.38
No. patients with Gd+ lesions - No. (%)			
0	32 (52.5%)	27 (44.3%)	
1–2	20 (32.8%)	23 (37.7%)	p = 0.36
≥3	9 (14.8%)	11 (18.0%)	
T2 lesion load (FLAIR sequences; mm³)			
Mean ± SD	15,284±16,466	10,283±11,696	p = 0.16
Median (range)	9,197 (338–73,226)	7,205 (326–61,025)	

Abbreviations: AZA, azathioprine; EDSS, Expanded Disability Status Scale; IFN, interferon; SD, standard deviation.
[1]P-values for AZA vs. IFN comparison were obtained through: χ^2 test with one or two degrees of freedom for sex, number of patients with previous histories of AZA/IFN treatment, number of patients with relapses with concomitant disease and with Gd+ lesions; t-test for age; Mann-Whitney test for duration of disease, number of relapses, EDSS score, number of Gd+ lesions and T2 lesion load.
[2]Protocol violations.
[3]Scores on the EDSS range from 0 to 10, with higher scores indicating greater degree of disability.
[4]The sum does not add up to the total because of some missing values.

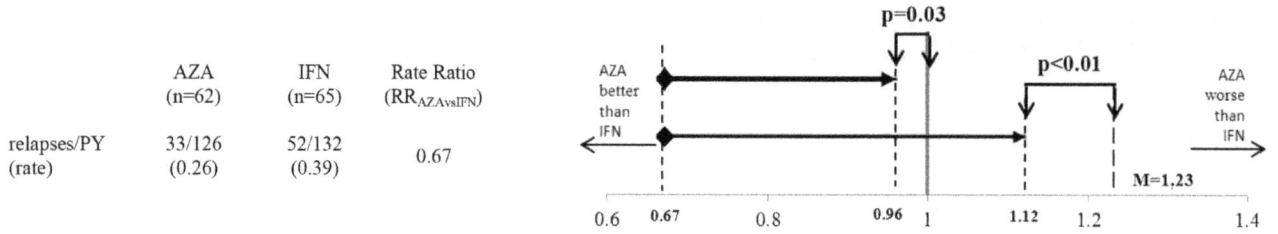

	AZA (n=62)	IFN (n=65)	Rate Ratio (RR$_{AZAvsIFN}$)
relapses/PY (rate)	33/126 (0.26)	52/132 (0.39)	0.67

Figure 2. Primary clinical outcome over 2 years: non-inferiority of effect of AZA vs. IFN, represented as annualized relapse rate ratio (RR$_{AZA/IFN}$) compared with the pre-established non-inferiority margin M (= 1.23) and with a margin M$_1$ = 1.0. One-sided 99% CI of the 0.67 ratio (upper-limit, U$_L$ = 1.12), represents an effect of AZA vs. IFNs equivalent to at least 75% of the effect of IFNs vs. Placebo. One-sided 95% CI of the same ratio (U$_L$ = 0.96), represents an effect of AZA vs. IFNs equivalent to at least 100% of the effect of IFNs vs. Placebo. Abbreviations: AZA, azathioprine; IFN, interferon; PY, person-years; RR, rate ratio.

at least 75% (99% CI) of that of IFNs, according to the CIs level selected. The effect size on new brain lesions (the main secondary outcome measure) was 1.1 with the upper CI levels (95%) indicating that in the worst case scenario efficacy of AZA vs. placebo could be estimated as at least 73% of that of the IFNs. The direct comparison of AZA and IFN efficacy therefore indicated a similar effect size, in reducing both relapses and new brain lesions. Both treatments were similarly efficacious in time to the first relapse, in slowing disability accumulation, and in the other secondary clinical and MRI outcome measures examined. Both medications showed better efficacy in the second year, probably for a delay in fully exerting their activity during the first months of treatment, at least in part determined by the initial dose titration. The observed lag of efficacy was similar for both treatments.

Similar efficacy of AZA and IFNs was observed both in the ITT and in the PP analysis and in the different sensitivity analyses performed. As in this study the comparator treatment included all the IFNs as a group, a sensitivity analysis excluding Avonex treated patients (probably the less efficacious of the IFNs [30]) confirmed the results of the main analysis.

AZA was compared to all the IFNs as a group because a centralized choice of one specific IFN could have raised allegation of conflict of interests, as in this academically driven independent study the medications were prescribed and charged to the NHS. In addition, under these experimental conditions, a centralized selection of a specific IFN could have reduced and distorted patient accrual in the participating centers.

The remarkable internal consistency between clinical and MRI data, between the ITT and the PP analysis and among the different sensitivity analyses, supported the robustness of the results. It must be pointed out that consistency between ITT and PP analysis is a critical requirement for reliability of non-inferiority studies [23–25].

The present study strengthens previous results of AZA vs. placebo [1–4] or vs. IFN [14–16], and expands previous available data as for the first time MRI was included as an outcome of AZA efficacy, thus allowing contemporary assessment of relapses and brain lesions accumulation. The previous MRI studies [17–18] indeed were informative for supporting the hypothesis of AZA efficacy on brain lesions, but were not aimed to assess clinical

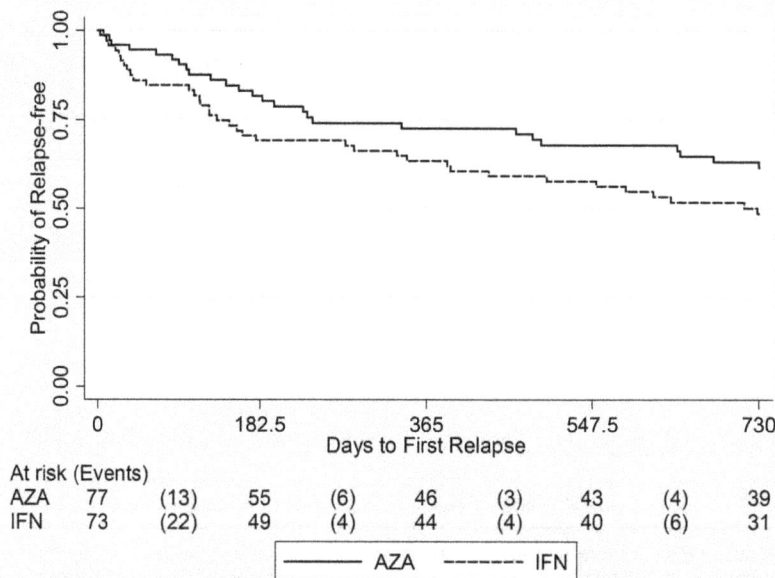

At risk (Events)									
AZA	77	(13)	55	(6)	46	(3)	43	(4)	39
IFN	73	(22)	49	(4)	44	(4)	40	(6)	31

Figure 3. Time to first relapse. Beneath the plot patients at risk and number of events (in brackets) by treatment were reported for each interval of 6 months. Abbreviations: AZA, azathioprine; IFN, interferon.

Table 2. Secondary clinical outcomes.

Outcome	1st Year			2nd Year			Overall (2 years of follow-up)		
	AZA (N=63)	IFN (N=68)	p-value[1]	AZA (N=62)	IFN (N=65)	p-value[1]	AZA (N=62)	IFN (N=65)	p-value[1]
Relapses									
Annualised relapse rate (95% CI)	0.37 (0.25–0.56)	0.47 (0.34–0.67)	p=0.37	0.18 (0.10–0.32)	0.29 (0.18–0.45)	p=0.19	0.26 (0.19–0.37)	0.39 (0.30–0.51)	p=0.07
Adjusted annualised relapse rate (95% CI)[2]	–	–	–	–	–	–	0.27 (0.19–0.38)	0.41 (0.31–0.54)	p=0.06
No. of patients with relapse - No. (%)									
0	45 (71.4%)	44 (64.7%)	p=0.63	52 (83.9%)	49 (75.4%)	p=0.42	39 (62.9%)	31 (47.7%)	p=0.22
1	14 (22.2%)	17 (25.0%)		9 (14.5%)	13 (20.0%)		15 (24.2%)	23 (35.4%)	
≥2	4 (6.4%)	7 (10.3%)		1 (1.6%)	3 (4.6%)		8 (12.9%)	11 (16.9%)	
No. of patients with relapses treated with corticosteroids – No. (%)									
0	–	–	–	–	–	–	40 (64.5%)	34 (52.3%)	p=0.22
1	–	–	–	–	–	–	16 (25.8%)	22 (33.9%)	
≥2	–	–	–	–	–	–	6 (9.7%)	9 (13.9%)	
Disability[3]									
Patients with no confirmed disability progression - % (95% CI)[4]	–	–	–	–	–	–	98.2 (91.5–99.9)	92.0 (81.8–97.4)	p=0.19
Change from baseline in EDSS score – Mean (95% CI)[5]	–	–	–	–	–	–	−0.08 (−0.31; 0.16)	0.22 (−0.03; 0.47)	p=0.08

Abbreviations: AZA, azathioprine; IFN, interferon.
[1] P-values for AZA vs. IFN comparison were obtained through χ^2 test with one degree of freedom for rate comparison, χ^2 test with two degrees of freedom for number of patients with relapses, Fisher's exact test for patients with no confirmed disability progression, and t-test for change in EDSS score.
[2] The analyses were adjusted for number of relapses during the previous two years, baseline EDSS score, and duration of disease from symptom onset.
[3] The analyses were based on 56 AZA and 50 IFN patients respectively, because of some missing values.
[4] A confirmed disability progression was defined as an increase of no less than one point of the EDSS score confirmed at least after six months; 95% CI were estimated through the exact method. All the patients, with the exception of two (who did not report a disability progression), had a baseline EDSS score between 1 and 5.
[5] Adjusted for baseline EDSS score.

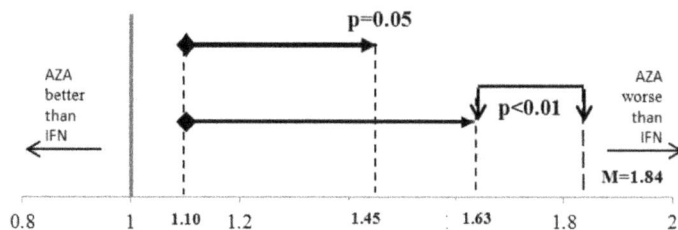

	AZA (n=50)	IFN (n=47)	Rate Ratio (RR$_{AZAvsIFN}$)
lesions/PY (rate)	76/100 (0.76)	65/94 (0.69)	1.10

Figure 4. Non-inferiority of the effect AZA vs. IFN on new T2 lesions over 2 years. One-sided 99% CI (upper-limit, U$_L$ = 1.63), and one-sided 95% CI (U$_L$ = 1.45), of the effect of AZA vs. IFNs as for annualized new T2 lesion rate ratio (RR$_{AZA/IFN}$), compared with the pre-established non-inferiority margin (M = 1.84), representing an effect of AZA vs. IFNs equivalent to the 73% of the effect of IFNs vs placebo. Abbreviations: AZA, azathioprine; IFN, interferon; PY, person-years; RR, rate ratio.

outcomes and were based on retrospective or open label designs [17–18].

It must be noted that the results of the present study were obtained administering AZA at the target dose of 3 mg/Kg/day, adjusted according to leuko/lymphocyte count. This approach was similar to that of the trials that also showed the most remarkable reduction in relapse rates induced by AZA [2–4,15], suggesting that appropriate dosage represents an important variable administering this treatment.

No unknown AEs occurred. Overall similar numbers of patients developed at least one AE. Leuko/lymphopenia in the AZA group was not associated with a higher incidence of infections and should be considered part of the desired mechanism of action. However, treatment discontinuations after AEs were significantly higher in the AZA group, mainly occurring during the first months of treatment. Most of the discontinuations for IFNs were in the

second year, confirming already known different temporal AE profile of each treatment.

Strengths and weaknesses of the study

The main limit of the study was probably the sample size, which resulted smaller than planned. This was due to difficulties in recruiting and retaining patients in the trial, particularly following the change in the Italian NHS reimbursement criteria that occurred during the recruitment period. Indeed, rational basis of a direct comparison and randomization between an old generic medication and a new approved drug were sometimes hard to explain both to neurologists and patients and contributed to these difficulties.

However, the sample size affected only the initial power estimate based on the conservative hypothesis of no difference between the means of the relapse rates. Indeed, the data obtained during the study, showing a difference favoring AZA, allowed a

Table 3. MRI outcomes. New brain lesions.

Outcome	Overall (2 years of follow-up)		
	AZA (N = 50)	IFN (N = 47)	p-value[1]
New T2 lesions			
Annualised new T2 lesion rate (95% CI)	0.76 (0.61–0.95)	0.69 (0.54–0.88)	p = 0.75
No. of patients with new T2 lesions - No. (%)			
0	27 (54.0%)	21 (45.0%)	
1–2	11 (22.0%)	18 (38.0%)	p = 0.41
≥3	12 (24.0%)	8 (17.0%)	
New Combined Unique (CE) lesions			
Annualised new CE lesion rate (95% CI)	0.78 (0.63–0.98)	0.70 (0.55–0.90)	p = 0.53
Gd+ lesions			
Gd+ lesion number			
Mean ± SD	0.20±0.50	0.40±1.35	
Median (range)	0 (0–2)	0 (0–5)	p = 0.52
No. patients with Gd+ lesions - No. (%)			
0	41 (84.0%)	43 (91.5%)	
1–2	8 (16.0%)	1 (2.0%)	p = 0.39
≥3	0 (0.0%)	3(6.5%)	
Missing data	1	0	

Abbreviations: AZA, azathioprine; IFN, interferon.
[1]P-values for AZA vs. IFN comparison were obtained through χ^2 test with one degree of freedom for rate comparison, χ^2 test with two degrees of freedom for number of patients with lesions, and Mann-Whitney test for Gd+ lesion number.

Table 4. Adverse Events.

Event	AZA (N$_{patients}$ = 69, N$_{events}$ = 308, PY = 108)	IFN (N$_{patients}$ = 77, N$_{events}$ = 241, PY = 136)	p-value[1]
All AEs[2]			
Patients – No./PY and rate (95%CI)	65/108	68/136	p = 0.28
	0.60 (0.47–0.77)	0.50 (0.40–0.64)	
AEs - No./PY and rate (95%CI)	308/108	241/136	p<0.01
	2.85 (2.54–3.19)	1.77 (1.56–2.01)	
Most frequently reported AEs[2]			
Influenza-like illness			
Patients – No./PY and rate (95%CI)	3/108	39/136	p<0.01
	0.03 (0.01–0.08)	0.29 (0.20–0.39)	
AEs - No./PY and rate (95%CI)	3/108	41/136	p<0.01
	0.03 (0.01–0.08)	0.30 (0.22–0.41)	
Fever			
Patients – No./PY and rate (95%CI)	2/108	19/136	p<0.01
	0.02 (0.00–0.07)	0.14 (0.08–0.22)	
AEs - No./PY and rate (95%CI)	2/108	20/136	p = 0.01
	0.02 (0.00–0.07)	0.15 (0.09–0.23)	
Local allergic reaction			
Patients – No./PY and rate (95%CI)	0/108	13/136	-
		0.10 (0.05–0.16)	
AEs - No./PY and rate (95%CI)	0/108	14/136	-
		0.10 (0.06–0.17)	
Systemic allergic reaction			
Patients – No./PY and rate (95%CI)	3/108	0/136	-
	0.03 (0.01–0.08)		
AEs - No./PY and rate (95%CI)	3/108	0/136	-
	0.03 (0.01–0.08)		
Nausea/vomiting			
Patients – No./PY and rate (95%CI)	30/108	1/136	p<0.01
	0.28 (0.19–0.40)	0.01 (0.00–0.04)	
AEs - No./PY and rate (95%CI)	35/108	1/136	p<0.01
	0.32 (0.23–0.45)	0.01 (0.00–0.04)	
Abnormal blood count			
Patients – No./PY and rate (95%CI)	46/108	24/136	p<0.01
	0.43 (0.31–0.57)	0.18 (0.11–0.26)	
AEs - No./PY and rate (95%CI)	106/108	39/136	p<0.01
	0.98 (0.80–1.19)	0.29 (0.20–0.39)	
Other abnormal blood tests[3]			
Patients – No./PY and rate (95%CI)	24/108	37/136	p = 0.44
	0.22 (0.14–0.33)	0.27 (0.19–0.37)	
AEs - No./PY and rate (95%CI)	46/108	54/136	p = 0.72
	0.43 (0.31–0.57)	0.40 (0.30–0.52)	
Other AE			
Patients – No./PY and rate (95%CI)	51/108	47/136	p = 0.12
	0.47 (0.35–0.62)	0.35 (0.25–0.46)	
AEs - No./PY and rate (95%CI)	70/108	54/136	p<0.01
	0.65 (0.51–0.82)	0.40 (0.30–0.52)	
Discontinued interventions due to AEs			
No. of patients with discontinued interventions due to AEs (%)	14 (20.3%)	6 (7.8%)	p = 0.03

Table 4. Cont.

Event	AZA		IFN		p-value[1]
	(N$_{patients}$ = 69, N$_{events}$ = 308, PY = 108)		(N$_{patients}$ = 77, N$_{events}$ = 241, PY = 136)		
Seriousness of AE[5]					
No. of events (%)[4]					
Minor/Moderate	291 (96.0%)		236 (98.3%)		p = 0.12
Major/Serious	12 (4.0%)		4 (1.7%)		
Correlation with study treatment					
No. of events (%)[4]					
Non-correlated/Unlikely	63 (20.7%)		49 (20.4%)		p = 0.95
Possible/Likely	242 (79.3%)		191 (79.6%)		

Abbreviations: AZA, azathioprine; IFN, interferon; PY, person-years.
[1]P-values for AZA vs. IFN comparison were obtained through χ^2 test with one degree of freedom for rate comparison, discontinued interventions due to adverse events, seriousness of adverse event, and correlation of event with treatment.
[2]All 95% CI were estimated using the exact method.
[3]Liver enzymes, thyroid function and bilirubin level.
[4]The sum does not add up to the total because of some missing values.
[5]Seriousness judged by the treating neurologist. SAEs classified according to the National Cancer Institute Common Terminology Criteria for AE [21] are reported in Table S1 in File S1.

power sufficient to establish non-inferiority at statistically robust levels of significance. Moreover, as documented by Schulz and Grimes [31] trials with low sample size might be acceptable if investigators use methodological rigor to eliminate bias and properly report to avoid misinterpretation.

Another possible limitation could be related to patient knowledge of the treatment. Indeed, out of the patients who refused the assigned treatment, all had been randomized to AZA. As this occurred before the first dose of AZA was administered, it was necessarily due to a different perception by the patients of this therapy with respect to the IFNs, which were specifically approved for MS. Successfully blinding of patients seemed unrealistic given the profoundly different side effects of AZA and IFNs of which the patients had been informed in detail. Indeed, analysis of blinding in previous studies revealed a strong tendency to treatment awareness in patients receiving IFNs [10,32].

Dropout rates was another possible issue in this study. Although the overall number of patients who withdrew the study was only 15%, a higher number of patients were lost to follow up in the AZA than in the IFN group, mainly during the first year. As this event may have diluted true differences between treatments, sensitivity analyses, based on two multiple imputation methods, were performed and no difference in the RR$_{AZA/IFN}$ estimate was observed, thus confirming the results obtained in the analysis of patients who completed the follow-up.

Finally, the different number of treatment discontinuations observed between the two groups (i.e., 39% of patients on AZA and 26% on IFN) could have impacted the study effect size. However, if only patients who began the treatment according to the study protocol are considered, a similar number of patients discontinued (32% on AZA and 25% on IFNs), suggesting similar compliance of the two medications over two years. The clear difference was that treatment interruptions were more frequent in the first year in the AZA group and in the second year in the IFN group.

Implications for clinical practice

The present study was the first independent RCT that directly compared efficacy of a generic medication (AZA) to a drug specifically approved for MS (IFN) using a non-inferiority design. The authors believe that the results of this study are robust, clinically meaningful and relevant for clinical practice, supporting AZA as a rational and effective alternative to IFNs in relapsing-remitting MS, particularly considering the convenience of oral administration and the cost, lower than the other available treatments. Nevertheless, the different side effect profiles of both medications have to be taken into account.

Supporting Information

Checklist S1 CONSORT checklist.

Protocol S1 Trial protocol.

Amendment S1 Amendment to the protocol.

File S1 Methods S1, Outcomes. Brain MRI: Scan acquisition specifications. **Table S1**, Serious Adverse Events (SAEs). **Table S2**, AEs – subtypes.

Acknowledgments

The authors wish to thank: The Italian Medicines Agency (Agenzia Italiana del Farmaco, AIFA) for the financial support; the Interdipartimental Center for Magnetic Resonance Imaging of University of Florence for the support in the MRI analysis; Paul Bowerbank for his help in reviewing the English of the manuscript.
Group information
The Multicenter Azathioprine Interferon-ß Non-Inferiority (M.A.I.N.) Trial Group and investigators are as follows: *Steering committee:* L Massacesi (Dipartimento di Neuroscienze, Psicologia, Farmaco e Salute del Bambino Università di Firenze, Italy; Neurologia 2, Azienda Ospedaliero-Universitaria Careggi, Firenze, Italy.), G Filippini, C Milanese, A Solari (Fondazione IRCCS Istituto Neurologico Carlo Besta, Milano), L La Mantia (Unità di Neurologia - Multiple Sclerosis Center, I.R.C.C.S. Santa Maria Nascente Fondazione Don Gnocchi, Milano), MD Benedetti (Dipartimento Universitario di Neurologia, Azienda Ospedaliera Universitaria Integrata, Verona), S Amoroso (Dipartimento di Neuroscienze,

Sezione di Farmacologia, Università Politecnica delle Marche, Ancona), G Mancardi (Dipartimento Neuroscienze, Università di Genova, Genova), D Orrico (Divisione di Neurologia, Ospedale Civile Santa Chiara, Trento), G Tedeschi (Clinica Neurologica, Università di Napoli), M Battaglia (AISM, FISM, Genova), MG Valsecchi (Centro di Biostatistica per l'Epidemiologia Clinica, Università Milano-Bicocca, Monza). *Study coordinators* C Milanese, L Massacesi. *Randomization centre* A Solari. *Data Coordination and Analysis:* G Filippini, I Tramacere (Fondazione IRCCS Istituto Neurologico Carlo Besta, Milano). *Image Analysis Centre:* L Massacesi, L Vuolo (Dipartimento di Neuroscienze, Azienda Ospedaliero-Universitaria Careggi, Firenze). *Independent data safety management committee (IDSMC)* G Tognoni (Istituto Mario Negri, Milano), R D'Alessandro (Clinica Neurologica, Università di Bologna), L Provinciali (Clinica Neurologica, Ospedali Riuniti, Ancona). *Pharmacologic surveillance Unit* S Amoroso (Dipartimento di Neuroscienze, Sezione di Farmacologia, Università Politecnica delle Marche, Ancona). *Study sites and hospitals (PI = Principal investigator)* **Dipartimento di Neuroscienze, Psicologia, Farmaco e Salute del Bambino Università di Firenze** and Neurologia 2, Azienda Ospedaliero-Universitaria Careggi, Firenze; L Massacesi (PI), A Repice, A Barilaro, L Vuolo. **Fondazione IRCCS Istituto Neurologico Carlo Besta**, **Milano**; C Milanese (PI), P Confalonieri. **Unità di Neurologia - Multiple Sclerosis Center, I.R.C.C.S. Santa Maria Nascente Fondazione Don Gnocchi, Milano**; L La Mantia, **Clinica Neurologica, Novara**; M Leone (PI), S Ruggerone, P Naldi. **Dipartimento di Scienze Neurologiche "La Sapienza", Roma**; C Pozzilli (PI), F De Angelis. **Policlinico "G. Rodolico", Azienda Ospedaliero-Universitaria, Catania**; F Patti (PI), S Messina. **Dipartimento di Neuroscienze, Clinica Neurologica 2, Genova**; G Mancardi (PI), E Capello. **Dipartimento Universitario di Neurologia, Azienda Ospedaliera Universitaria Integrata, Verona**; MD Benedetti (PI), A Gajofatto. **Centro Sclerosi Multipla, Clinica Neurologica, Ospedale Clinicizzato "Colle Dall'Ara", Chieti**; A Lugaresi (PI), G De Luca. **Clinica Neurologica, Università di Sassari**; G Rosati (PI), M Pugliatti. **Clinica Neurologica, Università di Napoli**; G Tedeschi (PI), S. Bonavita. **UO**

Neurologia, Ospedale S. Antonio, Padova; B Tavolato (PI). **Dipartimento di Neuroscienze, Clinica Neurologica, Modena**; P Sola (PI). **Ospedale Santa Maria, Reggio Emilia**; L Motti (PI). **Clinica Neurologica, Policlinico Universitario Mater Domini, Catanzaro**; A Quattrone (PI). **Clinica Neurologica, Ospedale S. Gerardo, Monza**; M Frigo (PI). **Clinica Neurologica, Azienda Ospedaliero-Universitaria S. Anna, Ferrara**; MR Tola (PI). **Clinica Neurologica, Ospedali Riuniti, Ancona**; M Danni (PI). **UO Neurologia, Istituto S. Raffaele "G. Giglio", Cefalù**; L Grimaldi (PI). **Dipartimento di Neuroscienze, Azienda Ospedaliero San Giovanni Battista, Università di Torino, Torino**; P Cavalla (PI). **UO Neurologia, Ospedale Sacro Cuore, Negrar**; F Marchioretto (PI), M Pellegrini. **Divisione Neurologia, Ospedale Santa Chiara, Trento**; D Orrico (PI). **Divisione di Neurologia, Ospedale Regionale, Bolzano**; R Schoenhuber (PI). **Azienda Ospedaliero-Universitaria Senese, Policlinico "Le Scotte", Siena**; M Ulivelli (PI). **UO Neurologia, Ospedale "Misericordia e Dolce", Prato**; M Falcini (PI). **Dipartimento di Neuroscienze, Sezione di Neurologia, Pisa**; A Iudice (PI). **UOC Neurologia, Policlinico "G. Martino", Messina**; C Messina (PI). **Dipartimento di Neuroscienze, Clinica Neurologica, Palermo**; G Savettieri (PI). **Dipartimento di Neuroscienze, Università Cattolica, Policlinico Gemelli, Roma**; AP Batocchi (PI). **Dipartimento Neuroriabilitativo ASL CN1, Cuneo**; F Perla (PI). **Ospedale S. Luigi Gonzagal, Orbassano**; A Bertolotto (PI).

Author Contributions

Conceived and designed the experiments: LM CM MDB LL GF AS. Performed the experiments: LM CM MDB GT. Analyzed the data: IT AR. Wrote the paper: GF IT LM. Critical revision of the manuscript for important intellectual content: SA MDB LL AS GT CM. Obtained funding: LM CM. Administrative, technical, and material support: MAB AR. Study supervision: LM CM.

References

1. The British, Dutch MSATG. (1988) Double-masked trial of azathioprine in multiple sclerosis. british and dutch multiple sclerosis azathioprine trial group. Lancet 2: 179–183.
2. Ellison GW, Myers LW, Mickey MR, Graves MC, Tourtellotte WW, et al. (1989) A placebo-controlled, randomized, double-masked, variable dosage, clinical trial of azathioprine with and without methylprednisolone in multiple sclerosis. Neurology 39: 1018–1026.
3. Goodkin DE, Bailly RC, Teetzen ML, Hertsgaard D, Beatty WW. (1991) The efficacy of azathioprine in relapsing-remitting multiple sclerosis. Neurology 41: 20–25.
4. Milanese C, La Mantia L, Salmaggi A, Eoli M. (1993) A double blind study on azathioprine efficacy in multiple sclerosis: Final report. J Neurol 240: 295–298.
5. Clegg A, Bryant J, Milne R. (2000) Disease-modifying drugs for multiple sclerosis: A rapid and systematic review. Health Technol Assess 4: i–iv, 1–101.
6. Yudkin PL, Ellison GW, Ghezzi A, Goodkin DE, Hughes RA, et al. (1991) Overview of azathioprine treatment in multiple sclerosis. Lancet 338: 1051–1055.
7. Goodin DS, Frohman EM, Garmany GP, Jr, Halper J, Likosky WH, et al. (2002) Disease modifying therapies in multiple sclerosis: Report of the therapeutics and technology assessment subcommittee of the American Academy of Neurology and the MS council for clinical practice guidelines. Neurology 58: 169–178.
8. IFNB MSG. (1993) Interferon beta-1b is effective in relapsing-remitting multiple sclerosis. I. clinical results of a multicenter, randomized, double-blind, placebo-controlled trial. the IFNB multiple sclerosis study group. Neurology 43: 655–661.
9. PRISMS. (1998) Randomised double-blind placebo-controlled study of interferon beta-1a in relapsing/remitting multiple sclerosis. PRISMS (prevention of relapses and disability by interferon beta-1a subcutaneously in multiple sclerosis) study group. Lancet 352: 1498–1504.
10. Jacobs LD, Cookfair DL, Rudick RA, Herndon RM, Richert JR, et al. (1996) Intramuscular interferon beta 1a for disease progression in relapsing multiple sclerosis. the multiple sclerosis collaborative research group (MSCRG). Ann Neurol 39: 285–294.
11. Paty DW, Li DK. (1993) Interferon beta-1b is effective in relapsing-remitting multiple sclerosis. II. MRI analysis results of a multicenter, randomized, double-blind, placebo-controlled trial. UBC MS/MRI study group and the IFNB multiple sclerosis study group. Neurology 43: 662–667.
12. Casetta I, Iuliano G, Filippini G. (2007) Azathioprine for multiple sclerosis. Cochrane Database Syst Rev (4): CD003982.

13. Filippini G, Munari L, Incorvaia B, Ebers GC, Polman C, et al. (2003) Interferons in relapsing remitting multiple sclerosis: A systematic review. Lancet 361: 545–552.
14. Palace J, Rothwell P. (1997) New treatments and azathioprine in multiple sclerosis. Lancet 350: 261.
15. Etemadifar M, Janghorbani M, Shaygannejad V. (2007) Comparison of interferon beta products and azathioprine in the treatment of relapsing-remitting multiple sclerosis. J Neurol 254: 1723–1728.
16. Milanese C, La Mantia L, Salmaggi A, Caputo D. (2001) Azathioprine and interferon beta-1b treatment in relapsing-remitting multiple sclerosis. J Neurol Neurosurg Psychiatry 70: 413–414.
17. Cavazzuti M, Merelli E, Tassone G, Mavilla L. (1997) Lesion load quantification in serial MR of early relapsing multiple sclerosis patients in azathioprine treatment. A retrospective study. Eur Neurol 38: 284–290.
18. Massacesi L, Parigi A, Barilaro A, Repice AM, Pellicano G, et al. (2005) Efficacy of azathioprine on multiple sclerosis new brain lesions evaluated using magnetic resonance imaging. Arch Neurol 62: 1843–1847.
19. McDonald WI, Compston A, Edan G, Goodkin D, Hartung HP, et al. (2001) Recommended diagnostic criteria for multiple sclerosis: Guidelines from the international panel on the diagnosis of multiple sclerosis. Ann Neurol 50: 121–127.
20. Kurtzke JF. (1983) Rating neurologic impairment in multiple sclerosis: An expanded disability status scale (EDSS). Neurology 33: 1444–1452.
21. CTC (2003). Cancer therapy evaluation program, common terminology criteria for adverse event, version 3.0, DCTD, NCI, NIH, DHHS.
22. Solari A, Filippini G, Mendozzi L, Ghezzi A, Cifani S, et al. (1999) Validation of Italian multiple sclerosis quality of life 54 questionnaire. J Neurol Neurosurg Psychiatry 67: 158–162.
23. Committee for medicinal product for human use (CHMP) (2005). Guideline on the choise of the non-inferiority margin. doc. ref. EMEA/CPMP/EWP/2158/99.
24. Piaggio G, Elbourne DR, Altman DG, Pocock SJ, Evans SJ, et al. (2006) Reporting of noninferiority and equivalence randomized trials: An extension of the CONSORT statement. JAMA 295: 1152–1160.
25. Sackett DL. (2004) Superiority trials, noninferiority trials, and prisoners of the 2-sided null hypothesis. ACP J Club 140: A11.
26. Rubin DB. (1987) Multiple imputation for nonresponse in surveys. New York: John Wiley & Sons.

27. Brand JPL. (1999) Development, implementation and evaluation of multiple imputation strategies for the statistical analysis of incomplete data sets, ph.D. thesis, erasmus university, rotterdam.

28. van Buuren S, Boshuizen HC, Knook DL. (1999) Multiple imputation of missing blood pressure covariates in survival analysis. Stat Med 18: 681–694.

29. Piaggio G, Elbourne DR, Pocock SJ, Evans SJ, Altman DG; CONSORT Group. (2012) Reporting of noninferiority and equivalence randomized trials: extension of the CONSORT 2010 statement. JAMA 308:2594–2604.

30. Filippini G, Del Giovane C, Vacchi L, D'Amico R, Di Pietrantonj C, et al. (2013) Immunomodulators and immunosuppressants for multiple sclerosis: A network meta-analysis. Cochrane Database Syst Rev 6: CD008933.

31. Schulz KF, Grimes DA. (2005) Sample size calculations in randomised trials: Mandatory and mystical. Lancet 365: 1348–1353.

32. The IFNB Multiple Sclerosis Study Group and The University of British Columbia MS/MRI Analysis Group. (1995) Interferon beta-1b in the treatment of multiple sclerosis: Final outcome of the randomized controlled trial. Neurology 45: 1277–1285.

20

Dll4 Blockade Potentiates the Anti-Tumor Effects of VEGF Inhibition in Renal Cell Carcinoma Patient-Derived Xenografts

Kiersten Marie Miles[1], Mukund Seshadri[2], Eric Ciamporcero[6], Remi Adelaiye[3], Bryan Gillard[2], Paula Sotomayor[4], Kristopher Attwood[5], Li Shen[1], Dylan Conroy[1], Frank Kuhnert[7], Alshad S. Lalani[7], Gavin Thurston[7], Roberto Pili[1,3]*

1 Genitourinary Program, Roswell Park Cancer Institute, Buffalo, New York, United States of America, 2 Department of Pharmacology & Therapeutics, Roswell Park Cancer Institute Division, University at Buffalo, Buffalo, New York, United States of America, 3 Department of Cancer Pathology & Prevention, Roswell Park Cancer Institute Division, University at Buffalo, Buffalo, New York, United States of America, 4 Department of Molecular and Cellular Biology, Roswell Park Cancer Institute Division, University at Buffalo, Buffalo, New York, United States of America, 5 Department of Biostatistics & Bioinformatics, Roswell Park Cancer Institute Division, University at Buffalo, Buffalo, New York, United States of America, 6 Medicine and Experimental Oncology, University of Turin, Turin, Italy, 7 Regeneron Pharmaceuticals, Inc., Tarrytown, New York, United States of America

Abstract

Background: The Notch ligand Delta-like 4 (Dll4) is highly expressed in vascular endothelium and has been shown to play a pivotal role in regulating tumor angiogenesis. Blockade of the Dll4-Notch pathway in preclinical cancer models has been associated with non-productive angiogenesis and reduced tumor growth. Given the cross-talk between the vascular endothelial growth factor (VEGF) and Delta-Notch pathways in tumor angiogenesis, we examined the activity of a function-blocking Dll4 antibody, REGN1035, alone and in combination with anti-VEGF therapy in renal cell carcinoma (RCC).

Methods and Results: Severe combined immunodeficiency (SCID) mice bearing patient-derived clear cell RCC xenografts were treated with REGN1035 and in combination with the multi-targeted tyrosine kinase inhibitor sunitinib or the VEGF blocker ziv-aflibercept. Immunohistochemical and immunofluorescent analyses were carried out, as well as magnetic resonance imaging (MRI) examinations pre and 24 hours and 2 weeks post treatment. Single agent treatment with REGN1035 resulted in significant tumor growth inhibition (36–62%) that was equivalent to or exceeded the single agent anti-tumor activity of the VEGF pathway inhibitors sunitinib (38–54%) and ziv-aflibercept (46%). Importantly, combination treatments with REGN1035 plus VEGF inhibitors resulted in enhanced anti-tumor effects (72–80% growth inhibition), including some tumor regression. Magnetic resonance imaging showed a marked decrease in tumor perfusion in all treatment groups. Interestingly, anti-tumor efficacy of the combination of REGN1035 and ziv-aflibercept was also observed in a sunitinib resistant ccRCC model.

Conclusions: Overall, these findings demonstrate the potent anti-tumor activity of Dll4 blockade in RCC patient-derived tumors and a combination benefit for the simultaneous targeting of the Dll4 and VEGF signaling pathways, highlighting the therapeutic potential of this treatment modality in RCC.

Editor: Natasha Kyprianou, University of Kentucky College of Medicine, United States of America

Funding: This research was supported in part by the National Cancer Institute, National Institutes of Health (P30CA016056) (RP), and by a research grant from Regeneron Pharmaceuticals, Inc. (RP). The funder provided support in the form of salaries for authors GT, ASL, FK, but did not have any additional role in the study design, data collection and analysis, decision to publish, or preparation of the manuscript.

Competing Interests: The authors have read the journal's policy and have the following competing interests: Employees from Regeneron: FK, ASL, GT. Research fundings from Regeneron: RP.

* Email: Roberto.Pili@RoswellPark.org

Introduction

Kidney cancer strikes close to 65,000 Americans every year and kills over 13,000 [1]. Renal cell carcinoma (RCC) is the most common type of kidney cancer, with 80% diagnosed as clear cell (cc) RCC. Treatment of localized RCC is usually centered on surgery and immunotherapy. Unfortunately, approximately 30–40% of kidney cancer patients eventually develop metastatic RCC and the current treatment options are limited. The well vascularized nature of RCC has generated considerable interest in the development of anti-angiogenic therapies for this disease.

Vascular endothelial growth factor (VEGF) is a protein that stimulates vasculogenesis and angiogenesis by initiating blood vessel sprouting and endothelial proliferation. Overexpression of VEGF is often associated with tumor growth and metastases and is a common target for cancer therapy [2]. Several anti-VEGF therapies, including tyrosine kinase inhibitors (TKIs), are currently used in the frontline management of RCC. Sunitinib is an oral, multi-targeted receptor TKI that is FDA approved for the treatment of RCC and GIST; and which has been shown to inhibit tumor vascularization by diminishing signaling through VEGF receptors 1 and 2, and platelet derived growth factor receptor (PDGFR). Ziv-aflibercept is a protein therapeutic that binds to all isoforms of VEGF-A, as well as VEGF-B and placental growth factor (PlGF) [3], [4]. In several types of tumor xenograft models, including RCC, ziv-aflibercept was found to inhibit tumor growth with an associated large reduction of tumor vasculature, with less promotion of changes in gene expression in normal organs than seen following receptor TKI treatment [5], [6]. Ziv-aflibercept was recently approved for use in combination with chemotherapy for the treatment of colon carcinoma in patients who previously failed oxaliplatin-based therapy [7]. Further, ziv-aflibercept is currently under exploratory clinical investigations in patients with clear cell RCC who are refractory to VEGF-tyrosine kinase inhibitors (NCI trial number E4805). Unfortunately, the clinical benefit associated with anti-VEGF therapies is often limited, as patients exhibit acquired tumor resistance to VEGF inhibition; thus there is great interest in identifying additional angiogenesis targets that, in combination with anti-VEGF therapies, can lead to more effective treatments for RCC.

The Dll4-Notch pathway is an evolutionarily conserved signaling pathway that functions as a key negative regulator of physiological and pathological angiogenesis downstream of VEGF [8]. Dll4 is a Notch ligand that is induced in endothelial tip cells of angiogenic sprouts and loss of expression has been shown to lead to excessive production of aberrant non-functional tumor vessels and associated reduced tumor growth [9], [10]. Dll4 is predominately found in the developing endothelium, with an almost 9-fold increased expression reported within the vasculature of ccRCC, as compared to normal kidneys [11]. Multiple tumor types have been found to express Dll4 and RCC, in particular, has been shown to be regulated by the Dll4/Notch pathway [12]. Accordingly, therapeutic targeting of Dll4 in the treatment of renal cell carcinoma may hold much promise.

The aim of this study was to explore the effects of Dll4 antibody therapy alone and in combination with approved VEGF inhibitors on tumor growth and perfusion in patient-derived xenograft (PDX) ccRCC models. In our experimental models, we observed considerable single agent activity of Dll4 antibody targeting stromal Dll4, and an enhancement of the anti-tumor effects by combination with VEGF inhibition. In both cases, the anti-tumor effects were associated with profound tumor vascular changes and reduction in tumor perfusion. In addition, the anti-tumor efficacy of anti-Dll4 and anti-VEGF combination therapy was also observed in a sunitinib resistant ccRCC model, which further highlights the great therapeutic potential of targeting these two pathways.

Materials and Methods

Compounds

REGN1035, REGN421 (also known as enoticumab), and ziv-aflibercept (also known as VEGF Trap) were produced by Regeneron Pharmaceuticals, Inc. (Tarrytown, NY). REGN1035 is a preclinical monoclonal mouse antibody that selectively binds and blocks murine Dll4. REGN421 is a fully human IgG1 monoclonal antibody that binds human Dll4 and is currently under clinical investigation in a Phase I study in patients with advanced solid tumor malignancies. Ziv-aflibercept is a fully human fusion protein comprised of the extracellular domains of

VEGFR1 and VEGFR2 fused to a human IgG1 constant domain. Sunitinib (Sutent) was purchased from LC Laboratories (Woburn, MA).

Xenograft models and treatment protocol

RP-R-01 is a xenograft model established from a skin metastasis from a patient with sporadic ccRCC, previously treated with sunitinib. VHL (von Hippel-Lindau) was not found to be expressed in RP-R-01 tumor cells. The establishment and characterization of this model was previously described [13]. RP-R-02 is a xenograft model also established from a skin metastasis, but from a patient with VHL syndrome and hereditary ccRCC, with no prior treatments. Importantly, both models were passaged only *in vivo*, thus minimizing the selection for growth and loss of cellular heterogeneity of the primary tumor often seen in cell culture. Collection of tumor samples was obtained via regulatory approval at the institution. The *in vivo* experiments were conducted once.

Immunodeficient SCID male mice purchased from Roswell Park Cancer Institute (RPCI) were utilized for these studies and all procedures were approved by The Institute Animal Care and Use Committee (IACUC). Mice were kept in a temperature controlled room on a 12/12 hours light/dark schedule with food and water *ad libitum*. Mice were implanted subcutaneously in the flank area with ~0.5 mm^3 size RP-R-01 or RP-R-02 ccRCC tumor tissue. Approximately 6 weeks later, when tumors reached an average volume of 68.0 mm^3, mice were divided into homogenous groups (7–8 mice/group) as determined by caliper measurements. Tumor volume was calculated as mm^3 ($\sqrt{}$(length × width))^3 ×0.5. Mice were treated with vehicle (hFc control protein, 4.89 mg/kg, s.q.), sunitinib (40 mg/kg, 5x/wk, orally), or ziv-aflibercept (5 mg/kg, 2x/wk, s.q.) and/or REGN1035 (5 mg/kg, 1x/wk, s.q.) for a period of five to six weeks.

A sunitinib resistant ccRCC model was established utilizing subcutaneous implantation of RP-R-01 tumor tissue. Mice with established tumors (average volume of 78.0 mm^3) were treated with sunitinib (40 mg/kg, 5x/wk, orally) for 4 weeks until tumor tissue was no longer responsive to treatment (tumor volume was ~6 times that of pretreatment volume). At which time, mice were treated with either sunitinib (40 mg/kg, 5x/wk, orally), ziv-aflibercept (5 mg/kg, 2x/wk, s.q.), REGN1035 (5 mg/kg, 1x/wk, s.q.) or the combination of ziv-aflibercept plus REGN1035 for a period of four weeks.

Mouse body weight and tumor caliper measurements were taken weekly. Body weight changes over the course of treatments are given in Table S1. Some weight loss was observed in mice treated with REGN1035 alone and in combination with sunitinib, ziv-aflibercept or REGN421. The vehicle group in 1 of 4 experiments also showed a reduction in weight, most likely due to tumor growth. At the time of harvest, it was noted that the livers of some (~40%) of the mice treated with REGN1035 alone and in combination with ziv-aflibercept appeared patchy. Upon histological examination, the livers showed evidence of heterogeneous septal fibrosis and vascular congestion (Fig. S1). These findings are in agreement with a previous report on the effects of Dll4 blockade on rodent liver histology [14]. Tumor tissue was harvested and weighed at the end of treatment, and fixed in 10% normal buffered formalin or zinc.

Immunohistochemistry

Formalin fixed and processed tissue sections were embedded in paraffin blocks and cut at 4 µm, placed on charged slides, and dried at 60°C for one hour. Slides were cooled to room temperature, deparaffinized in three changes of xylene, and rehydrated using graded alcohols. For antigen retrieval, slides were treated by citrate buffer (pH 6.0) (Biocare Medical) and heated in the microwave for 10 minutes, followed by a 15 minute cool down. Endogenous peroxidase was quenched with aqueous 3% H_2O_2 for 10 minutes and washed with PBS/T. Slides were loaded on a DAKO autostainer and serum free protein block (DAKO) was applied for 5 minutes, blown off, and the antibodies (Ki67, Thermo Scientific; CD31, Dianova) were applied for one hour. Biotinylated goat anti-rabbit IgG (Vector) secondary antibody was applied for 30 minutes, followed by the Elite ABC Kit (Vectastain), also for 30 minutes and the DAB chromogen (Dako) for five minutes, OR biotinylated goat anti-rat IgG (BD Pharmingen) secondary-thirty minutes, followed by ZSA-(Streptavidin Horseradish Peroxidase Conjugate (Invitrogen) for thirty minutes followed by the DAB chromogen for five minutes. Finally, the slides were counterstained with hematoxylin, dehydrated, cleared and cover slipped. Images were captured using a Scanscope XT system (Aperio Imaging) and analyzed using Imagescope software (Aperio). Necrosis (H&E), Ki67, and CD31 immunostaining quantification, approximately 4 randomly selected fields of 6 to 8 samples per treatment, was done in a blind manner using Image J software. Results are expressed as the average per treatment of positive area (H&E and CD31) and positive nuclei (Ki67) $\pm$ S.E.

Immunofluorescence

Tumor tissue was removed and fixed in formalin for 24 hours. Samples were dehydrated and paraffin embedded. Paraffin blocks were sectioned (6 μm), deparaffinized, and antigen retrieval was performed by boiling the slides for 15 minutes in citrate buffer (pH 6.0). Slides were blocked in 1% bovine serum albumin (Sigma-Aldrich), diluted in PBS for 30 minutes, and incubated overnight with the primary anti-mouse CD31 antibody (1/40, Dianova), followed by incubation with the secondary antibody Cy3-conjugated anti-rat IgG (1/400, Invitrogen). Sections were mounted using Vectashield (Vector Laboratories). CD31 immunostaining quantification, approximately 4 randomly selected fields of 6 to 8 samples per treatment, was done in a blind manner using Image J software. Background was subtracted to determine the percentage of positive area. Results are expressed as the average per treatment of CD31 positive area $\pm$ S.E.

Magnetic Resonance Imaging (MRI)

Experimental MRI examinations were carried out in a 4.7 T/33-cm horizontal bore magnet (GE NMR Instruments, Fremont, CA) incorporating AVANCE digital electronics (Bruker Biospec with ParaVision 3.0.2; Bruker Medical Inc., Billerica, MA) and a removable gradient coil insert (G060, Bruker Medical Inc., Billerica, MA) generating maximum field strength of 950 mT/m and a custom-designed 35-mm RF transmit-receive coil. Mice were placed on a form-fitted MR-compatible sled (Dazai Research Instruments, Toronto, Canada) and supplied with 2% isoflurane during image acquisition. Respiration rates and core-body temperature were monitored continuously while mice were in the scanner. Preliminary scout images were acquired on the sagittal and axial planes to assist in slice prescription for subsequent scans. Multislice non contrast-enhanced T2-weighted images were acquired on the axial planes with the following parameters: $TE_{eff} = 41$ ms, $TR = 2500$ ms, FOV $= 3.2 \times 3.2$ cm, matrix size $= 256 \times 192$, 25 slices, slice thickness 1 mm). T1-relaxation rates (R1) were measured using a saturation recovery, fast spin echo as described [15], [16]. A series of ten images (3 before contrast and 7 following administration of albumin-GdDTPA, 0.1 mmol/kg) were obtained to estimate changes in relative blood volume and permeability of tumors. MR angiog-

raphy was performed using a three-dimensional spoiled gradient echo sequence (matrix size $192 \times 96 \times 96$; FOV $4.8 \times 3.2 \times 3.2$ cm, flip angle $= 40°$, acquisition time $= 2$ m 18 s. Raw image sets were transferred to a processing workstation and converted into Analyze format (Analyze 7.0, Analyze Direct, Overland Park, KS, USA). Linear regression analysis of the normalized change in R1 versus time curve was carried out to compute the relative blood volume of tumors. T1 relaxation maps (R1 maps) of animals were calculated on a pixel-by-pixel basis in MATLAB (Math Works, Inc.). For each treatment group, T1 enhancement maps were generated by subtracting a postcontrast R1 map from the pre contrast R1 map of the same animal.

Statistical Analysis

Data are expressed as mean $\pm$ standard error (S.E). Tumor size is modeled as a function of time, experimental group and their interaction using linear mixed models, with tumor growth rates compared between experimental groups using the appropriate contrasts of estimated interaction terms. The association between end of treatment (EOT) outcomes and experimental group are evaluated using ANOVA models, with pairwise comparisons made using two-sample t-tests when appropriate. All tests are two-sided. All model assumptions were verified graphically and a log-transformation was found to be necessary for tumor size. All pairwise comparisons were adjusted using the Holm-Bonferroni method for controlling experiment wise error-rate. The analyses were conducted in Graph Pad Prism 5 (Graph Pad Software Inc.) and SAS v9.4 (Cary, NC) at a statistical significance level of 0.05.

Results

Potent anti-tumor activity of Dll4 blockade in RCC PDX models plus a significant combination benefit for combined inhibition of Dll4 and VEGF signaling

To assess the anti-tumor efficacy of anti-Dll4 and anti-Dll4/VEGF combination therapy, SCID mice were implanted with RP-R-01 or RP-R-02 ccRCC patient-derived xenograft tumors and treated with REGN1035 and/or sunitinib or ziv-aflibercept (Fig. 1A–C). Single agent treatment in the RP-R-01 tumor model reduced tumor growth by 38% (sunitinib); 46% (ziv-aflibercept); 36% and 55% (REGN1035), $p < 0.01$ vs. vehicle, and an even more significant effect on tumor growth was observed in combination treated groups (72% reduction with REGN1035 plus sunitinib; 80% reduction with REGN1035 plus ziv-aflibercept, $p < 0.01$ combination vs. vehicle, $p < 0.01$ combination vs. single agent; Table S1). Noteworthy, REGN1035 treatment combined with ziv-aflibercept resulted in not only an additive anti-tumor effect, but also regression of established RP-R-01 tumors (Fig. 1B). A similar observation was found in the treatment-naïve patient-derived RP-R-02 model, with 38% (sunitinib) and 55% (REGN1035) reduction of growth from single agent treatment and 72% reduction following combination treatment, $p < 0.01$ (Fig. 1C). At end of treatment (EOT), the average RP-R-01 tumor volume and weight following REGN1035 and/or sunitinib administration are shown in Figures 1A and 1D, respectively: vehicle (677.3 mm^3, 0.914 g), sunitinib (329.5 mm^3, 0.512 g), REGN1035 (204.3 mm^3, 0.271 g), and combination (144.6 mm^3, 0.210 g). Figures 1B and 1E show the average EOT tumor volume and weight, respectively, of RP-R-01 tissue treated with REGN1035 and/or ziv-aflibercept: vehicle (617.7 mm^3, 0.631 g), ziv-aflibercept (245.4 mm^3, 0.270 g), REGN1035 (307.9 mm^3, 0.353 g), and combination (52.5 mm^3, 0.056 g). RP-R-02 tumor volume and weight are shown in Figures 1C and 1F, respectively: vehicle (476.3 mm^3, 0.419 g), sunitinib

(149.3 mm^3, 0.251 g), REGN1035 (110.31 mm^3, 0.096 g), and combination (47.5 mm^3, 0.049 g). ANOVA analysis showed a significant association between treatment and EOT tumor weight, with all p values <0.05. The tumor growth rate was lower in the combination treatment than in single agent or vehicle. The single agents have no significant difference, but both have lower growth rates than the vehicle. Overall, all treatments were well tolerated. No overt signs of toxicity (i.e. extreme weight loss, lack of food consumption or diarrhea) were observed in either xenograft model following REGN1035 and/or sunitinib treatment. A 16% decrease in mouse body weight relative to vehicle was observed following REGN1035 plus ziv-aflibercept combination treatment in the RP-R-01 model. However, in that experiment the vehicle group also had a 10% decrease in body weight and the difference

with the combination group was not statistically significant (Table S2). The mice otherwise appeared healthy with no other signs of distress.

To examine the effects of treatment on tumor necrosis, end of treatment tumor tissue sections were stained with hematoxylin and eosin (H&E). As shown in Figures 2A–C, a modest reduction in viable tissue was observed following single agent treatment with anti-VEGF therapy (sunitinib, 3–21% necrosis), (ziv-aflibercept, 9% necrosis). Tumors treated with REGN1035 or combinations displayed a substantially increased percentage of necrosis than vehicle or VEGF inhibitor-treated tumors (vehicle, 7–11%; REGN1035, 44–52%; REGN1035 plus sunitinib, 41–57%; REGN1035 plus ziv-aflibercept, 86%, all p<0.05 vs. vehicle) (Fig. 2D–F).

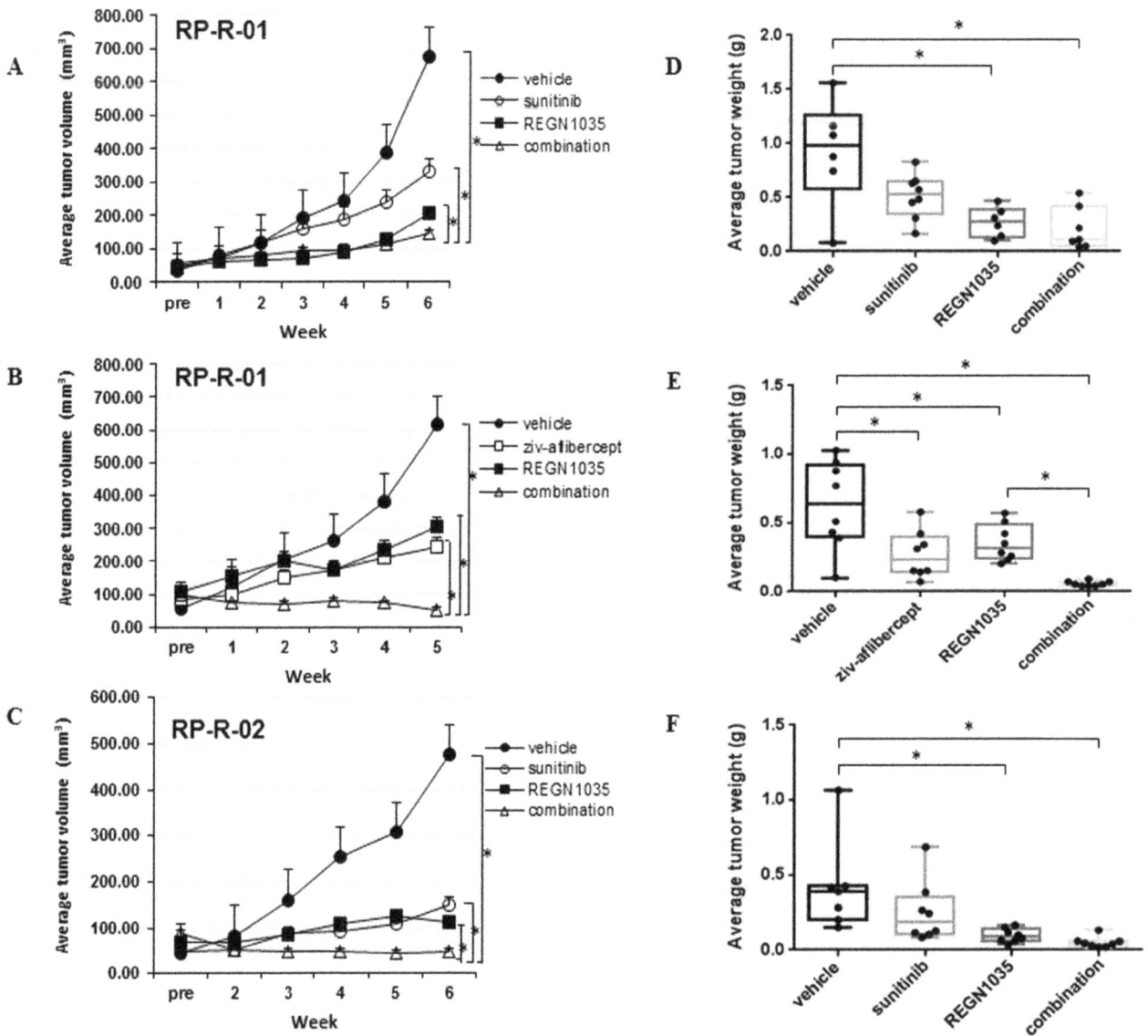

Figure 1. Anti-tumor efficacy of anti-Dll4 (REGN1035) and/or anti-VEGF (sunitinib or ziv-aflibercept) in RP-R-01 and RP-R-02 ccRCC patient derived xenografts. Mice (8 mice/group) were treated with vehicle, sunitinib, or ziv-aflibercept and/or REGN1035. Left panel: Tumor growth curves. (A) RP-R-01 REGN1035 and/or sunitinib treatment groups (B) RP-R-01 REGN1035 and/or ziv-aflibercept treatment groups (C) RP-R-02 REGN1035 and/or sunitinib treatment groups. Each line represents the average tumor volume (mm^3) of each treatment group ± S.E. (D, E, F) End point tumor weights (g). * p<0.05 using adjusted t-test analysis.

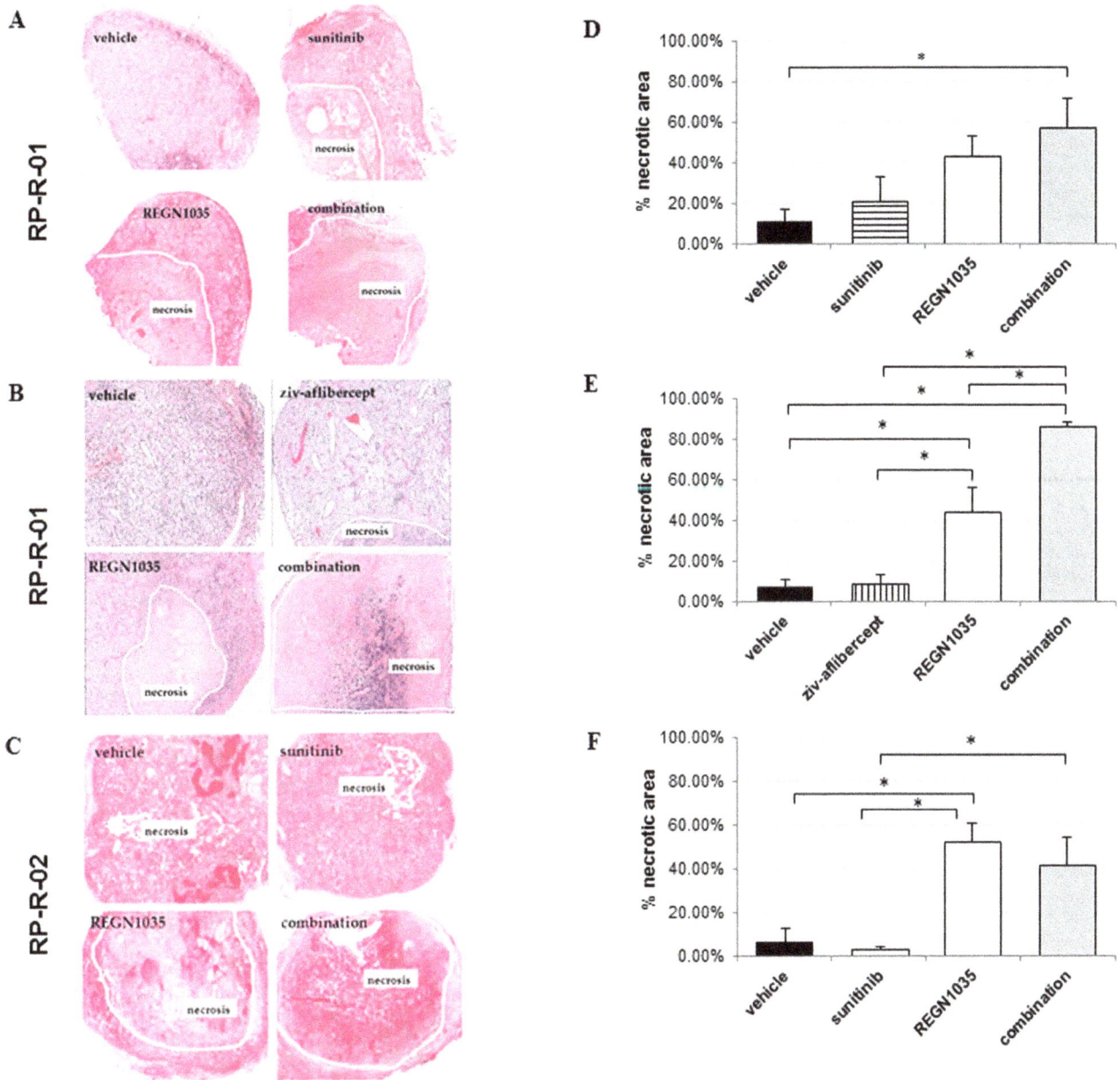

Figure 2. Effect of REGN1035 and/or anti-VEGF (sunitinib or ziv-aflibercept) treatment on tumor cell viability. Mice (8 mice/group) implanted with (A, B) RP-R-01 or (C) RP-R-02 tissues were treated with vehicle, sunitinib, or ziv-aflibercept and/or REGN1035. Tumors were harvested, processed, and tissue sections were stained for hematoxylin and eosin. Left panels: Representative images of tumor necrosis. (D, E, F) Quantitative analysis was done in a blinded fashion. Results are expressed as mean percentage necrotic area ± S.E. *$p < 0.05$ using adjusted t-test analysis.

We were also interested in assessing the effect of anti-Dll4 and anti-VEGF treatment on cellular proliferation. As shown in Figures 3A–B, single agent inhibition of Dll4 signaling with REGN1035 induced a modest increase of Ki67 expression in RP-R-01 tumor sections, presumably reflecting increased endothelial proliferation. In contrast, ziv-aflibercept and the combination with REGN1035 was associated with a significant decrease in cellular proliferation (ziv-aflibercept, 28% reduction, $p < 0.05$; combination, 42% reduction, $p < 0.01$, as compared to vehicle), which correlates with the inhibition of tumor growth shown in Figure 1B.

Dll4 blockade enhances the anti-vascular effects of VEGF inhibition

We assessed the anti-vascular effects of anti-Dll4 and anti-VEGF treatment in our RCC models using immunofluorescence, immunohistochemistry, and non-invasive magnetic resonance imaging (MRI). The panel of images shown in Figure 4 represents immunofluorescence staining of end-of-treatment tumor sections [RP-R-01 (A and B), RP-R-02 (C)] with anti-CD31 antibody. A reduction in vessel density was observed following single agent treatment with sunitinib (34% and 85% reduction in RP-R-01, $p < 0.01$ and RP-R-02, respectively) and ziv-aflibercept (14% reduction in RP-R-01) (Fig. 4D–F). Tumors treated with single agent REGN1035, in contrast, showed a statistically significant increase

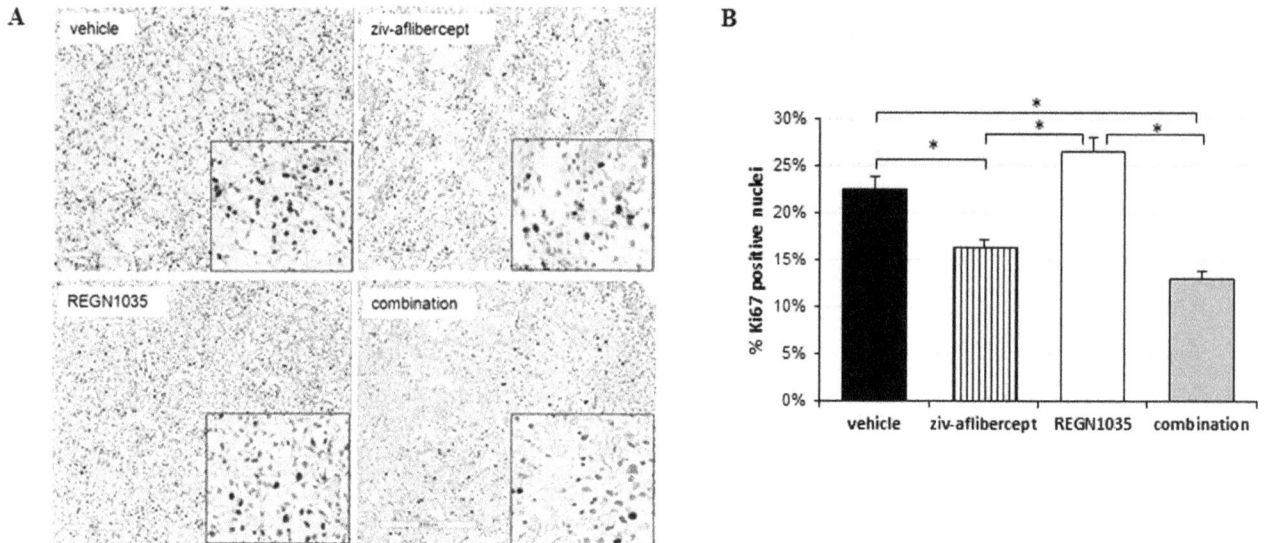

Figure 3. Effects of REGN1035 and/or ziv-aflibercept on tumor cell proliferation in RP-R-01 ccRCC xenograft. Mice were treated with vehicle, ziv-aflibercept and/or REGN1035. Tumors were harvested, processed, and tissue sections were stained for differential expression of Ki67. (A) Representative images. (B) Quantitative analysis was done in a blinded manner. Results are expressed as mean percentage positive nuclei ± S.E. *$p <$ 0.05 using adjusted t-test analysis.

in vascular structures, as compared to vehicle (111% and 180% increase in RP-R-01, $p<0.01$; 22% increase in RP-R-02). This increase in tumor microvascular density is consistent with the observed increase in Ki67 staining shown in Figure 3. In addition, REGN1035 treatment promoted structural changes within the tumor vasculature with the appearance of extensively unorganized aberrant networks of small, highly branched vessels. Combination treatment resulted in significantly less tumor vascularity (50% and 68% reduction in RP-R-01; 49% reduction in RP-R-02, $p<0.05$), with a great percentage of the tissue nearly devoid of vascular networks.

Next, we examined the effects of combined Dll4 and VEGF blockade on tumor vascular function using contrast-enhanced MRI. Tumors were imaged at 24 hours (early) and 2 weeks (late) after the start of treatment to characterize the vascular response of tumors to acute and chronic administration of both agents. Quantitative estimates of contrast agent concentration ($\Delta R1$) in tumors (n = 3 per group) and contralateral kidneys were obtained to compute changes in blood volume (Y-intercept) and permeability (slope). At 24 hours post treatment (Fig. 5A), a significant reduction in blood volume ($p<0.001$) in tumors treated with ziv-aflibercept alone (0.25 ± 0.06) or REGN1035 alone (0.72 ± 0.10) compared to control tumors (1.08 ± 0.09) was observed. Animals treated with the combination showed the greatest reduction in vascular volume compared to controls and either monotherapy ($p<0.0001$). Combination treatment resulted in durable anti-vascular activity with a significant ($p<0.0001$) reduction in blood volume (0.015 ± 0.06) at the two week time point (Fig. 5B) compared to controls (0.75 ± 0.05), ziv-aflibercept alone (0.14 ± 0.06) and REGN1035 alone (0.20 ± 0.04). No difference in perfusion ($\Delta R1$) of kidneys was observed with single agent or combination treatments at both time points (Fig. S2). The panel of images shown in Figure 5C represent contrast enhancement maps of three contiguous slices of a tumor in each group at the end of two week treatment period. While single agent treatments resulted in reduction in perfusion compared to control tumors, combination treatment resulted in marked reduction in tumor growth and

perfusion as evidenced by decreased contrast agent uptake in the tumor. Corresponding 3D MR angiography images of a representative tumor in all 4 groups is shown in Figure S3.

Dll4 blockade enhances the anti-vascular effects of VEGF blockade in a sunitinib resistant RCC model

To assess the anti-tumor efficacy of anti-Dll4 and anti-Dll4/VEGF combination therapy in a sunitinib resistant xenograft model, SCID mice were implanted subcutaneously with RP-R-01 tissue and treated with sunitinib until resistance was observed (when tumor size doubled that of pretreatment size). At which time, mice either continued to be treated with sunitinib or were switched to ziv-aflibercept, REGN1035 or the combination of ziv-aflibercept plus REGN1035. As shown in Figure 6A, only the combination of REGN1035 and ziv-aflibercept induced a significant tumor growth inhibition and even tumor regression, as compared to the group continued to be exposed to sunitinib. EOT tumor volume and weight are shown in Figures 6A and 6B, respectively: sunitinib (1010.5 mm^3, 0.823 g), ziv-aflibercept (661.8 mm^3, 0.600 g), REGN1035 (1075.3 mm^3, 0.827 g), and combination (308.9 mm^3, 0.311 g). The anti-tumor efficacy of the combination treated mice was found to be significantly different ($p<0.05$) from single agent sunitinib and REGN1035 treated mice, but not ziv-aflibercept treated mice. Interestingly, the greater anti-tumor effect in the combination group was not associated with greater inhibition of tumor blood vessel density (Fig. 6C–D). No overt signs of toxicity were observed, with only minimal weight loss was noted in the combination group (6.35%, ±1.28).

The potent anti-tumor activity of Dll4 blockade is dependent on targeting Dll4 in the tumor stroma

Species-specific Taqman RNA gene expression analysis was performed to determine the levels of Dll4 expression in the RP-R-01 model and to gain a better understanding of the anti-tumor mechanism of anti-Dll4 therapy. Mouse Dll4 was robustly expressed in the stroma of RP-R-01 tumors, consistent with the function of Dll4 as a critical regulator of tumor angiogenesis,

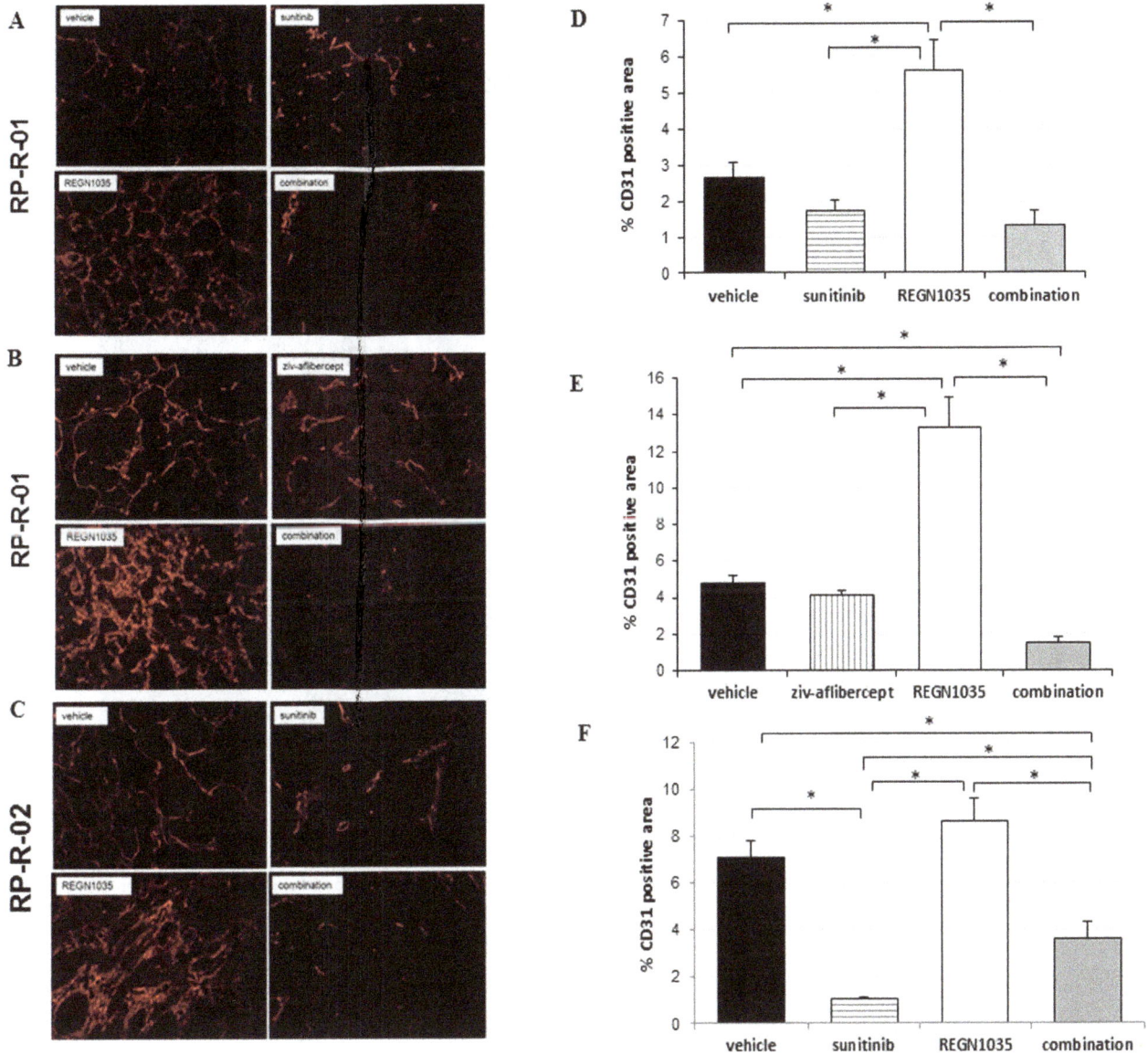

Figure 4. Effect of REGN1035 and/or anti-VEGF (sunitinib or ziv-aflibercept) on (A, B) RP-R-01 and (C) RP-R-02 tumor vasculature. Tumors from treated mice were harvested, processed, and tissue sections were stained for the differential expression of CD31 (red) for visualization of endothelial cells (left panels). (D, E, F) Blinded quantitative analysis of CD31 (right panels). Results are expressed as mean percentage positive stained area ± S.E. *$p<0.05$ using adjusted t-test analysis.

whereas the levels of tumor-cell expressed Dll4 (human) were very low, at the limit of detection (Fig. S4). To determine the relative contributions of blocking stromal (mouse) Dll4 vs. Dll4 expressed by tumor cells (human) to the overall anti-tumor activity, we treated RP-R-01 tumor-bearing SCID mice with the human Dll4-specific monoclonal antibody REGN421 (enoticumab), the mouse Dll4-specific antibody REGN1035, or the combination. As shown in Figures 7A and 7B, treatment with human Dll4-specific REGN421 showed only marginal anti-tumor efficacy, with no significant differences observed from the vehicle treated group. The mouse Dll4-specific REGN1035 treatment, on the other hand, resulted in significant RP-R-01 tumor growth inhibition (67%, $p<0.01$), consistent with results shown in Figure 1. Combination treatment of anti-human and anti-mouse Dll4 antibodies did not result in enhanced anti-tumor effects compared to single agent administration of REGN1035. These results

demonstrate that the anti-tumor activity of Dll4 blockade in the RP-R-01 RCC model is entirely dependent on targeting Dll4 in the tumor stroma as opposed to tumor cell-expressed Dll4, and furthermore highlights the lack of tumor growth-promoting autocrine Dll4-Notch tumor cell signaling in this model.

Discussion

The treatment options for patients with renal cell carcinoma have expanded considerably over the past decade, with five agents targeting VEGF signaling now approved for advanced disease. However, overcoming acquired resistance to frontline anti-VEGF therapies remains a challenge. Ample data in the literature indicate that Dll4 signaling plays a critical role in tumor angiogenesis and possibly in mediating resistance to anti-VEGF therapies, thus providing rationale for combined VEGF and Dll4

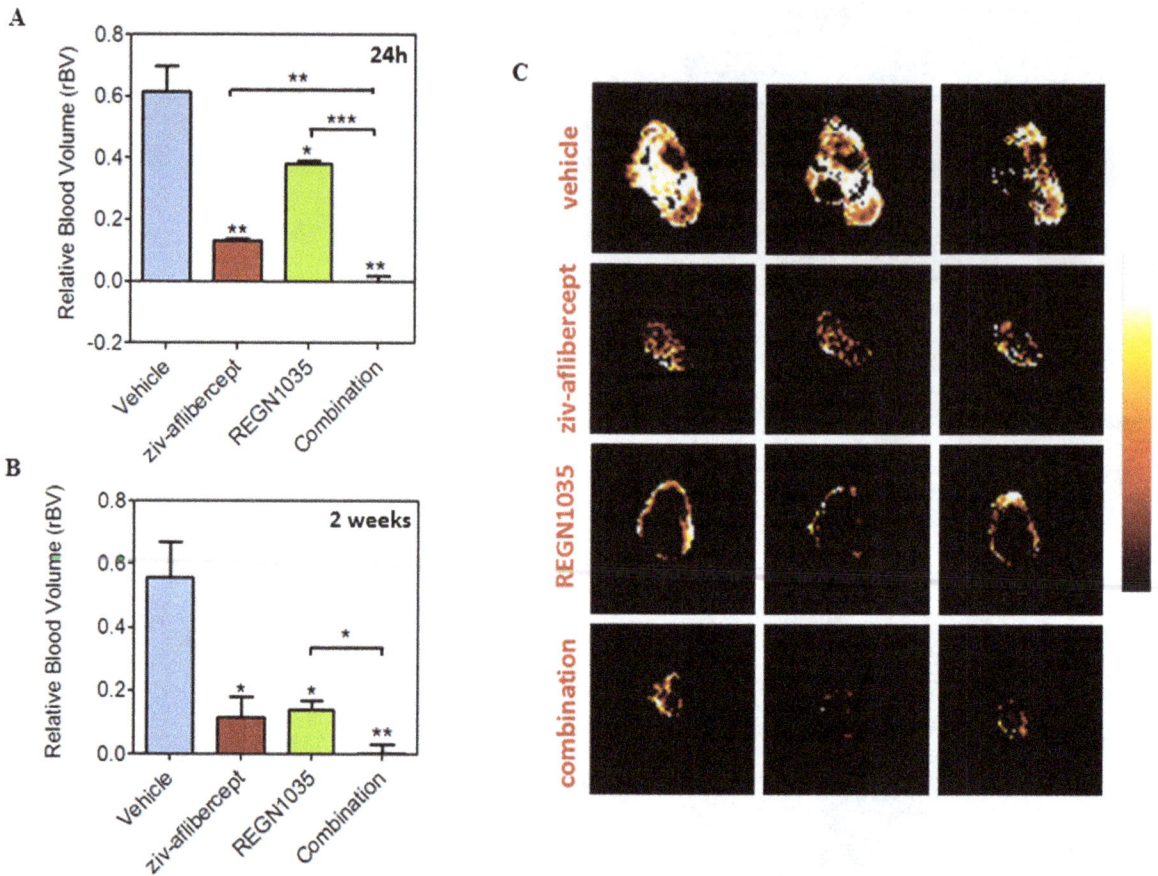

Figure 5. Vascular response of RP-R-01 tumors to combined DLL4-VEGF blockade. MRI-based estimates of relative blood volume estimates of RP-R-01 tumors at (A) 24 hours and (B) 2 weeks (C) Panel of images represent contrast enhancement maps of a representative tumor from each group 2 weeks post treatment. Three contiguous slices of the tumor are shown. All treatment groups showed significant reduction in rBV compared to controls. Combination treatment resulted in the greatest reduction in tumor perfusion. *$p<0.05$, **$p<0.01$, ***$p<0.001$.

inhibition. Blockade of the Dll4-Notch pathway in preclinical cancer models results in non-productive angiogenesis, that is, excessive production of aberrant non-functional tumor vascular structures associated with reduced tumor growth. Thus, it functions via a different mechanism of action than the targeting of the VEGF signaling pathway. In fact, some tumors resistant to anti-VEGF therapy have been shown to be responsive to anti-Dll4 [10], [17]; and the inhibition of the Dll4-Notch signaling pathway has been found to enhance the efficacy of VEGF inhibitors [18]. Furthermore, patients with low Dll4 expression treated with anti-VEGF therapy were found to exhibit significant prolongation of progression free survival over patients with higher levels of Dll4 expression [19]. Similarly, high expression of Dll4 by endothelial cells was shown to be a statistically significant adverse prognostic factor in breast and ovarian cancer patients [20], [21]; and elevated expression of both DLL4 and VEGF was found to be a significant overall survival disadvantage in nasopharyngeal carcinoma patients, as compared to those with dual low expression [22]. Taken together, these findings provide a strong rationale for the combined blockade of VEGF and Dll4-Notch signaling in renal cancer patients.

Herein, we analyzed the anti-tumor activity of blocking Dll4-Notch signaling alone and in combination with anti-VEGF agents in patient-derived ccRCC models. We found that treatment with the anti-mouse Dll4 monoclonal antibody REGN1035 produces potent single agent anti-tumor efficacy in these models. Impor-

tantly, combination treatment with REGN1035 and either VEGF pathway targeting agents results in enhanced anti-tumor effects and even produced tumor regression.

Our study highlights the angiogenic mechanism by which blockade of Dll4 results in inhibition of tumor growth and vessel functionality. Extensive tumor necrosis and non-functional angiogenesis were observed in RCC tumors in response to Dll4 blockade. More specifically, a decrease in tumor perfusion was observed following REGN1035 treatment by MRI imaging in spite of the marked increase in tumor vessel density observed in these samples, confirming that Dll4 inhibition produces non-productive tumor angiogenesis that is associated with the subsequent impairment in tumor growth. Combination treatment of anti-Dll4 antibody with either anti-VEGF agent resulted in reductions in tumor perfusion and markedly increased tumor necrosis compared to single agents. Of note, analysis of the tumor vasculature revealed that the combination treatments produced decreases in microvascular densities similar to or exceeding the anti-vascular effects observed for the VEGF pathway targeting agents alone, suggesting that in the models analyzed in this study, the anti-VEGF vascular 'pruning' effects were dominant over the endothelial hypersprouting phenotype associated with Dll4 blockade.

In a separate experiment, we tested whether Dll4 blockade in combination with continuous VEGF inhibition could also impair tumor growth in a sunitinib resistant PDX model. Interestingly,

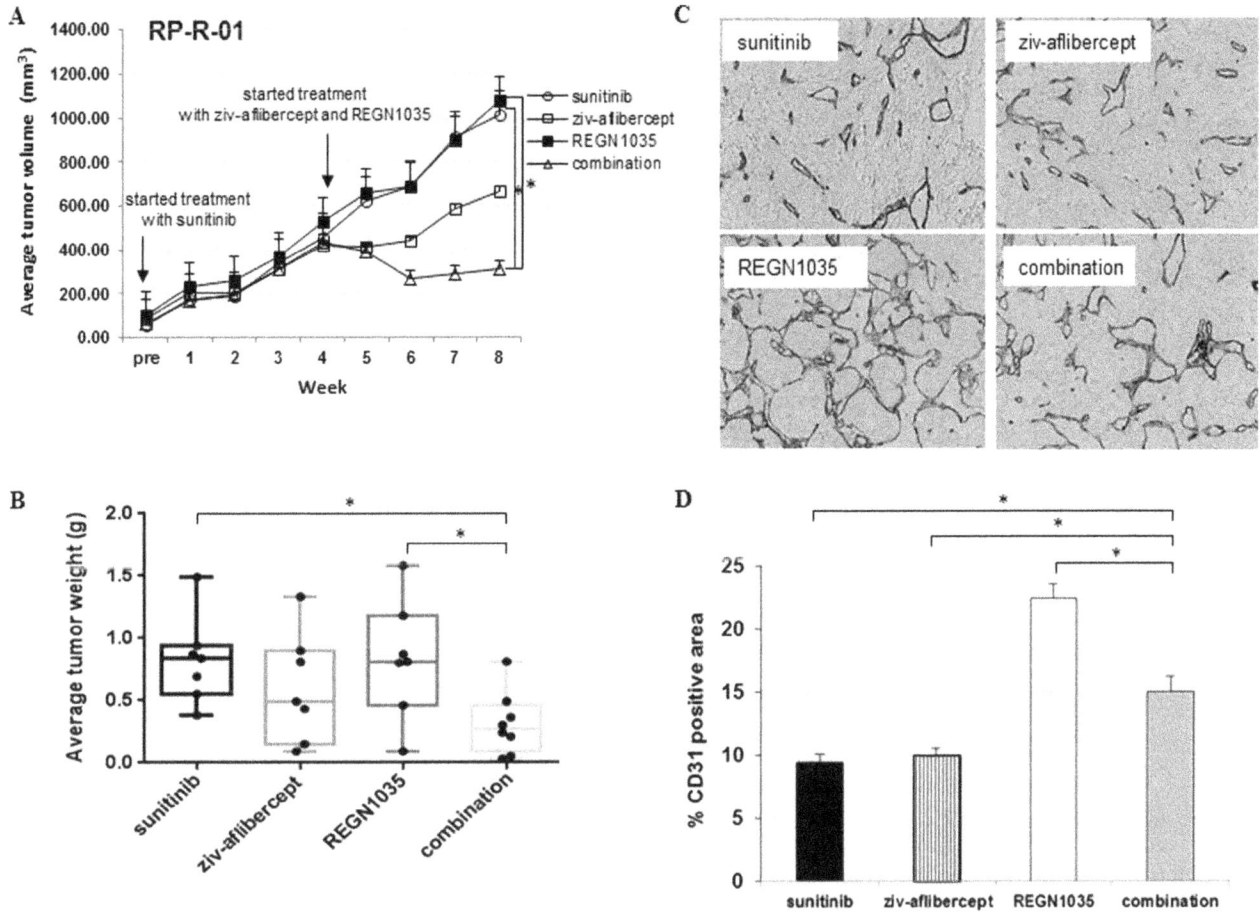

Figure 6. Anti-tumor efficacy of anti-Dll4 (REGN1035) and anti-VEGF (ziv-aflibercept) in a sunitinib resistant RP-R-01 ccRCC patient-derived xenograft model. Mice with established subcutaneous tumors were treated with sunitinib for 4 weeks until tumor tissue was no longer responsive to treatment (tumor volume was ~6 times that of pretreatment volume). At which time, mice were treated with either sunitinib, ziv-aflibercept, REGN1035 or the combination of ziv-aflibercept plus REGN1035 for a period of four weeks. (A) Tumor growth curve of average tumor volume (mm^3) ± S.E. (B) End point tumor weights (g). *$p < 0.05$, as compared to combination group using adjusted t-test analysis. *Effect of REGN1035 and/or anti-VEGF (ziv-aflibercept) on sunitinib resistant RP-R-01 tumor vasculature.* Sunitinib resistant tumors from treated mice were harvested, processed, and tissue sections were stained for the differential expression of CD31. (C) Representative pictures. (D) Blind quantitative analysis of CD31. Results are expressed as mean percentage positive stained area ± S.E. *$p < 0.05$, as compared to combination group using t-test analysis.

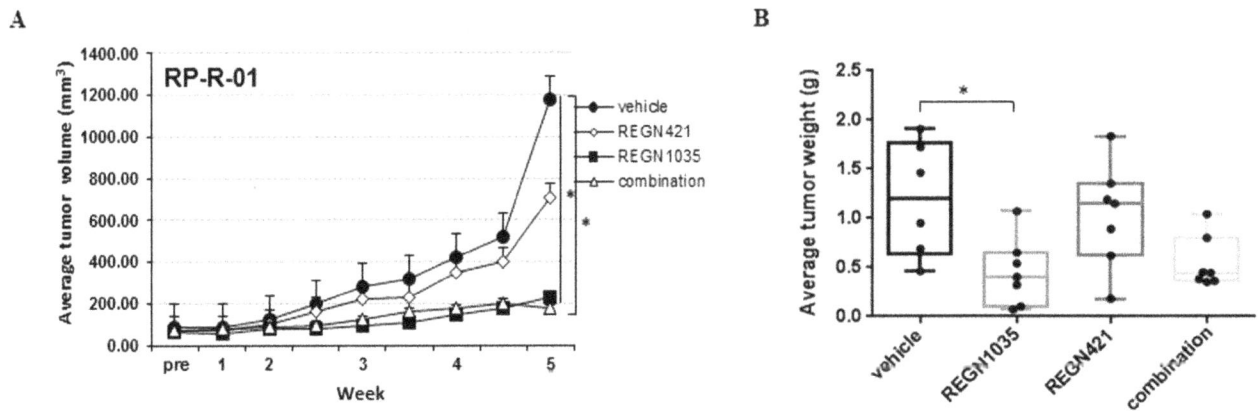

Figure 7. Effect of combined Dll4 blockade on RP-R-01 tumor and stromal cells. Mice were treated with vehicle, human Dll4-specific antibody REGN421 (10 mg/kg, 5x/wk, s.q.), mouse Dll4-specific antibody REGN1035 (5 mg/kg, 1x/wk, s.q.) or combination. (A) Tumor growth curve of treatment groups. Each line represents the average tumor volume (mm^3) of each treatment group ± S.E. (B) Average end point tumor weights. *$p < 0.05$, as compared to vehicle group; combination compared to single agents (REGN421, $p = 0.160$; REGN1035, $p = 0.691$) using adjusted t-test analysis.

despite clear blood vessel remodeling, Dll4 blockade did not have activity as a single agent in this sunitinib resistant PDX model, but it potentiated the anti-tumor effect of ziv-aflibercept by inducing tumor regression. However, the enhanced anti-tumor effect in the combination group was not associated with significant inhibition of blood vessel density as observed in the RP-R-01 sunitinib sensitive PDX model, suggesting, perhaps, that those tumor blood vessels, even if present, may be less functional. This additional observation supports the hypothesis that Dll4 blockade in the setting of effective VEGF inhibition may have clinical benefit also in tyrosine kinase inhibitor resistant ccRCC.

The Dll4-Notch signaling pathway has been implicated in regulating tumor initiating cells, also referred as cancer stem cells (CSCs) [23], [24]. This population of cells, which is reported to possess self renewal, tumor initiating, and differentiating properties, has been shown to play a role in tumor growth, metastasis, and tumor resistance [25]. In our experimental setting, we did not observe single agent anti-tumor activity for the selective targeting of human, tumor cell-expressed Dll4 or anti-tumor additivity for the concomitant blocking of human (tumor cells) and murine (endothelial cells) Dll4. Although, this finding does not rule out the possibility that targeting tumor (stem) cell-expressed Dll4 may contribute to the overall anti-tumor activity of Dll4 blockade in other settings, it suggests that the anti-tumor activity of Dll4 blockade in the employed RCC PDX model is dependent on targeting Dll4 in the tumor stroma, and the lack of tumor growth-promoting autocrine Dll4-Notch tumor cell signaling in this model.

Reports in the literature have raised some concern regarding the safety of chronic anti-Dll4 treatment [26], [27], but the majority of studies have shown it to be well tolerated. Dll4 expression is found to be extensive in the immature developing endothelium of neoplastic tissue, with low to undetectable levels in normal tissue, which constitutes the basis for the specific targeting of the tumor endothelium. While we observed some weight loss ($<$ 10%) in mice treated with REGN1035, sunitinib or REGN421 on an acute treatment schedule (See Table S2), the animals did not present overt signs of toxicity. We did observe a 16% body weight loss in the REGN1035-ziv-aflibercept combination group. However, it should be noted the vehicle group also had a 10% decrease in body weight and the difference with the combination group was not statistically significant (Table S2). Histological examination of treated livers revealed mild evidence of septal and periportal fibrosis and vascular congestion (Fig. S1). In addition, the observed increase in liver blood vessels induced by single agent REGN1035 was modest as compared to the effect on tumor blood vessels. Overall, our data suggest that this combinatorial treatment approach is relatively well tolerated in the preclinical models utilized, though we recognize that the time of drug exposure was limited to clearly define the toxicity of this combination. This is important in view of the fact that combinations of VEGF inhibitors with other targeted therapies (i.e. mTOR inhibitors) in RCC have been hampered by increased toxicity and lack of clear greater clinical benefit as compared to single agents. Dll4 blockade may represent an alternative target for therapeutic interventions in combination with either a VEGF blocker (i.e. bevacizumab or ziv-aflibercept) or a VEGF receptor tyrosine kinase inhibitor (i.e. sunitinib, pazopanib or axitinib) to delay the occurrence of acquired-resistance to approved VEGF inhibitors.

In conclusion, we report here the potent anti-tumor activity for the blockade of Dll4 as monotherapy and a benefit for the combined treatment of anti-Dll4 with VEGF pathway targeting agents in ccRCC PDX models. Our data provide support for combining anti-angiogenic therapies to achieve a more effective treatment response; and specifically warrant clinical investigation of anti-Dll4 therapies alone and in combination with VEGF targeting agents for the treatment of ccRCC.

Supporting Information

Figure S1 Liver H&E histology. (A) Mice inoculated with RP-R-02 tumor tissue were treated for 5 weeks with vehicle, REGN1035, or REGN1035 plus ziv-aflibercept combination. Livers were harvested, processed, and tissue sections were stained for hematoxylin and eosin. Representative image of (left) vehicle treated mice shows normal histology, (middle) REGN1035 treated shows mild septal fibrosis and vascular congestion, and (right) REGN1035 plus ziv-aflibercept also shows mild congestion, periportal fibrosis, and micro steatosis. *Effect of anti-Dll4 and/or anti-VEGF (ziv-aflibercept) on liver vasculature.* (B and C) RP-R-R01 bearing mice previously exposed to sunitinib were treated for 4 additional weeks with sunitinib, REGN1035, or REGN1035 plus ziv-aflibercept combination (See experiment in Fig. 6). Livers from treated mice were harvested, processed, and tissue sections were stained for the differential expression of CD31. Quantitative analysis of CD31 staining was performed in a blinded fashion. Results are expressed as mean percentage positive stained area $\pm$ S.E. *$p < 0.05$, as compared to single agent anti-Dll4 (REGN1035) group using t-test analysis.

Figure S2 Tumor and kidney perfusion. (A and B) Plots show the change in R1 (ΔR1) values of tumors 24 hours and 2 weeks post therapy, respectively. (C and D) No difference in perfusion (ΔR1) of kidneys (normal) was observed with single agent or combination treatments at both time points highlighting the selectivity of tumor vascular response to therapy.

Figure S3 Contrast-enhanced 3D MR angiography images of mice bearing RP-R-01 tumors (outlined in yellow) from all four treatment groups (vehicle, ziv-aflibercept, REGN1035, and combination) at both time points. Control tumors showed marked signal enhancement following contrast administration at both time points (24 hours and two weeks), indicative of the well vascularized nature of these tumors. Control tumors also showed increased growth over the two week period. While single agent treatment with ziv-aflibercept and REGN1035 resulted in moderate tumor growth inhibition and reduction in perfusion, combination treatment resulted in a significant reduction in tumor volume and perfusion as evidenced by a lack of contrast enhancement on the 3D angiography images.

Figure S4 Dll4 expression in RP-R-01 tumors. Dll4 expression in RP-R-01 tumors normalized to cyclophilin by TaqMan PCR. Mouse Dll4 is robustly expressed in the stroma of RP-R-01 tumors, while human Dll4 levels are at the limit of detection (mouse Dll4 mRNA is 780 times more abundant than human).

Table S1 Statistical analysis of the tumor growth data.

Table S2 Average percent body weight change. Mice were weighed weekly and the average percent change from baseline was calculated as follows: (End body weight - start body weight)/start body weight x 100$\pm$ S.E.

Acknowledgments

This study was previously presented in abstract form at the 2012 American Association for Cancer Research Annual Meeting. We would like to thank the MTMR and Pathology Core Facilities at Roswell Park Cancer Institute for animal handling and processing and staining of tissue samples.

Author Contributions

Conceived and designed the experiments: KMM MS FK ASL GT RP. Performed the experiments: KMM MS EC RA BG PS LS DC FK. Analyzed the data: KMM MS FK ASL GT RP KA. Contributed reagents/materials/analysis tools: FK ASL GT RP. Wrote the paper: KMM MS FK ASL GT RP.

References

1. National Cancer Institute at the National Institutes of Health. Available: http://www.cancer.gov/cancertopics/types/kidney. Accessed 2014 Jul 12.
2. Ellis LM, Hicklin DJ (2008) VEGF-targeted therapy: mechanism of anti-tumour activity. Nat Rev Cancer 8: 579–591.
3. Weis SM, Cheresh DA (2011) Box 3: Resistance to VEGF-targeted therapies. From: Tumor angiogenesis: molecular pathways and therapeutic targets. Nat Med 17: 1359–1370.
4. Fischer C, Jonckx B, Mazzone M, Zacchigna S, Loges S, et al. (2007) Anti-PlGF inhibits growth of VEGF(R)-inhibitor-resistant tumors without affecting healthy vessels. Cell 131: 463–475.
5. Verheul HM, Hammers H, van Erp K, Wei Y, Sanni T, et al. (2007) Vascular endothelial growth factor trap blocks tumor growth, metastasis formation, and vascular leakage in an orthotopic murine renal cell cancer model. Clin Cancer Res 13: 4201–4208.
6. Ioffe E, Burova E, Nandor S, Bai Y, Rudge JS, et al. (2012) Comparison of the effects of aflibercept (VEGF Trap) and small molecule kinase inhibitors on tumors and normal organs in mouse models. In: Proceedings of the 103rd Annual Meeting of the AACR 2012 Mar 31–Apr 4; Chicago, IL; Abstract 1023.
7. Gaya A, Tse V (2012) A preclinical and clinical review of aflibercept for the management of cancer. Cancer Treat Rev 38: 484–493.
8. Bridges E, Oon CE, Harris A (2011) Notch regulation of tumor angiogenesis. Future Oncol 7: 569–588.
9. Kuhnert F, Kirshner JR, Thurston G (2011) Dll4-Notch signaling as a therapeutic target in tumor angiogenesis. Vasc Cell 3: 20.
10. Noguera-Troise I, Daly C, Papadopoulos NJ, Coetzee S, Boland P, et al. (2006) Blockade of Dll4 inhibits tumour growth by promoting non-productive angiogenesis. Nature 444: 1032–1037.
11. Patel NS, Li JL, Generali D, Poulsom R, Cranston DW, et al. (2005) Up-regulation of delta-like 4 ligand in human tumor vasculature and the role of basal expression in endothelial cell function. Cancer Res 65: 8690–8697.
12. Aparicio LM, Villaamil VM, Gallego GA, Cainzos IS, Campelo RG, et al. (2011) Expression of Notch1 to -4 and their ligands in renal cell carcinoma: a tissue microarray study. Cancer Genomics Proteomics 8: 93–101.
13. Hammers HJ, Verheul HM, Salumbides B, Sharma R, Rudek M, et al. (2010) Reversible epithelial to mesenchymal transition and acquired resistance to sunitinib in patients with renal cell carcinoma: evidence from a xenograft study. Mol Cancer Ther 9: 1525–1535.
14. Yan M, Callahan CA, Beyer JC, Allamneni KP, Zhang G, et al. (2010) Chronic DLL4 blockade induces vascular neoplasms. Nature 463: E6–7.
15. Seshadri M, Mazurchuk R, Spernyak JA, Bhattacharya A, Rustum YM, et al. (2006) Activity of the vascular-disrupting agent 5,6-dimethylxanthenone-4-acetic acid against human head and neck carcinoma xenografts. Neoplasia 8: 534–542.
16. Ellis L, Shah P, Hammers H, Lehet K, Sotomayor P, et al. (2012) Vascular disruption in combination with mTOR inhibition in renal cell carcinoma. Mol Cancer Ther 11: 383–392.
17. Ridgway J, Zhang G, Wu Y, Stawicki S, Liang WC, et al. (2006) Inhibition of Dll4 signaling inhibits tumour growth by deregulating angiogenesis. Nature 444: 1083–1087.
18. Li JL, Sainson RC, Oon CE, Turley H, Leek R, et al. (2011) DLL4-Notch signaling mediates tumor resistance to anti-VEGF therapy in vivo. Cancer Res 71: 6073–6083.
19. Jubb AM, Miller KD, Rugo HS, Harris AL, Chen D, et al. (2011) Impact of exploratory biomarkers on the treatment effect of bevacizumab in metastatic breast cancer. Clin Cancer Res 17: 372–381.
20. Jubb AM, Soilleux EJ, Turley H, Steers G, Parker A, et al. (2010) Expression of vascular notch ligand delta-like 4 and inflammatory markers in breast cancer. Am J Pathol 176: 2019–2028.
21. Hu W, Lu C, Dong HH, Huang J, Shen DY, et al. (2011) Biological roles of the Delta family Notch ligand Dll4 in tumor and endothelial cells in ovarian cancer. Cancer Res 71: 6030–6039.
22. Zhang JX, Cai MB, Wang XP, Duan LP, Shao Q, et al. (2013) Elevated DLL4 expression is correlated with VEGF and predicts poor prognosis of nasopharyngeal carcinoma. Med Oncol 30: 390.
23. Gurney A, Hoey T (2011) Anti-DLL4, a cancer therapeutic with multiple mechanisms of action. Vasc Cell 3: 18.
24. Hoey T, Yen WC, Axelrod F, Basi J, Donigian L, et al. (2009) DLL4 blockade inhibits tumor growth and reduces tumor-initiating cell frequency. Cell Stem Cell 5: 168–177.
25. Hassan KA, Wang L, Korkaya H, Chen G, Maillard I, et al. (2013) Notch pathway activity identifies cells with cancer stem cell-like properties and correlates with worse survival in lung adenocarcinoma. Clin Cancer Res 19: 1972–1980.
26. Yan M (2011) Therapeutic promise and challenges of targeting DLL4/NOTCH1. Vasc Cell 3: 17.
27. Li JL, Jubb AM, Harris AL (2010) Targeting DLL4 in tumors shows preclinical activity but potentially significant toxicity. Future Oncol 6: 1099–1103.

21

Is MR Spectroscopy Really the Best MR-Based Method for the Evaluation of Fatty Liver in Diabetic Patients in Clinical Practice?

Daniella Braz Parente[1,2]*, Rosana Souza Rodrigues[1,2], Fernando Fernandes Paiva[1,4], Jaime Araújo Oliveira Neto[1], Lilian Machado-Silva[3], Valeria Lanzoni[5], Carlos Frederico Ferreira Campos[3], Antonio Luis Eiras-Araujo[1,2], Pedro Emmanuel Alvarenga Americano do Brasil[1], Philippe Garteiser[6], Marilia de Brito Gomes[3], Renata de Mello Perez[1,2,3]

1 D'Or Institute for Research and Education, Rio de Janeiro, Brazil, 2 Federal University of Rio de Janeiro, Rio de Janeiro, Brazil, 3 University of the State of Rio de Janeiro, Rio de Janeiro, Brazil, 4 Institute of Physics of São Carlos, University of São Paulo, São Carlos, Brazil, 5 Federal University of São Paulo, São Paulo, Brazil, 6 Université Paris Diderot Sorbonne, Paris, France

Abstract

Objective: To investigate if magnetic resonance spectroscopy (MRS) is the best Magnetic Resonance (MR)-based method when compared to gradient-echo magnetic resonance imaging (MRI) for the detection and quantification of liver steatosis in diabetic patients in the clinical practice using liver biopsy as the reference standard, and to assess the influence of steatohepatitis and fibrosis on liver fat quantification.

Methods: Institutional approval and patient consent were obtained for this prospective study. Seventy-three patients with type 2 diabetes (60 women and 13 men; mean age, 54 ± 9 years) underwent MRI and MRS at 3.0 T. The liver fat fraction was calculated from triple- and multi-echo gradient-echo sequences, and MRS data. Liver specimens were obtained in all patients. The accuracy for liver fat detection was estimated by receiver operator characteristic (ROC) analysis, and the correlation between fat quantification by imaging and histolopathology was analyzed by Spearman's correlation coefficients.

Results: The prevalence of hepatic steatosis was 92%. All gradient-echo MRI and MRS findings strongly correlated with biopsy findings (triple-echo, rho = 0.819; multi-echo, rho = 0.773; MRS, rho = 0.767). Areas under the ROC curves to detect mild, moderate, and severe steatosis were: triple-echo sequences, 0.961, 0.975, and 0.962; multi-echo sequences, 0.878, 0.979, and 0.961; and MRS, 0.981, 0.980, and 0.954. The thresholds for mild, moderate, and severe steatosis were: triple-echo sequences, 4.09, 9.34, and 12.34, multi-echo sequences, 7.53, 11.75, and 15.08, and MRS, 1.71, 11.69, and 14.91. Quantification was not significantly influenced by steatohepatitis or fibrosis.

Conclusions: Liver fat quantification by MR methods strongly correlates with histopathology. Due to the wide availability and easier post-processing, gradient-echo sequences may represent the best imaging method for the detection and quantification of liver fat fraction in diabetic patients in the clinical practice.

Editor: Ferruccio Bonino, University of Pisa, Italy

Funding: This work was funded by the D'Or Institute for Research and Education and by FAPERJ (Fundação Carlos Chagas Filho de Amparo à Pesquisa do Estado do Rio de Janeiro). The funders had no role in study design, data collection and analysis, decision to publish, or preparation of the manuscript.

Competing Interests: The authors have declared that no competing interests exist.

* Email: daniella.parente@gmail.com

Introduction

Non-alcoholic fatty liver disease (NAFLD) affects 10–30% of the general population across all ethnicities and age groups [1–5]. Obesity and diabetes are the primary risk factors. Worldwide, the prevalence of obesity, diabetes, and fatty liver is rising [1,3–5]. NAFLD is a clinicopathologic syndrome with a wide spectrum of histological abnormalities and clinical outcomes [1,2,4,6,7]. While some patients have isolated steatosis, others have non-alcoholic steatohepatitis (NASH), which can progress to cirrhosis, and are at increased risk for hepatocellular carcinoma [1,2,4,6,7]. Today, NAFLD is the third most common indication for liver transplantation in the United States and is on a trajectory to become the most common indication [8]. Therefore, early diagnosis is important for appropriate treatments and to prevent progression.

The prevalence of NAFLD in diabetic patients is approximately 70% [9–12]. Type 2 diabetes is an important risk factor for NAFLD and the disease follows a more aggressive course in these patients with necroinflammation and fibrosis [13–17]. The prevalence of NASH in diabetic patients is not well established

Table 1. Triple- and Multi-echo Sequences Parameters.

	Triple-echo	Multi-echo
TR (ms)/TE (ms)	180/2.3, 3.45, 4.6	180/1.15, 2.3, 3.45, 4.6, 5.75, 6.9, 8.05
Flip angle (degrees)	30	15
Slice thickness (mm)	6	6
Interslice gap (mm)	1	1
Matrix	116×117	116×117
Number of slices	33	33
FOV (mm)	350×350	350×350
NSA	1	1
Acquisition time (s)	43,6	43,6
Number/duration of breath holds (s)	2/21.8	2/21.8
Parallel imaging, acceleration factor	SENSE, 2	SENSE, 2

TR, repetition time; FOV, field of view; NSA, number of signals averaged; SENSE, sensitivity encoding.

[18], but has been estimated to be between 22% and 88% [11,19]. Diabetic patients commonly have comorbidities (e.g., obesity or coronary heart disease) and may be at higher risk of complications during liver biopsy [20]. Therefore, noninvasive methods to diagnose NAFLD, quantify liver fat, stage disease severity, and monitor patients over time is important.

Several imaging methods have been used in the diagnosis of NAFLD. Ultrasonography (US) is the most common and accurately detects moderate and severe NAFLD, but it is not sensitive to mild steatosis [21–23]. Interobserver agreement for the severity of NAFLD can be as low as 55% [24]. Therefore, US does not allow precise fat liver quantification for patient follow-up. Computed tomography (CT) is also limited for the detection of mild steatosis and ionizing radiation prevents its use for long-term monitoring [21–23,25]. Magnetic resonance imaging (MRI) and magnetic resonance spectroscopy (MRS) are considered excellent imaging methods for the noninvasive detection and quantification of liver fat [23,26–28]. However, the accuracy of MRI and MRS

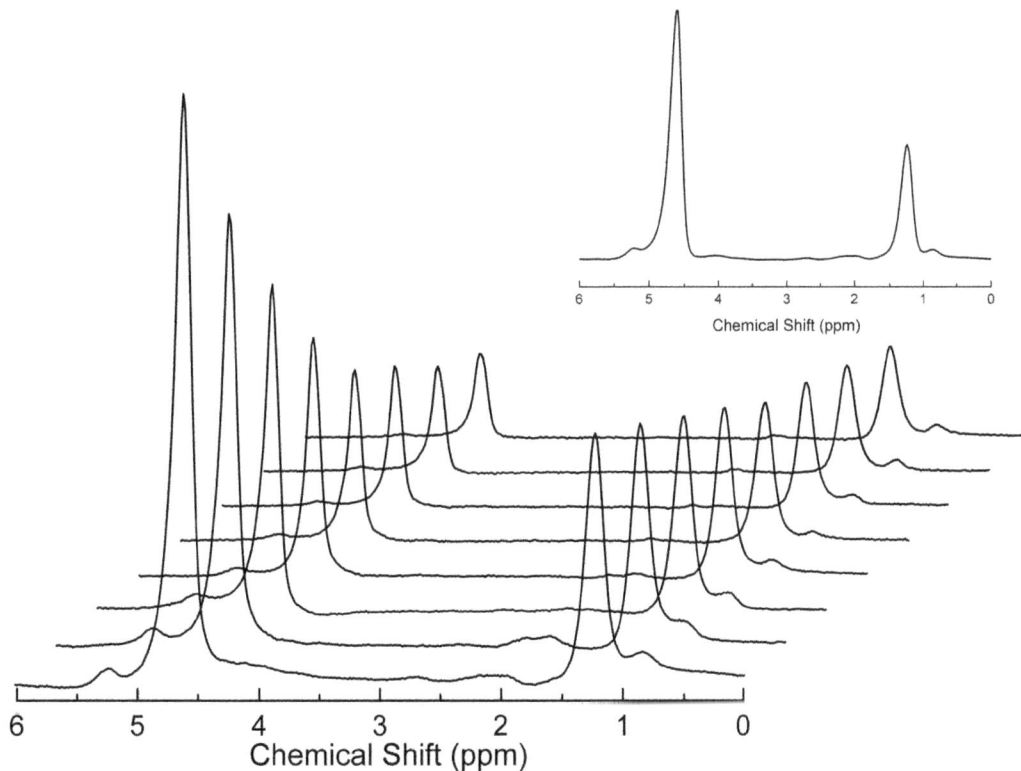

Figure 1. Representative MRS data obtained from a 62-year-old woman with type 2 diabetes and moderate steatosis. T2 estimation was done by fitting the multiecho dataset for both water and fat components considering the spectral modeling. Fat fraction was calculated as described in details throughout the text using the T2-corrected single echo datasets (shown in detail).

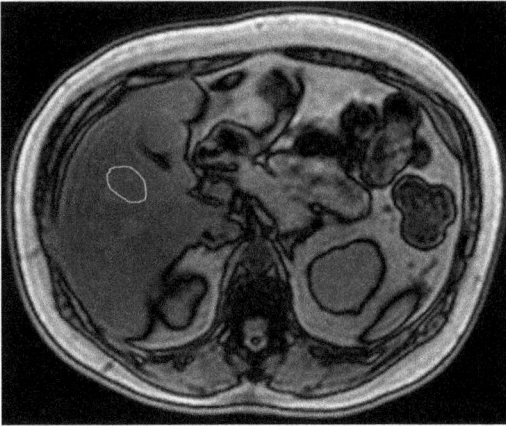

Figure 2. Representative out-of-phase MR images from a 62 year-old woman with type 2 diabetes and moderate steatosis. MR images obtained from breath-hold T1-weighted triple-echo spoiled gradient-echo sequence. ROI was manually drawn at the spectroscopic voxel location (segment V, colocalized with liver biopsy), as shown. ROI, region of interest.

in the detection and quantification of liver fat fraction, the thresholds for mild, moderate and severe steatosis, and the influence of steatohepatitis and fibrosis on the quantification of liver fat fraction are still unknown. Therefore, the goal of this study was to assess the diagnostic performance of triple- and multi-echo MRI, and 1H spectroscopy in the evaluation of hepatic steatosis, to determine the thresholds for different steatosis grades, and to assess if steatohepatitis and/or fibrosis changes MR quantification of liver steatosis using histologic assessment as the reference standard.

Materials and Methods

Patients

This prospective study was approved by the Institutional Ethics Committee of Pedro Ernesto University Hospital. Written informed consent was obtained from all patients. Between June 2010 and February 2012, type 2 diabetic patients at the University of the State of Rio de Janeiro, Brazil, between 18 and 70 years of age with clinical indications for liver biopsy to evaluate NAFLD were consecutively enrolled. In order to study a homogeneous population with NAFLD, patients with other chronic liver diseases were excluded, because some of them, like hepatitis C can be associated with fatty liver and with fibrosis. Exclusion criteria were: other possible causes of chronic liver disease (positive serology for hepatitis B or C), history of alcoholism (≥ 20 g of alcohol per day), severe or decompensated cardiopulmonary disease, renal failure (creatinine >1.5 mg/dL), coagulopathy disorders, medication that could cause NAFLD, contraindications to MRI (i.e., claustrophobia or metallic implants), or refusal of liver biopsy. Criteria for withdrawal from the study included other etiology for chronic liver disease upon liver biopsy or insufficient biopsy material for histological analysis.

MRI and MRS

MRI and MRS were performed during the same examination on a 3.0 T magnet (Philips Medical Systems, Eindhoven, Netherlands) with a Quasar dual gradient system with a peak gradient amplitude of 80 mT/m and slew rate of 200 mT/m/ms. A whole-body transmitter coil and an sixteen-element, receive-

only, phased-array coil were used. All patients were supine. Patients suspended respiration at the end of inspiration for breath-hold sequences and were instructed to breathe smoothly for the respiratory-triggered sequences. For correct positioning, coronal localizer images were acquired at maximum inspiration and expiration. Axial and coronal T2 images were obtained for anatomical reference.

Gradient echo sequences

The liver fat fraction was quantified using T1-weighted, 2D spoiled gradient-echo sequences. Low flip angles were used to minimize T1 effects. To estimate T2* effects, three and seven serial echoes were obtained at different echo times. Sequence parameters are summarized in Table 1.

MRS

Single-voxel MRS data were acquired from $30 \times 30 \times 30$ mm voxels obliquely positioned by a radiologist (D.B.P. with 10 years of experience with liver imaging) on the Couinaud segment V that corresponded to the location of the biopsy. Localizer sequences at maximum inspiration, maximum expiration, and during free breathing were used to ensure the voxel was inside the liver during the entire respiratory cycle. Care was taken to avoid liver edges, large hepatic vessels, and the biliary tree. Water suppression was not performed and automated shimming generated water line widths of 40–50 Hz.

Point -resolved spectroscopy sequences (PRESS) were used for MRS acquisition. For T2 correction, a multi-echo version was used and 8 spectra were collected at echo times (TE) of 40, 50, 60, 70, 80, 90, 100, and 110 ms. To minimize T1 effects, the repetition time (TR) was 2000 ms. The number of data points collected was 1024 across a 2000 Hz spectral window and measurements were the averages of 2 acquisitions (Figure 1). To estimate the fat fraction, single-echo, single-voxel MRS data were acquired using the same sequence with the following parameters: a TR of 4000 ms, a TE of 40 ms, a spectral window of 2000 Hz, the number of data points collected was 1024, and the number of acquisitions was 40 (Figure 1 - detail).

Gradient echo image analysis

All MR imaging results were interpreted by one radiologist (D.B.P. with 10 years of experience with liver imaging), who was blinded to spectroscopic results. Analysis was performed using a custom analysis package in Matlab (Mathworks, Natick, MA). The radiologist manually drew a region of interest (ROI) approximately 900 mm^2 in area and placed it at segment V of the liver, in the same region where MRS measurements and biopsies were performed (Figure 2). The fat fraction (including correction for T2* decay and noise bias) was obtained from average ROI values in magnitude images using a multipeak spectral model for fat detection [29,30].

MRS analysis

MRS data were analyzed by a MR physicist (F.F.P., 5 years of experience with MRS) who was blinded to imaging results. Analysis used the Advanced Method for Accurate, Robust, and Efficient Spectral (AMARES) algorithm included in jMRUI [31]. At each echo time, the water (4.7 ppm) and fat (0.5–3 ppm) peaks were measured. Each measurable peak area was individually corrected for T2 decay using nonlinear least-square fits to determine their relative proton density. The relative proton densities of the fat peaks located underneath the water peaks were determined according to Hamilton et al. [32]. The total fat

Flowchart of Patient Enrollment

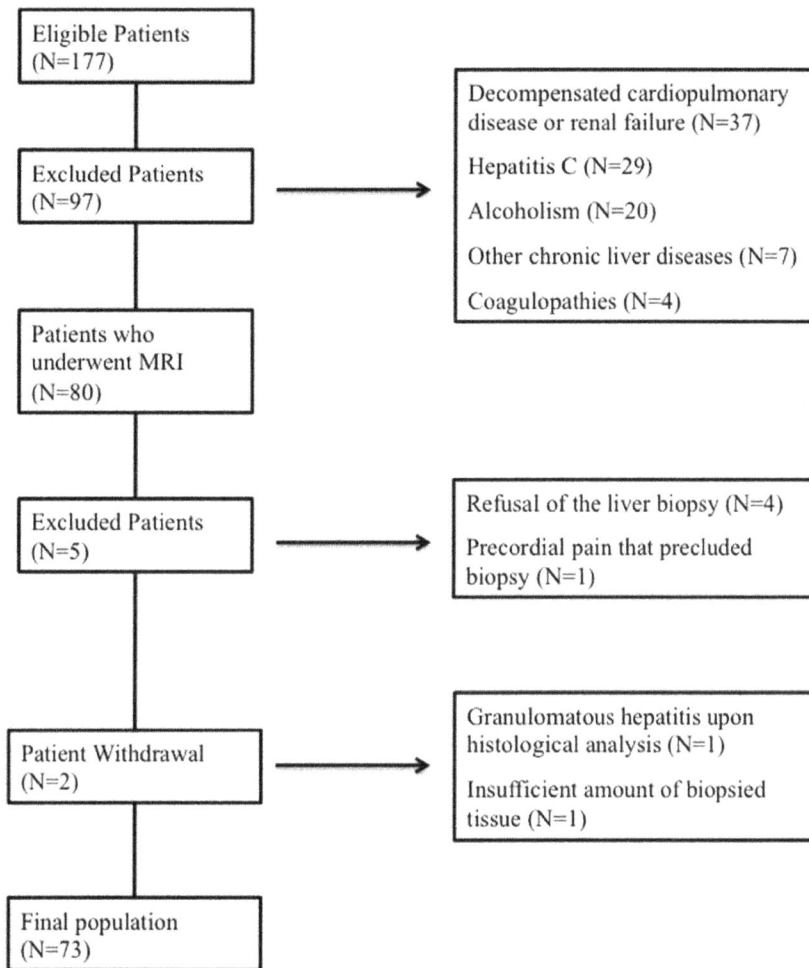

Figure 3. Flowchart of patient enrollment.

proton density was defined as the sum of all T2-corrected individual fat peaks. The proton density fat fraction (PDFF) was calculated as the ratio of the fat proton density to the sum of the fat and water proton densities.

Liver Biopsy and Evaluation

Liver specimens were obtained from all patients. Subcostal liver biopsies of the segment V of the liver were performed under US guidance using a 16-gauge Menghini biopsy needle. Specimens were 2 cm in length or longer, fixed in 10% formaldehyde solution, and then embedded in paraffin. The sections were then stained with hematoxylin and eosin, Masson's trichrome, and Perls' Prussian blue.

All biopsy slides were examined prospectively by a pathologist (V.L., 28 years of experience). Semiquantitative analysis of steatosis assessed the entire liver fragment and was performed by calculating the percentage of steatotic hepatocytes in the liver parenchyma. Results were classified into the following 4 groups according to the NASH Clinical Research Network (NASH-CRN) scoring system [33]: normal, <5%; mild, 5–33%; moderate, 33–66%; and severe, >66%. Steatosis measurements were scored in

increments of 5% for more precise assessment. The pathologist's diagnosis of steatohepatitis was based on the presence of steatosis, hepatocyte injury (ballooning), and lobular inflammation. Fibrosis was scored from F0 to F4 [33]. The presence of siderosis was also evaluated.

Statistical Analyses

Statistical analyses were performed in R-project (version 2.15). Spearman statistic was used to estimate correlations. Linear regression analyses were conducted to explore the influence of steatohepatitis and fibrosis in liver fat measurements. For the linear models the areas under ROC curve were estimated with the Obuchowski's method[34]. Areas under the ROC curves were estimated by the trapezoidal method for mild (5–33%), moderate (33–66%), and severe steatosis (>66%) as reference values in biopsy evaluations. Decision thresholds were estimated for each MR technique through the maximization of the Youden J index on smoothed robust ROC curves. The ROC curves were compared using a variety of methods with a two-sided test. P values <0.05 indicated significant differences.

Table 2. General characteristics of the patients.

	N = 73
Duration of diabetes (years)	11.07±8.12
ALT*	31.59±20.85
AST*	24.66±13.04
Alkaline Fosfatase*	143.19±73.57
Gama-Glutamil transferase*	53.77±41.18
Platelet*	251,616±59,678
Total cholesterol*	188.46±39.10
HDL*	49.28±15.49
Triglycerides*	145.59±69.75
Glucose*	164±63.61
HbA1c levels*	8.59±2.25
Macrovascular complications	5.5%
Microvascular complications	13.7%
Hypertension	75%
Metabolic Syndrome	93.2%
Hypercholesterolemia	45.1%
Statine use	43.1%
Metformine use	90.3%
Insuline use	54.8%

* Mean ± SD.

Results

Patients

A total of 177 patients were interviewed for this study. Ninety-seven patients were excluded: 37 had decompensated cardiopulmonary or renal failure, 29 had hepatitis C, 20 had alcoholism, 7 had other chronic liver diseases, and 4 had coagulopathies. Thus, 80 patients underwent MRI. Five patients were subsequently excluded: 4 refused liver biopsy and 1 had precordial pain that precluded biopsy. Then, two patients were withdrawal: one due to an insufficient amount of biopsied tissue and 1 for granulomatous hepatitis upon histological analysis (Figure 3). Therefore, the final population of the study included 73 patients (60 women [82%] and 13 men [18%]) aged 54±9 years. The mean body mass index

(BMI) was 31.4 kg/m^2 (range, 23.2–42.7 kg/m^2). Ninety-six percent (70 of 73) of patients were overweight (BMI>25 kg/m^2) and 62% (45 of 73) were obese (BMI>30 kg/m^2). MRI and MRS were performed during the same session and within 3 months after the liver biopsy. Thirty-six percent of all patients had elevated aminotransferase levels. Detailed demographic characteristics of the patients are included at Table 2.

Histological Analysis

Upon histology, the prevalence of steatosis (>5%) was 92% (67 patients). Mild steatosis was detected in 35 patients, moderate in 11 patients, and severe in 21 patients. Thirty-seven percent of the patients had steatohepatitis. Fibrosis was observed in 21 (29%) patients. The breakdown of NAFLD fibrosis scores among these

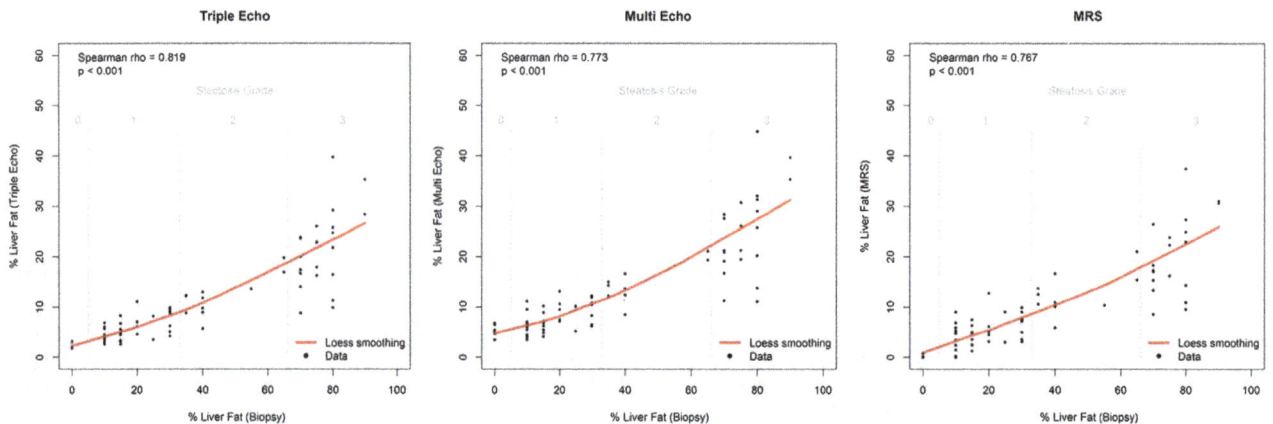

Figure 4. Correlations between triple- and multi-echo sequences and MR spectroscopy versus histopathology examination.

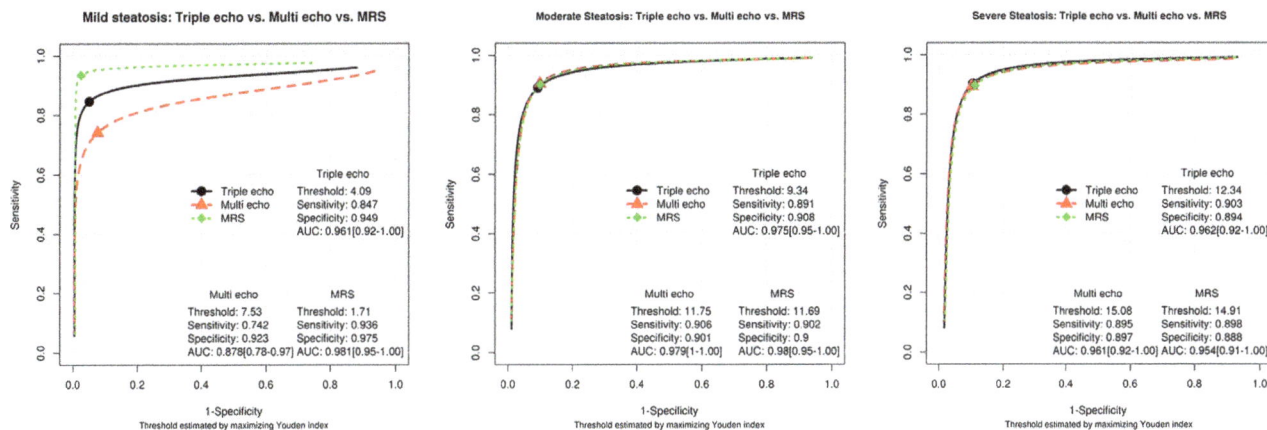

Figure 5. Diagnostic performance for triple- and multi-echo sequences, and MRS using histopathology as the gold standard. The best cut-off point was identified using the Youden index.

patients were: F1, 12 patients; F2, 6 patients; F3, 2 patients; and F4, 1 patient. Two patients had mild siderosis.

Correlations

Figure 4 shows correlations of the triple- and multi-echo sequences and MR spectroscopy with histopathology. Both MRI and MRS strongly correlated with liver biopsy findings (triple-echo: rho = 0.819, p<0.001; multi-echo: rho = 0.773, p<0.001; MRS: rho = 0.767, p<0.001). The correlation of PDFF in mild or moderate hepatic steatosis was found to be better than in severe steatosis.

Diagnostic Accuracy

The capability of each MR technique to diagnose steatosis was evaluated using histopathology for comparison. The sensitivities, specificities, thresholds, and AUC of each MR technique for mild, moderate, and severe steatosis are shown in figure 5. ROC curves were compared and a significant difference was observed for mild steatosis between multi-echo MRI and MRS (p = 0.033). However, no significant difference between triple-echo and multi-echo MRI (p = 0.093) or between triple-echo MRI and MRS (p = 0.42) was observed for mild steatosis. There was also no significant difference among the different MR methods for the ROC curves in moderate and severe steatosis.

The median fat fraction determined by the different MR methods for mild steatosis varies from 4.98 to 7.06, for moderate

steatosis from 10.84 to 14.27, and for severe steatosis from 18.26 to 27.75, and a progressive increase in the interquartile ranges using the same MR method is noted with no overlap (Table 3). Comparative analyses were performed in all groups, analyzed as paired comparisons between two groups to find out the differences between groups. All the comparative analyses showed p<0.05, suggesting that all the groups are different.

One may see that the overall performance measures of the linear models do not change much when a univariable (with imaging only) and multivariable (with steatohepatitis and fibrosis (F0 vs. F1–F4) are conducted in any of the MR technique (Table 4 and Table 5). Therefore, despite they are significant in the model, fibrosis and steatohepatitis contribute very little to the imaging results.

Discussion

Our study evaluated two MRI chemical shift techniques (triple- and multi-echo imaging) and MRS to diagnose steatosis and quantify fat in the livers of patients with type 2 diabetes. We compared these techniques to histopathological findings. Our results demonstrated that all MR techniques had high sensitivity and specificity for NAFLD diagnosis and strongly correlated with histopathology. In mild steatosis, a similar performance was observed between triple-echo sequences and MRS. In moderate

Table 3. Triple- and Multi-echo MRI and MRS medians for no steatosis, mild, moderate, and severe steatosis using biopsy evaluations as reference values.

	No Steatosis	Mild Steatosis	Moderate Steatosis	Severe Steatosis	Total	p value
	6	**35**	**11**	**21**	**73**	
Triple-echo median (IQR)	2.62 (2.11,3.08)	5.08 (3.56,7.05)	12.17 (9.32,13.25)	21.75 (16.36,25.68)	8.76 (4.45,16.19)	<0.001
Multi-echo median (IQR)	5.16 (4.77,6.24)	7.06 (5.76,10.12)	14.27 (12.28,17.41)	25.73 (19.48,30.74)	10.69 (6.48,19.14)	<0.001
MRS median (IQR)	0.12 (0.06,0.66)	4.98 (3.12,7.05)	10.84 (10.32,14.53)	18.26 (15.28,24.9)	7.53 (3.59,15.28)	<0.001

MRI, magnetic resonance imaging; MRS, magnetic resonance spectroscopy; IQR, interquartile range;
All the groups were compared by 2×2 independent sample tests and the p values were <0.05 in all the analyses.

Table 4. Univariable linear regressions analyses for each one of the imaging techniques.

Stats	Estimate	S.E.	Lower 0.95	Upper 0.95
Triple-echo model				
Triple-echo	33.829	2.256	29.33	38.327
R2	0.76	-	-	-
ROC AUC	0.865	0.015	-	-
Multi-echo model				
Multi-echo	32.891	2.291	28.322	37.46
R2	0.744	-	-	-
ROC AUC	0.848	0.018	-	-
MRS model				
MRS	33.318	2.33	28.673	37.963
R2	0.742	-	-	-
ROC AUC	0.845	0.019	-	-

S.E., standard error; ROC, receiver operating characteristic; AUC, area under the curve; MRS, magnetic resonance spectroscopy.

and severe steatosis there was no significant difference among triple- and multi-echo sequences and MRS.

Although steatosis measurements by MR and histology were correlated, the actual values were different because the parameters used to estimate liver fat are different. Pathologists quantify the percentage of hepatocytes containing fat, whereas MR measures the signal from fat protons. Idilman et al. [35] found that PDFF better correlated with mild or moderate hepatic steatosis than severe steatosis, which is consistent with our data (Figure 4). These results suggest that hepatocytes in severe steatosis contain varied

Table 5. Multivariable linear regressions analysis for each one of the imaging techniques.

Stats	Effect	S.E.	Lower 0.95	Upper 0.95
Triple-echo model				
Triple-echo	28.846	2.43	23.995	33.697
NASH = yes	12.55	4.056	4.453	20.647
fibrosis = 1	−0.512	4.31	−9.115	8.09
fibrosis = 2	16.376	6.004	4.391	28.361
fibrosis = 3 or 4	−5.499	7.306	−20.083	9.084
R2	0.841	-	-	-
ROC AUC	0.88	0.014	-	-
Multi-echo model				
Multi-echo	27.718	2.4	22.927	32.508
NASH = yes	14.533	4.076	6.398	22.668
fibrosis = 1	−1.147	4.412	−9.954	7.66
fibrosis = 2	15.11	6.114	2.906	27.315
fibrosis = 3 or 4	−7.03	7.426	−21.851	7.792
R2	0.835	-	-	-
ROC AUC	0.864	0.016	-	-
MRS model				
MRS	27.248	2.444	22.371	32.125
NASH = yes	14.645	4.173	6.316	22.975
fibrosis = 1	1.143	4.455	−7.749	10.036
fibrosis = 2	13.483	6.258	0.992	25.975
fibrosis = 3 or 4	−8.063	7.589	−23.212	7.085
R2	0.828	-	-	-
ROC AUC	0.864	0.016	-	-

S.E., standard error; ROC, receiver operating characteristic; AUC, area under the curve; NASH, non-alcoholic steatohepatitis; MRS, magnetic resonance spectroscopy.

quantities of fat, but are not distinguished from each other upon histopathology (each is counted as a fat-containing hepatocyte). However, MR methods quantify the amount of fat in tissue. The fat fraction can be >2 times greater by histopathological assessment than by MR techniques, suggesting that many hepatocytes contain little fat. However, MRI and MRS measurements are similar [36,37] to each other. Studies with larger numbers of patients should be performed to better understand the relationship between fat measurements by MR and histopathology.

Few studies have evaluated the influence of steatohepatitis or fibrosis in liver fat quantification [35,38]. Although Idilman et al. [45]. found that hepatic fibrosis reduced the correlation between biopsy results and liver fat fraction, our results are similar to the ones of Tang et al. [38], where the presence of steatohepatitis and/ or fibrosis did not affect MR steatosis measurements.

Our threshold values for the detection of steatosis were similar to those in other studies that used histopathology [36,37,39–42], but the appropriate thresholds have yet to be defined. In our study, the threshold for the detection of mild steatosis varied from 1.71 using MRS, to 4.09 using triple-echo sequence, to 7.53 using multi-echo MRI. Only a small overlap was observed between patients with no steatosis vs. mild steatosis for multi-echo sequence, where the IQR 75 for no steatosis was 6.24 and the IQR 25 for mild steatosis was 5.76. Neither other MR method nor other group had any overlap, suggesting that the technique may be able to accurately differentiate the patient groups. In addition, there were proportional increasing fat fraction medians for all MR techniques in patients with higher steatosis grades determined by histopathology. Thus, we believe that triple-echo, multi-echo, and MR spectroscopy are accurate non-invasive imaging methods for the diagnosis, grading, and follow-up of NAFLD.

Hepatic siderosis distorts the local magnetic field and causes loss of phase coherence and T2* shortening, which leads to signal loss at in-phase times compared to out-of-phase times [43,44]. The T2* relaxation time varies widely among patients and using theoretical T2* relaxation times may lead to incorrect interpretations [45]. The T2* relaxation time can be calculated for each patient using triple- and multi-echo MRI, and with T2* correction, may prevent misinterpretation in cases of hepatic siderosis, a condition that can be associated with NAFLD [46]. In this study, only 2 patients had hepatic siderosis. Thus, we could not evaluate its effects on liver fat quantification.

Gradient-echo MRI appears to be the most appropriate for routine clinical use. In moderate and severe steatosis, no significant difference was observed for all MR methods. In our study, triple-echo sequence showed excellent correlation to histopathology and was similar to MRS to detect and quantify the liver fat fraction in mild steatosis. In addition, gradient-echo MR imaging can measure the liver fat fraction throughout the liver, has a short acquisition time, can be performed as a breath-hold sequence, and does not require hardware upgrades. Furthermore, it allows individual T2* corrections and the post-processing is easier, faster, and less prone to misinterpretation than MRS.

Although MRS enables highly accurate liver fat quantification, it requires strong magnetic fields, data processing is more complex and time consuming, it requires a large team highly specialized personnel, and is much more prone to errors. Lastly, it evaluates only a single voxel, which can lead to misinterpretation in cases of heterogeneous steatosis.

This study has some limitations. First, MRS was performed using a PRESS sequence, which may be more sensitive to J coupling effects [47]. This could lead to a systematic underestimation of fat relaxation times and slightly overestimate PDFF. Also, data acquisition time could be reduced by employing a single signal acquisition. We averaged many MRS acquisitions to ensure high signal-to-noise ratios and minimize baseline variations. Therefore, MRS had to be performed during free breathing where voxels moved 2–3 cm in the longitudinal plane. To minimize motion-related bias, the protocol included a coronal sequence during maximal inspiration and another during maximal expiration to ensure voxels remained properly positioned in the liver during acquisition. The MRI and MRS analyses were performed only in segment V, in the location corresponding to the liver biopsy and other liver segments were not evaluated to maintain clinically reasonable scan times. MRS voxels could also be difficult to position because of the biliary tree, vessels, and magnetic susceptibility in other liver segments. The prevalence of NAFLD in our population was extremely high and this could have negatively influenced the specificity, but this is inherent in the studied population. To the best of our knowledge, this is the first study to compare fat quantification by MRI and histopathology in diabetic patients. In addition, our study evaluated the performance of triple- and multi-echo MRI and MRS, with individual T2* and T2 corrections, respectively, which are important steps to allow comparisons between different magnets at different institutions.

In summary, MR measurements may be useful to screen for NAFLD. Liver fat quantification by MRI and MRS strongly correlated with histopathology, even in the presence of steatohepatitis and fibrosis. Triple- and multi-echo MRI and MRS were highly accurate and may be used as a substitute for liver biopsy. Due to the wide availability and easier post-processing, gradient-echo MRI appears to be the most appropriate for routine clinical use in the evaluation of NAFLD in diabetic patients.

Acknowledgments

Debora Lima; Adriana Passos; Erica Samão; D'Or Institute for Research and Education; FAPERJ.

Author Contributions

Conceived and designed the experiments: DBP RSR FFP JAON RMP. Performed the experiments: DBP FFP JAON VL CFFC RMP. Analyzed the data: DBP RSR FFP JAON LMS VL CFFC PEAAB RMP. Contributed reagents/materials/analysis tools: DBP RSR FFP JAON LMS VL CFFC AEA PEAAB PG RMP. Wrote the paper: DBP RSR FFP JAON LMS VL CFFC AEA PEAAB PG MBG RMP.

References

1. Farrell GC, Larter CZ (2006) Nonalcoholic fatty liver disease: from steatosis to cirrhosis. Hepatology 43: S99–S112.
2. Ong JP, Younossi ZM (2007) Epidemiology and natural history of NAFLD and NASH. Clin Liver Dis 11: 1–16, vii.
3. Szczepaniak LS, Nurenberg P, Leonard D, Browning JD, Reingold JS, et al. (2005) Magnetic resonance spectroscopy to measure hepatic triglyceride content: prevalence of hepatic steatosis in the general population. Am J Physiol Endocrinol Metab 288: E462–468.
4. Angulo P (2002) Nonalcoholic fatty liver disease. N Engl J Med 346: 1221–1231.
5. Browning JD, Szczepaniak LS, Dobbins R, Nuremberg P, Horton JD, et al. (2004) Prevalence of hepatic steatosis in an urban population in the United States: impact of ethnicity. Hepatology 40: 1387–1395.
6. Brunt EM, Tiniakos DG (2010) Histopathology of nonalcoholic fatty liver disease. World J Gastroenterol 16: 5286–5296.
7. Tiniakos DG, Vos MB, Brunt EM (2010) Nonalcoholic fatty liver disease: pathology and pathogenesis. Annu Rev Pathol 5: 145–171.
8. Charlton MR, Burns JM, Pedersen RA, Watt KD, Heimbach JK, et al. (2011) Frequency and outcomes of liver transplantation for nonalcoholic steatohepatitis in the United States. Gastroenterology 141: 1249–1253.

9. Leite NC, Salles GF, Araujo AL, Villela-Nogueira CA, Cardoso CR (2009) Prevalence and associated factors of non-alcoholic fatty liver disease in patients with type-2 diabetes mellitus. Liver Int 29: 113–119.

10. Cusi K (2009) Nonalcoholic fatty liver disease in type 2 diabetes mellitus. Curr Opin Endocrinol Diabetes Obes 16: 141–149.

11. Williams CD, Stengel J, Asike MI, Torres DM, Shaw J, et al. (2011) Prevalence of nonalcoholic fatty liver disease and nonalcoholic steatohepatitis among a largely middle-aged population utilizing ultrasound and liver biopsy: a prospective study. Gastroenterology 140: 124–131.

12. Targher G, Bertolini L, Padovani R, Rodella S, Tessari R, et al. (2007) Prevalence of nonalcoholic fatty liver disease and its association with cardiovascular disease among type 2 diabetic patients. Diabetes Care 30: 1212–1218.

13. Loomba R, Abraham M, Unalp A, Wilson L, Lavine J, et al. (2012) Association between diabetes, family history of diabetes and risk of nonalcoholic steatohepatitis and fibrosis. Hepatology.

14. Neuschwander-Tetri BA, Clark JM, Bass NM, Van Natta ML, Unalp-Arida A, et al. (2010) Clinical, laboratory and histological associations in adults with nonalcoholic fatty liver disease. Hepatology 52: 913–924.

15. Silverman JF, O'Brien KF, Long S, Leggett N, Khazanie PG, et al. (1990) Liver pathology in morbidly obese patients with and without diabetes. Am J Gastroenterol 85: 1349–1355.

16. Wanless IR, Lentz JS (1990) Fatty liver hepatitis (steatohepatitis) and obesity: an autopsy study with analysis of risk factors. Hepatology 12: 1106–1110.

17. Harrison SA, Oliver D, Arnold HL, Gogia S, Neuschwander-Tetri BA (2008) Development and validation of a simple NAFLD clinical scoring system for identifying patients without advanced disease. Gut 57: 1441–1447.

18. Lazo M, Clark JM (2008) The epidemiology of nonalcoholic fatty liver disease: a global perspective. Semin Liver Dis 28: 339–350.

19. Gupte P, Amarapurkar D, Agal S, Baijal R, Kulshrestha P, et al. (2004) Nonalcoholic steatohepatitis in type 2 diabetes mellitus. J Gastroenterol Hepatol 19: 854–858.

20. Adams LA, Harmsen S, St Sauver JL, Charatcharoenwitthaya P, Enders FB, et al. (2010) Nonalcoholic fatty liver disease increases risk of death among patients with diabetes: a community-based cohort study. Am J Gastroenterol 105: 1567–1573.

21. Ma X, Holalkere NS, Kambadakone RA, Mino-Kenudson M, Hahn PF, et al. (2009) Imaging-based quantification of hepatic fat: methods and clinical applications. Radiographics 29: 1253–1277.

22. Qayyum A, Chen DM, Breiman RS, Westphalen AC, Yeh BM, et al. (2009) Evaluation of diffuse liver steatosis by ultrasound, computed tomography, and magnetic resonance imaging: which modality is best? Clin Imaging 33: 110–115.

23. Reeder SB, Cruite I, Hamilton G, Sirlin CB (2011) Quantitative Assessment of Liver Fat with Magnetic Resonance Imaging and Spectroscopy. J Magn Reson Imaging 34: spcone.

24. Strauss S, Gavish E, Gottlieb P, Katsnelson L (2007) Interobserver and intraobserver variability in the sonographic assessment of fatty liver. AJR Am J Roentgenol 189: W320–323.

25. Pickhardt PJ, Jee Y, O'Connor SD, del Rio AM (2012) Visceral adiposity and hepatic steatosis at abdominal CT: association with the metabolic syndrome. AJR Am J Roentgenol 198: 1100–1107.

26. Cassidy FH, Yokoo T, Aganovic L, Hanna RF, Bydder M, et al. (2009) Fatty liver disease: MR imaging techniques for the detection and quantification of liver steatosis. Radiographics 29: 231–260.

27. Schwenzer NF, Springer F, Schraml C, Stefan N, Machann J, et al. (2009) Non-invasive assessment and quantification of liver steatosis by ultrasound, computed tomography and magnetic resonance. J Hepatol 51: 433–445.

28. Reeder SB, Robson PM, Yu H, Shimakawa A, Hines CD, et al. (2009) Quantification of hepatic steatosis with MRI: the effects of accurate fat spectral modeling. J Magn Reson Imaging 29: 1332–1339.

29. Yokoo T, Bydder M, Hamilton G, Middleton MS, Gamst AC, et al. (2009) Nonalcoholic fatty liver disease: diagnostic and fat-grading accuracy of low-flip-angle multiecho gradient-recalled-echo MR imaging at 1.5 T. Radiology 251: 67–76.

30. Kuhn JP, Hernando D, Munoz del Rio A, Evert M, Kannengiesser S, et al. (2012) Effect of multipeak spectral modeling of fat for liver iron and fat quantification: correlation of biopsy with MR imaging results. Radiology 265: 133–142.

31. Stefan D, Di Cesare F, Andrasescu A, Popa E, Lazariev A, et al. (2009) Quantitation of magnetic resonance spectroscopy signals: the jMRUI software package. Measurement Science & Technology 20.

32. Hamilton G, Yokoo T, Bydder M, Cruite I, Schroeder ME, et al. (2011) In vivo characterization of the liver fat (1)H MR spectrum. NMR Biomed 24: 784–790.

33. Kleiner DE, Brunt EM, Van Natta M, Behling C, Contos MJ, et al. (2005) Design and validation of a histological scoring system for nonalcoholic fatty liver disease. Hepatology 41: 1313–1321.

34. Obuchowski NA (2006) An ROC-type measure of diagnostic accuracy when the gold standard is continuous-scale. Stat Med 25: 481–493.

35. Idilman IS, Aniktar H, Idilman R, Kabacam G, Savas B, et al. (2013) Hepatic steatosis: quantification by proton density fat fraction with MR imaging versus liver biopsy. Radiology 267: 767–775.

36. d'Assignies G, Ruel M, Khiat A, Lepanto L, Chagnon M, et al. (2009) Noninvasive quantitation of human liver steatosis using magnetic resonance and bioassay methods. Eur Radiol 19: 2033–2040.

37. Hussain HK, Chenevert TL, Londy FJ, Gulani V, Swanson SD, et al. (2005) Hepatic fat fraction: MR imaging for quantitative measurement and display-early experience. Radiology 237: 1048–1055.

38. Tang A, Tan J, Sun M, Hamilton G, Bydder M, et al. (2013) Nonalcoholic fatty liver disease: MR imaging of liver proton density fat fraction to assess hepatic steatosis. Radiology 267: 422–431.

39. van Werven JR, Marsman HA, Nederveen AJ, Smits NJ, ten Kate FJ, et al. (2010) Assessment of hepatic steatosis in patients undergoing liver resection: comparison of US, CT, T1-weighted dual-echo MR imaging, and point-resolved 1H MR spectroscopy. Radiology 256: 159–168.

40. Kim H, Taksali SE, Dufour S, Befroy D, Goodman TR, et al. (2008) Comparative MR study of hepatic fat quantification using single-voxel proton spectroscopy, two-point dixon and three-point IDEAL. Magn Reson Med 59: 521–527.

41. Lee SS, Park SH, Kim HJ, Kim SY, Kim MY, et al. (2010) Non-invasive assessment of hepatic steatosis: prospective comparison of the accuracy of imaging examinations. J Hepatol 52: 579–585.

42. Noworolski SM, Lam MM, Merriman RB, Ferrell L, Qayyum A (2012) Liver Steatosis: Concordance of MR Imaging and MR Spectroscopic Data with Histologic Grade. Radiology 264: 88–96.

43. Westphalen AC, Qayyum A, Yeh BM, Merriman RB, Lee JA, et al. (2007) Liver fat: effect of hepatic iron deposition on evaluation with opposed-phase MR imaging. Radiology 242: 450–455.

44. O'Regan DP, Callaghan MF, Wylezinska-Arridge M, Fitzpatrick J, Naoumova RP, et al. (2008) Liver fat content and T2*: simultaneous measurement by using breath-hold multiecho MR imaging at 3.0 T–feasibility. Radiology 247: 550–557.

45. Thomsen C, Becker U, Winkler K, Christoffersen P, Jensen M, et al. (1994) Quantification of liver fat using magnetic resonance spectroscopy. Magn Reson Imaging 12: 487–495.

46. Mashhood A, Railkar R, Yokoo T, Levin Y, Clark L, et al. (2012) Reproducibility of hepatic fat fraction measurement by magnetic resonance imaging. J Magn Reson Imaging.

47. Hamilton G, Middleton MS, Bydder M, Yokoo T, Schwimmer JB, et al. (2009) Effect of PRESS and STEAM sequences on magnetic resonance spectroscopic liver fat quantification. J Magn Reson Imaging 30: 145–152.

Permissions

All chapters in this book were first published in PLOS ONE, by The Public Library of Science; hereby published with permission under the Creative Commons Attribution License or equivalent. Every chapter published in this book has been scrutinized by our experts. Their significance has been extensively debated. The topics covered herein carry significant findings which will fuel the growth of the discipline. They may even be implemented as practical applications or may be referred to as a beginning point for another development.

The contributors of this book come from diverse backgrounds, making this book a truly international effort. This book will bring forth new frontiers with its revolutionizing research information and detailed analysis of the nascent developments around the world.

We would like to thank all the contributing authors for lending their expertise to make the book truly unique. They have played a crucial role in the development of this book. Without their invaluable contributions this book wouldn't have been possible. They have made vital efforts to compile up to date information on the varied aspects of this subject to make this book a valuable addition to the collection of many professionals and students.

This book was conceptualized with the vision of imparting up-to-date information and advanced data in this field. To ensure the same, a matchless editorial board was set up. Every individual on the board went through rigorous rounds of assessment to prove their worth. After which they invested a large part of their time researching and compiling the most relevant data for our readers.

The editorial board has been involved in producing this book since its inception. They have spent rigorous hours researching and exploring the diverse topics which have resulted in the successful publishing of this book. They have passed on their knowledge of decades through this book. To expedite this challenging task, the publisher supported the team at every step. A small team of assistant editors was also appointed to further simplify the editing procedure and attain best results for the readers.

Apart from the editorial board, the designing team has also invested a significant amount of their time in understanding the subject and creating the most relevant covers. They scrutinized every image to scout for the most suitable representation of the subject and create an appropriate cover for the book.

The publishing team has been an ardent support to the editorial, designing and production team. Their endless efforts to recruit the best for this project, has resulted in the accomplishment of this book. They are a veteran in the field of academics and their pool of knowledge is as vast as their experience in printing. Their expertise and guidance has proved useful at every step. Their uncompromising quality standards have made this book an exceptional effort. Their encouragement from time to time has been an inspiration for everyone.

The publisher and the editorial board hope that this book will prove to be a valuable piece of knowledge for researchers, students, practitioners and scholars across the globe.

List of Contributors

Julnar Usta, Khaled Rida, Omar El-Rifai and Tamar Majarian
Department of Biochemistry and Molecular Genetics; Faculty of Medicine, American University of Beirut, Beirut, Lebanon

Antonios Wehbeh and Theresa Alicia Estiphan
Faculty of Medicine, American University of Beirut Medical Center, Beirut, Lebanon

Kassem Barada
Division of Gastroenterology, Department of Internal Medicine, American University of Beirut Medical Center, Faculty of Medicine, Beirut, Lebanon

Wenzhi Wang, Yumin Hu, Peiou Lu, Yingci Li, Yunfu Chen, Mohan Tian and Lijuan Yu
Center of PET/CT-MRI, Cancer Hospital of Harbin Medical University, Harbin, 150081, China

Giordano Valente, Lorenzo Pitto and Fulvia Taddei
Medical Technology Laboratory, Rizzoli Orthopaedic Institute, Bologna, Italy

Debora Testi
BioComputing Competence Centre, SCS s.r.l., Bologna, Italy

Ajay Seth
Department of Bioengineering, Stanford University, Stanford, California, United States of America

Scott L. Delp
Department of Bioengineering, Stanford University, Stanford, California, United States of America
Department of Mechanical Engineering, Stanford University, Stanford, California, United States of America

Rita Stagni
Department of Electrical, Electronic and Information Engineering, University of Bologna, Bologna, Italy

Marco Viceconti
Department of Mechanical Engineering and INSIGNEO Institute for In Silico Medicine, University of Sheffield, Sheffield, United Kingdom

Gadi Goelman and Noam Gordon
MRI/MRS Lab, The Human Biology Research Center, Department of Medical Biophysics, Hadassah Hebrew University Medical Center, Jerusalem, Israel

Omer Bonne
Department of Psychiatry, Hadassah Hebrew University Medical Center, Jerusalem, Israel

Max Seidensticker, Ricarda Seidensticker, Robert Damm, Konrad Mohnike and Jens Ricke
Universitätsklinik Magdeburg, Klinik für Radiologie und Nuklearmedizin, Magdeburg, Germany
International School of Image-Guided Interventions, Deutsche Akademie für Mikrotherapie, Magdeburg, Germany

Maciej Pech
Universitätsklinik Magdeburg, Klinik für Radiologie und Nuklearmedizin, Magdeburg, Germany
International School of Image-Guided Interventions, Deutsche Akademie für Mikrotherapie, Magdeburg, Germany
Medical University of Gdansk, 2nd Department of Radiology, Gdansk, Poland

Bruno Sangro
Clinica Universidad de Navarra, Liver Unit, Department of Internal Medicine, Pamplona, Spain

Peter Hass and Günther Gademann
Universitätsklinik Magdeburg, Klinik für Strahlentherapie, Magdeburg, Germany

Peter Wust
Charité Universitätsmedizin Berlin, Klinik für Radioonkologie und Strahlentherapie, Berlin, Germany

Siegfried Kropf
Universitätsklinik Magdeburg, Institut für Biometrie und Medizinische Informatik, Magdeburg, Germany

Muireann Irish
School of Psychology, the University of New South Wales, Sydney, Australia
Neuroscience Research Australia, Randwick, Sydney, Australia
Australian Research Council Centre of Excellence in Cognition and its Disorders, Sydney, Australia

Michael Hornberger
Neuroscience Research Australia, Randwick, Sydney, Australia
School of Medical Sciences, the University of New South Wales, Sydney, Australia
Department of Clinical Neuroscience, University of Cambridge, Cambridge, United Kingdom

Shadi El Wahsh, Sharpley Hsieh, John R. Hodges and Olivier Piguet
Neuroscience Research Australia, Randwick, Sydney, Australia
School of Medical Sciences, the University of New South Wales, Sydney, Australia
Australian Research Council Centre of Excellence in Cognition and its Disorders, Sydney, Australia

Bonnie Y. K. Lam
Neuroscience Research Australia, Randwick, Sydney, Australia
School of Medical Sciences, the University of New South Wales, Sydney, Australia

Suncica Lah
Australian Research Council Centre of Excellence in Cognition and its Disorders, Sydney, Australia, School of Psychology, the University of Sydney, Sydney, Australia

Laurie Miller
Australian Research Council Centre of Excellence in Cognition and its Disorders, Sydney, Australia, Neuropsychology Unit, Royal Prince Alfred Hospital, and Central Clinical School, University of Sydney, Sydney, Australia

Noemi Pavo, Georg Strebinger, Gerald Maurer and Mariann Gyöngyösi
Department of Cardiology, Medical University of Vienna, Vienna, Austria

Andras Jakab
Department of Biomedical Imaging and Image-guided Therapy, Medical University of Vienna, Vienna, Austria

Maximilian Y. Emmert, Petra Wolint and Simon P. Hoerstrup
Swiss Centre for Regenerative Medicine, University of Zürich, Zürich, Switzerland, Division of Surgical Research, University Hospital of Zürich, Zürich, Switzerland
Clinic for Cardiovascular Surgery, University Hospital of Zürich, Zürich, Switzerland

Matthias Zimmermann
Department of Thoracic Surgery, Medical University of Vienna, Vienna, Austria

Hendrik Jan Ankersmit
Christian Doppler Laboratory for Cardiac and Thoracic Diagnosis and Regeneration, Vienna, Austria

Christopher R. Heier and Alfredo D. Guerron
Center for Genetic Medicine Research, Children's National Medical Center, Washington, D.C., United States of America

Alexandru Korotcov and Stephen Lin
Department of Radiology, Howard University College of Medicine, Washington, D.C., United States of America

Heather Gordish-Dressman, Kanneboyina Nagaraju and Eric P. Hoffman
Center for Genetic Medicine Research, Children's National Medical Center, Washington, D.C., United States of America
Department of Integrative Systems Biology, George Washington University School of Medicine and Health Sciences, Washington, D.C., United States of America

Stanley Fricke
Department of Diagnostic Imaging and Radiology, Children's National Medical Center, Washington, D.C., United States of America

Raymond W. Sze
Department of Radiology, Children's National Medical Center, Washington, D.C., United States of America

Paul Wang
Department of Radiology, Howard University College of Medicine, Washington, D.C., United States of America
Department of Electrical Engineering, Fu Jen Catholic University, Taipei, Taiwan

Miho Sasaki, Misa Sumi, Sato Eida, Ikuo Katayama, Yuka Hotokezaka and Takashi Nakamura
Department of Radiology and Cancer Biology, Nagasaki University School of Dentistry, Nagasaki, Japan

Haruyasu Yamada, Osamu Abe, Takashi Shizukuishi, Junko Kikuta and Hiroki Haradome
Department of Radiology, Nihon University School of Medicine, Tokyo, Japan

Takahiro Shinozaki, Ko Dezawa and Yoshiki Imamura
Department of Oral Diagnostic Sciences, Nihon University School of Dentistry, Tokyo, Japan

Akira Nagano and Masayuki Matsuda
Department of Radiological Technology, Nihon University Itabashi Hospital, Tokyo, Japan

Ann-Marie Bintu Munda Jah-Kabba, Guido Matthias Kukuk, Dariusch Reza Hadizadeh, Frank Träber, Hans Heinz Schild and Winfried Albert Willinek
University of Bonn, Dept. of Radiology, Germany

Arne Koscielny, Mustapha Sundifu Kabba and Frauke Verrel
University of Bonn, Dept. of Surgery, Germany

Ana Virel, Erik Faergemann and Ingrid Strömberg
Department of Integrative Medical Biology, Umea° University, Umeå, Sweden

Greger Orädd
Department of Radiation Sciences, Umea° University, Umeå, Sweden

Maria Engström
Division of Radiology, Department of Medical and Health Sciences, Linköping University, Linköping, Sweden
Center for Medical Image Science and Visualization (CMIV), Linköping University, Linköping, Sweden

Jan B. M. Warntjes
Center for Medical Image Science and Visualization (CMIV), Linköping University, Linköping, Sweden
Division of Cardiovascular Medicine, Department of Medical and Health Sciences, Linköping University, Linköping, Sweden
SyntheticMR AB, Linköping, Sweden

Anders Tisell and Peter Lundberg
Center for Medical Image Science and Visualization (CMIV), Linköping University, Linköping, Sweden
Division of Radiation Physics, Department of Medical and Health Sciences, Linköping University, Linköping, Sweden

Anne-Marie Landtblom
Center for Medical Image Science and Visualization (CMIV), Linköping University, Linköping, Sweden
Division of Neurology, Department of Clinical and Experimental Medicine, Linköping University, Linköping, Sweden

David Seelig, An-Li Wang and Daniel Romer
Annenberg Public Policy Center, Annenberg School for Communication, University of Pennsylvania, Philadelphia, Pennsylvania, 19104, United States of America

Daniel D. Langleben
Annenberg Public Policy Center, Annenberg School for Communication, University of Pennsylvania, Philadelphia, Pennsylvania, 19104, United States of America
Department of Psychiatry, School of Medicine, University of Pennsylvania, Philadelphia, Pennsylvania, 19104, United States of America

Kanchana Jaganathan, James W. Loughead, Shira J. Blady and Anna Rose Childress
Department of Psychiatry, School of Medicine, University of Pennsylvania, Philadelphia, Pennsylvania, 19104, United States of America

Angel Soto-Hermida, Mercedes Fernández-Moreno, Natividad Oreiro, Carlos Fernández-López, Estefania Cortés-Pereira, Ignacio Rego-Pérez and Francisco J. Blanco
Grupo de Genómica, Servicio de Reumatología, Instituto de Investigación Biomédica de A Coruña (INIBIC), Complexo Hospitalario Universitario de A Coruña (CHUAC),

Sergas, Universidade da Coruña (UDC), A Coruña, España Sonia Pértega
Unidad de Epidemiología Instituto de Investigacion Biomedica de A Coruña (INIBIC), Complexo Hospitalario Universitario de A Coruña (CHUAC), Sergas, Universidade da Coruña (UDC), A Coruña, España

Shu-Xun Hou, Jia-Liang Zhu, Dong-Feng Ren, Zheng Cao and Jia-Guang Tang
Department of Orthopaedics, The First Affiliated Hospital of General Hospital of Chinese PLA, Beijing, China

Feng Shuang
Department of Orthopaedics, The First Affiliated Hospital of General Hospital of Chinese PLA, Beijing, China
Department of Orthopedics, The 94th Hospital of Chinese PLA, Nanchang, China

Chun-Chuan Chen, Kai-Syun Syue and Kai-Chiun Li
Graduate Institute of Biomedical Engineering, National Central University, Jhongli city, Taoyuan County, Taiwan

Shih-Ching Yeh
Department of Computer Science and Information Engineering, National Central University, Jhongli city, Taoyuan County, Taiwan

Gareth J. Barker
Institute of Psychiatry, King's College London, London, United Kingdom

Steve C. R. Williams
Institute of Psychiatry, King's College London, London, United Kingdom
National Institute for Health Research Biomedical Research Centre for Mental Health at South London and Maudsley NHS Foundation Trust and Institute of Psychiatry, King's College London, London, United Kingdom

Amanda Worker, Flavio Dell'Acqua, Andrew Simmons and Richard G. Brown
Institute of Psychiatry, King's College London, London, United Kingdom
National Institute for Health Research Biomedical Research Centre for Mental Health at South London and Maudsley NHS Foundation Trust and Institute of Psychiatry, King's College London, London, United Kingdom

National Institute for Health Research Biomedical Research Unit for Dementia at South London and Maudsley NHS Foundation Trust and Institute of Psychiatry, King's College London, London, United Kingdom

K. Ray Chaudhuri
Institute of Psychiatry, King's College London, London, United Kingdom
National Institute for Health Research Biomedical Research Centre for Mental Health at South London and Maudsley NHS Foundation Trust and Institute of Psychiatry, King's College London, London, United Kingdom
National Institute for Health Research Biomedical Research Unit for Dementia at South London and Maudsley NHS Foundation Trust and Institute of Psychiatry, King's College London, London, United Kingdom
King's College Hospital, London, United Kingdom

Camilla Blain
Institute of Psychiatry, King's College London, London, United Kingdom
King's College Hospital, London, United Kingdom

Jozef Jarosz
King's College Hospital, London, United Kingdom

P. Nigel Leigh
Trafford Centre for Biomedical Research, Brighton and Sussex Medical School, University of Sussex, Falmer, Brighton, United Kingdom

Luca Massacesi
Dipartimento di Neuroscienze, Psicologia, Farmaco e Salute del Bambino Universita` di Firenze, Firenze, Italy
Neurologia 2, Azienda Ospedaliero-Universitaria Careggi, Firenze, Italy

Anna Repice
Neurologia 2, Azienda Ospedaliero-Universitaria Careggi, Firenze, Italy

Irene Tramacere, Graziella Filippini Alessandra Solari and Clara Milanese
Fondazione IRCCS Istituto Neurologico Carlo Besta, Milano, Italy

Salvatore Amoroso
Dipartimento di Neuroscienze, Sezione di Farmacologia, UniversitàPolitecnica delle Marche, Ancona, Italy

Mario A. Battaglia
Associazione Italiana Sclerosi Multipla (AISM), Fondazione Italiana Sclerosi Multipla (FISM), Genova, Italy

Maria Donata Benedetti
Dipartimento Universitario di Neurologia, Azienda Ospedaliera Universitaria Integrata di Verona, Verona, Italy

Loredana La Mantia
Unitádi Neurologia - Multiple Sclerosis Center, I.R.C.C.S. Santa Maria Nascen Fondazione Don Gnocchi, Milano, Italy

Gioacchino Tedeschi
Clinica Neurologica, Universitádi Napoli, Napoli, Italy

Kiersten Marie Miles, Li Shen and Dylan Conroy
Genitourinary Program, Roswell Park Cancer Institute, Buffalo, New York, United States of America,

Roberto Pili
Genitourinary Program, Roswell Park Cancer Institute, Buffalo, New York, United States of America

Mukund Seshadri and Bryan Gillard
Department of Pharmacology & Therapeutics, Roswell Park Cancer Institute Division, University at Buffalo, Buffalo, New York, United States of America,

Remi Adelaiye
Department of Cancer Pathology & Prevention, Roswell Park Cancer Institute
Division, University at Buffalo, Buffalo, New York, United States of America

Paula Sotomayor
Department of Molecular and Cellular Biology, Roswell Park Cancer Institute Division, University at Buffalo, Buffalo, New York, United States of America

Kristopher Attwood
Department of Biostatistics & Bioinformatics, Roswell Park Cancer Institute Division, University at Buffalo, Buffalo, New York, United States of America

Eric Ciamporcero
Medicine and Experimental Oncology, University of Turin, Turin, Italy

Frank Kuhnert, Alshad S. Lalani and Gavin Thurston
Regeneron Pharmaceuticals, Inc., Tarrytown, New York, United States of America

Jaime Araújo Oliveira Neto and Pedro Emmanuel Alvarenga Americano do Brasil
D'Or Institute for Research and Education, Rio de Janeiro, Brazil

Daniella Braz Parente, Rosana Souza Rodrigues and Antonio Luis Eiras-Araujo
D'Or Institute for Research and Education, Rio de Janeiro, Brazil
Federal University of Rio de Janeiro, Rio de Janeiro, Brazil

Renata de Mello Perez
D'Or Institute for Research and Education, Rio de Janeiro, Brazil
Federal University of Rio de Janeiro, Rio de Janeiro, Brazil
University of the State of Rio de Janeiro, Rio de Janeiro, Brazil

Fernando Fernandes Paiva
D'Or Institute for Research and Education, Rio de Janeiro, Brazil
Institute of Physics of São Carlos, University of São Paulo, São Carlos, Brazil

Lilian Machado-Silva, Carlos Frederico Ferreira Campos and Marilia de Brito Gomes
University of the State of Rio de Janeiro, Rio de Janeiro, Brazil

Valeria Lanzoni
Federal University of São Paulo, São Paulo, Brazil

Philippe Garteiser
Université Paris Diderot Sorbonne, Paris, France

Index

www.ingramcontent.com/pod-product-compliance
Lightning Source LLC
Chambersburg PA
CBHW061259190326
41458CB00011B/3715